Theories of Borderline Personality Disorder

Mojgan Salavati • Edward A. Selby

Theories of Borderline Personality Disorder

Concepts and Empirical Base

Springer

Mojgan Salavati
Psychology
Iran University of Medical Sciences
Tehran, Iran

Edward A. Selby
Psychology
Rutgers, The State University of New Jersey
Piscataway, NJ, USA

ISBN 978-3-031-75502-6 ISBN 978-3-031-75503-3 (eBook)
https://doi.org/10.1007/978-3-031-75503-3

This Springer imprint is published by the registered company Springer Nature Switzerland AG
The registered company address is: Gewerbestrasse 11, 6330 Cham, Switzerland

"As someone deeply invested in understanding the complexities of mental health, I find this book to be an essential resource for anyone looking to comprehend the intricacies of Borderline Personality Disorder. It offers a nuanced, multi-faceted approach to understanding BPD, blending decades of research with practical, real-world insights. The authors have masterfully woven together cognitive-behavioral theories, developmental perspectives, and therapeutic interventions to provide a comprehensive view of this often misunderstood disorder. Whether you're a clinician, researcher, or someone with a personal connection to BPD, this book equips you with the knowledge and empathy necessary to make a meaningful impact. I highly recommend it to anyone seeking to deepen their understanding and support of those affected by BPD."

–Ted Bender, PhD, MBA, Chief Operating Officer, *Applied Behavioral Analysis (ABA) Centers of America*

Introduction

Borderline Personality Disorder (BPD) is one of the most intricate and challenging diagnoses faced by modern mental health clinicians and researchers, one that has intrigued and perplexed clinicians, researchers, and those directly affected by it for decades. This often-misunderstood condition is characterized by potentially chronic symptoms such as intense emotional instability or mood swings, chaotic relationships, behavioral impulsivity, and at times, a deep-seated fear of abandonment. The impact of these symptoms is felt daily by both the individual with the diagnosis and those around them, who often struggle to respond effectively or empathetically with these interpersonally challenging situations. For clinicians, it presents a unique set of challenges, as patients with BPD often struggle to maintain consistent therapeutic relationships and may experience rapid shifts in mood and behavior that are difficult to predict or manage. This disorder not only impacts the individual but also reverberates through their relationships with family, friends, and society at large. For those who live with it, BPD can be a source of profound emotional pain, one that leads the BPD diagnosis to have high associations with substance use overdose and suicidal behavior. The high mortality level and public health burden resulting from the BPD diagnosis makes it vital to have a clear understanding of the causal and maintenance factors perpetuating the disorder.

Despite being one of the most researched personality disorders, BPD remains one of the most stigmatized and misunderstood. The complexity of BPD has led to a wide array of theories aimed at understanding its origins, manifestations, and potential treatments. Over decades, these theories have evolved significantly, often reflecting broader changes in psychology, psychiatry, and neuroscience. From the early psychoanalytic perspectives that attributed BPD to developmental failures in early childhood, to more contemporary cognitive-behavioral approaches that emphasize dysfunctional thought patterns and emotional regulation difficulties, each theoretical framework has offered unique insights into the nature of the disorder. However, the diversity of these theories also highlights the inherent challenges in fully comprehending BPD. No single theory can encompass all aspects of the disorder, which is why a multifaceted approach is necessary. This book is dedicated to exploring several modern, primarily cognitive and behavioral theories that have shaped our understanding of BPD.

Although in the early days of clinical theorizing surrounding BPD, psychodynamic theories dominated diagnostic formulations and treatment approaches, in the last 30–40 years the bulk of modern research has explore the cognitive-behavioral roots of BPD. Whereas the original psychodynamic formulations of BPD focused on key childhood experiences in the development of BPD, which tend to be more integrated into developmental theories of BPD now, cognitive-behavioral theories, focus on the patterns of thought and behavior that maintain the disorder. Although the past is very important, especially in the case of BPD diagnoses, it is most important to understand how these factors shaped current cognitive, social interaction, self-perception, and identity patterns that exist at present to create what we now recognize as BPD.

This book strives to present an intensive examination of the theoretical processes that instantiate BPD over several layers of functioning: neurobiological, developmental, behavioral, cognitive, and self-actuation. Although the book does not delve into the depths of intensive neurophysiological examination of BPD, of which there are a growing number of advances and theories, several advances arising from neurophysiological research are incorporated throughout the book. It is our perspective that various biological vulnerabilities exist in the eventual development of BPD, but that these vulnerabilities are compounded by various psychosocial and environmental that we have chosen to focus on throughout the book. We believe that this higher order, integrative focus on the disorder will be most helpful for individuals, clinicians, students, advocates, and educators trying to develop an understanding of BPD in ways that allow for them to better shape and improve the lives of those with BPD.

This book seeks to weave together these diverse cognitive-behavioral theoretical perspectives, offering a comprehensive overview of the many ways in which BPD has been understood and treated over the years. By exploring the historical context of these theories, as well as their current applications and limitations, we hope to provide readers with a deep and nuanced understanding of BPD. In the start of the book, we focus on key foundations in understanding the BPD diagnosis. Chapter 1 introduces the concept of BPD as well as historical considerations in the modern presentation of the diagnosis. Chapter 2 focuses on foundational issues in the diagnosis of BPD, including heterogeneous presentation and alternative diagnostic conceptualizations of BPD diagnostic assessment (e.g., DSM-5 alternative personality disorders model and the Hierarchical Taxonomy of Psychopathology (HiTOP)).

In Chap. 3 we explore developmental processes and research focusing on the roles of parenting styles and how such early interactions can be connected to eventual BPD diagnosis. Parenting styles associated with the development of BPD often include behaviors like emotional invalidation, reward/punishment inconsistency, or emotional neglect. Although the impact of parenting on BPD development can be clear in cases of abuse or domestic violence, at times the impact of parenting styles can be more nuanced, with many of those diagnosed with BPD coming from supportive family environments as well. Invalidation, for example, happens when a child's feelings or life events are belittled (on purpose or inadvertently), criticized, ignored, or overlooked, leading the child to believe their emotions are incorrect or insignificant. Likewise, inconsistent parenting, where the caregivers' reactions are erratic across similar situations, can lead to confusion and insecurity, making it hard for the child to establish a consistent and healthy self-identity. Such problematic parenting methods can play a key role in the emotional instability, fear of being left behind, and issues with self-identity that are typical of BPD. Finally, in Chap. 4 we build on this prior discussion and explore the impact of aversive childhood experiences and maltreatment as experiences that set the stage for later development of BPD through the instigation of several maladaptive developmental processes.

In Chaps. 5, 6, 7, 8, and 9 we explore advances in our understanding of emotion regulation and dysregulation in BPD. One of the most heavily explored areas of modern BPD research involves emotion regulation, which refers broadly to one's ability to attend to emotional experiences, clearly label and understand them, and behave in ways that facilitate improvement of negative emotions and endurance of positive emotions. Emotion dysregulation, on the other hand, refers to various factors that make emotional experiences more distressing, painful, and difficult to control. In this book, Chap. 5 presents a general overview of various emotion regulation and dysregulation concepts as theoretically applied to BPD, and subsequent chapters build on this foundation with more in-depth emotion regulation-based theories of BPD.

Next, one of the most successful treatments for BPD to date is Marsha Linehan's (1993) Dialectical Behavior Therapy (DBT) for BPD. However, DBT is not just an effective treatment for BPD, as it includes one of the most comprehensive and empirically explored theories for understanding BPD. This is why two chapters have been dedicated to the theory. Chapter 6 provides an overview of DBT theory, while Chap. 7 presents a developmental perspective of DBT theory. At the heart of DBT theory is the idea that individuals with BPD have a biological predisposition to emotional dysregulation. This means they are biologically more sensitive to emotional stimuli, experience emotions more intensely, and take longer to return to a stable emotional state after an emotional episode. In essence, people with BPD are wired to experience emotions more acutely and for prolonged periods compared to others. In addition to this biological vulnerability, Linehan emphasizes the role of an invalidating environment. An invalidating environment is one where a person's emotional experiences are consistently dismissed, trivialized, or punished by caregivers or significant others. This can manifest in various ways, such as ignoring the person's emotions, criticizing them for expressing feelings, or responding unpredictably to their emotional displays. Over time, this environment teaches the individual that their emotions are wrong or unacceptable, making it difficult for them to trust and regulate their emotional experiences. Linehan's theory posits that the interaction between these two factors—biological vulnerability and an invalidating environment—leads to the development of BPD. DBT integrates cognitive-behavioral techniques with mindfulness practices, which are specifically designed to address the emotional dysregulation and impulsivity common in BPD. It equips patients with practical skills for managing distress, improving interpersonal relationships, and reducing self-destructive behaviors. Over time, individuals who undergo DBT often experience significant reductions in symptoms, leading to improved emotional stability, better coping mechanisms, and enhanced quality of life. Although delving into the full literature on scientific support for the efficacy of this intervention is beyond the scope of this book, we present two intensive chapters on the underlying theory behind DBT.

In Chap. 8, the Emotional Cascade Theory of BPD (Selby and Joiner Jr 2009) is introduced. This is a psychological model that strives to explain the intense emotional experiences and behavioral dysregulation characteristic of the disorder. The theory posits that individuals with BPD are prone to "emotional cascades," where negative emotions, such as anger, sadness, or anxiety, trigger a self-perpetuating cycle of rumination and heightened emotional distress. According to the theory, when a person with BPD experiences a negative emotional event, they tend to engage in rumination—repetitively and passively focusing on the distressing feelings and the causes or consequences of those feelings. This rumination amplifies the intensity of the negative emotion, leading to an escalation of emotional distress. The heightened emotional state can become so overwhelming that the individual feels compelled to engage in impulsive or self-destructive behaviors, such as self-harm, substance abuse, or reckless actions, to distract from or cope with the overwhelming emotions. Therapeutic interventions, such as mindfulness-based therapies and cognitive-behavioral strategies, can help individuals with BPD interrupt the cascade by reducing rumination and promoting more adaptive emotional regulation techniques. By breaking the cycle of emotional escalation, these treatments can help alleviate the severity of emotional distress and reduce the likelihood of impulsive, self-destructive behaviors. Finally, emotional cascade theory extends our understanding of the nature of BPD into the realm of complex dynamic systems theory, which can help us understand BPD as an "emergent" complex phenomenon.

Following the prior chapters on emotion regulation in BPD, in Chap. 9 we explore more specific cognitive factors involved in BPD, namely *schemas*. Schema Theory (Young et al. 1996) has also been applied to understanding BPD. This conceptual framework provides a structure for comprehending the development and maintenance of deep-seated, unhealthy patterns of thought, emotion, and action in people with BPD. Schema Theory suggests that individuals with BPD often acquire early, harmful patterns of thinking, which are widespread and persistent, originating from childhood experiences and reinforced over time. These patterns emerge from unmet emotional needs during crucial developmental stages, such as the desire for safety, consistency, affection, and approval. Schema Theory also introduces the idea of "modes," which are various mental states that people with BPD might switch to in reaction to their patterns. Frequently observed modes in BPD include the "Vulnerable Child" state, characterized by feelings of fear and helplessness, the "Angry Child" state, characterized by anger and irritation, and the "Detached Protector" state, where the individual emotionally withdraws to avoid discomfort. In "Schema Therapy," the objective is to assist individuals with BPD in recognizing and confronting their harmful patterns, understanding their origins, and cultivating more constructive ways of thinking, feeling, and acting. By tackling the underlying causes of these unhealthy patterns, Schema Therapy seeks to alleviate the emotional volatility, social challenges, and self-destructive tendencies linked to BPD, leading to a more stable and rewarding life.

In Chap. 10 we explore the experience of dissociation in BPD. Although dissociation is not a form of emotion dysregulation per se, dissociation frequently occurs during times of high emotional distress. Dissociative experiences can involve a temporary disconnect from reality, where individuals may feel detached from their thoughts, emotions, or surroundings. Such experience can manifest as feeling "numb," as if the individual is observing themselves from outside their body or experiencing a sense of unreality. Because dissociative episodes often occur during times of emotional distress, they are often thought of as a coping mechanism to manage overwhelming emotions. However, although dissociation may provide temporary relief, it can also exacerbate feelings of confusion and instability, contributing to the overall sense of disconnection, identity disturbance, and chaos often seen in BPD.

In Chap. 11 we present perspectives on Acceptance and Commitment Focused (ACT) therapy for BPD. ACT represents a recent conceptualization of various diagnoses, including BPD, in which the primary aspects of dysfunction and distress arise from non-acceptance and behaviors inconsistent with personal values. ACT encourages individuals to embrace their thoughts and feelings without criticism or suppression, even when these experiences are hard or upsetting. These acceptance processes are enhanced by additional dedication to engage in activities that are in line with the person's principles, instead of being fueled by the instant desire to flee from pain. ACT's focus on embracing can break the pattern of dodging emotions and impulsive actions that worsen the condition. Through learning to watch and accept their inner experiences, individuals can lessen their emotional reactiveness and achieve a stronger sense of control over their actions. The dedication aspect of ACT assists people with BPD to concentrate on long-term aims and values, which can direct them towards actions and choices that are more beneficial.

In the final stretch of the book, Chaps. 12, 13, 14, 15, and 16, we explore the theoretical foundations of comorbidity that exist between BPD other psychiatric diagnoses. BPD is known for being a highly comorbid condition, and the better we can understand these comorbidity patters, the better we can understand the core elements of the BPD diagnosis. Chapter 12 focuses on nonsuicidal self-injury (NSSI) and suicidal behavior in BPD, which are very common among those with the diagnosis. Indeed, suicidal and NSSI behavior are among the most provocative, frightening, and stigmatized behaviors experienced by those with BPD, and they can result in intense and often negative reactions from those around them.

Chapter 13 focuses on the comorbidity between BPD and posttraumatic and other traumatic stress disorders. Many individuals with BPD have experienced early-life trauma such as physical and/or sexual abuse, molestation, neglect, or chronic emotional abuse. In recognition of the key role that trauma can have in the development of BPD, Chap. 13 is dedicated to issues of trauma and how trauma is oriented into conceptualizations of BPD and complex PTSD (c-PTSD). Traumatic experiences, especially during key developmental stages, can lead to emotional dysregulation, unstable relationships, and a fragile sense of self—core features of BPD. Trauma disrupts the development of healthy coping mechanisms, often resulting in impulsive or self-destructive behaviors to manage overwhelming emotions. It also contributes to distorted thinking and a persistent fear of abandonment. In treatment, addressing trauma is essential for helping individuals with BPD heal and develop healthier coping strategies, and in doing so, individuals with BPD can work through the emotional and relational instability caused by their traumatic past.

Chapter 14 explores the connection between BPD and eating disorders. BPD and eating disorders co-occur frequently in clinical settings, sharing common features such as emotional dysregulation, impulsivity, and a distorted sense of self. Major eating disorders associated with BPD include anorexia nervosa (both binge-purge and restricting subtypes), bulimia nervosa, and binge eating disorder. Individuals with BPD may use disordered eating behaviors, such as bingeing, purging, or restrictive eating, as a way to cope with intense emotions or feelings of emptiness. The impulsivity seen in BPD can also contribute to erratic eating patterns, binge eating, self-starvation, and suicidal behavior. Eating disorders also seem to work in synergistic fashion with BPD, with the presence of one diagnosis exacerbating the symptoms of the other, leading to even more severe emotional and behavioral difficulties than a single diagnosis would cause.

Next, in Chap. 15 we discuss the overlap between BPD and a key developmental disorder: Attention-Deficit Hyperactivity Disorder (ADHD). A growing level of research indicates that many individuals diagnosed with one disorder also meet diagnostic criteria for the other. Both BPD and ADHD share symptoms like impulsivity, emotional dysregulation, and difficulties with attention and focus. Some studies suggest that ADHD, particularly when left untreated, may increase the risk of developing BPD, as chronic impulsivity and emotional instability can contribute to the relational and identity disturbances characteristic of BPD. However, ongoing questions remain regarding the biological versus behavioral interplay of BPD and ADHD symptoms. Finally, the co-occurrence of these disorders often leads to more severe symptoms and challenges in treatment, highlighting the need for integrated approaches that address both conditions.

In our final analysis, Chap. 16, we present several additional comorbidities associated with BPD, including major depressive disorder and bipolar disorders, anxiety disorders, and substance use disorders. Each class of diagnoses represents a unique overlap with BPD symptoms, and highlights how challenging the BPD diagnosis is when understanding diagnostic overlap. Do some disorders have shared vulnerabilities with BPD, like bipolar disorder, or do some disorders result from difficulty managing emotions or impulsivity, like substance use disorders? The answer appears to be nuanced and multifaceted across these diagnoses, further complicating theoretical formulations of BPD in the process.

On a final note, although this book does not provide intensive coverage of the implementation or techniques involved in psychosocial interventions for BPD, most chapters address the impact of relevant theoretical approaches on therapeutic interventions and impact for those with BPD. In our view, the better we understand the theoretical formulations of BPD, the more effective and efficient we can make our treatments, ultimately reducing the suffering and facilitating flourishing for those impacted by this difficult diagnosis.

Whether you are a mental health professional, a student, a researcher, or someone with a personal connection to BPD, this book aims to equip you with the knowledge and insights needed to approach this disorder with empathy, respect, and an informed perspective. By critically analyzing the theories that have influenced our comprehension of BPD, we aim to enhance your understanding of the disorder while encouraging you to engage in thoughtful reflection regarding the practical application of these theories. Our goal is to foster a more compassionate and effective methodology for treating and supporting individuals with BPD, thereby enhancing their quality of life and the standard of care they receive.

As we navigate through the diverse theoretical frameworks that have sought to define BPD, we will examine the implications of each theory for clinical practice, the ways in which various theories may complement or contradict one another, and the persistent challenges associated with treating such a complex and multifaceted disorder. Through this investigation, we strive to illuminate a constructive path forward, providing hope, empathy, and understanding to those impacted by BPD and to those dedicated to helping them.

References

Linehan M. Cognitive-behavioral treatment of borderline personality disorder. Guilford Press; 1993.

Selby EA, Joiner Jr TE. Cascades of emotion: the emergence of borderline personality disorder from emotional and behavioral dysregulation. Rev Gen Psychol. 2009;13(3):219–29.

Young JE, McGinn L, Salkovskis P. Schema-focused therapy. Springer Ser Comp Treat Psychol Disord. 1996;291.

Contents

1 **Borderline Personality Disorder: Definition and History** 1

2 **Diagnostic Perspectives of Borderline Personality Disorder** 13

3 **Parenting Styles and Borderline Personality Disorder** 37

4 **Childhood Maltreatment and Borderline Personality Disorder** 57

5 **Emotion Regulation and Dysregulation in Borderline Personality Disorder** 95

6 **Linehan's Biosocial Model and Borderline Personality Disorders** 121

7 **A Developmental Biospecial Model of Borderline Personality Disorder** 145

8 **The Emotional Cascade Model of Borderline Personality Disorder** 165

9 **The Schema Model of Borderline Personality Disorder** 205

10 **Dissociation in Borderline Personality Disorder** 225

11 **Acceptance and Commitment Model of Borderline Personality Disorder** 247

12 **Nonsuicidal Self-Harm and Suicide in Borderline Personality Disorder** 267

13 **Post-Traumatic Stress Disorder (PTSD)/Complex Post-Traumatic Stress Disorder (C-PTSD) and Borderline Personality Disorder** 351

14 **Eating Disorders and Borderline Personality Disorder** 377

15 Attention-Deficit/Hyperactivity Disorder (ADHD) and Borderline Personality Disorder 399

16 Other Psychiatric Comorbidities and Borderline Personality Disorder 421

Index 449

Chapter 1
Borderline Personality Disorder: Definition and History

Introduction

Borderline personality disorder (BPD) is a chronic psychiatric disorder that is presented as one of the most prevalent mental health issues in clinical settings (DSM-5-TR, APA 2022; Kulacaoglu and Kose 2018). BPD is a severely complicated and heterogenous mental disorder featured by disturbed patterns of identity diffusion, disturbed interpersonal relationships, affective instability, chronic feeling of emptiness, and severe impulsive behaviors and self-destructive behaviors such as suicidal behaviors (APA 2022). Disturbances in managing emotion, behavior, interpersonal relationships, and identity presented four "quadrants of BPD" which contribute to destabilizations in main domains of functioning and cascade into interruption of developmental life opportunities, as well as toward impaired physical and mental health (Choi-Kain et al. 2022). Although BPD is typically first diagnosed in adulthood, its evolution emerges in the early stages of life. Negative affectivity and impulsivity anticipate severely harsh parenting styles, which contribute to elevated risk for later BPD diagnosis in the presence of exposure to various social adversities (Stepp et al. 2016a, b; Winsper et al. 2017). Experiencing significant social and functional disturbances, lower levels of academic and occupational achievement, higher use of medical and psychiatric services, and lower levels of stability in social support are marked issues in individuals with BPD (Winograd et al. 2008; Choi-Kain and Sharp 2021).

In line with findings, BPD is often presented as a female-predominant disorder in both research and clinical contexts (Qian et al. 2022), which means it is found more frequently in the female gender in clinical samples (Bozzatello et al. 2024). However, some authors hypothesized the presence of bias in the diagnostic criteria thresholds, in the population sampling (community versus clinical), in instruments of evaluation (clinical versus self-report measurements), and in the diagnostic construct of BPD, which suggest higher frequency among females compared to males

E. A. Selby, M. Salavati, *Theories of Borderline Personality Disorder*,
https://doi.org/10.1007/978-3-031-75503-3_1

(Bozzatello et al. 2024; Boggs 2005; Qian et al. 2022). In accordance with a scoping review, Qian et al. (2022) pointed out that males with BPD are more likely to exhibit externalizing symptoms such as aggressiveness, as well as comorbid disorders such as substance use, while women with BPD display more internalizing symptoms such as emotional instability and comorbid disorders such as mood and eating disorders (Qian et al. 2022). Population and epidemiological studies have indicated that males are more likely to manifest aggression and display high novelty seeking (Barnow et al. 2007; Staniloiu and Markowitsch 2012), whereas females are inclined to show greater levels of harm avoidance and lower novelty seeking (Barnow et al. 2007; Deng et al. 2023), and also, females are more vulnerable to express and talk about their emotions (Liddon et al. 2018). In line with studies, it has been shown that *men* were more likely to indicate the criteria "intense and inappropriate anger" (Tadić et al. 2009; Michonski et al. 2013), " more to be diagnosed antisocial personality" (Bender et al. 2003), and "impulsivity and impulsive behaviors" (Zanarini et al. 2011); *women* reported the criteria "chronic feelings of emptiness" (Zanarini et al. 2011), "anxiety and eating disorders" (Krueger et al. 1998), "affective instability" (Zanarini et al. 2011; Tadić et al. 2009), "identity disturbances" (De Moor et al. 2023; Johnson et al. 2012), and "unstable relationship" (De Moor et al. 2023), but not "suicidality/self-harm behaviors" (Zanarini et al. 2011; De Moor et al. 2023; Marchetto 2006). Moreover, higher levels of hypersensitivity to external stimuli, contributing to anxiety and avoidance, and also greater levels of alexithymia with higher tendency to despair were reported among women (Amerio et al. 2023). According to Cloninger's psychological model, some investigators propose various differences in temperamental dimensions between genders, especially high levels of novelty-seeking, neuroticism and agreeableness among women, whrereas high levels of dissocial behaviors among men (Barnow et al. 2007; Banzhaf et al. 2012).

According to DSM-5, based on the National Comorbidity Survey Replication, the estimated prevalence of BPD was 1.4%, as well as, in accordance with the National Epidemiologic Survey, the prevalence of BPD was reported 5.9%. Moreover, the prevalence of BPD was estimated 6% for primary care settings, 10% in outpatient mental health clinics, 20% among psychiatric populations (APA 2022), and 1–2% in general population (Sadock et al. 2017; Biskin and Paris 2012). Women account for 70% of populations with BPD in clinical settings (Gunderson et al. 2018). Based on epidemiological findings in the USA, the lifetime prevalence of BPD was nearly 6%, and in the UK, a large national sample indicated a community prevalence of 0.7% (Coid et al. 2006). In primary care settings, approximately a range from 4% to 6% (Gross et al. 2002), and also, a heightened prevalence to 9.3% in community outpatient clinics and nearly 20% among inpatient settings were estimated (Zimmerman et al. 2005). BPD influences 1%–3% of general adolescent and adult population, 9% of all emergency department visits, 50% of suicidal patients in emergency rooms, and 20%–25% of psychiatric inpatients (Pascual et al. 2007; Hong et al. 2017; Zimmerman et al. 2008, 2013, 2015, 2023; Soeteman et al. 2008). Ten Have et al. (2016) studied the prevalence of different numbers of BPD symptoms in the general population and its co-occurrence with other mental disorders. In addition, they evaluated to what extent mental disability is associated with the number of BPD symptoms. The results indicated that among total population, 69.9% reported no BPD symptoms, while 25.2% showed 1–2 symptoms, 3.8% had 3–4 symptoms, and 1.1% had >5 BPD symptoms. The number of BPD symptoms found was indicated to be positively related to not living with a partner, with no paid job, having a comorbid mood, anxiety, or substance use disorder. Additionally, positive associations were found in using services for dealing with mental health problems (Ten Have et al. 2016). During last decades, BPD has been placed in the center of experts' debates and numerous investigations have been done to clarify its psychopathology, to elucidate its etiology, and to provide effective therapeutic interventions for this complicated and controversial personality disorder (e.g., Baryshnikov et al. 2017, 2024; Gabbard 2005; Gunderson et al. 2018; Maldonato et al. 2018; Cavelti et al. 2024). Especially, its substantial clinical heterogeneity, highly extensive comorbidity, lack of diagnostic reliability and validity, optional criterion cutoffs, and temporal characteristics and comorbidities with other personality disorders contributed to considering BPD as the most controversial personality disorder (Calvo et al. 2016; Maldonato et al. 2018).

Furthermore, the severely intense stigma surrounding BPD has resulted in substantial controversy when it comes to matters of diagnosis (Campbell et al. 2020), such as the diagnosis of BPD among adolescents (Cavelti et al. 2024; Schmeck et al. 2022), overlap with trauma-related disorders, and a general critique about scientific issues of BPD (Tyrer et al. 2022), which may be led to non-diagnosis of BPD or misdiagnosis of other psychiatric disorders (Kernberg and Yeomans 2013; Lewis and Grenyer 2009). In accordance with a recent systematic review, it was explored that individuals with BPD, who received health services, reported a mixture of negative and positive experiences. Negative experiences comprised having no crucially adequate information about their diagnosis, resulting in resistance of their diagnosis, feeling hopelessness due to perceiving BPD as "untreatable" disorder. However, positive experiences encompass a clearer understanding of themselves and their problems, which contribute to lesser feelings of loneliness and promote the sense of relief (Lester et al. 2020). Tedesco et al. (2024) studied the complex reality of living with BPD among 15 BPD participants to explore topics of illness onset, insight, experience of diagnosis, and treatment. Individuals' explanations for BPD emergence were different from biological, psychological, and social factors. The findings showed that any benefits of diagnosis such as improving insight and decreasing withdrawal were contrasted with challenges like stigma and treatment unavailability. In addition, delay in diagnosis was a common problem, and no participants reported receiving a diagnosis of BPD during adolescence, while 85% of them believed that they would have benefited from a diagnosis in adolescence. Twenty-seven percent of participants felt highly supported in the diagnosis process. The participants suggested an ideal four-step diagnosis procedure, encompassing: (1) explain the process; (2) assess completely; (3) explore how the manifestations are active in daily life; and (4) connect diagnosis to evidence-based therapeutic planning (Tedesco et al. 2024).

Historical Perspective of BPD

A historical viewpoint can assist us in developing a holistic understanding of BPD. As Linehan (1993) mentioned, the formal concept of BPD is relatively new in the field of psychopathology. The concept of BPD did not emerge in the *Diagnostic and Statistical Manual of Mental Disorders* (DSM) published by the American Psychiatric Association until the publication of DSM-III in 1980 (Linehan 1993). Phenomenological descriptions of individuals with BPD date back to the late nineteenth and early twentieth centuries (Stone 1981, 2000, 2016, 2019; Feinstein 2021). Although a particular constellation of traits comprising the diagnostic entity was recognized much earlier, much of the current interest in this population has resulted from its recently gained official status. That status was not achieved without much controversy and dispute. The "official" nomenclature and diagnostic criteria have been arrived at both through political compromise and attention to empirical data (Linehan 1993). Finally, an important cautionary note is that some of the historical descriptions that will be provided are now considered archaic, inconsistent with modern scientific advances in understanding mental health, and potentially stigmatizing; however, modern work on BPD is striving to reduce stigmatized and unfair views of this challenging diagnosis.

Before 1970, the recognition of "borderline" stemmed from an era when the psychoanalytic viewpoint was dominant in psychology and emerging diagnostic classification systems. Borderline was identified based on psychoanalytic theoretical formulations and was presented as patients experiencing neurosis, considered as targetable and treatable, simultaneously with psychosis, considered as untreatable. This perspective was influenced by the construct on "*borderline personality organization*", which was mentioned by Kernberg (1975). *Borderline*, when used adjectivally, suggests something that is in the close proximity to something else. The term "borderline" was first described by the psychoanalyst Stern in 1938 (Biskin and Paris 2012; Gunderson et al. 2011). The term borderline was introduced originally when clinicians met a group of clients with a combination of psychotic and neurotic features, which made the diagnosis difficult. These groups were labeled as "the borderline of psychosis and neurosis" (Stern 1938; Kaufman et al. 2017). These individuals were often recognized by clinicians as individuals with milder forms of psychosis. For instance, Kraepelin presented individuals with dementia praecox (psychosis) and manic-depression, as well as identified patients with milder symptoms of each of these conditions who were between these two (Kraepelin 1921). The term "borderline personality" was not applied until 1938, when Stern suggested a group of individuals assigned "neither into the psychotic nor into the psychoneurotic group in terms of symptoms." (Stern 1938). In line with Stone (2005), the word *borderline* was used in psychiatry to identify a group of people who have either (a) a condition that approximated another, already well-established disorder, or (b) a condition that placed a region between two rather indistinct boundary levels of mental functioning.

Stern (1938) drew attention to the simultaneous idealization and devaluation of the analyst and of the other person important in the life of the patient. An inability of borderline patients to deal with adequately stressful situation was named "psychic bleeding" by Stern (1938), and overreaction to mild criticism was another feature, which was called "negative therapeutic reaction" (Zanarini 2005). Deutsch (1942) used the term "as if" instead of the word "borderline", who are characterized by a lack of warmth and a mild depersonalization that are matched with a subset of people with BPD, encompassing an individual who remarked "*I am so empty! …I have no feeling*." (Deutsch 1942). Deutsch (1942) described borderline condition as depersonalization, narcissistic identifications with others, a fully maintained grasp on reality, poverty of object relations, a masking of all aggressive tendencies by passivity, and inner emptiness. Deutsch resembled borderline to some forms of emotional disturbance and their relationship to schizophrenia, and reported cases, whose emotional relationship to the outside world and to his own ego appears impoverished or absent, and emphasized that such disturbances of emotional life take various forms. Individuals, who complained of their inner experiences and their disturbances, might be transitory and fleeting and indicate a fluctuated nature. Deutsch also added that the emotional difficulties and disorders may be perceived as existing personality or it may be projected onto the outside world (Deutsch 1942).

The place of borderline personality disorder (BPD) in psychiatric nosology has long been a point of contention (Zanarini et al. 1998, 2007). In line with Zanarini (2005), another feature mentioned in Stern's work is "projective mechanisms". It means that borderline patients tend to externalize and assign blame to outsiders. Masochism and depression, as well as issues in reality testing, especially in interpersonal sphere, are more frequent in these groups of people (Zanarini 2005). This feature referred as "splitting" in Kernberg's theory is manifested by idealizing and devaluating people in their relationships. In other words, borderline cases attribute positive and awesome qualities to their partner, and abruptly with no reason or illogical ration, their attitudes alter in a way that leads to the development of immensely awful attitudes and hostile behaviors toward people.

In 1947, Schmideberg conceptualized borderline patients as a series of symptoms, including the inability to tolerate routine and regularity, tendency to break many regulations of social convention, such as being late for appointments and unreliable about payment, unable to be focused on the process of psychotherapy during sessions, poor motivation for treatment, failures to develop meaningful insight, having a chaotic life, engaging in petty criminal acts, and inability to establish emotional contact. Schmideberg (1947) claimed that the majority of her patients suffered neither from a classical neurosis nor a definite psychosis. They were "difficult" and might or might not had circumscribed neurotic symptoms. Most of them would probably be diagnosed as "psychopaths" or "borderline cases". Hoch and Polatin (1947) preambled that there were a group of clients not to be distinguished clinically as psychoneurosis. They emphasized that many of these patients had been analyzed for a considerable period of time and the suspicion had never been raised that they were not psychoneurotic.

Based on Hoch and Polatin (1947), some psychiatrists conceded that the clinical and psychodynamic structure of these cases differs from the neurosis—although retaining a great deal of resemblance to the neurotic disturbances—and called them "borderline cases." Classifying these patients with the schizophrenic reactions was justified because many of the basic mechanisms in these cases were very similar to those commonly known in schizophrenia (Polatin and Hoch 1947; Gunderson et al. 2011). Knight (1953) concentrated on primitive defense mechanisms lurking behind the higher-level defenses in borderline cases and on the fragility of their hold on reality. Instead of focusing on the concept of schizophrenia, he concentrated on schizophrenia and provided a broad view to comprehend borderline, it did not dwell overly long on the point. For the first time, Knight (1953) suggested that describing borderline just through definition and similarities with schizophrenia cannot assist clinician to understand "borderline". Whereas he has accentuated for achieving a clearer picture of borderline, it is more useful and practical to consider borderline like an entity into itself. Knight (1953) argued that the term "borderline state" had achieved almost no official status in psychiatrics nomenclature and conveyed no diagnostic illumination of a case other than the implication that the patient is quite sick but not frankly psychotic. Rado (1957) tried to describe borderline as "extractive disorder", a complex of various symptoms: impatience and intolerance of frustration, rage outbursts, irresponsibility, excitability, parasitism, hedonism, depressive spells, and "affect hunger". Moreover, Esser and Lesser (1965) introduced borderline as a "hysteroid disorder" consisting of irresponsibility, erratic work history, chaotic and unfulfilling relationships that never become profound or lasting, early childhood history of emotional problems and disturbed habit patterns, and chaotic sexuality. The other group of researchers who contributed a description of borderline were Grinker et al. (1968). According to their description, there are a series of common characteristics in all borderline and also, they categorized borderline to four subtypes.

Kernberg (1975) updated Stern's definition of the term "borderline" by suggesting the term "borderline personality organization", featured by a certain complex of symptoms and clinical characteristics encompassing intact relationship to reality, use of defense mechanisms (splitting and idealization), and identity diffusion such as object relations (Kernberg 1967, 1971; Biskin and Paris 2012; Gunderson et al. 2011). Core concept of BPD in Kernberg's model (1975, Clarkin & Kernberg, 2015) includes mental representations that are originated from internalization of attachment relationship with caregivers. The degree of differentiation and integration of mentioned representations of self and other with their emotional valence contribute to personality organization. Kernberg (1975) proposed that the concepts of pre-schizophrenic, personality structure, borderline states, psychotic characters, and borderline personality have emerged in clinical practices with patients who were seriously disturbed and multisymptomatic. Kernberg (1975) identified these patients in a specific psychologically pathological structure, who were varied from neurotic and psychotic patients, and named them as having "borderline personality organization" (BPO). These patients were prone to lack of reality testing and delusional idea contributing to defensive splitting (Feinstein 2021; Jacobson 1954, 1957, 1964; Kilen 1946). Kernberg described these patients as descriptive pathology and the level of structural organization, engaging lack of anxiety tolerance, impaired impulse control, disturbances in the development of sublimatory channels, ego weakness, and internalized object relations. Based on object relation theory (Yeomans et al. 2015), a psychological structure has been recognized as a stable and tolerant pattern of psychological functions that organized the person's behavior, perceptions, and subjective experience. The nature and degree of integration of the sense of self and other have been shown as the most remarkable psychological structures among patients with severe personality diosrders in the nature and degree of integration of the sense of self and others. In line with this conceptualization, individuals with BPO experience severely intense emotions that are not related to each other internally, which contributes to being overwhelmed subjectively by severe emotions at the moment and disturbed ability to cognitively appraise situations precisely. According to this view, the term borderline is used to describe most serious forms of character pathology. Two main aspects of BPD include affect and self-regulating. Negative affect, especially hostility and aggression, with the lowest level of positive emotion, as well as poor self-regulation comprising impulsivity and impulsive aggression is presented as core pathological aspect in BPD (Kernberg 1985; Gunderson et al. 2011). Patients with BPO are manifested by the disintegrated nature of identity, application of primitive defenses, fragile reality testing, disturbed affect regulation and sexual and aggressive expression, inconsistent internalized values, and poor quality of relations with others. This pathological structure comprises of a disturbed integration of the primitive positive (idealized) and negative (persecutory) segments of early object relations (Yeomans et al. 2015).

Another conceptualization, which flourished in the 1960s and 1970s, focused on the propensity of borderline patients to have transient psychotic or psychotic-like experience. In this view, borderline personality was thought of as being a schizophrenia spectrum disorder (Wender 1977). Between 1970–1980, following the initial attempts of Grinker et al. (1968), borderline syndrome was suggested which contributed to officially entering the DSM-III (1980) as "*borderline personality disorder*." (Gunderson et al. 1984, 2011, 2018; Biskin and Paris 2012; APA 1980) and received more attention from clinical research (Feinstein 2021). Other conceptualizations, which organized much of clinical care and empirical research in the 1980s, focused on the chronic dysphoria and affective lability of borderline patients. In this view, borderline personality was thought of as being an affective spectrum disorder (Akiskal 1981; Stone 1981; Zanarini and Frankenburg 2007). Gunderson et al. (1984) described a specific form of personality disorder that can be distinguished from a substantial number of other axis II disorders, particularly those in the "odd" and "anxious". BPD was officially identified as personality disorder diagnosis in third edition of the DSM-III and has become a focused subject for numerous researches and experts to allocate higher attention for debating and studying BPD clinically and empirically (Samuel et al. 2012).

References

Akiskal HS. Subaffective disorders: dysthymic, cyclothymic and bipolar II disorders in the "borderline" realm. Psychiatr Clin. 1981;4(1):25–46.

American Psychiatric Association. Diagnostic and statistical manual of mental disorders. 3rd ed. Washington, DC: American Psychiatric Association; 1980.

American Psychiatric Association. Diagnostic and statistical manual of mental disorders. 5th ed. Text Revised (DSM-5-TR); 2022.

Amerio A, Natale A, Gnecco GB, Lechiara A, Verrina E, Bianchi D, Fusar-Poli L, Costanza A, Serafini G, Amore M, Aguglia A. The role of gender in patients with borderline personality disorder: differences related to hopelessness, alexithymia, coping strategies, and sensory profile. Medicina. 2023;59(5):950.

Banzhaf A, Ritter K, Merkl A, Schulte-Herbrüggen O, Lammers CH, Roepke S. Gender differences in a clinical sample of patients with borderline personality disorder. J Personal Disord. 2012;26(3):368–80.

Barnow S, Herpertz SC, Spitzer C, Stopsack M, Preuss UW, Grabe HJ, Kessler C, Freyberger HJ. Temperament and character in patients with borderline personality disorder taking gender and comorbidity into account. Psychopathology. 2007;40(6):369–78.

Baryshnikov I, Joffe G, Koivisto M, Melartin T, Aaltonen K, Suominen K, Rosenström T, Näätänen P, Karpov B, Heikkinen M, Isometsä E. Relationships between self-reported childhood traumatic experiences, attachment style, neuroticism and features of borderline personality disorders in patients with mood disorders. J Affect Disord. 2017;210:82–9.

Baryshnikov I, Rosenström TH, Isometsä ET. Psychological pain as a risk factor for suicidal ideation: an ecological momentary assessment study on inpatients with depression with and without comorbid borderline personality disorder. J Clin Psychiatry. 2024;85(2):54110.

Bender DS, Farber BA, Sanislow CA, Dyck IR, Geller JD, Skodol AE. Representations of therapists by patients with personality disorders. Am J Psychother. 2003;57(2):219–36.

Biskin RS, Paris J. Management of borderline personality disorder. CMAJ. 2012;184(17):1897–902.

Boggs CD. Clinical overlap between posttraumatic stress disorder and borderline personality disorder in male veterans. Texas A&M University; 2005.

Bozzatello P, Blua C, Brandellero D, Baldassarri L, Brasso C, Rocca P, Bellino S. Gender differences in borderline personality disorder: a narrative review. Front Psych. 2024;15:1320546.

Calvo N, Valero S, Sáez-Francàs N, Gutiérrez F, Casas M, Ferrer M. Borderline personality disorder and personality inventory for DSM-5 (PID-5): dimensional personality assessment with DSM-5. Compr Psychiatry. 2016;70:105–11.

Campbell K, Clarke KA, Massey D, Lakeman R. Borderline personality disorder: to diagnose or not to diagnose? That is the question. Int J Ment Health Nurs. 2020;29(5):972–81.

Cavelti M, Blaha Y, Lerch S, Hertel C, Berger T, Reichl C, Koenig J, Kaess M. The evaluation of a stepped care approach for early intervention of borderline personality disorder. Borderl Personal Disord Emot Dysregul. 2024;11(1):12.

Choi-Kain LW, Sharp C, editors. Handbook of good psychiatric management for adolescents with borderline personality disorder. American Psychiatric Pub; 2021.

Choi-Kain LW, Sahin Z, Traynor J. Borderline personality disorder: updates in a postpandemic world. Focus. 2022;20(4):337–52.

Clarkin JF, Kernberg OF. Transference-focused psychotherapy for borderline personality disorder: a clinical guide. American Psychiatric Pub; 2015.

Coid J, Yang MI, Tyrer P, Roberts A, Ullrich S. Prevalence and correlates of personality disorder in Great Britain. Br J Psychiatry. 2006;188(5):423–31.

De Moor EL, Klimstra TA, Van Doeselaar L, Branje S. Who am I? studying autobiographical reasoning, identity commitment and exploration processes, and narrative content in unison. J Early Adolesc. 2023:02724316231216388.

Deng W, Yan S, Xu Y, Lu Z, Liu L, Zhou Y, Chen M. Effects of BPD tendencies and subjective well-being on NSSI in adolescents with PTSD. Front Psych. 2023;14:1152352.

Deutsch H. Some forms of emotional disturbance and their relationship to schizophreniapsychosis. 1942;Q11:301–21.
Esser R, Lesser S. Hysterical personality. A reevaluation. Psychoanal. 1965.
Feinstein R. Personality disorders. Oxford University Press; 2021.
Gabbard GO. Mind, brain, and personality disorders. Am J Psychiatry. 2005;162(4):648–55.
Grinker R, Webble B, Drye R. The borderline syndrome. A behavioral study of ego-functions. New York: Basic Books; 1968.
Gross R, Olfson M, Gameroff M, Shea S, Feder A, Fuentes M, Lantigua R, Weissman MM. Borderline personality disorder in primary care. Arch Intern Med. 2002;162(1):53–60.
Gunderson JG, Frank AF, Katz HM, Vannicelli ML, Frosch JP, Knapp PH. Effects of psychotherapy in schizophrenia: II. Comparative outcome of two forms of treatment. Schizophr Bull. 1984;10(4):564–98.
Gunderson JG, Stout RL, McGlashan TH, Shea MT, Morey LC, Grilo CM, Zanarini MC, Yen S, Markowitz JC, Sanislow C, Ansell E. Ten-year course of borderline personality disorder: psychopathology and function from the collaborative longitudinal personality disorders study. Arch Gen Psychiatry. 2011;68(8):827–37.
Gunderson JG, Herpertz SC, Skodol AE, Torgersen S, Zanarini MC. Borderline personality disorder. Nat Rev Dis Primers. 2018;4(1):1–20.
Hong M, Cho HN, Kim AR, Hong HJ, Kweon YS. Suicidal deaths in elementary school students in Korea. Child Adolesc Psychiatry Ment Health. 2017;11:1–5.
Jacobson E. Contribution to the metapsychology of psychotic identifications. J Am Psychoanal Assoc. 1954;2:239–62.
Jacobson E. Denial and repression. J Am Psychoanal Assoc. 1957;5:61–92.
Jacobson E. The self and the object world. New York: International Universities Press; 1964.
Johnson MD, Morgeson FP, Hekman DR. Cognitive and affective identification: Exploring the links between different forms of social identification and personality with work attitudes and behavior. Journal of Organizational Behavior. 2012 Nov;33(8):1142–67.
Kaufman EA, Puzia ME, Mead HK, Crowell SE, McEachern A, Beauchaine TP. Children's emotion regulation difficulties mediate the association between maternal borderline and antisocial symptoms and youth behavior problems over 1 year. J Personal Disord. 2017;31(2):170–92.
Kernberg O. Borderline personality organization. J Am Psychoanal Assoc. 1967;15(3):641–85.
Kernberg O. Further contributions to the treatment of narcissistic personalities: A reply to the discussion by Paul H. Ornstein. The International journal of psycho-analysis. 1975;56:245.
Kernberg OF. Prognostic considerations regarding borderline personality organization. J Am Psychoanal Assoc. 1971;19(4):595–635.
Kernberg OF. Borderline conditions and pathological narcissism. 1985.
Kernberg OF, Yeomans FE. Borderline personality disorder, bipolar disorder, depression, attention deficit/hyperactivity disorder, and narcissistic personality disorder: practical differential diagnosis. Bull Menn Clin. 2013;77(1):1–22.
Kilen M. Notes on some schizoid mechanisms. Int J Psychoanal. 1946;27(Pt 3–4):99–110.
Knight RP. Borderline states. In: Joint Session of the American Psychoanalytic Association and the Section on Psychoanalysis of the American Psychiatric Association, May, 1952. Read at the aforementioned conference. Atlantic City: International Universities Press; 1953.
Kraepelin E. Bismarcks Persönlichkeit, Ungedruckte persönliche Erinnerungen. Südd Monatsh. 1921;19:105–22.
Krueger RF, Moffitt TE, Caspi A, Bleske A, Silva PA. Assortative mating for antisocial behavior: developmental and methodological implications. Behav Genet. 1998;28:173–86.
Kulacaoglu F, Kose S. Borderline personality disorder (BPD): in the midst of vulnerability, chaos, and awe. Brain Sci. 2018;8(11):201.
Lester R, Prescott L, McCormack M, Sampson M, North West Boroughs Healthcare, NHS Foundation Trust. Service users' experiences of receiving a diagnosis of borderline personality disorder: a systematic review. Personal Ment Health. 2020;14(3):263–83.

Lewis KL, Grenyer BF. Borderline personality or complex posttraumatic stress disorder? An update on the controversy. Harv Rev Psychiatry. 2009;17(5):322–8.
Liddon L, Kingerlee R, Barry JA. Gender differences in preferences for psychological treatment, coping strategies, and triggers to help-seeking. Br J Clin Psychol. 2018;57(1):42–58.
Linehan M. Cognitive-behavioral treatment of borderline personality disorder. Guilford Press; 1993.
Maldonato NM, Sperandeo R, Moretto E, Dell'Orco S. A non-linear predictive model of borderline personality disorder based on multilayer perceptron. Front Psychol. 2018;9:447.
Marchetto MJ. Repetitive skin-cutting: parental bonding, personality and gender. Psychol Psychother Theory Res Pract. 2006;79(3):445–59.
Michonski JD, Sharp C, Steinberg L, Zanarini MC. An item response theory analysis of the DSM-IV borderline personality disorder criteria in a population-based sample of 11-to 12-year-old children. Personal Disord Theory Res Treat. 2013;4(1):15.
Pascual JC, Córcoles D, Castaño J, Ginés JM, Gurrea A, Martín-Santos R, Garcia-Ribera C, Pérez V, Bulbena A. Hospitalization and pharmacotherapy for borderline personality disorder in a psychiatric emergency service. Psychiatr Serv. 2007;58(9):1199–204.
Polatin P, Hoch P. Diagnostic evaluation of early schizophrenia. J Nerv Ment Dis. 1947;105(3):221–30.
Qian X, Townsend ML, Tan WJ, Grenyer BF. Sex differences in borderline personality disorder: a scoping review. PLoS One. 2022;17(12):e0279015.
Rado S. Narcotic bondage: a general theory of the dependence on narcotic drugs. Am J Psychiatry. 1957;114(2):165–70.
Sadock BJ, Sadock VA, Ruiz P. Comprehensive textbook of psychiatry. 10th ed. Wolters Kluwer; 2017.
Samuel DB, Miller JD, Widiger TA, Lynam DR, Pilkonis PA, Ball SA. Conceptual changes to the definition of borderline personality disorder proposed for DSM-5. J Abnorm Psychol. 2012;121(2):467.
Schmeck K, Kumperscak HG, Birkhölzer M, Goth K. Dimensional assessment of personality disorders in young people: a closer look on personality functioning in younger ages, different cultures, and various clinical settings. Front Psych. 2022;13:1082189.
Schmideberg M. The treatment of psychopaths and borderline patients. Am J Psychother. 1947;1(1):45–70.
Soeteman DI, Verheul R, Busschbach JJ. The burden of disease in personality disorders: diagnosis-specific quality of life. J Personal Disord. 2008;22(3):259–68.
Staniloiu A, Markowitsch HJ. Towards solving the riddle of forgetting in functional amnesia: recent advances and current opinions. Front Psychol. 2012;3:403.
Stepp SD, Lazarus SA, Byrd AL. A systematic review of risk factors prospectively associated with borderline personality disorder: taking stock and moving forward. Personal Disord Theory Res Treat. 2016a;7(4):316.
Stepp SD, Scott LN, Jones NP, Whalen DJ, Hipwell AE. Negative emotional reactivity as a marker of vulnerability in the development of borderline personality disorder symptoms. Dev Psychopathol. 2016b;28(1):213–24.
Stern A. Psychoanalytic investigation of and therapy in the border line group of neuroses. Psychoanal Q. 1938;7(4):467–89.
Stone MH. Borderline syndromes: a consideration of subtypes and an overview, directions for research. Psychiatr Clin. 1981;4(1):3–24.
Stone MH. Clinical guidelines for psychotherapy for patients with borderline personality disorder. Psychiatr Clin N Am. 2000;23(1):193–210.
Stone MH. Borderline personality disorder: history of the concept. Med Psychiatry. 2005;31(1)
Stone MH. Long-term course of borderline personality disorder. Psychodyn Psychiatry. 2016;44(3):449–74.
Stone MH. Borderline personality disorder: clinical guidelines for treatment. Psychodyn psychiatry. 2019;47(1):5–26.

Tadić A, Wagner S, Hoch J, Başkaya Ö, Von Cube R, Skaletz C, Lieb K, Dahmen N. Gender differences in axis I and axis II comorbidity in patients with borderline personality disorder. Psychopathology. 2009;42(4):257–63.

Tedesco V, Day NJ, Lucas S, Grenyer BF. Diagnosing borderline personality disorder: reports and recommendations from people with lived experience. Personal Ment Health. 2024;18(2):107–21.

Ten Have M, Verheul R, Kaasenbrood A, van Dorsselaer S, Tuithof M, Kleinjan M, de Graaf R. Prevalence rates of borderline personality disorder symptoms: a study based on The Netherlands Mental Health Survey and Incidence Study-2. BMC Psychiatry 2016;16:1–0.

Tyrer P, Tyrer H, Yang M. The influence of personality disorder in predicting suicidal behaviour in common mental disorders: a 30-year study. Personal Ment Health. 2022;16(2):111–9.

Wender PH. The scope and validity of the schizophrenic spectrum concept. In: Psychiatric diagnosis. London: Palgrave Macmillan; 1977. p. 109–27.

Winograd G, Cohen P, Chen H. Adolescent borderline symptoms in the community: prognosis for functioning over 20 years. J Child Psychol Psychiatry. 2008;49(9):933–41.

Winsper C, Tang NK, Marwaha S, Lereya ST, Gibbs M, Thompson A, Singh SP. The sleep phenotype of borderline personality disorder: a systematic review and meta-analysis. Neurosci Biobehav Rev. 2017;73:48–67.

Yeomans EE, Clarkin JF, Kernberg OF. Transference-focused psychotherapy for borderline personality disorder: a clinical guide. American Psychiatric Association; 2015.

Zanarini MC, editor. Borderline personality disorder. CRC Press; 2005.

Zanarini MC, Frankenburg FR. The essential nature of borderline psychopathology. J Personal Disord. 2007;21(5):518–35.

Zanarini MC, Frankenburg FR, Dubo ED, Sickel AE, Trikha A, Levin A, Reynolds V. Axis I comorbidity of borderline personality disorder. Am J Psychiatry. 1998;155(12):1733–9.

Zanarini MC, Frankenburg FR, Reich DB, Silk KR, Hudson JI, McSweeney LB. The subsyndromal phenomenology of borderline personality disorder: a 10-year follow-up study. Am J Psychiatry. 2007;164(6):929–35.

Zanarini MC, Horwood J, Wolke D, Waylen A, Fitzmaurice G, Grant BF. Prevalence of DSM-IV borderline personality disorder in two community samples: 6,330 English 11-year-olds and 34,653 American adults. J Personal Disord. 2011;25(5):607–19.

Zimmerman M, Rothschild L, Chelminski I. The prevalence of DSM-IV personality disorders in psychiatric outpatients. Am J Psychiatry. 2005;162(10):1911–8.

Zimmerman SM, Phelps E, Lerner RM. Positive and negative developmental trajectories in US adolescents: where the positive youth development perspective meets the deficit model. Res Hum Dev. 2008;5(3):153–65.

Zimmerman M, Morgan TA. The relationship between borderline personality disorder and bipolar disorder. Dialogues in clinical neuroscience. 2013 Jun 30;15(2):155–69.

Zimmerman M. Borderline personality disorder: a disorder in search of advocacy. The Journal of nervous and mental disease. 2015 Jan 1;203(1):8–12.

Zimmerman M, Becker L. The hidden borderline patient: patients with borderline personality disorder who do not engage in recurrent suicidal or self-injurious behavior. Psychological medicine. 2023 Aug;53(11):5177–84.

Chapter 2
Diagnostic Perspectives of Borderline Personality Disorder

Introduction

Borderline Personality Disorder (BPD) is a severe mental health condition represented by pervasive patterns of instability in self-image and identity, affective-emotional regulation difficulties, instability in mood, dysfunctional interpersonal relationships, and marked impulsivity (APA 2022). Based on DSM-5, BPD symptomatology encompasses four main domains: (1) affective and emotional dysregulation; (2) behavioral dysregulation dimensions, comprising impulsivity and suicidal behaviors; (3) interpersonal instability featured by fear of abandonment and intense unstable relationship; and (4) cognitive and self-disturbance including paranoid ideation, dissociative symptoms, and identity impairments (APA 2022). Individuals with BPD demonstrate substantial morbidity contributing to complicated medical care in comparison to other people (Kulacaoglu and Kose 2018). The onset of BPD is initially during adolescence and continues into adulthood (Chanen 2015). Moreover, it has been proposed specifically as a diagnosis emerges in adolescents based on DSM-5 (APA 2022).

Diagnostic and Statistical Manual of Mental Disorders, Fifth Edition (DSM-5)

BPD is a challenging diagnosis due to its heterogenous phenotype, its extensively substantial overlap with other psychiatric disorders, and its debated diagnostic validity and reliability (Garland and Miller 2020; Jablensky 2016). BPD is proposed as a severely chronic psychiatric disorder composed of heterogenous and psychological and neurobiological adversities (Herzog et al. 2022) and a constellation of symptoms encompassing 9 categorical criteria (Bach and Sellbom 2016),

E. A. Selby, M. Salavati, *Theories of Borderline Personality Disorder*,
https://doi.org/10.1007/978-3-031-75503-3_2

comprising diverse patterns of maladaptive characteristics, including: (1) fluctuating affective states and emotional instability pictured by severe emotional responses, rapid and intense mood fluctuations, and an inability to manage anger; (2) identity issues, a sense of purposelessness, emptiness, boringness, and continuous complaining from life situation; (3) severe interpersonal relationship difficulties, frequent conflicts with others, experiencing high levels of hostility in relationship, repeated thoughts of being betrayed and abandoned, and experiencing extremely intense negative emotions in relationships; (4) self-destructive and self-harm behaviors, impulsivity, aggression, risky sexual behaviors, and high tendency toward engaging in self-injurious behaviors to reduce negative emotions; and (5) dissociative experiences and stress-induced paranoia (DSM-5-TR, APA 2022; Sadock et al. 2017; Bach et al. 2016a; Kendler et al. 2010). The hallmark of BPD includes an excessively pervasive instability of affect, self-image, interpersonal relationships, and impulsivity (Sadock et al. 2017). Common among individuals with BPD are self-destructive behaviors and dysregulated behaviors (Selby et al. 2022), such as binge and purging (American Psychiatric Association 2013), substance use issues (Khosravi 2020; Miller et al. 2018, 2021), reckless driving (Bornovalova et al. 2005), nonsuicidal self-harm (NSSH), and suicidal behaviors (Howard et al. 2021; Brickman et al. 2014; Selby and Gardner 2015; Johns et al. 2023). BPD is a severe, debilitating mental disorder characterized by considerable problematic behaviors especially deliberate self-harm and suicidal behaviors and patterns of dysfunctional instability across emotional, behavioral, cognitive, and interpersonal domains (Stead et al. 2019; Sharp and Wall 2018). Table one shows the diagnostic criteria for BPD (Table 2.1).

Table 2.1 Diagnostic criteria for borderline personality disorders

Diagnostic criteria
A pervasive pattern of instability of interpersonal relationships, self-image, and effects and marked impulsivity, beginning by early adulthood and present in a variety of contexts, as indicated by five (or more) of the following:
1. Frantic efforts to avoid real or imagined abandonment. (Note: Do not include suicidal or self-mutilating behavior covered in criterion 5).
2. A pattern of unstable and intense interpersonal relationships characterized by alternating between extremes of idealization and devaluation.
3. Identity disturbance: markedly and persistently unstable self-image or sense of self.
4. Impulsivity in at least two areas that are potentially self-damaging (e.g., spending, sex, substance abuse, reckless driving, being eating). (Note: Do not include suicidal or self-mutilating behavior covered in criterion 5).
5. Recurrent suicidal behavior, gestures, or threats, or self-mutilating behavior.
6. Affective instability due to marked reactivity to mood (e.g., intense episodic dysphoria, irritability, or anxiety usually lasting a few hours and only rarely more than a few days).
7. Chronic feelings of emptiness.
8. Inappropriate, intense anger or difficulty controlling anger (e.g., frequent displays of temper, constant anger, recurrent physical fights).
9. Transient, stress-related paranoid ideation, or severe dissociative symptoms.

Based on DSM-5-TR, the essential characteristic of BPD includes a pervasively serious pattern of instability in interpersonal relationships, self-image, and emotions, exhibited by remarkable impulsivity that appears by early adulthood and is manifested in a variety of contexts. *Criterion 1* proposes a perception of imminent separation or rejection, which contributes to substantial alterations in self-image, emotion, cognition, and behavior. These people exhibit fear of abandonment, inappropriate anger, sensitivity to environmental conditions, and frantic attempts to avoid abandonment comprising impulsive behaviors such as self-harm and suicidal behaviors. *Criterion 2* states that individuals with BPD reveal a pattern of instability and issues in interpersonal relationships, in which they idealize people and see people as perfect and good; and they may switch quickly from idealizing other people to devaluating them and see them as bad or even evil. *Criterion 3* mentions that individuals with BPD experience identity disturbances manifested by remarkable and persistent instability in self-image or sense of self which contribute to sudden dramatic alterations in self-image, lack of a meaningful relationship, nurturing, and support. Individuals with BPD experience enduring identity issues that contribute to maladaptive patterns of behaviors which generate repetitive patterns of difficult relationships. *Criterion 4* emphasizes on impulsive behaviors which lead to potentially self-damaging and various self-destructive behaviors. *Criterion 5* proposes that individuals with BPD exhibit recurrent suicidal behavior, gestures, or threats, or self-harm behaviors. *Criterion 6* cites that those individuals with BPD display affective instability because of a considerable mood reactivity such as irritability, intense episodic dysphoria, and periods of anger, panic, and anxiety. *Criterion 7* points out that individuals with BPD experience chronic feelings of emptiness occurring with painful feelings of loneliness contributing to frequently seeking excitement. *Criterion 8* states that BPD individuals display extreme expression of inappropriately intense anger and have issues in controlling their anger occurred with outbursts of anger. *Criterion 9* proposes that patients with BPD experience periods of extreme stress, transient paranoid ideation, or dissociative symptoms which may last minutes to hours. Some individuals with BPD revealed periods of transient psychotic symptoms during stress. A meta-analysis of 3543 participants demonstrated that BPD symptomatology was related to less frequent use of adaptive emotion regulation strategies such as cognitive reappraisal, problem solving, and acceptance and more frequent use of maladaptive strategies such as suppression, rumination, and avoidance (Leichsenring et al. 2024).

Recent evidence and empirical investigations have highlighted that internalizing and externalizing psychopathology often emerge before the onset of BPD in adolescents. Internalizing psychopathology encompasses depression, anxiety, obsessive-compulsive disorder, separation anxiety disorder and social phobia, dissociation, and suicidality including suicidal ideation and behaviors, while externalizing psychopathology mainly comprises conduct disturbances, oppositional defiant disorder, attention-deficit/hyperactivity disorder, impulsive/aggressive behaviors, self-injurious behaviors, and substance use disorder (Chanen et al. 2008, 2017; Ha et al. 2014; Fonagy et al. 2015; Fonagy and Luyten 2016; Kaess et al. 2014). Moreover, based on a substantial body of literature, it has been demonstrated that in the context of the interaction between predisposing biological vulnerabilities, invalidating environment and stressful life events can be considered predisposing conditions to develop mental issues and pathological personality traits during adolescence (Linehan 1993; Livesley 2000; Sharp and Wall 2018; Stepp et al. 2014a, c, 2016). Stepp et al. (2013) examined the influence of contributive interaction of negative emotionality and internalizing psychopathology on early onset of BPD (Stepp et al. 2013). In a longitudinal study, Cramer (2016) pointed out that childhood personality traits, including impulsivity and nonconformity/aggression, can contribute to adult BPD features (Cramer 2016). Conway et al. (2018) evaluated the impacts of various environmental stressful factors, comprising happening of acute and chronic stressors in individual, family, peer, and academic contexts, as well as personal characteristics to develop a contribution to the hypothesis suggesting BPD as the result of complicated interaction between pathogenic environments and individuals' vulnerabilities. The findings indicated that adolescent internalizing psychopathology and traits of negative emotionality preceded borderline pathology (Conway et al. 2018). Through a 2-year longitudinal study in a community population, Tragesser et al. (2010) indicated that negative affect strongly predicts the most BPD symptoms in the future, but no predictive role was found for future impulsive behaviors (Tragesser et al. 2010). Based on a cross-sectional study, Tragesser and Robinson (2009) revealed that both affective instability and impulsivity uniquely were associated with BPD features (Tragesser and Robinson 2009). Bo and Kongerslev (2017) demonstrated that remarkably high level of psychopathology, including internalizing and externalizing, impaired mentalizing abilities, and attachment issues, were considerably associated with BPD in adolescents in comparison to other psychiatric disorders (Bo and Kongerslev 2017). In a longitudinal study, Carlson et al. (2009) showed that endogenous and environmental history in early childhood contribute to impairments of child functioning in middle childhood and early adolescence which can lead to BPD symptoms in adulthood (Carlson et al. 2009). A substantial body of investigations have revealed highly significant associations between externalizing and internalizing pathologies and early onset of BPD (Belsky et al. 2012; Bornovalova et al. 2018; Bo and Kongerslev 2017), such as childhood ADHD and BPD (Miller et al. 2018; Thatcher et al. 2005), dissociation and BPD (Krabbendam et al. 2015), adolescents' self-injurious behaviors and BPD (Koenig et al. 2017), depression and early BPD symptoms (Stepp et al. 2013; Ramklint et al. 2003; Thatcher et al. 2005), early BPD substance use disorder (Stepp et al. 2013; Bornovalova et al. 2018; Ramklint et al. 2003; Thatcher et al. 2005), oppositional defiant disorder in childhood and BPD (Ha et al. 2014; Stepp et al. 2012, 2014b), and adolescents' psychotic-like symptoms and BPD (Thompson et al. 2018, 2020).

As mentioned in numerous scientific writings, BPD is a heterogenous mental disorder consisting of various clinically meaningfully variants of BPD that can be described through both a variable-centered and a person-centered approach (Smits et al. 2017). The majority of these studies relied on the growing empirical and clinical need to recognize appropriate treatment work for patients with BPD (McGlashan et al. 2000). Recognizing both discrete and subtle subtypes of BPD can contribute to identifying more effective treatments for patients with BPD (Smits et al. 2017). Lewis et al. (2012) proposed that there are 256 possible combinations which can be used to make a diagnosis of BPD and any two individuals with the same diagnosis might only display one shared criterion (Lewis et al. 2012). This remarkable heterogeneity in BPD presentation has caused numerous challenges and debates in clinical practice with regard to therapeutic approach (Yeomans et al. 2012; Clarkin et al. 2007; Luyten et al. 2021). Variable-centered approaches attempt to diminish the wide variety of BPD criteria into more concise number of basic dimensions, including two-factor or four-factor solutions: interpersonal/relational, and identity stability; impulsivity and affective instability comprising different complexes of the nine BPD diagnostic criteria (Blais et al. 1999; Clarkin et al. 1993; Sanislow et al. 2012). To elaborate this approach, it was assumed that BPD might be sufficiently recognized by a one-dimensional model encompassing factors manifesting different degrees of severity on the underlying spectrum (Fossati et al. 1999; Trull et al. 2011). A person-centered approach presents clusters which can differentiate between (1) individuals with few or no BPD criteria or low probability of BPD pathology, and (2) patients with a great number of BPD criteria or high probability of BPD pathology (Fossati et al. 1999; Clifton et al. 2007) which lead to identifying differences in the presence and severity of BPD psychopathology (Smits et al. 2017). Numerous subtypes of BPD have been presented, for instance, two separated subtypes based on interpersonal functioning were introduced by Leihener et al. (2003) comprising *autonomous* and *dependent*; five subtypes based on the characteristics of interpersonal patterns presented by Salzer et al. (2013) including *vindicative, moderate submissive, nonassertive, exploitable, and socially avoidant*; and also, based on a contrast analysis of clinician-rated affect experience and affect regulation, three subtypes were recognized by Zittel Conklin and Westen (2005) encompassing *internalizing dysregulated, externalizing/dysregulated,* and *histrionic-impulsive.* Moreover, four subtypes were identified: *high-functioning internalizing, histrionic, depressive internalizing,* and *angry externalizing* in sample of adolescents (Bradley et al. 2005). Caligor and Kernberg (2005) presented three subtypes of BPD: the first group was manifested by *low levels of antisocial, paranoid, and aggressive features*; the second group was characterized by *elevated paranoid features*; and the third group was featured by *heightened antisocial and aggressive presentations* (Caligor et al. 2007). Hallquist and Pilkonis (2012) mentioned four subtypes which varied in terms of anger/aggressiveness/antisocial behavior and mistrustfulness: *angry-aggressive* type (high levels of aggression, antisocial behavior, and dysfunctional interpersonal relationships); an *angry/mistrustful* type (remarkable concerns about being abused in relationships and inappropriate anger); a *poor identity/low angry* type (poor sense of self and self-injurious behaviors and low aggressiveness); and *prototypical* type (moderate levels of anger, and low levels of aggression, antisocial behavior, and mistrustfulness). According to a cluster-analytic approach, Smits et al. (2017) recognized three clusters of BPD patients with discrete profiles. The largest cluster included patients featured by "core BPD" with no remarkable increases in other PD dimensions. The second cluster comprised of "Extravert/externalizing" patients manifested by great levels of histrionic, narcissistic, and antisocial features. The third cluster was "Schizotypal/paranoid" presented by patients with considerable schizotypal and paranoid manifestations (Smits et al. 2017).

Dimensional Versus Categorical Perspective

The modern conceptualization of personality disorders (PDs) first emerged with the publication of DSM-III in 1980 and identified PDs as constellations of personality traits that are inflexible and manipulative, contribute to remarkable functional disturbances or subjective distress, and are pervasive, chronic, and resistant to treatment (Diagnostic 1980). In DSM-III-R (APA 1987) and DSM-IV (APA 1994), a substantial attempt was devoted to redefining the criteria for personality disorders and developing a more reliable diagnosis (Trull and Durrett 2005). Recent editions of the *Diagnostic and Statistical Manual of Mental Disorders* (DSM-5) have formulated personality disorders as categorical constructs; yet, remarkable personality disorder co-occurrence proposes underlying latent dimensions. Additionally, various BPD criteria are like Criterion A of the new DSM-5 Sect. 3 general criteria for personality pathology (Sharp et al. 2015). "The greatest challenge that the extensive comorbidity data pose to current nosological system concerns the validity of the diagnostic categories themselves-do these disorders constitute distinct clinical perspectives" (Mineka et al. 1998, p.380).

The classification of psychiatric disorders has been generally debated by several theorists, researchers, experts, and clinicians from various disciplines, such as psychiatry, psychology, and philosophy. Categorical viewpoints present various mental issues as separate types that comprise an expansive heterogenous group of individuals with clear phenotypical symptoms. However, dimensional perspectives address limitations of traditional categorical modes (Markon et al. 2011; Regier et al. 2013) and propose that mental disorders are extreme variants of one or more psychological attributes contributing to a diagnosis, considering each person on a spectrum ranging from normal to abnormal behaviors (Schierenbeck 2023); dimensional perspectives consider that there should be no discrete boundaries between disorders and provide significant information about the subthreshold traits of personality disorders (Trull and Durrett 2005). There are several debates about choosing a categorical or dimensional system. Combined approaches integrate categorical and dimensional components, addressing different types of mental disorders and their severity dimensionally (Schierenbeck 2023). The categorical classification of psychiatric disorders stems from medical taxonomy, while dimensional systems consider an individual on one or more psychological dimensions (Millon et al. 2011, 2012). The question of whether BPD should be considered in a categorical or dimensional style is really prominent (Gunderson et al. 2018). Numerous studies have been investigated to determine whether BPD should be conceptualized as a dimensional variable which is more accurate, or is it more precise if BPD is formulated based on a categorical system (Trull et al. 2011, 2018). In spite of amassing steady criticism (Ekselius et al. 1993; Frances 1982), categorical models of personality disorders have demonstrated considerable benefits in classification of personality disorders, which contributed to providing a mechanism for organizing, research, and treatment (Monaghan and Bizumic 2023). On the other hand, dimensional models of PDs specifically address two main criteria: *severity* and *style.* Severity considers the major distress which is common to all PDs, which influence the individuals' self-direction, identity, and interpersonal functioning, besides individuals' capability to develop close relationships and have empathy with other people (Clark et al. 2018; Conway et al. 2018, 2019; Wright et al. 2016; Hopwood et al. 2013). Severity is the core element for diagnosing PDs (Bach and Tracy 2022; Tyrer et al. 2019) and indicates the range of dysfunctions and impaired outcomes in PDs (Monaghan and Bizumic 2023). Style describes the stylistic characteristics of the presentation which is remarkably associated with some derivation of the Five-Factor Model (FFM) of personality (Goldberg 1993; Costa and McCrae 1999).

One of the most contested questions which has been presented is whether a construct like BPD is stable or not (Conway et al. 2019). Albeit stability and pervasive inflexibility have been considered generally for criteria in all personality disorders, BPD is manifested by instability in various domains comprising interpersonal behaviors, affect, and identity (Hopwood et al. 2009). In line with numerous investigations, a dimensional conceptualization has been proposed to present personality disorders as maladaptive variants of normal personality traits (Livesley and Jang 2005; Clark 2007; Widiger and Lowe 2008; Trull and Durrett 2005). This dimensional approach presents a quantitative estimation of the degree to which associated personality traits are manifested in every person. The advantages of this dimensional approach consist of providing an explanation for symptom heterogeneity and lack of precise borders between various categorical diagnoses, as well as providing significant information about subthreshold traits and symptoms of clinical and experimental studies. Additionally, dimensional model of personality disorders provides an integrated scientific finding regarding the distribution of personality traits and related maladaptivity into a classification system (Trull et al. 2008, 2018). Trait-state-occasion modeling, a confirmatory factor analytic technique, decomposes psychological constructs into *trait* and *occasion* dimensions (Cole et al. 2008, 2009). This model categorizes BP pathology into time-invariant such as traitand time varying such as situational elements (Chritopher et al. 2018). Based on this model, a state factor exhibits an individual's standing on a BPD dimension at a specific point of time which is composed of time-invariant-varying processes. A *state* represents the common variance in the manifest of BPD indicators, including the nine BPD diagnostic criteria in DSM. On the other hand, the trait factor is an unchangeably enduring core of borderline pathology, called borderline proneness, which is completely fixed over the time and exhibits chronic susceptibility to symptoms. The *trait* is presented as a combination of genetic predispositions to BPD, long-standing personality features, and obstinate social-environmental conditions (Distel et al. 2009; Gunderson et al. 2011). The occasion factors are time-specific impacts on BPD and are proposed as the reasons that BPD state factors are not completely stable during the time. These factors are situational in nature and are considered transitory biological, social, and psychological determinants of BPD, which are somewhat persistent over time (Ciesla and Roberts 2007; Ciesla et al. 2011).

In line with a body of studies, there appears to be little evidence that endorsed the categorical perspective of BPD (e.g., Clark 2007; Livesley 2003; Trull and Durrett 2005). Several studies applied taxometric analysis to evaluate whether BPD is best manifested as a discrete clinical entity or a dimensional structure, and all of them endorsed a dimensional conceptualization, despite various criticisms about such methodology (e.g., Ayer et al. 2013; Trull et al. 1990; Rothschild et al. 2003; Edens et al. 2008; Arntz et al. 2009). Moreover, a substantial number of explanatory and confirmatory factor analytic investigations have demonstrated a remarkable support for the multifactorial conceptualization of BPD (Mullins-Sweatt et al. 2012), except one study which did not endorse these findings (Fossati et al. 2001). In summary, it seems that the more beneficial approach to provide a conceptualization of BPD is to consider BPD as a set of maladaptive personality traits instead of as a discrete, homogenous category, which would contribute to recognizing certain components of BPD, allowing for clinician to concentrate on a specific element (Mullins-Sweatt et al. 2012).

In 2001, Lynam and Widiger (2001) presented the FFM as an alternative dimensional model of personality disorders, encompassing a broad domain of *neuroticism* (emotional instability vs stability), *extraversion* (vs introversion), *openness* (or unconventionality), *agreeableness* (vs antagonism), and *conscientiousness* (or constraint vs. disinhibition). FFM has demonstrated a strong resistance toward numerous criticisms across the time and contributed to meaningful inferences about individual differences based on hereditable genetic underpinnings (Bouchard and Loehlin 2001) combined with biological systems (Harkness et al. 2014) and generated a notable candidate for elucidating all personality variation (Widiger and Costa 2013). In accordance with personality science literature, BPD was presented as an engaging high level of neuroticism and low levels of agreeableness and conscientiousness, and BPD was also positively associated with openness to emotions and actions yet unrelated to openness to values. In other words, according to FFM, BPD is considered a reflection of a specific set of core personality attributes (Hopwood et al. 2012). In one study, Hopwood et al. (2012) compared the stability of FFM traits in individuals with BPD to that in individuals with other PDs among 432 participants with BPD and other PDs. The findings showed no difference in structural stability across groups. Differential stability was reported lower for FFM traits in the BPD group, as well as the strongest consistency observed for neuroticism and conscientiousness. In addition, growth curve models indicated that neuroticism and conscientiousness elevated faster among individuals with BPD, and the BPD group exhibited higher individual-level instability for neuroticism and conscientiousness in these models. Moreover, lesser instability in terms of the ipsative configuration of FFM facet-level profiles was found in individuals with BPD in comparison with other personality disorder diagnoses over time (Hopwood et al. 2012). Distel et al. (2009) evaluated the phenotypic and genetic association between BPD and FFM personality traits. In line with the results, broad-sense heritability estimated for neuroticism, agreeableness, conscientiousness, extraversion, openness to experience, and BPD was 43%, 36%, 47%, 54%, and 45%, respectively. Phenotypic correlations between personality and FFM personality traits ranged from 0.06% for openness to experience to 0.68% for neuroticism. In addition, multiple regression indicated that there was a combination of high neuroticism and low agreeableness which predicted BPD strongly. Further, multivariate genetic analyses demonstrated that the genetic factors that impact individual differences in neuroticism, conscientiousness, agreeableness, and extraversion elucidated all genetic lability to BPD (Distel et al. 2009).

Widiger and Samuel (2005) proposed that BPD comprises all six facets of Neuroticism, low trust and compliance from Agreeableness, low competence from conscientiousness, low self-conscientiousness, and impairments in sense of self (Widiger 2012; Widiger and Rojas 2015; Widiger et al. 2002). Samuel and Widiger (2008) reported positive associations between BPD and the Neuroticism facets of anxiousness, angry hostility, depressiveness, self-consciousness, impulsiveness, and vulnerability. In addition, negative relationships were found between BPD and the Extraversion facets of warmth and positive emotions, the Agreeableness facets of trust, straightforwardness, and compliance, as well as conscientiousness facets of competence, dutifulness, self-discipline, and deliberation (Samuel and Widiger 2008). Lynam and Widiger (2001) and Chritopher et al. (2018) examined the probability that BPD has both stable and dynamic components among 668 adult psychiatric patients. The findings indicated that less than half of BPD variability (45%) was time-invariant during the study timeframe. Moreover, it was demonstrated that borderline proneness showed very close association with a previously validated FFM trait compound of borderline characteristics. Additionally, the trait versus situational elements indicated a pattern of discrimination validity in association with various putative causal agents of BPD such as environmental and temperamental dimensions. Based on their conclusion, borderline pathology encompasses a stable core and sizable situational elements, and both components associate systematically to normative personality dimensions and risk factors (Chritopher et al. 2018). Through a confirmatory factor analysis, Andión et al. (2011) compared the FFM, a Three-factor Model, and a unidimensional model of BPD diagnosis criteria in 338 patients with BPD. The results of confirmatory factor analysis endorsed both the hypothesized unidimensional and the Three-Factor Model; however, the Three-Factor Model showed better fitness than the unidimensional model. Additionally, the Five-Factor Model was not confirmed. Based on their conclusion, the DSM-IV BPD criteria formalize BPD as a unidimensional construct, the results revealed that the Three-Factor Model can provide an elaborated understanding of etiopathogenesis of BPD (Andión et al. 2011). Based on a cross-sectional study design, Amini et al. (2014) evaluated the association between the FFM and DSM-5 pathological traits among 130 individuals with BPD who were prisoned. The findings demonstrated a significant positive association between neuroticism with emotional lability ($r = 0.34, p < 0.01$), anxiousness ($r = 0.286, p < 0.01$), and impulsivity ($r = 0229$, $p < 0.05$). Moreover, a substantially significant association was found between openness and emotional lability ($r = 0.316$, $p < 0.01$) and risk taking ($r = 0.193$, $p < 0.05$). Further, a negative was obtained between openness and impulsivity

($r = -0.244$, $p < 0.01$), separation insecurity ($r = -0.194$, $p < 0.05$), and depressivity ($r = -0.19$, $p < 0.05$). The results revealed a considerable positive relationship between FFM and DSM-5 personality traits with DSM-IV-TR BPD symptoms (Amini et al. 2014). Koster et al. (2020) examined the correlations between the FFM personality traits and BPD manifestations in a sample of 162 adolescents. The results supported previous studies and have indicated that BPD dimensions were greatly associated with high neuroticism, low conscientiousness, low agreeableness, and lesser extent with low extraversion (Koster et al. 2020). In accordance with the theoretical literature, experimental investigations, and surveys of clinicians and researchers, 11 facets from FFM were recognized which have been associated to the description of BPD: (1) high anxiousness; (2) angry-hostility; (3) depressiveness; (4) self-consciousness; (5) impulsivity; (6) vulnerability from Neuroticism; (7) high fantasy from Openness to Experience; (8) low trust; (9) straightforwardness; (10) compliance from Agreeableness; and (11) low deliberation from Conscientiousness. Widiger and Samuel (2005) assessed these 11 facets using 10-item scales to identify FFM components of BPD, encompassing anxious uncertainty (the BPD variant of FFM anxiousness), dysregulated anger (the BPD variant of FFM anger hostility), despondence (FFM depressives), self-disturbance (FFM self-consciousness), behavioral dysregulation (FFM impulsivity), emotional dysregulation (the BPD variant of FFM vulnerability), fragility (the BPD variant of FFM vulnerability), dissociative tendencies (FFM openness to fantasy), distrustfulness (low FFM trust), manipulativeness (low FFM straightforwardness), oppositional (low FFM compliance), and rashness (low FFM deliberation) (Samuel and Widiger 2006). Mullins-Sweatt et al. (2012) studied the psychometric data of a self-report measure of BPD from the viewpoint of FFM and demonstrated good internal consistency, convergent, discriminant, and incremental validity among its subscales (Mullins-Sweatt et al. 2012).

Alternative DSM-5 Model for Personality Disorders

The alternative DSM-5 model for personality disorders (AMPD, listed in Sect. 3) was presented to consider the scientific issues associated with personality disorder classifications, providing a more comprehensive understanding of the extant studies on personality psychopathology, consisting of BPD (Morey et al. 2022; APA 2022; Zimmerman et al. 2019; Monaghan and Bizumic 2023; Choi-Kain et al. 2022). AMPD dimensionally defines personality pathology based on severity of dysfunction and maladaptive style (Bilton and Shepard 2022). Several researchers and clinical experts have debated the construct of BPD as maintained in DSM-5 Sect. 2 because of issues such as within diagnosis heterogeneity, remarkably excessive overlap with other psychiatric disorders, and optional diagnostic boundaries (Widiger and Trull 2007; Bach and Sellbom 2016; Torres-Soto et al. 2019). To achieve a clarified elucidation for these issues, the alternative DSM-5 model for personality disorders (PDs) has been provided in Sect. 3 in order to develop a better understanding of the extant research on personality psychopathology, comprising BPD (APA 2022; Morey et al. 2022). The alternative DSM-5 model has been provided as an alternative to the extent of personality disorders classification in Sect. 2 which emphasized on disturbances in personality functioning along with 5 higher-order and 25 lower-order dimensional personality traits establishing 6 categorical PDs, consisting of BPD (Monaghan and Bizumic 2023; Bach and Sellbom 2016; APA 2022; Torres-Soto et al. 2019; Bach et al. 2016a, b). In this hybrid dimensional-categorical model in Sect. 3, personality disorders have been defined in terms of impairments in personality functioning and pathological personality traits (APA 2022). This model includes two required determinants: (1) the level of impairment in personality functioning (criterion A), comprising *self-* and *interpersonal* functioning; and (2) pathological personality traits level (criterion B), consisting of *Negative Affectivity, Detachment, Antagonism, Disinhibition, and Psychoticism.* The disturbances in personality functioning and personality traits manifestations are partially inflexible and pervasive across a broad range of personal and social situations (Criterion C), including *identity, self-direction, empathy, and intimacy*; nearly stable across time, with an onset during adolescent and early adulthood (Criterion D); not better elucidated by other mental health difficulties (Criterion E); cannot be attributed to the physiological impacts or other mental conditions (Criterion F); and can be explained as a normal individuals' developmental stage or sociocultural environment (Criterion G) (APA 2022; Bach and Sellbom 2016; Krueger and Hobbs 2020).

Numerous investigations on the Sect. 3 model have claimed that specific BPD traits substantially demonstrate conceptually anticipated associations with its DSM-5 Sect. 2 counterpart (Clark et al. 2018; Yam and Simms 2014; Morey et al. 2022; Miller et al. 2014; Jopp and South 2015). The proposed diagnostic criteria for BPD are as follows: (A) impairments in personality functioning exhibited by *disturbances in identity* such as impoverished, poorly developed self-images, self-criticism, and feeling of emptiness; disturbances in self-direction such as unstable goal-settings and career plans; disturbances in empathy such as selectively biased attributes toward others; and disturbances in intimacy such as fear of abandonment and chaotic interpersonal relationships, as well as (B) seven pathological personality traits including **Emotional Lability** (from Negative affectivity aspect) such as unstable emotional experiences and frequent mood changes; **Anxiousness** (from Negative affectivity aspect) such as nervousness and fearful apprehension by uncertainty; and **Separation Insecurity** (from Negative Affectivity aspect) such as fear of rejection and separation; **Depressivity** (from Detachment aspect) such as hopelessness, pessimism about future, and suicidal thoughts and behaviors; **Impulsivity** (from Disinhibition aspect) such as acting out and self-harming behaviors; **Risk taking** (from Disinhibition aspect) such as risky and potentially self-damaging activities and lack of concern for one's limitations; **Hostility** (from Antagonism aspect) such as feelings of anger and irritability (APA 2022; Bach and Sellbom 2016; Anderson 2020; Sellbom et al. 2014; Yam and Simms 2014; Hopwood et al. 2012; Monaghan and Bizumic 2023). Especially, studies concentrating on BPD have demonstrated a considerable overlap between latent representations of Sects. 2 and 3 BPD models (Sellbom et al. 2014), as well as it has been shown that the BPD Sect. 3 trait profile explains a range of internalizing and externalizing behaviors related to traditional Sect. 2 BPD operationalization (Anderson et al. 2014). Moreover, it has been recognized that difficulties in cognitive and perceptual regulation and suspiciousness raise this anticipation through mapping onto the two major elements of stress-induced symptoms of BPD including dissociation and paranoia (Zanarini et al. 2013). Bach and Sellbom (2016) evaluated the experimental associations between DSM-5 Sect. 3 traits and all nine DSM-IV Axis II/DSM-5 Sect. 2 dichotomous criteria variable among 142 individuals with BPD. The results indicated an association between categorical BPD criteria and conceptually related DSM-5 Sect. 3 traits, except for the criterion of chronic feelings of emptiness. Additionally, they revealed that Emotional Lability, Anxiousness, Separation Insecurity, Depressivity, Impulsivity, Risk taking, and Hostility conceptually were coherent with BPD categorical criteria; however, a strong association was found between Suspiciousness and BPD criteria. Further, it was shown that Emotional Lability, Impulsivity, and Suspiciousness can be considered as unique predictors of BPD (Bach and Sellbom 2016). In another study, Bach et al. (2016a, b) explored the utility of DSM-5 Sect. 3 personality traits in distinguishing individuals with BPD ($n = 101$) from individuals with other personality disorders ($n = 101$) and healthy controls ($n = 101$), and also in determining which traits are most unique to individuals with BPD. The findings showed that Emotional Lability, Risk Taking, and Suspiciousness specifically distinguish individuals with BPD from other PDs, while Emotional Lability, Depressivity, and Suspiciousness uniquely differentiated from healthy controls (Bach et al. 2016a, b).

Gamache et al. (2021) pointed out four AMPD profiles for BPD: (a) borderline traits, (b) moderate pathology with impulsivity; (c) moderate pathology with identity issues and depressivity; and (d) severe pathology (Bilton and Shepard 2022). Identifying major components of BPD is substantially crucial. Through a factor analysis to recognize these elements for BPD, four core elements were found: *painful incoherence* (remarkable intense emotional pain represented a fragmented sense of self, the most significant factor); *role absorption* (loss of identity); *inconsistency*; and *lack of commitment* (the least significant factor) (Meares et al. 2011). Bassett (2012) proposed that although significant characteristics of BPD, including fear of abandonment, impulsivity, recurrent self-inflicted behaviors, emotional instability and rapid fluctuations of mood elicited by daily events, episodic outburst of anger and explosive rage, and episodic psychotic manifestations are clearly remarkable, they are not considered as core features (Bassett 2012). In accordance with a factor analysis, Clifton et al. (2007) reported three core features of BPD, encompassing impaired relatedness (identity disturbance, chronic perceptions of internal emptiness, interpersonal relationship difficulties), behavioral dysregulation (self-harm behaviors, impulsivity), and emotional dysregulation (inappropriate anger, efforts to avoid abandonment). In line with such findings, these factors showed notable correlation with each other contributing to one statistically comprehensive construct (Clifton et al. 2007). Bassett (2012) suggested "emotionally noxious sense of self", recognized as an emotionally painful disruption of self-identity, a recurrent fear of abandonment and emptiness, as the most significant core entity in BPD (Bassett 2012). Zanarini et al. (2007) suggested that the interaction of emotionally noxious sense of self with kindling life events develops the predisposition into a full clinical syndrome. Calvo et al. (2016) examined the use of the presented traits in Sect. 3 of the DSM-5 for BPD diagnosis among BPD sample ($n = 84$) and non-BPD sample ($n = 45$). The findings showed significantly greater scores in BPD group, as well as notably higher traits of emotional instability, restricted affectivity, and impulsivity were associated with BPD.

A Hierarchical Taxonomy of Psychopathology (HiTOP) Primer for BPD

Given evidence has been supported the multidimensional structure of personality pathology (Mullins-Sweatt et al. 2020; Hopwood 2018). Traditional diagnostic taxonomies, such as DSM (American Psychiatric Association 2013) and ICD (World Health Organization 2020), provide numerous benefits in psychiatry and offer a shared language from researchers and clinicians, although as mentioned earlier, they have seriously remarkable limitations (Walton et al. 2024; Mullins-Sweatt et al. 2020). First, traditional taxonomies address psychiatric disorders to be distinct categories rather than considering mental issues and psychopathologies in a continuum with normality (Carragher et al. 2015; Haslam et al. 2012, 2020; Walton et al. 2024), and therefore, contribute to missing substantially clinically significant data (Markon et al. 2013). Notably, some patients do not meet the threshold number of diagnostic criteria to be diagnosed with a specific mental disorder, however experiencing clinically considerable disturbances (Walton et al. 2024). Second, dichotomous diagnoses indicate limited reliability over time and across clinicians (Chmielewski et al. 2011; Markon et al. 2013). Third, numerous diagnoses are heterogeneous and include diverse features (Watson et al. 2006; Zimmerman and Morgan 2013; Zimmerman 2015; Zimmerman and Becker 2023). The Hierarchical Taxonomy of Psychopathology (HiTOP) was developed to consider these limitations (Martin et al. 2023; Walton et al. 2024; Mullins-Sweatt et al. 2020) and offer solution for these issues by evaluating psychopathology as a constellation of continuous dimensions (Walton et al. 2024). Moreover, HiTOP addresses these limitations by modeling psychopathology dimensionally (Markon et al. 2013; Chmielewski et al. 2017; Samuel 2015) and decomposing wider syndromes into homogenous dimensions at lower level of the hierarchy (Walton et al. 2024). Additionally, HiTOP addresses comorbidity directly, and its structure represents empirical patterns of correlations (Kotov et al. 2011; Watson and Clark 2023), as well as HiTOP as a theoretical model of psychopathology which provides a bridge to pass the gaps within the treatment outcome investigations (Mullins-Sweatt et al. 2020). HiTOP is an experimentally originated, dimensional model of the core dimensions of mental health and psychological symptoms and functioning (Martin et al. 2023; Conway et al. 2023). HiTOP is a dimensional of psychopathology that comprises mood, anxiety, psychotic, substance use, personality, and other psychiatric disorders (Kotov et al. 2011; Walton et al. 2024). This model proposes an alternative research paradigm which has various association with categorical rubrics (Conway et al. 2023). HiTOP provides a constellation of empirically derived hierarchal traits that are shared across continuums of psychiatric conditions (Kotov et al. 2021). The main purposes of HiTOP are to promote the use and consider the limitations of traditional diagnosis, such as arbitrary thresholds of severity, within-disorder heterogeneity, and low reliability (Martin et al. 2023). HiTOP diminishes the limitations of traditional classification by: (a) providing a definition of pathology in terms of spectrum ranging from normative to maladaptive; (b) drawing continuum based on observed covariation in signs, symptoms, and syndromes; and (c) arranging spectrum in a hierarchy, ranging from narrow and specific such as clusters of symptoms to broadly general such as spectra of interrelated diagnostic phenomena (Latzman et al. 2021). HiTOP encompasses six broad spectrums: *internalizing, detachment, antagonistic externalizing, disinhibited externalizing, thought disorders, and somatoform* (Latzman et al. 2021; Choi-Kain et al. 2022; Kotov et al. 2011, 2018; Krueger et al. 2018). In other words, the HiTOP comprises six spectra that are conceptualized as three superspectra: *psychosis* (combination of thought disorder and detachment); *externalizing* (subsuming disinhibited and antagonistic forms of psychopathology); and *emotional dysfunction* (modeling the commonality between internalizing and somatoform) (Walton et al. 2024). The highest level is a single general factor of psychopathology, and three broad domains of internalizing, externalizing, and thought disorder are beneath this level (Forbes et al. 2021; Lahey 2021). Moreover, broad spectrums are combined into more expansive superspectra: emotional dysfunction (internalizing and somatoform), externalizing (disinhibited and antagonistic), and psychosis (thought disorder and detachment) (Anderson et al. 2014; Forbes et al. 2021; Krueger et al. 2007; Patrick et al. 2013). HiTOP model identifies a general psychopathology factor (Caspi and Moffitt 2018; Lahey 2021; Latzman et al. 2021). BPD has been presented as a personality pathology comprised of patterns featured by instability, disturbed self-esteem and self-direction, and chaotic interpersonal relationships, accompanied by characteristics of impulsivity, hostility, and self-destructive behaviors (APA 2022; Paris 2015). Dimensionally, traits of affective lability, anxiousness, separation insecurity, depressivity, impulsivity and self-destructive behaviors, risk-taking behaviors, and hostility are all manifested in BPD (APA 2022; Bach et al. 2016a, b; Calvo et al. 2016; Fowler et al. 2020; Latzman et al. 2021; Samuel et al. 2012). According to the HiTOP model, the BPD conceptualization integrates traits of the internalizing spectrum, certain to the subfactor of Distress, comprising Anxiousness, Emotional Lability, Hostility, Perseveration, Low Restricted Affectivity, Separation Insecurity, Submissiveness, Identity Problems, Negative Relationships, Fragility, Ineptitude, Low Invulnerability, Antagonistic Externalizing Spectrum such as Rudeness, Flirtatiousness, and Low Timorousness (Kotov et al. 2011, Carvalho et al. 2018).

References

American Psychiatric Association (1987). Diagnostic and statistical manual of mental disorders (3rd ed., Revised (DSM-III-R)). Washington DC: American Psychiatric Press.

American Psychiatric Association. Diagnostic and statistical manual of mental disorders. 5th ed. Arlington: American Psychiatric Association; 2022.

American Psychiatric Association DS. Diagnostic and statistical manual of mental disorders: DSM-5. Washington, DC: American Psychiatric Association; 2013.

Amini M, Sadat Safavi N, Mirzaeyan Bahnamiri R, Mirzaei Omran M, Amini M. Development of an instrument for assessing the impact of environmental context on adoption of cloud computing for small and medium enterprises. Aust J Basic Appl Sci. 2014;8(10):129–35.

Anderson G. Pathoetiology and pathophysiology of borderline personality: role of prenatal factors, gut microbiome, mu-and kappa-opioid receptors in amygdala-PFC interactions. Prog Neuro-Psychopharmacol Biol Psychiatry. 2020;98:109782.

Anderson J, Snider S, Sellbom M, Krueger R, Hopwood C. A comparison of the DSM-5 section II and section III personality disorder structures. Psychiatry Res. 2014;216(3):363–72.

Andión Ó, Ferrer M, Gancedo B, Calvo N, Barral C, Torrubia R, Casas M. Confirmatory factor analysis of borderline personality disorder symptoms based on two different interviews: the structured clinical interview for DSM-IV axis II disorder and the revised diagnostic interview for borderlines. Psychiatry Res. 2011;190(2–3):304–8.

Arntz A, Bernstein D, Oorschot M, Schobre P. Theory of mind in borderline and cluster-C personality disorder. J Nerv Ment Dis. 2009;197(11):801–7.

Ayer L, Greaves-Lord K, Althoff RR, Hudziak JJ, Dieleman GC, Verhulst FC, van der Ende J. Blunted HPA axis response to stress is related to a persistent dysregulation profile in youth. Biol Psychol. 2013;93(3):343–51.

Bach B, Sellbom M. Continuity between DSM-5 categorical criteria and traits criteria for borderline personality disorder. Can J Psychiatry/La Rev Can Psychiatr. 2016;61(8):489–94. https://doi.org/10.1177/0706743716640756.

Bach B, Tracy M. Clinical utility of the alternative model of personality disorders: a 10th year anniversary review. Personal Disord Theory Res Treat. 2022;13(4):369.

Bach B, Sellbom M, Sune B, Simonsen E. Utility of DSM-5 section III personality traits in differentiating borderline personality disorder from comparison groups. Eur Psychiatry. 2016a;37(9):22. https://doi.org/10.1016/j.eurpsy.2016.04.006.

Bach B, Maples-Keller JL, Bo S, Simonsen E. The alternative DSM–5 personality disorder traits criterion: a comparative examination of three self-report forms in a Danish population. Personal Disord Theory Res Treat. 2016b;7(2):124.

Bassett D. Borderline personality disorder and bipolar affective disorder. Spectra or spectre? A review. Aust N Z J Psychiatry. 2012;46(4):327–39.

Belsky DW, Caspi A, Arseneault L, Bleidorn W, Fonagy P, Goodman M, Houts R, Moffitt TE. Etiological features of borderline personality related characteristics in a birth cohort of 12-year-old children. Dev Psychopathol. 2012;24(1):251–65.

Bilton DT, Shepard WD. Rhithrops capensis gen. Et sp. nov., a new aquatic dryopid beetle from the Western cape of South Africa (Coleoptera: Dryopoidea: Dryopidae). Zootaxa. 2022;5195(6):539–53.

Blais MA, Hilsenroth MJ, Fowler JC, Conboy CA. A Rorschach exploration of the DSM-IV borderline personality disorder. J Clin Psychol. 1999;55(5):563–72.

Bo S, Kongerslev M. Self-reported patterns of impairments in mentalization, attachment, and psychopathology among clinically referred adolescents with and without borderline personality pathology. Bord Personal Disord Emot Dysregul. 2017;4:1.

Bornovalova MA, Lejuez CW, Daughters SB, Rosenthal MZ, Lynch TR. Impulsivity as a common process across borderline personality and substance use disorders. Clin Psychol Rev. 2005;25:790–812.

Bornovalova MA, Verhulst B, Webber T, McGue M, Iacono WG, Hicks BM. Genetic and environmental influences on the co-development among borderline personality disorder traits, major depression symptoms, and substance use disorder symptoms from adolescence to young adulthood. Dev Psychopathol. 2018;30(1):49–65.
Bouchard TJ, Loehlin C. Genes, evolution, and personality. Behav Genet. 2001;31(3):243–73. https://doi.org/10.1023/A:1012294324713.
Bradley R, Zittel Conklin C, Westen D. The borderline personality diagnosis in adolescents: gender differences and subtypes. J Child Psychol Psychiatry. 2005;46(9):1006–19.
Brickman LJ, Ammerman BA, Look AE, Berman ME, McCloskey MS. The relationship between nonsuicidal self-injury and borderline personality disorder symptoms in a college sample. Bord Personal Disord Emot Dysregul. 2014;1:14. http://www.bpded.com/content/1/1/14
Caligor E, Kernberg OF. Major theories of personality disorder; 2005. p. 114.
Caligor E, Kernberg OF, Clarkin JF. Handbook of dynamic psychotherapy for higher level personality pathology. American Psychiatric Pub; 2007.
Calvo N, Valero S, Sáez-Francàs N, Gutiérrez F, Casas M, Ferrer M. Borderline personality disorder and personality inventory for DSM-5 (PID-5): dimensional personality assessment with DSM-5. Compr Psychiatry. 2016;70:105–11.
Carlson EA, Egeland B, Sroufe LA. A prospective investigation of the development of borderline personality symptoms. Dev Psychopathol. 2009;21(4):1311–34.
Carvalho LF, Sette CP, Ferrari BL. Problematic smartphone use relationship with pathological personality traits: systematic review and meta-analyzes. Cyberpsychol J Psychosoc Res Cyberspace. 2018;12(3):5.
Carragher N, Krueger RF, Eaton NR, Slade T. Disorders without borders: current and future directions in the meta-structure of mental disorders. Soc Psychiatry Psychiatr Epidemiol. 2015;50:339–50.
Caspi A, Moffitt TE. All for one and one for all: mental disorders in one dimension. Am J Psychiatry. 2018;175(9):831–44. https://doi.org/10.1176/appi.ajp.2018.17121383.
Chanen AM. Borderline personality disorder in young people: are we there yet? J Clin Psychol. 2015;71:778–91. PMID: 26192914. https://doi.org/10.1002/jclp.22205.
Chanen AM, Jackson HJ, McCutcheon LK, et al. Early intervention for adolescents with borderline personality disorder using cognitive analytic therapy: randomised controlled trial. Br J Psychiatry. 2008;193:477–84.
Chanen A, Sharp C, Hoffman P, et al. Prevention and early intervention for borderline personality disorder: a novel public health priority. World Psychiatry. 2017;16:215–6.
Chmielewski M, Bagby RM, Quilty LC, Paxton R, Ng SA. A (re)-evaluation of the symptom structure of borderline personality disorder. Can J Psychiatry. 2011;56(9):530–9.
Chmielewski M, Ruggero CJ, Kotov R, Liu K, Krueger RF. Comparing the dependability and associations with functioning of the DSM–5 section III trait model of personality pathology and the DSM–5 section II personality disorder model. Personal Disord Theory Res Treat. 2017;8(3):228.
Choi-Kain LW, Sahin Z, Traynor J. Borderline personality disorder: updates in a post-pandemic world. Focus. 2022;20(4):337–52.
Chritopher M, Hunsinger M, Goerling LRJ, et al. Mindfulness-based resilience training to reduce health risk, stress reactivity, and aggression among law enforcement officers: a feasibility and preliminary efficacy trial. Psychiatry Res. 2018;264:104–15. https://doi.org/10.1016/j.psychres.2018.03.059.
Ciesla JA, Roberts JE. Rumination, negative cognition, and their interactive effects on depressed mood. Emotion. 2007;7(3):555.
Ciesla JA, Felton JW, Roberts JE. Testing the cognitive catalyst model of depression: does rumination amplify the impact of cognitive diatheses in response to stress? Cogn Emot. 2011;25(8):1349–57.
Clark LA. Assessment and diagnosis of personality disorder: perennial issues and an emerging reconceptualization. Annu Rev Psychol. 2007;58:227–57.

Clark LA, Nuzum H, Ro E. Manifestations of personality impairment severity: comorbidity, course/prognosis, psychosocial dysfunction, and 'borderline' personality features. Curr Opin Psychol. 2018;21(21):117.

Clarkin JF, Hull JW, Cantor J, Sanderson C. Borderline personality disorder and personality traits: a comparison of SCID-II BPD and NEO-PI. Psychol Assess. 1993;5(4):472.

Clarkin JF, Levy KN, Lenzenweger MF, Kernberg OF. Evaluating three treatments for borderline personality disorder: a multiwave study. Am J Psychiatry. 2007;164(6):922–8.

Clifton A, Pilkonis PA, McCarty C. Social networks in borderline personality disorder. J Personal Disord. 2007;21(4):434–41.

Cole PM, Hall SE, Hajal NJ. Emotion dysregulation as a risk factor for psychopathology. Child Adolesc Psychopathol. 2008;2:341–73.

Cole PM, Llera SJ, Pemberton CK. Emotional instability, poor emotional awareness, and the development of borderline personality. Dev Psychopathol. 2009;21(4):1293–310.

Conway CC, Boudreaux M, Oltmanns TF. Dynamic associations between borderline personality disorder and stressful life events over five years in older adults. Personal Disord Theory Res Treat. 2018;9(6):521.

Conway CC, Forbes MK, Forbush KT, Fried EI, Hallquist MN, Kotov R, Mullins-Sweatt SN, Shackman AJ, Skodol AE, South SC, Sunderland M. A hierarchical taxonomy of psychopathology can transform mental health research. Perspect Psychol Sci. 2019;14(3):419–36.

Conway C, Naragon-Gainey K, Lopez MM. Defining distress tolerance in a structural model of big five personality domains. J Pers. 2023; https://doi.org/10.31234/osf.io/gpnwq

Costa PT, McCrae RR. The five-factor model of personality: theoretical perspectives, vol. 2. New York: Guilford; 1999. p. 51–87.

Cramer P. Childhood precursors of adult borderline personality disorder features: a longitudinal study. J Nerv Ment Dis. 2016;204(7):494–9.

Distel MA, Trull TJ, Willemsen G, Vink JM, Derom CA, Lynskey M, Martin NG, Boomsma DI. The five-factor model of personality and borderline personality disorder: a genetic analysis of comorbidity. Biol Psychiatry. 2009;66(12):1131–8.

Diagnostic AP. Statistical manual of mental disorders. Washington DC: American Psychiatric Association; 1987/1980.

DSM-IV. Diagnostic and statistical manual of mental disorders, 4th ed. Washington: by the American Psychiatric Association, APA; 1994. Psychol Med. 1996;26(3):651–2.

Edens JF, Marcus DK, Ruiz MA. Taxometric analyses of borderline personality features in a large-scale male and female offender sample. J Abnorm Psychol. 2008;117(3):705.

Ekselius L, Lindström E, von Knorring L, Bodlund O, Kullgren G. Personality disorders in DSM-III-R as categorical or dimensional. Acta Psychiatr Scand. 1993;88(3):183–7.

Fonagy P, Luyten P. A multilevel perspective on the development of borderline personality disorder. In: Cicchetti D, editor. Developmental psychopathology, vol. 3. New York: Wiley; 2016. p. 726–92.

Fonagy P, Luyten P, Allison E. Epistemic petrification and the restoration of epistemic trust: a new conceptualization of borderline personality disorder and its psychosocial treatment. J Personal Disord. 2015;29(5) https://doi.org/10.1521/pedi.2015.29.5.575.

Forbes MK, Sunderland M, Rapee RM, Batterham PJ, Calear AL, Carragher N, Ruggero C, Zimmerman M, Baillie AJ, Lynch SJ, Mewton L. A detailed hierarchical model of psychopathology: from individual symptoms up to the general factor of psychopathology. Clin Psychol Sci. 2021;9(2):139–68.

Fossati A, Madeddu F, Maffei C. Borderline personality disorder and childhood sexual abuse: a meta-analytic study. J Personal Disord. 1999;13(3):268–80.

Fossati A, Donati D, Donini M, Novella L, Bagnato M, Maffei C. Temperament, character, and attachment patterns in borderline personality disorder. J Personal Disord. 2001;15(5):390–40.

Fowler J, Gullo MJ, Elphinston RA. Impulsivity traits and Facebook addiction in young people and the potential mediating role of coping styles. Personal Individ Differ. 2020;161:109965.

Frances A. Categorical and dimensional systems of personality diagnosis: a comparison. Compr Psychiatry. 1982;23(6):516–27.

Gamache D, Savard C, Leclerc P, Payant M, Côté A, Faucher J, Lampron M, Tremblay M. Latent profiles of patients with borderline pathology based on the alternative DSM-5 model for personality disorders. Bord Personal Disord Emot Dysregul. 2021;8:1–3.
Garland J, Miller S. Borderline personality disorder: part 1 – assessment and diagnosis. BJPsych Adv. 2020;26:159–72. https://doi.org/10.1192/bja.2019.76.
Goldberg LR. The structure of phenotypic personality traits. Am Psychol. 1993;48(1):26.
Gunderson JG, Herpertz SC, Skodol AE, Torgersen S, Zanarini MC. Borderline personality disorder. Nat Rev Dis Primers. 2018;4(1):1–20.
Gunderson JG, Stout RL, McGlashan TH, Shea MT, Morey LC, Grilo CM, Zanarini MC, Yen S, Markowitz JC, Sanislow C, Ansell E. Ten-year course of borderline personality disorder: psychopathology and function from the Collaborative Longitudinal Personality Disorders study. Arch Gen Psychiatry. 2011;68(8):827–37.
Ha C, Balderas JC, Zanarini MC, Oldham J, Sharp C. Psychiatric comorbidity in hospitalized adolescents with borderline personality disorder. J Clin Psychiatry. 2014;75(5):15864.
Hallquist MN, Pilkonis PA. Refining the phenotype of borderline personality disorder: diagnostic criteria and beyond. Personal Disord Theory Res Treat. 2012;3(3):228.
Harkness AR, Reynolds SM, Lilienfeld SO. A review of systems for psychology and psychiatry: adaptive systems, personality psychopathology five (PSY–5), and the DSM–5. J Pers Assess. 2014;96(2):121–39.
Haslam N, Holland E, Kuppens P. Categories versus dimensions in personality and psychopathology: a quantitative review of taxometric research. Psychol Med. 2012;42(5):903–20.
Haslam N, McGrath MJ, Viechtbauer W, Kuppens P. Dimensions over categories: a meta-analysis of taxometric research. Psychol Med. 2020;50(9):1418–32.
Herzog P, Kube T, Fassbinder E. How childhood maltreatment alters perception and cognition – the predictive processing account of borderline personality disorder. Psychol Med. 2022;52(14) https://doi.org/10.1017/S0033291722002458.
Hopwood CJ. Interpersonal dynamics in personality and personality disorders. Eur J Personal. 2018;32(5):499–524.
Hopwood CJ, Newman DA, Donnellan MB, Markowitz JC, Grilo CM, Sanislow CA, Ansell EB, McGlashan TH, Skodol AE, Shea MT, Gunderson JG. The stability of personality traits in individuals with borderline personality disorder. J Abnorm Psychol. 2009;118(4):806.
Hopwood CJ, Thomas KM, Zanarini MC. Hyperbolic temperament and borderline personality disorder. Personal Ment Health. 2012;6(1):22–32.
Hopwood CJ, Schade N, Krueger RF, Wright AG, Markon KE. Connecting DSM-5 personality traits and pathological beliefs: toward a unifying model. J Psychopathol Behav Assess. 2013;35:162–72.
Howard J, De Jesu´ s-Romero R, Peipert A, Riley T, Rutter LA, Lorenzo-Luaces L. The significance of anxiety symptoms in predicting psychosocial functioning across borderline personality traits. PloS one. 2021 Jan 27;16(1):e0245099.
Jablensky A. Psychiatric classifications: validity and utility. World Psychiatry. 2016;15(1) https://doi.org/10.1002/wps.20284.
Johns L, Zhong C, Mezuk B. Understanding suicide over the life course using data science tools within a triangulation framework. J Psychiatr Brain Sci. 2023;8(1):e230003. https://doi.org/10.20900/jpbs.20230003.
Jopp AM, South SC. Investigating the personality inventory for DSM-5 using self and spouse reports. J Personal Disord. 2015;29(2):193–214.
Kaess M, Brunner R, Chanen A. Borderline personality disorder in adolescence. Pediatrics. 2014;34:782–93.
Kendler KS, Myers J, Reichborn-Kjennerud T. Borderline personality disorder traits and their relationship with dimensions of normative personality: a web-based cohort and twin study. Acta Psychiatr Scand. 2010;123(5):349–59. https://doi.org/10.1111/j.1600-0447.2010.01653.x.
Khosravi M. Eating disorders among patients with borderline personality disorder: understanding the prevalence and psychopathology. J Eat Disord. 2020;8:38. License CC BY 4.0. https://doi.org/10.21203/rs.3.rs-19823/v3.

Koenig J, Rinnewitz L, Parzer P, Resch F, Thayer JF, Kaess M. Resting cardiac function in adolescent nonsuicidal self-injury: the impact of borderline personality disorder symptoms and psychosocial functioning. Psychiatry Res. 2017;248:117–20.

Koster N, Laceulle OM, Van der Heijden PT, Klimstra T, De Clercq B, Verbeke L, De Caluwé EA, Van Aken MA. A psychometric evaluation of a reduced version of the PID-5 in clinical and non-clinical adolescents. Eur J Psychol Assess. 2020;36(5):758–66.

Kotov R, Ruggero CJ, Krueger RF, Watson D, Yuan Q, Zimmerman M. New dimensions in the quantitative classification of mental illness. Arch Gen Psychiatry. 2011;68(10):1003–11.

Krabbendam AA, Colins OF, Doreleijers TA, van der Molen E, Beekman AT, Vermeiren RR. Personality disorders in previously detained adolescent females: a prospective study. Am J Orthopsychiatry. 2015;85(1):63.

Kotov R, Krueger RF, Watson D. A paradigm shift in psychiatric classification: the Hierarchical Taxonomy of Psychopathology (HiTOP). World Psychiatry. 2018;17(1):24.

Kotov R, Krueger RF, Watson D, Cicero DC, Conway CC, DeYoung CG, Eaton NR, Forbes MK, Hallquist MN, Latzman RD, Mullins-Sweatt SN. The Hierarchical Taxonomy of Psychopathology (HiTOP): a quantitative nosology based on consensus of evidence. Annu Rev Clin Psychol. 2021;17(1):83–108.

Krueger RF, Markon KE, Patrick CJ, Benning SD, Kramer MD. Linking antisocial behavior, substance use, and personality: an integrative quantitative model of the adult externalizing spectrum. J Abnorm Psychol. 2007;116(4):645.

Krueger RF, Kotov R, Watson D, Forbes MK, Eaton NR, Ruggero CJ, Simms LJ, Widiger TA, Achenbach TM, Bach B, Bagby RM. Progress in achieving quantitative classification of psychopathology. World Psychiatry. 2018;17(3):282–93.

Krueger RF, Hobbs KA. An overview of the DSM-5 alternative model of personality disorders. Psychopathology. 2020;53(3–4):126–32.

Kulacaoglu F, Kose S. Borderline personality disorder (BPD): in the midst of vulnerability, chaos, and awe. Brain Sci. 2018;8:201. https://doi.org/10.3390/brainsci8110201.

Lahey BB. Dimensions of psychological problems: replacing diagnostic categories with a more science-based and less stigmatizing alternative. Oxford University Press; 2021.

Latzman RD, Krueger RF, DeYoung CG, Michelini G. Connecting quantitatively derived personality–psychopathology models and neuroscience. Personal Neurosci. 2021;4:e4.

Leichsenring F, Fonagy P, Heim N, Kernberg OF, Leweke F, Luyten P, Salzer S, Spitzer C, Steinert C. Borderline personality disorder: a comprehensive review of diagnosis and clinical presentation, etiology, treatment, and current controversies. World Psychiatry. 2024;23(1):4–25. https://doi.org/10.1002/wps.21156.

Leihener F, Wagner A, Haaf B, Schmidt C, Lieb K, Stieglitz R, Bohus M. Subtype differentiation of patients with borderline personality disorder using a circumplex model of interpersonal behavior. J Nerv Ment Dis. 2003;191(4):248–54.

Lewis K, Caputi P, Grenyer BF. Borderline personality disorder subtypes: a factor analysis of the DSM-IV criteria. Personal Ment Health. 2012;6(3):196–206.

Linehan M. Cognitive-behavioral treatment of borderline personality disorder. Guilford Press; 1993.

Livesley WJ. A practical approach to the treatment of patients with borderline personality disorder. Psychiatric Clinics of North America. 2000 Mar 1;23(1):211–32.

Livesley WJ. Practical management of personality disorder. Guilford Press; 2003.

Livesley WJ, Jang KL. Differentiating normal, abnormal, and disordered personality. Eur J Personal. 2005;19(4):257–68.

Luyten P, Campbell C, Fonagy P. Rethinking the relationship between attachment and personality disorder. Curr Opin Psychol. 2021;37:109–13.

Lynam DR, Widiger TA. Using the five-factor model to represent the DSM-IV personality disorders: an expert consensus approach. J Abnorm Psychol. 2001;110(3):401.

Markon KE, Chmielewski M, Miller CJ. The reliability and validity of discrete and continuous measures of psychopathology: a quantitative review. Psychol Bull. 2011;137(5):856.

Markon KE, Quilty LC, Bagby RM, Krueger RF. The development and psychometric properties of an informant-report form of the personality inventory for DSM-5 (PID-5). Assessment. 2013;20(3):370–83.

Martin JA, Tarantino DM, Levy KN. Investigating gender-based differential item functioning on the McLean screening instrument for borderline personality disorder (MSI-BPD): an item response theory analysis. Psychol Assess. 2023;35(5):462.

McGlashan TH, Grilo CM, Skodol AE, Gunderson JG, Shea MT, Morey LC, Zanarini MC, Stout RL. The collaborative longitudinal personality disorders study: baseline axis I/II and II/II diagnostic co-occurrence. Acta Psychiatr Scand. 2000;102(4):256–64.

Meares R, Gerull F, Stevenson J, Korner A. Is self-disturbance the core of borderline personality disorder? An outcome study of borderline personality factors. Aust N Z J Psychiatry. 2011;45(3):214–22.

Miller JD, McCain J, Lynam DR, Few LR, Gentile B, MacKillop J, Campbell WK. A comparison of the criterion validity of popular measures of narcissism and narcissistic personality disorder via the use of expert ratings. Psychol Assess. 2014;26(3):958.

Miller CE, Lewis KL, Huxley E, Townsend ML, Grenyer BFS. A 1-year follow-up study of capacity to love and work: what components of borderline personality disorder most impair interpersonal and vocational functioning? Personal Ment Health. 2018;12(4):334–44. https://doi.org/10.1002/pmh.1432.

Miller CE, Townsend ML, Grenyer BFS. Understanding chronic feelings of emptiness in borderline personality disorder: a qualitative study. Bord Personal Disord Emot Dysregul. 2021;8(1):24. https://doi.org/10.1186/s40479-021-00164-8.

Millon T, Millon CM, Meagher SE, Grossman SD, Ramnath R. Personality disorders in modern life. Wiley; 2012.

Millon T. Disorders of personality: introducing a DSM/ICD spectrum from normal to abnormal. Wiley; 2011.

Mineka S, Watson D, Clark LA. Comorbidity of anxiety and unipolar mood disorders. Annu Rev Psychol. 1998;49(1):377–412.

Monaghan C, Bizumic B. Dimensional models of personality disorders: challenges and opportunities. Front Psych. 2023;14:1098452.

Morey LC, McCredie MN, Bender DS, Skodol AE. Criterion A: level of personality functioning in the alternative DSM–5 model for personality disorders. Personal Disord Theory Res Treat. 2022;13(4):305.

Mullins-Sweatt SN, Shannon M, Sauer-Zavala, Lynam D, Miller JD, Widiger TA. Five-factor measure of borderline personality traits. J Pers Assess. 2012;94(5):475–87. https://doi.org/10.1080/00223891.2012.672504. Epub 2012 Apr 10.

Mullins-Sweatt SN, Hopwood CJ, Chmielewski M, Meyer NA, Min J, Helle AC, Walgren MD. Treatment of personality pathology through the lens of the hierarchical taxonomy of psychopathology: developing a research agenda. Personal Ment Health. 2020;14(1):123–41.

Patrick CJ, Venables NC, Yancey JR, Hicks BM, Nelson LD, Kramer MD. A construct-network approach to bridging diagnostic and physiological domains: application to assessment of externalizing psychopathology. J Abnorm Psychol. 2013;122(3):902.

Paris J. Stepped care and rehabilitation for patients recovering from borderline personality disorder. J Clin Psychol. 2015;71(8):747–52.

Ramklint M, Ramklint M, Ramklint M. Child and adolescent psychiatric disorders predicting adult personality disorder: a follow-up study. Nord J Psychiatry. 2003;57(1):23–8.

Regier DA, Narrow WE, Clarke DE, Kraemer HC, Kuramoto SJ, Kuhl EA, Kupfer DJ. DSM-5 field trials in the United States and Canada, part II: test-retest reliability of selected categorical diagnoses. Am J Psychiatry. 2013;170(1):59–70.

Rothschild L, Cleland C, Haslam N, Zimmerman M. A taxometric study of borderline personality disorder. J Abnorm Psychol. 2003;112(4):657.

Sadock E, Perrin PB, Grinnell RM, Rybarczyk B, Auerbach SM. Initial and follow-up evaluations of integrated psychological services for anxiety and depression in a safety net primary care clinic. Journal of clinical psychology. 2017 Oct;73(10):1462–81.

Salzer S, Streeck U, Jaeger U, Masuhr O, Warwas J, Leichsenring F, Leibing E. Patterns of interpersonal problems in borderline personality disorder. J Nerv Ment Dis. 2013;201(2):94–8.

Samuel DB. A review of the agreement between clinicians' personality disorder diagnoses and those from other methods and sources. Clin Psychol Sci Pract. 2015;22(1):1.

Samuel DB, Widiger TA. Clinicians' judgments of clinical utility: a comparison of the DSM-IV and five-factor models. J Abnorm Psychol. 2006;115(2):298.

Samuel DB, Widiger TA. A meta-analytic review of the relationships between the five-factor model and DSM-IV-TR personality disorders: a facet level analysis. Clin Psychol Rev. 2008;28(8):1326–42.

Samuel DB, Miller JD, Widiger TA, Lynam DR, Pilkonis PA, Ball SA. Conceptual changes to the definition of borderline personality disorder proposed for DSM-5. J Abnorm Psychol. 2012;121(2):467.

Sanislow CA, Marcus KL, Reagan EM. Long-term outcomes in borderline psychopathology: old assumptions, current findings, and new directions. Curr Psychiatry Rep. 2012;14:54–61.

Schierenbeck N. The historical transformation of the classification of personality disorders. Eur Psychiatry. 2023;66(S1):S147.

Selby EA, Gardner K. A latent profile analysis of suicidal and self-injurious behavior, other dysregulated behaviors, and borderline personality disorder symptoms. J Exp Psychopathol. 2015;6(4):356–368 ISSN 2043-8087. https://doi.org/10.5127/jep.034913.

Selby EA, Harnedy LE, Hiner M, Kim J. Developmental and momentary dynamics in the onset and maintenance of nonsuicidal self-injurious behavior and borderline personality disorder. Curr Psychiatry Rep. 2022;24:897–909.

Sellbom M, Smid W, De Saeger H, Smit N, Kamphuis JH. Mapping the personality psychopathology five domains onto DSM–IV personality disorders in Dutch clinical and forensic samples: implications for DSM–5. J Pers Assess. 2014;96(2):185–91.

Sharp C, Wall K. Personality pathology grows up: adolescence as a sensitive period. Curr Opin Psychol. 2018;21:111–6.

Sharp C, Wright AG, Fowler JC, Frueh BC, Allen JG, Oldham J, Clark LA. The structure of personality pathology: both general ('g') and specific ('s') factors? J Abnorm Psychol. 2015;124(2):387.

Smits ML, Feenstra DJ, Bales DL, de Vos J, Lucas Z, Verheul R, Luyten P. Subtypes of borderline personality disorder patients: a cluster-analytic approach. Bord Personal Disord Emot Dysregul. 2017;4:1–5.

Stead VE, Boylan K, Schmidt LA. Longitudinal associations between nonsuicidal self-injury and borderline personality disorder in adolescents: a literature review. Bord Personal Disord Emot Dysregul. 2019;6:3. https://doi.org/10.1186/s40479-019-0100-9.

Stepp SD, Whalen DJ, Pilkonis PA, Hipwell AE, Levine MD. Children of mothers with borderline personality disorder: identifying parenting behaviors as potential targets for intervention. Personal Disord Theory Res Treat. 2012;3(1):76.

Stepp SD, Olino TM, Klein DN, Seeley JR, Lewinsohn PM. Unique influences of adolescent antecedents on adult borderline personality disorder features. Personal Disord Theory Res Treat. 2013;4(3):223.

Stepp SD, Keenan K, Hipwell AE, Krueger RF. The impact of childhood temperament on the development of borderline personality disorder symptoms over the course of adolescence. Bord Personal Disord Emot Dysregul. 2014a;1:1.

Stepp SD, Whalen DJ, Scott LN, Zalewski M, Loeber R, Hipwell AE. Reciprocal effects of parenting and borderline personality disorder symptoms in adolescent girls. Dev Psychopathol. 2014b;26(2):361–78.

Stepp SD, Scott LN, Morse JQ, Nolf KA, Hallquist MN, Pilkonis PA. Emotion dysregulation as a maintenance factor of borderline personality disorder features. Compr Psychiatry. 2014c;55(3):657–66.

Stepp SD, Lazarus SA, Byrd AL. A systematic review of risk factors prospectively associated with borderline personality disorder: taking stock and moving forward. Personal Disord Theory Res Treat. 2016;7(4):316.

Thatcher DL, Cornelius JR, Clark DB. Adolescent alcohol use disorders predict adult borderline personality. Addict Behav. 2005;30(9):1709–24.
Thompson KN, Allen NB, Chong S, Chanen AM. Affective startle modulation in young people with first-presentation borderline personality disorder. Psychiatry Res. 2018;263:166–72.
Thompson KN, Jackson H, Cavelti M, Betts J, McCutcheon L, Jovev M, Chanen AM. Number of borderline personality disorder criteria and depression predict poor functioning and quality of life in outpatient youth. J Personal Disord. 2020;34(6):785–98.
Torres-Soto JF, Moya-Faz FJ, Giner-Alegría CA, Oliveras-Valenzuela MA. The PID-5 inventory: the dimensional profile of DSM5 to guide diagnosis and therapeutic needs in personality disorders. An Psicol. 2019;35(1):47–57.
Tragesser SL, Robinson RJ. The role of affective instability and UPPS impulsivity in borderline personality disorder features. J Personal Disord. 2009;23(4):370–83.
Tragesser SL, Bruns D, Disorbio JM. Borderline personality disorder features and pain: the mediating role of negative affect in a pain patient sample. Clin J Pain. 2010;26(4):348–53.
Trull TJ, Durrett CA. Categorical and dimensional models of personality disorder. Annu Rev Clin Psychol. 2005;1:355–80.
Trull TJ, Widiger TA, Guthrie P. Categorical versus dimensional status of borderline personality disorder. J Abnorm Psychol. 1990;99(1):40.
Trull TJ, Solhan MB, Tragesser SL, Jahng S, Wood PK, Piasecki TM, Watson D. Affective instability: measuring a core feature of borderline personality disorder with ecological momentary assessment. J Abnorm Psychol. 2008;117(3):647.
Trull TJ, Distel MA, Carpenter RW. DSM-5 borderline personality disorder: at the border between a dimensional and a categorical view. Curr Psychiatry Rep. 2011;13:43–9.
Trull TJ, Freeman LK, Vebares TJ, Choate AM, Helle AC, Wycoff AM. Borderline personality disorder and substance use disorders: an updated review. Bord Personal Disord Emot Dysregul. 2018;5:1–2.
Tyrer P, Mulder R, Kim YR, Crawford MJ. The development of the ICD-11 classification of personality disorders: an amalgam of science, pragmatism, and politics. Annu Rev Clin Psychol. 2019;15:481–502.
Watson S, Chilton R, Fairchild H, Whewell P. Association between childhood trauma and dissociation among patients with borderline personality disorder. Aust N Zealand J Psychiatry. 2006;40(5):478–81.
Walton CJ, Rasmussen A, Villatte M, Viera RV, Irwin L, Rossiter R. A relational frame approach to perspective taking in persons with borderline personality disorder. J Contextual Behav Sci. 2024;18:100777.
Watson D, Clark LA. Comorbidity and heterogeneity: two challenges for personality pathology research. Personal Disord Theory Res Treat. 2023;14(1):39.
Widiger TA, editor. The Oxford handbook of personality disorders. Oxford: Oxford University Press; 2012.
Widiger TA, Costa PT Jr. Personality disorders and the five-factor model of personality: rationale for the. 3rd ed. American Psychological Association; 2013.
Widiger TA, Lowe JR. A dimensional model of personality disorder: proposal for DSM-V. Psychiatr Clin N Am. 2008;31(3):363–78.
Widiger TA, Rojas SL. Personality disorders. Psychiatry. 2015;23:1706–48.
Widiger TA, Samuel DB. Evidence-based assessment of personality disorders. Psychol Assess. 2005;17(3):278.
Widiger TA, Trull TJ. Plate tectonics in the classification of personality disorder: shifting to a dimensional model. Am Psychol. 2007;62(2):71.
Widiger TA, Trull TJ, Clarkin JF, Sanderson C, Costa PT Jr. A description of the DSM-IV personality disorders with the five-factor model of personality. American Psychological Association; 2002.
World Health Organization. Mental health and psychosocial considerations during the COVID-19 outbreak, 18 March 2020. World Health Organization; 2020.

Wright AG, Zalewski M, Hallquist MN, Hipwell AE, Stepp SD. Developmental trajectories of borderline personality disorder symptoms and psychosocial functioning in adolescence. J Personal Disord. 2016;30(3):351–72.

Yam WH, Simms LJ. Comparing criterion-and trait-based personality disorder diagnoses in DSM-5. J Abnorm Psychol. 2014;123(4):802.

Yeomans F, Kenneth N, Meehan K. Treatment approaches for borderline personality disorder. Psychotherapy. 2012;2(6):42–6.

Zanarini MC, Frankenburg FR, Reich DB, Silk KR, Hudson JI, McSweeney LB. The subsyndromal phenomenology of borderline personality disorder: a 10-year follow-up study. Am J Psychiatry. 2007;164(6):929–35.

Zanarini MC, Frankenburg FR, Fitzmaurice G. Defense mechanisms reported by patients with borderline personality disorder and axis II comparison subjects over 16 years of prospective follow-up: description and prediction of recovery. Am J Psychiatry. 2013;170(1):111–20.

Zimmerman M, Morgan TA. The relationship between borderline personality disorder and bipolar disorder. Dialogues Clin Neurosci. 2013;15(2):155–69.

Zimmerman M. Borderline personality disorder: a disorder in search of advocacy. J Nerv Ment Dis. 2015;203(1):8–12.

Zimmerman M, Becker L. The hidden borderline patient: patients with borderline personality disorder who do not engage in recurrent suicidal or self-injurious behavior. Psychol Med. 2023;53(11):5177–84.

Zimmerman M, Balling C, Dalrymple K, Chelminski I. Screening for borderline personality disorder in psychiatric outpatients with major depressive disorder and bipolar disorder. J Clin Psychiatry. 2019;80(1):8448.

Zittel Conklin C, Westen D. Borderline personality disorder in clinical practice. Am J Psychiatry. 2005;162(5):867–75.

Chapter 3
Parenting Styles and Borderline Personality Disorder

Introduction

Borderline personality disorder (BPD) is a severely pervasive mental health issue characterized by emotional instability, negative affect, impulsivity, and interpersonal difficulties (APA 2022), which can be directly influenced by parenting styles. Parenting has a substantial influence on a child's life and development because parents are the most important part in the life of children. Numerous lines of evidence posit that individuals with BPD would expose frequent challenges in parenting which may result in detrimental impact on the child's development (Stepp et al. 2011). Parenting styles have significant associations with BPD (Hernández Orduña et al. 2022), and maladaptive parenting styles are considered well-established psychosocial risk factors for the development of BP pathology (Steele et al. 2019); these maladaptive parenting styles also magnify the risk of a wide range of emotional and behavioral difficulties in children (Stepp et al. 2011). Parents with BPD report a number of various emotional and behavioral difficulties in their parenting roles, especially fluctuations in mental well-being, issues with expressing suitable empathetic responses, keeping a stable and safe environment, parentification of children, parent-child role disturbances, and interpersonal conflict. All of these difficulties interfere with the parents' daily challenges (Barnow et al. 2006). Parental mental problems, such as depression (Taraban and Shaw 2018), bipolar disorders (Arman and Haghshenas 2022), anxiety disorders (Turner et al. 2003), substance-use disorders (Chassin et al. 2019), and personality disorders (Steele et al. 2019), especially BPD (Florange and Herpertz 2019; Musser et al. 2018; Petfield et al. 2015), contribute to impaired parenting behaviors, which subsequently result in an increased risk of psychopathology across life span (Seeger et al. 2023). Substantial body of studies have demonstrated an association between parental personality and problematic parenting. These findings emphasize the predictive role of maladaptive parenting in later personality issues in offspring and also a relation between parental

E. A. Selby, M. Salavati, *Theories of Borderline Personality Disorder*,
https://doi.org/10.1007/978-3-031-75503-3_3

personality and personality symptoms in offspring (e.g., Berg-Nielsen et al. 2002; Cohen et al. 2005; Johnson 2009). Taraban and Shaw (2018) have proposed a model by joining gender, cognitions, emotions, stress response, genetics, emotion regulation, family structure, and culture and clustering them into three domains: (1) parent characteristics, (2) child characteristics, and (3) family and social environment (Taraban and Shaw 2018). This model suggests parenting as a buffered system, in a way a risk factor may be compensated for by another positive or supportive influencing factors, such as resilience factor, across domains (Seeger et al. 2023).

According to a growing body of empirical investigations and clinical reports, maladaptive parenting has been demonstrated as a substantial etiological factor contributing to the development of various personality disorders in general, but especially borderline personality disorder (Steele et al. 2019; Barroso et al. 2018; Taraban and Shaw 2018; McLaughlin et al. 2012; Reupert and Maybery 2016). It has also been found to be a predictor of BPD features and diagnosis in later adolescence and adulthood (Zanarini 2000; Florange and Herpertz 2019; Petfield et al. 2015; Zalewski et al. 2015). The significant role of maladaptive parenting in the development of borderline personality pathology has been shown in various studies (Winsper 2018). These studies have conceptualized influencing factors that contributed to BPD as parenting personality (Steele et al. 2019), parental developmental history (Neppl et al. 2009), social relationships (Wittchen et al. 2011), work-ability and socioeconomic status (Wittchen et al. 2011), cognition, affect, stress response, and emotion regulation (Gross and Cassidy 2019). Furthermore, significant cognitive, emotional, or social prerequisites for positive parenting treatment, including attention, emotion regulation, or impulse control, are disturbed by personality disorders or mental issues in parents (Steele et al. 2019; Gross and Jazaieri 2014; Johnston and Sullivan 2020).

It should be mentioned that a disproportionately significant number of women presenting to a mother-baby unit met the diagnosis of BPD (Yelland et al. 2015). It has been suggested that women with BPD are overwhelmed by the demands of caring for an infant, especially when in interaction with distressed child (Geerling et al. 2019; Newman et al. 2015). Mothers with BPD are suggested to indicate mis-attitude speech and behaviors with their infants, encompassing critical, intrusive, and frightening comments and behaviors and escalated role confusion in comparison to mothers with depression and healthy group (Steele et al. 2020; Hobson et al. 2009). When the capability for a higher controlled thinking style is disturbed, mothers with BPD recruit defense mechanisms, including hypervigilance to abandonment and rejection, negative expectations of others, and a fragile self-esteem during stressful interactions with their infants (Donegan et al. 2003; Agrawal et al. 2004). This condition is pointed out as an oscillation from controlled mentalization, a conscious and reflective process, to automatic mentalization, provoked by nonconscious defense mechanisms developed during attachment (Fonagy and Luyten 2009). Consequently, these defense mechanisms are connected to a notable number of detrimental parental behaviors in mothers with BPD (Stepp et al. 2011), which lead to the impairment of mothers' capability to shape a healthy attachment with their offspring (Hobson et al. 2005). Kiel et al. (2011, 2023) demonstrated that mothers with BPD take a longer time to respond to their infant's distress, and they tend to do so with less positive emotion and comforting behaviors (Kiel et al. 2011, 2023). These mothers have been labeled as "less engaged" (Crandell et al. 2003), which are manifested as less smiling, mirroring, and less initiation (White et al. 2011). Moreover, studies have proposed that children of mothers with BPD exhibit substantially higher levels of emotional and behavioral issues in comparison with children of mothers with depression only, children of mothers without psychiatric disorders, or children of mothers with cluster C personality traits and disorders (Barnow et al. 2006).

Based on several investigations, it has been revealed that vulnerability from mother to children can be transmitted through maladaptive parenting and maternal emotional dysfunction; such mothers who are diagnosed BPD have problematic interactions with their children including insensitive, overprotective, and hostility in comparison with non-BPD mothers (Eyden et al. 2024). These maladaptive interactions contribute to developing psychopathology in children such as BPD symptoms, depressive disorders (Goodman et al. 2011; Beardslee et al. 2011), externalizing and internalizing problems (Pinquart 2017; Van Loon et al. 2014), insecure attachment patterns (Flowers et al. 2018), and emotion dysregulation (Eyden et al. 2024; Van Santvoort et al. 2015; Rasic et al. 2014; Bödeker et al. 2019). The features of BPD, encompassing emotional dysregulation and chaotic interpersonal relationships, generate deleterious consequences on the shaping of a healthy attachment between mothers with BPD and their children, which cause several developmental difficulties in their offsprings (Eyden 2021). Negatively chaotic parent-child interaction results in increasing both the internalizing and externalizing symptoms among youth with difficulties in emotion regulation (Feinberg et al. 2007). It should be highlighted that the parent-child relationship is considered as a primary core context in which BPD emerges (Winsper 2018), and the most severe stage of BPD symptoms happens during child-rearing years (Florange and Herpertz 2019). According to prospective studies, offspring BPD symptoms have been revealed to be related to prior harsh treatment and punishment (Hallquist et al. 2015), parental criticism (Whalen et al. 2015), overprotection (Schuppert et al. 2015), hostility (Carlson et al. 2009), maternal withdrawal and isolation (Lyons-Ruth et al. 2013), low parental warmth (Infurna et al. 2016a, b), and role reversal or boundary dissolution (Winsper et al. 2015). A great body of literature has demonstrated that children of mothers with BPD are more vulnerable to experiencing emotional dysregulation, suicidal ideation, insecure attachment styles, depressive symptoms, externalizing difficulties and internalizing issues, poorer general psychopathology, and unstable self-image (Barnow et al. 2006; Blankley et al. 2015; Macfie and Swan 2009; Schacht et al. 2013; White et al. 2011; Florange and Herpertz 2019). Investigations have shown that mothers with BPD cause various types of psychiatric disorders among infants (Kiel et al. 2017), children (Stepp et al. 2011), adolescents (Barnow et al. 2013), and adults (Khoury et al. 2019). These mothers may shift between over-involvement and under-involvement, intrusive behaviors and withdrawn, and avoidant behaviors (Stepp et al. 2011).

It has been indicated that mothers with BPD were manifested as intrusively insensitive in their speech and behaviors compared to healthy control (Crandell et al. 2003), and these mothers exhibit dysregulated affective relationships with their infant, comprising critical and intrusive behaviors, role confusion, frightened/frightening behaviors, and disorienting behaviors (Hobson et al. 2009). Moreover, it has been found that mothers with BPD may discourage their toddler, which can lead to disturbed autonomy, and also frighten their children to abandon them resulting role-reversal in children (Macfie and Swan 2009). In line with various studies, it has been proposed that mothers with BPD display less sensitivity and less structuring in mother-child interactions compared to healthy control. In addition, these mothers show various perceptions in their parenting capability, reporting less satisfaction, less competency, and more distress in their parenting abilities (Newman-Morris et al. 2020). Children of mothers with BPD are considered as a high-risk group due to high levels of impaired psychosocial outcomes (Stepp et al. 2011; Johnson 2009). These children have been assumed to be at the higher risk of developing various types of psychopathologies (Zalewski et al. 2015; Eyden et al. 2024; Florange and Herpertz 2019) and higher rates of functional and psychological disturbances (Stepp et al. 2011). In line with scientific literature, emotional instability, hostility, and impulsivity in mothers with BPD might be characterized as mood-dependent behaviors, comprising harsh punishment, invalidating responses, and coercive/controlling behaviors (Suveg et al. 2011). Feldman et al. (1995) found more BPD symptoms, ADHD symptoms, and other disruptive behaviors during childhood among children of BPD mothers in comparison with controls (Feldman et al. 1995). In addition, Barnow et al. (2006) indicated that adolescents of mothers with BPD, aged 11–18 years, displayed higher levels of attention problems, delinquency, and aggression compared to adolescents of mothers without any psychiatric disorders. Also, adolescents of mothers with BPD demonstrated greater levels of anxiety, depression, and low self-esteem compared with adolescents of mothers with depression and other personality disorders and healthy controls (Barnow et al. 2006).

Based on the contemporary etiological models, several interactive inherited-genetic pathways have emerged in BPD psychopathology, including genetic, neural, behavioral, family, and social pathways (Winsper 2018). Remarkable numbers of these pathways merge within the parent-offspring relationships, and this interaction has been considered a considerable context for the pathogenesis of BPD (Steele et al. 2019). In line with family investigations, a 4- to 20-fold upscale in BPD diagnosis and traits has been exhibited among first-degree relatives in comparison to the general population (Barnow et al. 2006; Zanarini et al. 1989). Additionally, in accordance with findings, it has been found that children of parents with BPD can inherit genes making them vulnerable to temperamental issues, emotional reactivity, and impulsivity (Steele et al. 2019; Stepp et al. 2011). The findings from population-based investigations propose a partially strong impact for both genetic and certain environmental experiences to explain the variation in BPD manifestations (Stepp et al. 2011). Diathesis-stress models of BPD psychopathology propose that inherited or biological predisposing (such as interpersonal hypersensitivity) has an interaction with environmental stressors to magnify the risk of the expression of BPD symptoms (Linehan 1998; Gunderson and Lyons-Ruth 2008; Zanarini 2000), and it has been assumed that these invalidated environments may mediate the relation between BPD symptomatology in parents and their children (Eyden et al. 2024). In other words, theoretical models propose that the transaction between invalidating parenting and child's genetic predisposing leads to an increased risk for poor psychosocial outcomes, encompassing BPD and other types of psychopathologies (Linehan 1993; Fruzzetti et al. 2005). According to Linehan (1993), BPD develops as a result of interaction between child vulnerabilities, including impulsivity and emotional sensitivity, and an invalidating social environment (Linehan 1993).

In line with a body of evidence, validating parenting, comprising emotional support and involvement, has a protective role in the development of BPD (Franssens et al. 2021). Problematic parenting, such as emotional withdrawal, parental inconsistencies, and invalidation of thoughts and emotions, contributes to the development of borderline features (Ball and Links 2009; Boucher et al. 2017; Infurna et al. 2015; Schuppert et al. 2015; Vanwoerden et al. 2017, 2022, 2023; Whalen et al. 2015). Parental invalidation may contribute to the development of BP psychopathology and BPD symptoms (Hope and Chapman 2019; Gill and Warburton 2014). Parental invalidation has been proposed as a core component in etiological models of BPD (Vanwoerden et al. 2017, 2022, 2023), and is defined as neglecting or ignoring the expression of emotion, dismissing or minimizing emotional experiences, and/or punishing the emotional expression (Vanwoerden et al. 2017, 2022, 2023; Garside et al. 2002). Parental emotional invalidation may lead to difficulties in the child's social problem-solving abilities and cognitive impairments such as splitting (Selby et al. 2008). Based on a dynamic approach, Vanwoerden et al. (2022) assessed parents' validating and invalidating behavior and its influence on youth BPD symptom expression in daily life, while accounting for parent-perceived helpfulness of these behaviors and youth-perceived support among 162 early adolescents. The findings indicated that at the between-person level, invalidating behaviors were associated with more BPD symptoms in daily life, while ignoring behaviors were related to fewer BPD symptoms. Youth-perceived support anticipated fewer BPD symptoms (Vanwoerden et al. 2022). In addition, in line with evidence, it was found that the experience of childhood emotional invalidation might interfere with the development of social problem-solving abilities, which increase the vulnerability toward later development of BPD and subsequent issues in romantic relationships (Bray et al. 2007). Moreover, parental emotional invalidation may cause cognitive impairments where a fluctuation between dichotomies (good and bad) would occur in the perceptions of others (Selby et al. 2008). Selby et al. (2008) recognized the influence of BPD symptomatology and current romantic relationships, and also, explored whether perceived childhood emotional invalidation mediates the association between BPD features and current romantic relationship dysfunction among a sample of 758 young adults. The results indicated that individuals with BPD features experience dysfunctional relationships which cannot be elucidated by comorbid depression, which suggests that perceived childhood emotional invalidation might lead to greater issues in romantic relationships (Selby et al. 2008).

Based on variations in warmth and control, four parenting dimensions have been presented: Authoritative (high warmth–high control), Authoritarian (low warmth–high control), and Indulgent/Permissive (high warmth–low control), and Neglectful (low warmth–low control) (Maccoby et al. 1984). Concentrating on parenting, it has been revealed that BPD symptoms are associated with psychological and behavioral control of children manifesting as invalidating responses, coercive behaviors, harsh punishment (Zalewski et al. 2014), invalidation, over-involvement, overprotection, lack of care, conflictual and inconsistent relationships, emotional withdrawal or unavailability, and role reversal (Boucher et al. 2017). In line with evidence-based literature, it has been approved that increased parenting stress and low warmth contribute to poor long-term outcomes for children, such as behavioral problems (Barroso et al. 2018). Parenting stress, a negative mental reaction to the normal actions and responsibilities as a parent, may lead to tiredness, frustration, or confusion (Barroso et al. 2018), and also, emotion-focused coping strategies and dysregulated negative emotions which are directed toward children (Le et al. 2020). These high levels of parenting stress are exhibited as a harsh or hostile parenting style (Le et al. 2020). Through a cross-sectional study, Steele et al. (2020) investigated the association between parents' subjective rating of stress and competence and issues in the parents' life, comprising their personality and other mental health issues, their attachment, reflective capacity, and recalled experiences from early family environment among a sample of 284 parents. The findings revealed that individuals with more BPD symptoms reported experiences of higher stress and lower competence in their parenting role in comparison with those with lower BPD manifestations. Moreover, more personality vulnerabilities and poor psychological well-being were found in these parents, as well as, recalling greater traumatic experiences in their childhood, more probability to endorse insecure attachment styles, and poorer reflective capacity. Further, parenting stress and competence showed an association with personality traits, general psychological wellbeing, recalled trauma history, attachment style, and reflective capacity variables. A strong association was found between parental reflective capacity and parenting stress, satisfaction, efficacy, the perception of having a difficult child and a difficult parent-child relationship, and psychological wellbeing, and parenting distress (Steele et al. 2020).

Another parenting dimension is warmth, conceptualized as a combination of levels of interactive interaction and positive emotion during such interactions with a child (Alegre et al. 2014; Lengua et al. 2013). Warm and accepting parenting can protect a child from negative outcomes connected to genetic and physiological vulnerabilities (Eley et al. 2004). Lack of warmth contributes to being rejecting, unresponsiveness, or sensitive toward children (Pinquart 2017) and is indicated by harsh reactions to children's negative emotions, which leads to intense expressions of emotion and lowered social competence in children (Fabes et al. 2001). Armour et al. (2023) explored the associations between perceived parenting and BPD in a sample of 270 adolescents. The findings demonstrated that controlling, rejecting, and chaotic parenting all can anticipate BPD, and all mentioned parenting elements were substantially associated with at least one BPD feature. Results suggested that chaotic parenting seems to have a prominent role in early BPD (Armour et al. 2023).

Family environment, history of psychopathology in parents, and history of abuse can independently predict BPD (Bradley et al. 2005). Problematic and maladaptive parenting has been demonstrated as a predictor for BPD features and diagnosis in later adolescence and adulthood (Eyden et al. 2024), and based on findings, more than 84% of individuals with BPD retrospectively reported experiences of bi-parent neglect and emotional abuse before the age of 18 (Zanarini et al. 2002). It has been demonstrated that mothers with substantially higher levels of BPD symptomatology reported greater levels of stress, lower competence, and indicated lower satisfaction with parenting roles compared to a control group (Petfield et al. 2015; Zalewski et al. 2015). Based on mother-child interaction studies, it was found that mothers with BPD symptoms considered their children as highly stressful, angry, and sad (Florange and Herpertz 2019). Elevated parenting stress has correlation with low levels of warmth among mothers with BPD. According to evidence-based findings, it has been proposed that psychological and behavioral control generally indicated by mothers with BPD can generate a higher rate of externalizing issues in their children (Petfield et al. 2015; Zalewski et al. 2015; Florange and Herpertz 2019). Whalen et al. (2015) studied the link between maternal BPD symptoms and discrepancies between mother-reported and observed infant expression of fear and anger. The results showed that maternal BPD symptoms, especially interpersonal symptoms, have associations with higher convergence of mother-reported and observed infant anger expression. Moreover, maternal symptoms did not indicate any relation with discrepancies between mother-reported and observed infant expressions and maternal BPD symptoms associated with both low and high levels of fear expression. Additionally, BPD behavioral symptoms demonstrated an association with higher convergence of mother-reported and observed infant fear expressions (Whalen et al. 2015). Dittrich et al. (2018) indicated that diagnosis of maternal BPD was indirectly related to increased abuse potential scores and mediated by severity of difficulties in emotion regulation among mothers with BPD (Dittrich et al. 2018).

Furthermore, in line with numerous findings, it has been indicated that maladaptive parenting may contribute to impairments in emotion regulation strategies (Hughes et al. 2012, 2020) and the transmission of social knowledge (Fonagy et al. 2017), which cause difficulties in major psychological processes, including emotional regulation and social cognition (Winsper 2018), and lead to increased vulnerabilities for various clinical disorders such as BPD in adolescence and adulthood (Steele et al. 2019). Substantial associations have been found between maternal BPD and lower levels of sensitivity, emotion recognition, parenting satisfaction and efficacy, as well as greater intrusiveness, overprotection, hostility, and parenting stress/distress, in comparison to maternal depressive disorder, other personality disorders, and healthy controls (Elliot et al. 2014; Newman-Morris et al. 2020; Frankel-Waldheter et al. 2015; Hobson et al. 2009). Evidence proposes that maternal BPD influences infant affect and early markers of self- and emotion regulation skills (Hobson et al. 2005; Newman-Morris et al. 2020). Based on cross-sectional study, Kim et al. (2014) examined attachment disturbance and emotion dysregulation manifesting in the psychopathology of BPD, as well as exploring two classes of cognitive emotion regulation strategies connected to psychopathology of BPD. The results revealed that positive and negative emotion regulation strategies were differentially implicated in the relation between attachment security and BPD characteristics. It was found that attachment security has a function as a buffer against BPD due to promoting positive emotion regulation strategies, while negative emotion regulation strategies attenuate the protective influence of attachment and positive emotion regulation strategies (Kim et al. 2014). Mothers with severe BPD symptoms tend to respond to an infant's negative emotions with high levels of intolerance, impatience, minimization, and invalidating behaviors (Florange and Herpertz 2019). Robin et al. (2021) studied the distinct influence of parental adversity and stressful life events on BPD emotional symptoms and the role of attachment and alexithymia in these emotional processes. The results demonstrated that dysfunctional parental interactions were associated with emotional symptoms, hopelessness, and anxious attachment in healthy controls, but not in the BPD group. Furthermore, stressful life events showed a positive correlation with emotional symptoms and avoidant attachment indicated negative correlation in the BPD group. Multivariate regression analysis displayed that among individuals with BPD, emotional symptoms were independent of dysfunctional parenting yet dependent on attachment. Moreover, raising the numbers of stressful life events decreased emotional symptoms in individuals with BPD, independently of parental interactions or attachment, and showed association with the growing use of operative thinking (Robin et al. 2021). Newman et al. (2007) demonstrated that infants of mothers with BPD (aged 3–36 months) exhibited lesser attention and lesser interest in interactions with their mother during a free-play interaction compared to healthy controls, which may be contributed to the development of avoidant interaction patterns between children and their mother (Newman et al. 2007). Mothers with marked levels of BPD symptoms manifest an interaction with their children featured by low sensitivity and high intrusiveness, with a hostile and incohesive family environment (Florange and Herpertz 2019; Petfield et al. 2015). Through a systematic review and qualitative synthesis concentrated on the psychosocial risk factors for BPD, five vulnerability factors were recognized, encompassing (1) childhood trauma/abuse; (2) unfavorable parenting; (3) object relations; (4) insecure attachment/loss; and (5) symbolization/reflectiveness capacity (Keinan et al. 2012). In another systematic review and qualitative synthesis in 40 cross-sectional and longitudinal studies conducted to identify the parent-child relationship associated with the development of BPD, it was pointed out that BPD participants reported higher rate of dysfunctional parent-child relationship in comparison to healthy controls. Parents retrospectively presented their BPD child as being unusually sensitive with a difficult temperament and having a remarkably chaotic relationship characterized by verbal abuse and antisocial behaviors. Furthermore, family perspective findings showed lesser parental care in BPD daughters, higher maternal overprotection, and inconsistent parental values and norms (Boucher et al. 2017). Hobson et al. (1998) observed that individuals with BPD manifested disturbed moment-to-moment relatedness with their psychotherapist, such as hostility and severe idealizing and devaluating exchanges, which resemble the patterns of their interactions with their mother (Hobson et al. 1998). In a meta-analysis study of 61 retrospective cross-sectional and prospective studies, Winsper et al. (2016) found significant maternal hostility, verbal abuse, and neglect among adults and youth with BPD (Winsper et al. 2016). Through a 33-person case-control, cross-sectional, and cohort quantitative study conducted to examine the parenting behaviors and attitudes of mothers with BPD, mother-child interactions, and offspring outcomes, Eyden et al. (2016) proposed that mothers with BPD appeared to be less sensitive, less engaged, more intrusive, more overprotective, more hostile, and more likely to have maladaptive interactions with their children. Additionally, their children revealed a wide range of psychological problems including depression, internalizing/externalizing difficulties, general psychopathology, low self-esteem, interpersonal issues, home difficulties, and general dysfunctions. In line with their findings, the most potentially core mechanisms underpinning the transmission of proneness in mother-child interaction comprised maladaptive parenting, maternal emotional impairments, and offspring characteristics (Eyden et al. 2016). Based on 17 cross-sectional studies that evaluated mothers with BPD, Petfield et al. (2015) found an association between maternal BPD and differences in parenting outcomes, encompassing decreased sensitivity and elevated intrusive toward child; issues in unstructured activities and poorer levels of family organization; family environments feature by remarkable levels of hostility and low levels of cohesion; heightened overprotection; poor mindedness; less competence and satisfaction in parenting role; and intensified parenting stress. Moreover, less satisfying interactions and difficulties in mother-child interactions, more cognitive-behavioral risk factors, and poor mental health were reported (Petfield et al. 2015). Boxberger (2020) examined the pathway through which increased symptoms of maternal BPD have association with greater levels of externalizing problems in their children by focusing on maternal warmth and parenting stress. The findings pointed out that heightened maternal BPD symptoms are related to remarkably higher levels of child externalizing difficulties and also to greater levels of parenting stress (Boxberger 2020). Williams et al. (2023a, b) examined mother-adolescent interactions and their association with adolescent BPD traits in a sample of 38 adolescents and their mothers compared to 35 healthy control group. Considering results, BPD groups displayed a substantially lower quality of maternal behaviors in comparison with the healthy control group. Maternal and adolescent behavior was anticipated by BPD traits alone; however, dyadic behavior was impacted by general adolescent psychopathology (Williams 2019).

BPD symptoms associated with interpersonal dysregulation may result in issues in parenting. Studies propose that relational patterns among BPD are featured by intense rejection sensitivity and frantic attempts to avoid abandonment. Therefore, mothers with BPD may fear desertion by their adolescent daughters, as well as they respond to their adolescent daughters' increasing autonomy with intrusive, coercive, and controlling behaviors. These mothers may seek excessive reassurance and soothing from their adolescent daughters not to be abandoned, hence, contributing to role reversals and efforts to control the adolescent daughters' behavior through guilt (Zalewski et al. 2014). Zalewski et al. (2014) studied relations between maternal BPD symptoms and parenting in 1598 adolescent girls and their mothers. The results indicated that maternal BPD symptoms were related to aspects of psychological and behavioral control, even after controlling for maternal depression and alcohol use severity. It was found that affective/behavioral dysregulation, but not interpersonal dysregulation or identity impairment, uniquely accounted for parenting (Zalewski et al. 2014). Moreover, based on a series of experimental and theoretical elaborations, it has been debated that relational aggression might be considered a developmental precursor of BPD. Relational aggression is concentrated on behaviors in which a person seeks to manipulate or disturb relationships (Crick and Grotpeter 1995). Early aggression and parenting experiences may vary in their long-term prediction of aggression or borderline features. Through a decayed longitudinal study among preschool children (84 boys and 84 girls), Nelson et al. (2014) indicated that preschool relational aggression in girls anticipated adolescent relational aggression. Preschool aversive parenting, such as authoritarian, permissive, and psychological controlling forms, remarkably predicted aggression and borderline manifestations in adolescent females. For adolescent males, preschool authoritative parenting was a protective factor against aggression and borderline features, while authoritarian parenting was suggested as a risk factor for later aggression (Nelson et al. 2014).

One of the most documented factors demonstrating a significantly psychogenic role in BPD is childhood traumatic experiences and insecure attachment (Zanarini and Wedig 2014; Baryshnikov et al. 2017, 2024; Gratz et al. 2022). Zanarini and Wedig (2014) have reviewed a series of studies which were done to assess the impact of parental separation or loss and disturbed parental involvement. They concluded that through this revision, four conclusions have emerged: (1) protracted childhood separations are both common and discriminating for individuals with BPD; (2) the majority of BPD cases usually describe their interaction and relationships with their mother as a hostile, conflict, faraway, distant, and in some cases in a overprotective manner; (3) the father's failure to be present and involved is an even more discriminating aspect of these families than the mother's problems; (4) inappropriate relationships, especially disturbed mental and emotional interactions with both parents, may be more specific and distinguishable for BPD and can affect more in development of BPD psychopathology in comparison to cases which include conflict just with one parent (Zanarini and Wedig 2014). Perez et al. (2020) indicated an association between father and NSSI in individuals with BPD with a history of childhood abuse, neglect, and maltreatment among 127 BPD patients through a cross-sectional study (Perez et al. 2020).

According to attachment theory, the child's early experiences with significant others, especially caregiver, impact the child's relationships over the years of their lifespan (Bowlby 1969; Stagaki et al. 2022). The most important point that should be mentioned is that the shaping of a person's basic assumptions, core beliefs, and expectations about themselves, others, and the environment during early experiences will contribute to developing romantic behaviors in adulthood (Stagaki et al. 2022). Individuals with BPD frequently exhibit attachment styles categorized as disorganized and unresolved (Levy et al. 2005), which impact the way in which a mother relates to her child. Mothers with higher level of unresolved trauma may have a relationship with their children in a manner that sways between hostility and passivity (Hesse and Main 2000). Through an open-ended narrative representation, Macfie and Swan (2009) evaluated mother-children attachment relationships in preschool and early school-aged children (ages 4–7) of mothers with BPD. The results revealed poor emotion regulation in the children's narrative as manifested by elevated probability to talk about fantasies and also material of a traumatic nature. Among children of mother with BPD, role reversal was significantly more to be present in their narratives. Moreover, higher fears of abandonment, in the case of resolving a predicted loss in their stories, were reported. Remarkably higher rates of negative parent-child relationship expectations, such as the relationships featured by unpredictability and danger, were revealed in the preschooler's narratives and shameful self-representations were found among the narratives of children of BPD mothers (Macfie and Swan 2009).

Pursuant to notes by Zanarini and Wedig (2014), parental separation or loss is one of the most crucial factors in the development of BPD, which leads to increased experience of chaotic and adverse environments in childhood and adolescence. Through assessing several studies in this subject, they found out that the majority of BPD in inpatient and outpatient settings had histories of parent loss because of divorce or death. Many of those patients reported that they came from broken families with highly conflictual relationships with their mothers and fathers. Taken together, many studies have shown that parental separation or loss due to divorce, death, and serious illness of their parents were higher than non-BPD cases (Soloff and Millward 1983; Akiskal 1994). In other words, experiencing the loss of parents was more common in BPD than the other clinical or nonclinical patients (Zanarini and Wedig 2014). Two major concepts which play main role in these difficulties composed of childhood trauma and attachment (Crowell et al. 2009). There are numerous associations between the severity of facial emotion in individuals with BPD including hypo- and hypersensitivity of emotions which indicate the attempts of individuals with BPD to identify early signs of threat or, in contrast, protection from actual trauma (Frick et al. 2012; Crowell et al. 2009; Nicol 2014; Van Heel et al. 2019). Derks et al. (2017) demonstrated a moderate association between low emotional awareness and difficulties in identifying and describing emotion and BPD. Derks et al. (2017) posited that during childhood, a series of emotional concepts are acquired which continue through obtaining synthetic emotional concepts during adulthood. These learning processes are dependent on early life experiences, environmental stability, and habitual patterns of selective attention (Smith and South 2020).

In line with a longitudinal study, it has been indicated that the experience of attachment disorganization and parental hostility in early childhood was associated with various dysfunctions in several domains, including attention, emotion, behavior, relationships, and self-representation, in middle childhood and early adolescence which finally contributed to development of different symptoms of BPD (Carlson et al. 2009). Zhang et al. (2021) examined whether adverse childhood experiences are associated with young adults' risky behaviors, including physical fighting, drinking problems, smoking problems, substance use, early sexual behaviors, digital media overuse, and suicidal ideation, among 1091 Chinese rural youth.

The findings demonstrated that accumulating exposure to adverse childhood experiences contributed to escalating the possibility of being involved in a variety of high-risk behaviors in young individuals, as well as the function of this association is partially through perceived stress (Zhang et al. 2021). There is a long history of research on psychopathology among family members of individuals with BPD. Childhood maltreatment and intimate partner violence are the most common types of family violence which are associated with a wide range of subsequences compromised of morbidity and fatality (McTavish et al. 2024). Experiences of one kind of family violence elevate the risk of experiencing other types of violence in families, especially childhood maltreatment (Oram et al. 2014; Godbout et al. 2019; Capaldi et al. 2012).

To sum, BPD is presented as a pervasively psychological problem featured by emotional-behavioral and interpersonal problems, which can be directly impacted by parenting styles. As shown, numerous empirical and clinical studies have demonstrated significant associations between maladaptive parenting styles and the development of BPD. Furthermore, a substantial number of findings indicated the presence of different mental state difficulties among BPD parents contributing to adverse dysfunctional interaction between individuals with BPD and their parents, especially difficulties in expressing empathetic responses and providing a valid and safe environment. Moreover, mothers with BPD are proposed to demonstrate misbehaviors with children leading to feeling of abandonment and rejection and fragile self-esteem in children. As mentioned, parental invalidation, including emotional and behavioral invalidating, has been presented as a major element in etiological models of BPD which led to issues in the child's social problem-solving abilities and cognitive impairments, as well as greater issues in romantic relationships in adulthood such as severe rejection sensitivity and frantic efforts to avoid abandonment. In addition, experiencing attachment disorganization and parental hostility in early childhood has shown several dysfunctional abilities in cognitive, emotional, behavioral, and interpersonal competence in middle childhood and early adolescence contributing to development of BPD.

References

Agrawal HR, Gunderson J, Holmes BM, Lyons-Ruth K. Attachment studies with borderline patients: a review. Harv Rev Psychiatry. 2004;12(2):94–104.

Akiskal HS. The temperamental borders of affective disorders. Acta Psychiatr Scand. 1994;89:32–7.

Alegre A, Benson MJ, Pérez-Escoda N. Maternal warmth and early adolescents' internalizing symptoms and externalizing behavior: mediation via emotional insecurity. J Early Adolesc. 2014;34(6):712–35. https://doi.org/10.1177/0272431613501408.

American Psychiatric Association. Diagnostic and statistical manual of mental disorders. 5th ed. Text Revised (DSM-5-TR); 2022.

Arman S, Haghshenas M. Metabolic effects of adding Topiramate on aripiprazole in bipolar patients aged between 6–18 years, a randomized, double-blind, placebo-controlled trial. J Res Med Sci. 2022;27(1):23.

Armour JA, Joussemet M, Mageau GA, Varin R. Perceived parenting and borderline personality features during adolescence. Child Psychiatry Hum Dev. 2023;54:927–38.

Ball JS, Links PS. Borderline personality disorder and childhood trauma: evidence for a causal relationship. Curr Psychiatry Rep. 2009;11(1):63–8.

Barnow S, Spitzer C, Grabe HJ, Kessler C, Freyberger HJ. Individual characteristics, familial experience, and psychopathology in children of mothers with borderline personality disorder. J Am Acad Child Adolesc Psychiatry. 2006;45(8):965–72.

Barnow S, Aldinger M, Arens EA, Ulrich I, Spitzer C, Grabe HJ, Stopsack M. Maternal transmission of borderline personality disorder symptoms in the community-based Greifswald family study. J Personal Disord. 2013;27(6):806–19.

Barroso NE, Mendez L, Graziano PA, Bagner DM. Parenting stress through the lens of different clinical groups: a systematic review & meta-analysis. J Abnorm Child Psychol. 2018;46:449–61.

Baryshnikov I, Rosenström TH, Isometsä ET. Psychological pain as a risk factor for suicidal ideation: an ecological momentary assessment study on inpatients with depression with and without comorbid borderlin personality disorder. J Clin Psychiatry. 2024;85(2):54110.

Baryshnikov I, Joffe G, Koivisto M, Melartin T, Aaltonen K, Suominen K, Rosenström T, Näätänen P, Karpov B, Heikkinen M, Isometsä E. Relationships between self-reported childhood traumatic experiences, attachment style, neuroticism and features of borderline personality disorders in patients with mood disorders. J Affect Disord. 2017;210:82–9.

Berg-Nielsen TS, Vikan A, Dahl AA. Parenting related to child and parental psychopathology: a descriptive review of the literature. Clin Child Psychol Psychiatry. 2002;7(4):529–52.

Beardslee WR, Gladstone TR, O'Connor EE. Transmission and prevention of mood disorders among children of affectively ill parents: a review. J Am Acad Child Adolesc Psychiatry. 2011;50(11):1098–109.

Blankley G, Galbally M, Snellen M, Power J, Lewis AJ. Borderline personality disorder in the perinatal period: early infant and maternal outcomes. Australas Psychiatry. 2015;23(6):688–92.

Bödeker K, Fuchs A, Führer D, Kluczniok D, Dittrich K, Reichl C, Reck C, Kaess M, Hindi Attar C, Möhler E, Neukel C. Impact of maternal early life maltreatment and maternal history of depression on child psychopathology: mediating role of maternal sensitivity? Child Psychiatry Hum Dev. 2019;50:278–90.

Boucher MÈ, Pugliese J, Allard-Chapais C, Lecours S, Ahoundova L, Chouinard R, Gaham S. Parent–child relationship associated with the development of borderline personality disorder: a systematic review. Personal Ment Health. 2017;11(4):229–55.

Bowlby J. Attachment and loss. Random House; 1969.

Boxberger A. Associations of maternal borderline personality disorder symptoms with parenting stress, maternal warmth, and child externalizing problems (Doctoral dissertation, University of Oregon); 2020.

Bradley R, Zittel Conklin C, Westen D. The borderline personality diagnosis in adolescents: gender differences and subtypes. J Child Psychol Psychiatry. 2005;46:1006–19.

Bray S, Barrowclough C, Lobban F. The social problem-solving abilities of people with borderline personality disorder. Behav Res Ther. 2007;45(6):1409–17.

Capaldi DM, Knoble NB, Shortt JW, Kim HK. A systematic review of risk factors for intimate partner violence. Partn Abus. 2012;3(2):231.

Carlson EA, Egeland B, Sroufe LA. A prospective investigation of the development of borderline personality symptoms. Dev Psychopathol. 2009;21(4):1311–34.

Chassin L, Hussong AM, Rothenberg WA, Sternberg A. Parenting and substance use disorder. In: Handbook of parenting. Milton: Routledge; 2019. p. 483–516.

Cohen LH, Gunthert KC, Butler AC, O'Neill SC, Tolpin LH. Daily affective reactivity as a prospective predictor of depressive symptoms. J Pers. 2005;73(6):1687–714.

Crandell LE, Patrick MPH, Hobson RP. Still-face' interactions between mothers with borderline personality disorder and their 2-month-old infants. Br J Psychiatry. 2003;183(3):239–47. https://doi.org/10.1192/bjp.183.3.239.

Crick NR, Grotpeter JK. Relational aggression, gender, and social-psychological adjustment. Child Dev. 1995;66(3):710–22.
Crowell SE, Beauchaine TP, Linehan MM. A biosocial developmental model of borderline personality: elaborating and extending Linehan's theory. Psychol Bull. 2009;135(3):495.
Derks YP, Westerhof GJ, Bohlmeijer ET. A meta-analysis on the association between emotional awareness and borderline personality pathology. J Personal Disord. 2017;31(3):362–84.
Dittrich K, Boedeker K, Kluczniok D, Jaite C, Hindi Attar C, Fuehrer D, et al. Child abuse potential in mothers with early life maltreatment, borderline personality disorder and depression. Br J Psychiatry. 2018;213(1):412–8. https://doi.org/10.1192/bjp.2018.74.
Donegan NH, Sanislow CA, Blumberg HP, Fulbright RK, Lacadie C, Skudlarski P, Gore JC, Olson IR, McGlashan TH, Wexler BE. Amygdala hyperreactivity in borderline personality disorder: implications for emotional dysregulation. Biol Psychiatry. 2003;54(11):1284–93.
Elliot RL, Campbell L, Hunter M, Cooper G, Melville J, McCabe K, Newman L, Loughland C. When I look into my baby's eyes... Infant emotion recognition by mothers with borderline personality disorder. Infant Ment Health J. 2014;35(1):21–32.
Eley TC, Sugden K, Corsico A, Gregory AM, Sham P, McGuffin P, Plomin R, Craig IW. Gene–environment interaction analysis of serotonin system markers with adolescent depression. Mol Psychiatry. 2004;9(10):908–15.
Eyden J. Mothers with borderline personality disorder: parenting knowledge, perceptions, and emotional availability (Doctoral dissertation, University of Warwick); 2021.
Eyden J, Winsper C, Wolke D, Broome MR, MacCallum F. A systematic review of the parenting and outcomes experienced by offspring of mothers with borderline personality pathology: potential mechanisms and clinical implications. Clin Psychol Rev. 2016;47:85–105.
Eyden J, MacCallum F, Bornstein MH, Broome M, Wolke D. Parenting knowledge and parenting self-efficacy of mothers with borderline personality disorder and depression: "I know what to do but think I am not doing it". Dev Psychopathol. 2024;36(2):648–59.
Fabes RA, Leonard SA, Kupanoff K, Martin CL. Parental coping with childrens negative emotions: relations with childrens emotional and social responding. Child Dev. 2001;72(3):907–20. https://doi.org/10.1111/1467-8624.00323.
Feinberg ME, Kan ML, Hetherington EM. The longitudinal influence of coparenting conflict on parental negativity and adolescent maladjustment. J Marriage Fam. 2007;69(3):687–702.
Feldman RB, Zelkowitz P, Weiss M, Vogel J. A comparison of the families of mothers with borderline and nonborderline personality disorders. Compr Psychiatry. 1995;36:157–63. https://doi.org/10.1016/S0010-440X(95)90110-8.
Florange JG, Herpertz SC. Parenting in patients with borderline personality disorder, sequelae for the offspring and approaches to treatment and prevention. Curr Psychiatry Rep. 2019;21:1–8.
Flowers AG, McGillivray JA, Galbally M, Lewis AJ. Perinatal maternal mental health and disorganised attachment: a critical systematic review. Clin Psychol. 2018;22(3):300–16.
Fonagy P, Luyten P. A developmental, mentalization-based approach to the understanding and treatment of borderline personality disorder. Dev Psychopathol. 2009;21(4):1355–81.
Fonagy P, Luyten P, Allison E, Campbell C. What we have changed our minds about: part 1. Borderline personality disorder as a limitation of resilience. Bord Personal Disord Emot Dysregul. 2017;4:1–1.
Frankel-Waldheter M, Macfie J, Strimpfel JM, Watkins CD. Effect of maternal autonomy and relatedness and borderline personality disorder on adolescent symptomatology. Personal Disord Theory Res Treat. 2015;6(2):152.
Franssens R, Abrahams L, Brenning K, Van Leeuwen K, De Clercq B. Unraveling prospective reciprocal effects between parental invalidation and pre-adolescents' borderline traits: between-and within-family associations and differences with common psychopathology-parenting transactions. Res Child Adolesc Psychopathol. 2021;49(10):1387–401.
Frick C, Lang S, Kotchoubey B, Sieswerda S, Dinu-Biringer R, Berger M, Veser S, Essig M, Barnow S. Hypersensitivity in borderline personality disorder during mindreading. PLoS One. 2012;7(8):e41650.

Fruzzetti AE, Shenk C, Hoffman PD. Family interaction and the development of borderline personality disorder: a transactional model. Dev Psychopathol. 2005;17(4):1007–30.

Garside R, Ayres R, Owen M, Pearson VA, Roizen J. Anonymity and confidentiality: rural teenagers' concerns when accessing sexual health services. J Family Plann Reprod Health Care. 2002;28:23–33.

Geerling I, Roberts RM, Williams AS. Impact of infant crying on mothers with a diagnosis of borderline personality disorder: a qualitative study. Infant Ment Health J. 2019;40(3):405–21. https://doi.org/10.1002/imhj.21776.

Gill D, Warburton W. An investigation of the biosocial model of borderline personality disorder. J Clin Psychol. 2014;70(9):866–73.

Godbout N, Daspe MÈ, Runtz M, Cyr G, Briere J. Childhood maltreatment, attachment, and borderline personality–related symptoms: gender-specific structural equation models. Psychol Trauma Theory Res Pract Policy. 2019;11(1):90.

Goodman M, Hazlett EA, Avedon JB, Siever DR, Chu KW, New AS. Anterior cingulate volume reduction in adolescents with borderline personality disorder and co-morbid major depression. J Psychiatr Res. 2011;45(6):803–7.

Gratz KL, Kiel EJ, Mann AJ, Tull MT. The prospective relation between borderline personality disorder symptoms and suicide risk: the mediating roles of emotion regulation difficulties and perceived burdensomeness. J Affect Disord. 2022;313:186–95.

Gross JT, Cassidy J. Expressive suppression of negative emotions in children and adolescents: theory, data, and a guide for future research. Dev Psychol. 2019;55(9):1938.

Gross JJ, Jazaieri H. Emotion, emotion regulation, and psychopathology: an affective science perspective. Clin Psychol Sci. 2014;2(4):387–401. https://doi.org/10.1177/2167702614536164.

Gunderson JG, Lyons-Ruth K. BPD's interpersonal hypersensitivity phenotype: a gene-environment-developmental model. J Pers Disord. 2008;22(1):22–41. https://doi.org/10.1521/pedi.2008.22.1.22.

Hallquist MN, Hipwell AE, Stepp SD. Poor self-control and harsh punishment in childhood prospectively predict borderline personality symptoms in adolescent girls. J Abnorm Psychol. 2015;124(3):549.

Hernández Orduña O, Arango I, Miranda Terres E, Muñoz Toledo C, Rodríguez Delgado A, Robles GR. Adaptation of a DBT intervention to reduce self-harm in borderline personality disorder. Int J Psychol Psychol Ther. 2022;22(3):277–87.

Hesse E, Main M. Disorganized infant, child, and adult attachment: collapse in behavioral and attentional strategies. J Am Psychoanal Assoc. 2000;48(4):1097–127.

Hobson RP, Patrick MPH, Valentine JD. Objectivity in psychoanalytic judgements. Br J Psychiatry. 1998;173(2):172–7.

Hobson PR, Patrick M, Crandell L, García-Pérez R, Lee A. Personal relatedness and attachment in infants of mothers with borderline personality disorder. Dev Psychopathol. 2005;17:329–47.

Hobson RP, Patrick MPH, Hobson JA, Crandell L, Bronfman E, Lyons-Ruth K. How mothers with borderline personality disorder relate to their year-old infants. Br J Psychiatry. 2009;195(4):325–30.

Hope NH, Chapman AL. Difficulties regulating emotions mediates the associations of parental psychological control and emotion invalidation with borderline personality features. Personal Disord Theory Res Treat. 2019;10(3):267.

Hughes AE, Crowell SE, Uyeji L, Coan JA. A developmental neuroscience of borderline pathology: emotion dysregulation and social baseline theory. J Abnorm Child Psychol. 2012;40:21–33.

Hughes DJ, Kratsiotis IK, Niven K, Holman D. Personality traits and emotion regulation: a targeted review and recommendations. Emotion. 2020;20(1):63.

Infurna MR, Reichl C, Parzer P, Schimmenti A, Bifulco A, Kaess M. Associations between depression and specific childhood experiences of abuse and neglect: a meta-analysis. J Affect Disord. 2015;190:47–55.

Infurna MR, Reichl C, Parzer P, Schimmenti A, Bifulco A, Kaess M. Associations between depression and specific childhood experiences of abuse and neglect: a meta-analysis. J Affect Disord. 2016a;190:47–55.

Infurna MR, Brunner R, Holz B, Parzer P, Giannone F, Reichl C, et al. The specific role of childhood abuse, parental bonding, and family functioning in female adolescents with borderline personality disorder. J Personal Disord. 2016b;30:177–92.
Johnson DR. Goal-directed attentional deployment to emotional faces and individual differences in emotional regulation. J Res Pers. 2009;43(1):8–13.
Johnston JR, Sullivan MJ. Parental alienation: in search of common ground for a more differentiated theory. Fam Court Rev. 2020;58(2):270–92.
Keinan G, Shrira A, Shmotkin, D. The association between cumulative adversity and mental health: considering dose and primary focus of adversity. Qual Life Res 2012;21:1149–58.
Khoury JE, Pechtel P, Andersen CM, Teicher MH, Lyons-Ruth K. Relations among maternal withdrawal in infancy, borderline features, suicidality/self-injury, and adult hippocampal volume: a 30-year longitudinal study. Behav Brain Res. 2019;374:112139.
Kiel EJ, Buss KA. Prospective relations among fearful temperament, protective parenting, and social withdrawal: the role of maternal accuracy in a moderated mediation framework. J Abnorm Child Psychol. 2011;39(7):953–66.
Kiel EJ, Viana AG, Tull MT, Gratz KL. Emotion socialization strategies of mothers with borderline personality disorder symptoms: the role of maternal emotion regulation and interactions with infant temperament. J Personal Disord. 2017;31(3):399–416. https://doi.org/10.1521/pedi_2016_30_256.
Kiel EJ, Jones LB, Tull MT, Gratz KL. Mothers' borderline personality disorder symptom severity and accuracy in predicting infant distress. Personal Disord Theory Res Treat. 2023;14(2):161.
Kim S, Sharp C, Carbone C. The protective role of attachment security for adolescent borderline personality disorder features via enhanced positive emotion regulation strategies. Personal Disord Theory Res Treat. 2014;5(2):125.
Le H, Hashmi A, Czelusta KL, Matin A, Moukaddam N, Shah AA. Is borderline personality disorder a serious mental illness? Psychiatr Ann. 2020;50(1):8–13.
Lengua LJ, Kiff C, Moran L, Zalewski M, Thompson S, Cortes R, Ruberry E. Parenting mediates the effects of income and cumulative risk on the development of effortful control. Soc Dev. 2013;23(3):631–49. https://doi.org/10.1111/sode.12071.
Levy KN, Meehan KB, Weber M, Reynoso J, Clarkin JF. Attachment and borderline personality disorder: implications for psychotherapy. Psychopathology. 2005;38(2):64–74.
Linehan MM. Skills training manual for treating borderline personality disorder. Guilford Press; 1993.
Linehan MM. An illustration of dialectical behavior therapy. Sess Psychother Pract Psychother Pract. 1998;4(2):21–44.
Lyons-Ruth K, Bureau JF, Holmes B, Easterbrooks A, Brooks NH. Borderline symptoms and suicidality/self-injury in late adolescence: prospectively observed relationship correlates in infancy and childhood. Psychiatry Res. 2013;206(2–3):273–81.
Maccoby EE, Snow ME, Jacklin CN. Children's dispositions and mother–child interaction at 12 and 18 months: a short-term longitudinal study. Dev Psychol. 1984;20(3):459.
Macfie J, Swan SA. Representations of the caregiver–child relationship and of the self, and emotion regulation in the narratives of young children whose mothers have borderline personality disorder. Dev Psychopathol. 2009;21(3):993–1011.
McLaughlin KA, Green JG, Gruber MJ, Sampson NA, Zaslavsky AM, Kessler RC. Childhood adversities and first onset of psychiatric disorders in a national sample of US adolescents. Arch Gen Psychiatry. 2012;69(11):1151–60.
McTavish JR, McHolm A, Niec A, Pietrantonio AM, McKee C, MacMillan HL. Case conceptualization in child welfare: an underused resource to improve child, family, and provider outcomes. Front Psych. 2024;14:1292690.
Musser N, Zalewski M, Stepp S, Lewis J. A systematic review of negative parenting practices predicting borderline personality disorder: are we measuring biosocial theory's 'invalidating environment'? Clin Psychol Rev. 2018;65:1–6.

Nelson DA, Coyne SM, Swanson SM, Hart CH, Olsen JA. Parenting, relational aggression, and borderline personality features: associations over time in a Russian longitudinal sample. Dev Psychopathol. 2014;26(3):773–87.

Neppl TK, Conger RD, Scaramella LV, Ontai LL. Intergenerational continuity in parenting behavior: mediating pathways and child effects. Dev Psychol. 2009;45(5):1241.

Newman LK, Stevenson CS, Bergman LR, Boyce P. Borderline personality disorder, mother–infant interaction and parenting perceptions: preliminary findings. Aust N Z J Psychiatry. 2007;41(7):598–605.

Newman L, Sivaratnam C, Komiti A. Attachment and early brain development–neuroprotective interventions in infant–caregiver therapy. Transl Dev Psychiatry. 2015;3(1):28647.

Newman-Morris V, Simpson K, Gray KM, Perry N, Dunlop A, Newman LK. Evaluation of early relational disturbance in high-risk populations: borderline personality disorder features, maternal mental state, and observed interaction. Infant Ment Health J. 2020;41(6):793–810.

Nicol K. Social and emotional processing in borderline personality disorder; 2014.

Oram S, Khalifeh H, Trevillion K, Feder G, Howard LM. Perpetration of intimate partner violence by people with mental illness: Siân Oram. Eur J Pub Health. 2014;24(suppl_2):cku162–047.

Perez S, Lorca F, Marco JH. Dissociation, posttraumatic stress symptoms, emotional dysregulation, and invalidating environments as correlates of NSSI in borderline personality disorder patients. J Trauma Dissociation. 2020;21(5):520–35.

Petfield L, Startup H, Droscher H, Cartwright-Hatton S. Parenting in mothers with borderline personality disorder and impact on child outcomes. Evid Based Ment Health. 2015;18(3):67–75. https://doi.org/10.1136/eb-2015-102163.

Pinquart M. Associations of parenting dimensions and styles with externalizing problems of children and adolescents: an updated meta-analysis. Dev Psychol. 2017;53(5):873–932. https://doi.org/10.1037/dev0000295.

Rasic D, Hajek T, Alda M, Uher R. Risk of mental illness in offspring of parents with schizophrenia, bipolar disorder, and major depressive disorder: a meta-analysis of family high-risk studies. Schizophr Bull. 2014;40(1):28–38.

Reupert A, Maybery D. What do we know about families where parents have a mental illness? A systematic review. Child Youth Serv. 2016;37(2):98–111.

Robin M, Douniol M, Pham-Scottez A, Gicquel L, Delvenne V, Nezelof S, Speranza M, Falissard B, Silva J, Corcos M. Specific pathways from adverse experiences to bpd in adolescence: a criteria-based approach of trauma. J Personal Disord. 2021;35(Supplement B):94–110.

Schacht JP, Anton RF, Myrick H. Functional neuroimaging studies of alcohol cue reactivity: a quantitative meta-analysis and systematic review. Addict Biol. 2013;18(1):121–33.

Schuppert HM, Albers CJ, Minderaa RB, Emmelkamp PM, Nauta MH. Severity of borderline personality symptoms in adolescence: relationship with maternal parenting stress, maternal psychopathology, and rearing styles. J Personal Disord. 2015;29(3):289–302.

Seeger K, Minderhoud PS, Peffeköver A, Vogel A, Brückner H, Kraas F, Oo NW, Brill D. Assessing land elevation in the Ayeyarwady Delta (Myanmar) and its relevance for studying sea level rise and delta flooding. Hydrol Earth Syst Sci. 2023;27(11):2257–81.

Selby EA, Braithwaite SR, Joiner TE Jr, Fincham FD. Features of borderline personality disorder, perceived childhood emotional invalidation, and dysfunction within current romantic relationships. J Fam Psychol. 2008;22(6):885.

Smith M, South S. Romantic attachment style and borderline personality pathology: a meta-analysis. Clin Psychol Rev. 2020;75:101781.

Soloff PH, Millward JW. Developmental histories of borderline patients. Compr Psychiatry. 1983;24(6):574–88.

Stagaki M, Nolte T, Feigenbaum J, King-Casas B, Lohrenz T, Fonagy P, Montague PR, Personality and Mood Disorder Research Consortium. The mediating role of attachment and mentalising in the relationship between childhood maltreatment, self-harm and suicidality. Child Abuse Negl. 2022;128:105576.

Steele KR, Townsend ML, Grenyer BF. Parenting and personality disorder: an overview and meta-synthesis of systematic reviews. PLoS One. 2019;14(10):e0223038.
Steele KR, Townsend ML, Grenyer BF. Parenting stress and competence in borderline personality disorder is associated with mental health, trauma history, attachment and reflective capacity. Bord Personal Disord Emot Dysregul. 2020;7:1–4.
Stepp SD, Whalen DJ, Pilkonis PA, Hipwell AE, Levine MD. Children of mothers with borderline personality disorder: identifying parenting behaviors as potential targets for intervention. Personal Disord. 2011;3(1):76–91. https://doi.org/10.1037/a0023081.
Suveg C, Shaffer A, Morelen D, Thomassin K. Links between maternal and child psychopathology symptoms: mediation through child emotion regulation and moderation through maternal behavior. Child Psychiatry Hum Dev. 2011;42:507–20. https://doi.org/10.1007/s10578-011-0223-8.
Sved Williams A, Hill R. The management of perinatal borderline personality disorder. J Clin Med. 2023;12(21):6850.
Taraban L, Shaw DS. Parenting in context: revisiting Belsky's classic process of parenting model in early childhood. Dev Rev. 2018;48:55–81.
Turner SM, Beidel DC, Roberson-Nay R, Tervo K. Parenting behaviors in parents with anxiety disorders. Behav Res Ther. 2003;41(5):541–54.
Van Heel M, Luyten P, De Meulemeester C, Vanwalleghem D, Vermote R, Lowyck B. Mentalizing based on external features in borderline personality disorder compared with healthy controls: the role of attachment dimensions and childhood trauma. J Personal Disord. 2019;33(6):736–50.
Van Loon LM, Van de Ven MO, Van Doesum KT, Witteman CL, Hosman CM. The relation between parental mental illness and adolescent mental health: the role of family factors. J Child Fam Stud. 2014;23:1201–14.
Van Santvoort F, Hosman CM, Janssens JM, Van Doesum KT, Reupert A, Van Loon LM. The impact of various parental mental disorders on children's diagnoses: a systematic review. Clin Child Fam Psychol Rev. 2015;18:281–99.
Vanwoerden S, Kalpakci A, Sharp C. The relations between inadequate parent-child boundaries and borderline personality disorder in adolescence. Psychiatry Res. 2017;257:462–71.
Vanwoerden S, Byrd AL, Vine V, Beeney JE, Scott LN, Stepp SD. Momentary borderline personality disorder symptoms in youth as a function of parental invalidation and youth-perceived support. J Child Psychol Psychiatry. 2022;63(2):178–86.
Vanwoerden S, McLaren V, Stepp SD, Sharp C. Are we thinking about the same disorder? A trifactor model approach to understand parents' and their adolescents' reports of borderline personality pathology. J Pers Assess. 2023;105(4):487–98.
Whalen DJ, Kiel EJ, Tull MT, Latzman RD, Gratz KL. Maternal borderline personality disorder symptoms and convergence between observed and reported infant negative emotional expressions. Personal Disord. 2015;6(3):229–38.
White H, Flanagan TJ, Martin A, Silvermann D. Mother–infant interactions in women with borderline personality disorder, major depressive disorder, their co-occurrence, and healthy controls. J Reprod Infant Psychol. 2011;29(3):223–35.
Williams LH. Thinking through death and employment: the automatic yet temporary use of schemata in everyday reasoning. Eur J Cult Stud. 2019;22(1):110–27.
Williams R, Chiesa M, Moselli M, Frattini C, Casini M, Fonagy P. The relationship between mood disorders, personality disorder and suicidality in adolescence: does general personality disturbance play a significant role in predicting suicidal behavior? Bord Personal Disord Emot Dysregul. 2023a;10(1):32.
Williams K, Fleck L, Fuchs A, Koenig J, Kaess M. Mother–child interactions in adolescents with borderline personality disorder traits and the impact of early life maltreatment. Child Adolesc Psychiatry Ment Health. 2023b;17(1):96.
Winsper C. The aetiology of borderline personality disorder (BPD): contemporary theories and putative mechanisms. Curr Opin Psychol. 2018;21:105–10.

Winsper C, Marwaha S, Lereya ST, Thompson A, Eyden J, Singh SP. Clinical and psychosocial outcomes of borderline personality disorder in childhood and adolescence: a systematic review. Psychol Med. 2015;45(11):2237–51.

Winsper C, Lereya ST, Marwaha S, Thompson A, Eyden J, Singh SP. The aetiological and psychopathological validity of borderline personality disorder in youth: a systematic review and meta-analysis. Clin Psychol Rev. 2016;44:13–24.

Wittchen HU, Jacobi F, Rehm J, Gustavsson A, Svensson M, Jönsson B, Olesen J, Allgulander C, Alonso J, Faravelli C, Fratiglioni L. The size and burden of mental disorders and other disorders of the brain in Europe 2010. Eur Neuropsychopharmacol. 2011;21(9):655–79.

Yelland C, Girke T, Tottman C, Williams AS. Clinical characteristics and mental health outcomes for women admitted to an Australian Mother-Baby Unit: a focus on borderline personality disorder and emotional dysregulation? Australas Psychiatry. 2015;23(6):683–7. https://doi.org/10.1177/1039856215590251. Epub 2015 Jun 11.

Zalewski M, Stepp SD, Scott LN, Whalen DJ, Beeney JF, Hipwell AE. Maternal borderline personality disorder symptoms and parenting of adolescent daughters. J Personal Disord. 2014;28(4):541–54.

Zalewski M, Stepp SD, Whalen DJ, Scott LN. A qualitative assessment of the parenting challenges and treatment needs of mothers with borderline personality disorder. J Psychother Integr. 2015;25(2):71–89. https://doi.org/10.1037/a0038877.

Zanarini MC. Childhood experiences associated with the development of borderline personality disorder. Psychiatr Clin N Am. 2000;23:89–101. https://doi.org/10.1016/S0193-953X(05)70145-3.

Zanarini MC, Wedig MM. Childhood adversity and the development of borderline personality disorder. In: Handbook of borderline personality disorder in children and adolescents. New York: Springer New York; 2014. p. 265–76.

Zanarini MC, Gunderson JG, Frankenburg FR, Chauncey DL. The revised diagnostic interview for borderlines: discriminating BPD from other axis II disorders. J Personal Disord. 1989;3(1):10–8.

Zanarini MC, Yong L, Frankenburg FR, Hennen J, Reich DB, Marino MF, Vujanovic AA. Severity of reported childhood sexual abuse and its relationship to severity of borderline psychopathology and psychosocial impairment among borderline inpatients. J Nerv Ment Dis. 2002;190(6):381–7.

Zhang D, Lee EK, Mak EC, Ho CY, Wong SY. Mindfulness-based interventions: an overall review. Br Med Bull. 2021;138(1):41–57.

Chapter 4
Childhood Maltreatment and Borderline Personality Disorder

Introduction

A child is a human being with his/her own personality characteristics and perceptions. Childhood is a risky and quickly moving phase of human development in all cognitive, emotional, behavioral, and social facets. Every aspect of the child, including physical and psychological, needs to be accepted, validated, noticed, nurtured, and cherished by the child's major caregiver or parents. Irreverence, hostility, or violence toward the value of these fundamental aspects of a child's psychosocial being can often be represented by the categories of childhood maltreatment and neglect (Barnet et al. 1999; Fayaz 2019). Adverse childhood experiences (ACEs) are described as experiencing repeatedly notorious experiences that are manifested by a deviation from the expected environment and require adaptation (Antoniou et al. 2023; Turecki et al. 2014; Merrick et al. 2020a), encompassing physical, sexual, and emotional abuse, parallel illness, criminality, violence, neglect, and poverty (Antoniou et al. 2023; Turecki et al. 2014; Merrick et al. 2020b; McLaughlin et al. 2015; Kruger et al. 2018). The construct of ACEs includes potentially traumatic negative experiences and events that happen in childhood and adolescence under 18 years of age (Crouch et al. 2019; Tzouvara et al. 2023) and consists of experiencing violence; physical, emotional, and sexual abuse or neglect, and household dysfunctions such as be the witness of severe and repeated domestic violence; and having a family member with various types of dangerous behaviors and attempt or die by suicide (Burgin and Daniel 2024). Furthermore, ACEs are composed of different aspects of the environments where the child engaged should be provided with a sense of safety, stability, and bonding, but that instead include various forms of difficulties such as substance misuse, mental health issues, or instability because of parental separation or legal issues such as incarceration of a parent, sibling, or other member of the household. Adverse childhood experiences can be emotionally distressing and contribute to long-term negative effects over lifespan (Division of

E. A. Selby, M. Salavati, *Theories of Borderline Personality Disorder*,
https://doi.org/10.1007/978-3-031-75503-3_4

Violence Prevention National Center for Injury Prevention and Control, CDC 2019). An expanded range of individuals, family, and community elements can influence a child's likelihood of experiencing ACEs, for instance, living in a house with an unstable situation, having parents with a history of experiencing ACEs, and or experiencing several social and environmental dysfunctions during childhood and adolescence (CDC 2021; Trygg et al. 2021; Hargreaves et al. 2019; Walsh et al. 2019). Various terminologies have been used for "ACEs" by writers for centuries dating back, such as "battered child syndrome" (Kempe 1962), which increased stronger interest and concern for this hidden harmful matter. Between 1963 and 1967, the obligatory child abuse reporting regulation was passed in every state in the United States. In addition, the term "child abuse" was added to the MEDLINE system, with 12 categorized articles under this keyword, expanding to 600 articles in 2006 (Jenny 2010; Brewer-Smyth 2022). ACEs are highly prevalent (Bellis et al. 2019; Kessler et al. 2017; Bürgin et al. 2023; Brewer-Smyth 2022) and negatively influence individuals' physical and psychological well-being and interpersonal and social functioning (Tzouvara et al. 2023; Antoniou et al. 2023; Tzouvara et al. 2023) and revictimization as well (Gama et al. 2021; Brewer-Smyth 2022). Moreover, ACEs are related to epigenetic age acceleration (EAA) (Wolf et al. 2018), due to its association with poor health (Janusek et al. 2017). ACEs not only can lead to intensifying the risk of long-term consequences for society (Burgin and Daniel 2024; Heck et al. 2024; Hughes et al. 2021; Bellis et al. 2019; Brewer-Smyth 2022), but also can highly lead to health-risk issues (Lovis-Schmidt et al. 2022; Ross et al. 2020), such as chronic pain (Burke et al. 2017), heightened risk factor for fibromyalgia in later life (Low and Schweinhardt 2012), and poor immune system (Gill et al. 2020), as well as including mental health problems, major disease, diseases of aging, even, and premature mortality (Bellis et al. 2019; Clemens et al. 2021; Hughes et al. 2021; Sahle et al. 2021; Johnson et al. 2022; Burgin and Daniel 2024; Elovainio et al. 2012; Mathur et al. 2018; Schneider et al. 2020). In line with the majority of clinical and empirical consensus, one of the most prominent factors in the development of mental problems is composed of the experience of early childhood adversity and the experience of chronic and uncontrollable stressful events (e.g., Shonkoff et al. 2012; Ehrlich et al. 2016). Adverse childhood experiences are assumed to be potentially traumatic experiences that occurred before the age of 18. Adverse childhood experiences are considered as extremely severe and traumatic experiences composed of experiencing violence, child abuse and neglect, domestic violence and several forms of intense household dysfunctions such as domestic violence, alcohol/substance abuse, different types of community and collective violence, witnessing violence in the home or community, or having a suicidal family member who attempts frequently or died by suicide (WHO 2012; Redfield 2019; Matjasko et al. 2022). Ongoing studies are important to clarify the major risk and protective factors involved in adverse childhood experiences and explore the negative outcomes that children are exposed to during these adverse events (Matjasko et al. 2022).

Despite broad consensus that childhood adversity is a substantial societal issue, a long history of disagreement among investigators, lawmakers, and clinicians exists as to what exactly constitutes childhood adversity and maltreatment.

Experiences of childhood maltreatment, child abuse, and neglect are a pervasive public physical and psychological health adversity associated with serious cognitive, psychological, emotional, and behavioral problems (Toth and Manly 2019; Amédée 2020; Hughes et al. 2017, 2020a) and are associated with morbidity, mortality, and various forms of psychopathology across lifespan (Gruhn and Compas 2020; Norman 2017; Hughes et al. 2017). Child abuse is a severe and pervasive issue around the world, with child physical abuse reported as 22–25% and sexual abuse as 8% of men and 18% of women (Stoltenborgh et al. 2011, 2013). In comparison to other types of traumatic and neglective life experiences, it has been revealed that childhood maltreatment and abuse can have the greatest potential impact throughout the lifespan for psychological, emotional, developmental, and behavioral matters. This is due to the destructive impact of the abusive acts, as well as the potential concomitant interference with all aspects of cognitive and mental development (Tanaka et al. 2015; Veitch Wolfe and Kelly 2018). Childhood maltreatment is a globally widespread mental and physical health matter affecting a substantial range of children worldwide (Chamberlain et al. 2019a, b; Khoury et al. 2022) and has a detrimental impact on the lives of millions of children and adolescents (Gama et al. 2021). Investigations have documented that childhood maltreatment contributes to the development of various mental health difficulties in the victims of abuse (Reyes et al. 2019a, b, 2024; Bellis et al. 2019), and among several identified risk factors, the most influential component is exposure to detrimental childhood experience composed of emotional, physical, and sexual abuse (Mainali et al. 2020).

Based on the Centers for Disease Control and Prevention (CDC; Leeb 2008), childhood maltreatment is "any kind of act or series of acts of commission or omission by a parent or caregiver that leads to harm, potential for harm, or threat of harm to a child," and includes neglect, physical and sexual abuse, and emotional and psychological maltreatment, irrespective of intent (Veitch Wolfe and Kelly 2019). Childhood maltreatment and neglect is a substantial public health (Matjasko et al. 2022), physically and mentally, that influences millions of children and families every year (Swenson and Schaeffer 2018). Childhood maltreatment has become a major concern in the scientific associations (Almeida et al. 2023). According to the CDC (2012), childhood adversity contributes to elevated risk for developing short-term and long-term negative physical and psychological consequences (CDC 2012). Childhood maltreatment is the most significant childhood adversity which has the most considerable pathogenic influence on mental health of adolescence and adulthood (McLaughlin et al. 2012; Bellis et al. 2019) and is associated with different mental problems in adulthood (e.g., Wu et al. 2022, 2023a, b; Baldwin et al. 2019; Gruhn and Compas 2020). Based on United Nations Convention on the Rights of the Child (UNCRC), any person under the age of 18 is considered a child. In line with available figures in 2013, nearly 3.9 million children were identified as the victims of child abuse or neglect in the USA (Jaffee 2017). Child abuse is a public issue considered as a major concern in mental health settings, which according to some estimates results in five to six children dying due to frequent domestic violence, physical maltreatment, sexual trauma, or neglect (Oswald et al. 2010, 2014).

Childhood maltreatment occurs in all ages, and based on reports, 27% of victims are younger than three years and 20% are aged three or four years (Mainali et al. 2020). Approximately, 7.5 million children have been reported as victims of childhood maltreatment in the USA annually, including 74.9% victims of neglect, 18.3% victims of physically abused, 8.6% sexually abused, and 7.1% of emotionally psychologically maltreatment (Mainali et al. 2020). Through systematic reviews and meta-analyses of self-report studies, rates of 12.7% for sexual abuse, 22.6% for physical abuse, 36.6% for emotional abuse, 16.3% for physical neglect, and 18.4% for emotional neglect have been illustrated (Mehta et al. 2021; Stoltenborgh et al. 2015).

Childhood Adversity and Maltreatment

The definition of childhood maltreatment is crucial to understand in terms of its characteristics, prevalence, incidence, and consequences, as well as for planning and interventions to prevent it. Based on the scientific literature, the definition of childhood maltreatment has been considered in a broad spectrum from active "acts of commission" to passive "acts of omission". The active is usually named "*child abuse*" and passive is called "*child neglect*" (Laajasalo et al. 2023). Childhood trauma is any kind of maltreatment, abuse, or neglect that contributes to physical, emotional, and sexual hurt for a child (You et al. 2022; Norman 2017). In line with a growing body of investigations, childhood trauma impacts the progress of child's emotional, cognitive, social, and behavioral abilities, as well as physical growth can be affected by this unbearable psychological and social issue throughout childhood and later life (Cicchetti 2016; Mello et al. 2009; You et al. 2022). Childhood maltreatment and early life adversity create biological, neurobiological, and psychological problems in children and adolescents which lead to negative adulthood outcomes, such as disturbed mental and physical health (Mersky et al. 2017; Jones et al. 2018), depression (Mansueto et al. 2021; Klumparendt et al. 2019), higher levels of dysfunctions in all aspects of life, such as lower-level occupations (Metzler et al. 2017; Liu et al. 2021; Wang et al. 2022), and greater rates of crime victimization (Ports et al. 2016; Cheng et al. 2022). Child abuse and childhood adversity are serious mental health problems, which contribute to severe short-term and long-term destructive impacts on physical and mental health, opportunity, and well-being later in life (National Center for Injury Prevention and Control 2022; Abbott and Slack 2021; D'arcy-Bewick et al. 2022). Based on mythological advances and empirical investigations, childhood maltreatment has been categorized to four groups, including *physical abuse*, *sexual abuse*, *neglect*, and *emotional maltreatment* (Wolfe and Kelly 2019), and other *exploitation* (Palusci 2022; The United Convention on the Rights of the Child, CRC 1989; Tobin and Cashmore 2020).

Physical Abuse Regarding clinical report and experimental data, physical abuse is defined as any actual or potential physical harm caused by an interaction or lack of an interaction, which is notably in the field of parental or caregiver's control, responsibility, or power (WHO 1999; Palusci 2022). Any kind of intentional physical injury to a child, which involves a broad range from minor buries to severe fracture or death due to doing destructive and forbidden acts against a child, such as punching, beating, kicking, throwing, burning, and so on, which are done by caregiver, parents, or others who have responsibility for the child has been defined as physical abuse (APA, DSM-5-TR 2022). As mentioned, the definitions of child abuse, including all types of this issue, are influenced by cultural-contextual considerations. For instance, in some countries, slapping or canning is a common method of physical punishment. Physical abuse refers to observable physical harm; otherwise, is considered as physical chastisement. Physical abuse can be happened in conjunction with other forms of abuse, especially sexual abuse, or can be intrafamilial or institutional (Carr et al. 2020).

Sexual Abuse Sexual abuse is considered as a severe physical and psychological toxic experience for a child. There are several forms of sexual abuse, consisting of "sexual exploitation refers to the use of individuals for profit such as pornography", "sexual violence refers to the violent aspects of specific sexual acts", and "incest refers to intrafamilial abuse" (Rey-Salmon et al. 2020). Sexual abuse has been defined as any physical contact with a child for sexual purposes without (or even with) the child's meaningful consent; in such cases, the perpetrator effectively takes ownership of the child's body (Cloitre et al. 2020). Based on DSM-5-TR (2022), sexual abuse encompasses any type of sexual behavior composing of a child who is the object to provide sexual satisfaction and gratification to a caregiver, parent, or others who have responsibility for the child (APA, DSM-5-TR 2022). "Sexual abuse includes activities such as fondling a child's genitals, penetration, incest, rape, sodomy, and indecent exposure, noncontact exploitation of a child by a parent or caregiver- for example, forcing, tricking, enticing, threatening, or pressuring a child to participate in acts for the sexual gratification of others, without direct physical contact between child and abuser" (APA, DSM-5-TR 2022, p.992). The documented role of child trauma in the development of BPD is well established, and research has shown that among all traumas, sexual trauma plays a significant, severe role in the development of BPD and is the type of abuse most related to developing a BPD diagnosis in adulthood (e.g., Dadomo et al. 2022).

Child psychological abuse/emotional maltreatment includes using inappropriate behaviors in a way that destroys a child's emotional/ psychological development, sense of worth, self-esteem, and sense of identity by parent or caregivers (Fayaz 2019). Based on DSM-5-TR (2022), child psychological abuse consists of "berating, disparaging, or humiliating the child; threatening, harming/abandoning; confining the child; egregious scapegoating of the child; coercing the child to inflict Pin on himself or herself; and disciplining the child excessively through physical or nonphysical means" (DSM-5-TR 2022, p.994). Emotional maltreatment is defined as pervasive and extreme frustrating of child's basic emotional needs (White et al. 1993) which is considered as a "pathogenic relational experience" (Cicchetti and Toth 2016) with a lack of emotional satisfaction of child's emotional demand due to the absence of efficient caregivers (White et al. 2015). Emotional maltreatment or psychological abuse is often a hidden subtype of childhood maltreatment, which can be difficult to define and detect (Baker and Brassard 2019; Hart et al. 2017); there is also a great tendency to underestimate emotional maltreatment in caregiver and mental health reports (Baker et al. 2021). Furthermore, there are several issues regarding the patterns of clinically associated diagnostic results of emotional maltreatment and also being age-dependent (Cicchetti and Toth 2016; Schlensog-Schuster et al. 2024).

Neglect and Childhood Deprivation Presenting an exact definition for neglect is difficult, especially one that does not result in misspecification, especially in family poverty situation. Neglect has been defined as any established or doubtful visible acts or elimination by a child's parent or other caregiver which contribute to depriving the child's age-associated basic needs, and therefore, contribute to physical or psychological harm. According to the WHO, neglect is defined as the failure of a parent to provide child's need including emotional development, health, education, nutrition, shelter, and security and safety, where he/she is responsible for (Balençon et al. 2018). Based on DSM-5-TR (2022), child neglect includes abandonment, deprivation from suitable supervision and vital education, lack of parental attention to emotional and psychological needs, and failure to provide basic physical-somatic needs such as medical care, nutrition, shelter, and clothing (APA, DSM-5-TR). Neglect can be categorized as physical neglect, medical neglect, educational neglect, and emotional neglect (Fayaz 2019).

The Association Between Childhood Maltreatment and Development of Borderline Personality Disorder

Borderline personality disorder (BPD) is a remarkably prevalent personality disorder among clinical and community samples emerging by late adolescence and early adolescence (DSM-5-TR 2023; Martín-Blanco et al. 2017; Gunderson et al. 2018; Baptista et al. 2023). BPD consists of a wide range of symptoms including emotional instability, chaotic interpersonal relationships, fear of abandonment, emotion dysregulation, chronic dysphoria or depression, and feeling of emptiness (DSM-5-TR 2023) accompanying with behavioral disturbances, impaired psychological functions, emotional instability (Dadomo et al. 2016, 2018, 2020), problematic interpersonal relationships and self-image issues (De Panfilis et al. 2019; Lieb et al. 2004), self-inflicted self-injury (e.g., Gibson K, Morgan 2013; Morgan et al. 2022) and suicide attempts (Aouidad et al. 2020), and other self-destructive behaviors, substance use (e.g., Kaufman et al. 2020), sexual risk-taking (e.g., Brüne et al. 2017; Sansone and Sansone 2011), impulsiveness (e.g., Crowell et al. 2009;

Mortensen et al. 2010; Lapomarda et al. 2021), and strong feelings of severely deep inadequacy, dissociative experiences (Zanarini et al. 1999; Koenigsberg et al. 2002; Bateman et al. 2023). Personality development is influenced by early-life experiences and adverse childhood experiences (Congdon et al. 2012; Reyes et al. 2019a, b, 2023), such as high tendency toward self-criticism and self-blame (Baetens et al. 2015), lower self-esteem, and high levels of impulsivity and aggression (Di Pierro et al. 2012). Furthermore, adverse childhood experiences can lead to the development of problematic and pathological personality traits and various types of personality disorders. Specific categories of adverse childhood experiences, composed of physical abuse, sexual abuse, emotional neglect, and verbal abuse, are associated to escalated risk for pathologic personality traits and personality (Nederlof et al. 2010a, b; Zhang et al. 2021). Moreover, punishment and guilt are prevalent and unwanted emotions among victims of childhood maltreatment and abuse are considered as mediators that lead to nonsuicidal self-injury (NSSI) in abused individuals (Glassman et al. 2007).

A history of emotional abuse, physical abuse, sexual abuse, and neglect in childhood has shown substantial associations with BPD (Stepp et al. 2016a, b). A body of research has emphasized on the maliciously pervasive role of childhood adversities and negative experiences, especially child abuse and maltreatment in the development of BPD, as well as based on a growing number of experimental and clinical studies, it has been documented that these aversive and traumatic experiences cause profound and burdensome consequences resulting in the development of a wide range of psychiatric disorders and personality disorders, especially BPD (See e.g., Turner et al. 2020, 2018; Afifi and MacMilan 2011; Crowell et al. 2013; Selby and Yen 2014; Gratz et al. 2017, 2019, 2022; Zanarini and Wedig 2014; Chamberlain et al. 2019a, b). In compliance with diathesis-stress theories of BPD (Battle et al. 2004), inherited vulnerability, especially temperament and genetic polymorphisms, and adverse traumatic experiences, specifically child abuse and neglect, have a synergic role to develop BP pathology. The body of work has shown that child maltreatment and different types of child abuse can contribute to the development of BPD (see e.g., Fruzzetti et al. 2005; Grove and Crowell 2019, Jaffee 2017; Zanarini and Wedig 2014; Gratz et al. 2011; Bornovalva et al. 2013; Zanarini et al. 1989). Emotionally invalidating environment, in which child's inner emotional experiences are responded by parents via ignoring, punishing, dismissed, and regarded (Elzy et al. 2013; Linehan 1993), contextual risk factors especially child maltreatment and abuse (Grove and Crowell 2019; Gratz et al. 2011; Bornovalva et al. 2013), and sociocultural invalidation (Grove and Crowell 2019) are different types of invalidating environments where caregivers have the most significant roles.

In addressing the issue of childhood adversity, Crowell et al. (2022) noted that there are numerous invalidating environments described in BPD cases. Crowell et al. (2022) posit "at one extreme, clients describe chronic abuse, neglect, sexual exploitation, loss of a parent, exposure to substance use, caregiver instability, or other negative experiences that severely compromised their upbringing. At another extreme, many clients describe a stable and fairly typical upbringing, ye one where they always felt inadequate, out place, or like the "problem child" in the family"."

Focusing on this issue further, Crowell et al. (2022) explored several BPD case reports of invalidating environment outside of their family, for instance, bullying and being physically annoyed at school, sexual assault by peers or trusted individuals, being under emotional abuse such as rejection and ridicule, and even in some cases experiencing trauma (Crowell et al. 2022).

In line with theories of invalidating environment, the overlapping factors that combined the other environmental and biological components lead to the genesis of BPD, and the role of cumulative influences of traumatic experiences exacerbates the severity of borderline personality features (Hecht et al. 2014; Winsper et al. 2012; Ibrahim et al. 2018; Bozzatello et al. 2021). Childhood adversity and maltreatment is a transdiagnostic risk factor for psychiatric disorders (Struck et al. 2020a, b; Bellis et al. 2019), has a considerable generalized role in the development of personality disorders (Afifi and MacMilan 2011; Battle et al. 2004; Bellis et al. 2019), and BPD in particular (Quenneville et al. 2020; Wota et al. 2014). Intrapsychic factors comprising temperamental characteristics and personality traits in childhood and adolescence have been considered as main contributing components for the development of BPD. In keeping with general consensus, temperamental vulnerabilities, encompassing affective instability, negative affectivity, negative emotionality, inappropriate anger, poor emotional control, impulsivity, and aggression, combined with traumatic adverse childhood experiences, have a major role in the development of borderline pathology (Bozzatello et al. 2019; Linehan 1993; Belsky et al. 2012; Hecht et al. 2014; Cloninger et al. 1993). Among environmental factors, the most substantial factors identified as predisposing condition for early BPD involved familial maltreatment and parent-child conflicting relationship (Bozzatello et al. 2021). Through a longitudinal study using a discordant twin design and biometric modeling, Bornovalova et al. (2013) examined the causal relationship between childhood maltreatment (sexual, emotional, and physical abuse) before age 18 and BPD traits at age 24, as well as the mediating and moderating influences of symptoms of childhood externalizing and internalizing disorders on the association between child abuse and BPD traits. The results of discordant twin analyses and biometric modeling revealed little to no evidence that is consistent with a causal impact of childhood maltreatment on BPD traits. In turn, pursuant to the findings, it was found that the association between childhood abuse and BPD traits originates from common genetic effects and showed an overlap with externalizing and internalizing disorders as well (Bornovalova et al. 2013).

In line with experimental and clinical studies, it has been documented that among people with a history of childhood maltreatment and abuse, various forms of mental health issues incline to emerge earlier with notably greater severity, escalated rate of comorbidity, and lower desirable responses to pharmaceutical and psychological treatment in comparison with non-maltreated individuals (Alvarez-Tomás et al. 2017; Gruhn and Compas 2020). In line with Redfield (2019), negative general and mental health consequences are associated with aversive childhood experiences and childhood maltreatment, including injury, mental health difficulties, chronic diseases, and risky behaviors (Redfield 2019). Several recent studies have highlighted the immediate risk of psychological difficulties and psychiatric disorders following maltreatment in early childhood (e.g., Winter et al. 2022); some work has emphasized on delayed effects (Anderson et al. 2016), as well as severe influences of maltreatment during adolescence (e.g., Thornberry et al. 2010). Adverse childhood experiences and childhood maltreatment lead to increasing proneness to suffering from various types of physical and mental health issues (Reyes et al. 2019a, b, 2024; Lee and Choi 2023; Turner et al. 2021, 2018), and both clinical and community samples confirm the role of adverse childhood experiences in the etiology of psychiatric disorders and mental issues (Wu et al. 2022, 2023a, b; Marshall et al. 2020; Vial et al. 2021), such as *interpersonal and intimate relationships* (Krause-Utz et al. 2021a, b), *anxiety and mood disorders* (Fletcher et al. 2014; Widom et al. 2018; Stapp et al. 2020; Raposo et al. 2014; Wu et al. 2022, 2023a, b; Norman 2017; Steine et al. 2020), *PTSD* and *CPTSD* (Haj-Yahia et al. 2021; Kaess et al. 2013; Kolthof et al. 2022; Ford and Courtois 2021; Lee and Choi 2023; Cloitre et al. 2014), *depressive episodes and major depressive disorder* (Kealy et al. 2020; Struck et al. 2020a, b; Abbott and Slack 2021; Baetens et al. 2015; Gardner et al. 2019; Steine et al. 2020; Antoniou et al. 2023), *chronic pain* (Antoniou et al. 2023), *loneliness* (Wong et al. 2020; Narita et al. 2020; Hyland et al. 2019), *hopelessness* (Coutney et al. 2008; Klonsky et al. 2013; FrankLin et al. 2017, 2022; Franklin and Smeaton 2018; Berardelli et al. 2019), *attention deficit hyperactivity disorder* (Humphreys et al. 2020; Clayton et al. 2018), *psychosis* (Wu et al. 2022, 2023a, b; Narita et al. 2020; Huang et al. 2019), *substance and alcohol disorders* (Douglas et al. 2010; Norman 2017), *personality disorders* (Tyrka et al. 2009; Waxman et al. 2014; Wu et al. 2022, 2023a, b), *borderline personality disorder* (Pietrek et al. 2013; Herzog et al. 2022; Lee and Choi 2023; Ibrahim et al. 2018; Porter et al. 2020), *self-destructive risky behaviors and impulsivity* (Widom et al. 2018; Zhang et al. 2021), such as *suicidal ideation* (Prokopez et al. 2020; Agnew and Danese 2016), *suicidal behaviors* (Norman 2017; Dube et al. 2001; Stagaki et al. 2022; Xei et al. 2018; Wan et al. 2019; Forester et al. 2020), *deliberate nonsuicidal self-harm* (Liu et al. 2018; kaess et al. 2013; Bunting et al. 2023; Xu Peh et al. 2017; Muehlenkamp et al. 2010, 2017, 2023; Stagaki et al. 2022; Franzke et al. 2015; Forester and McKibbon 2020), *early smoking initiation* (Edwards et al. 2007), *Alcohol use* (Turniansky et al. 2019), *sleep difficulties* (Beilharz et al. 2020), *dissociative symptoms* (Ford and Gómez 2015; Mueller-Pfeiffer et al. 2013), and *internalizing/externalizing behaviors* (Geselowitz et al. 2021; Bornovalova et al. 2013).

Exposure to childhood maltreatment may result in deficiency in emotion regulation skills and socio-emotional competencies (Trickett et al. 2011; Steenkamp et al. 2022), the development of negative self-perceptions of being inadequate, undeserving of care and deserving to be punished, and feelings of self-loathing, helplessness, and shame (Lange and Sharma-Patel 2011). According to cumulative risk models, repeated and constant exposure to aversive stressful experiences among children and adolescents, such as childhood maltreatment, predicts different forms of mental health disorders in adulthood (Appleyard et al. 2005), especially experiencing childhood adversities may lead to the insufficient adaptive strategies to cope with stressful life events resulting in potentially amplified risk for the development of several mental disorders (Compas et al. 2017). In line with a growing body of research, adverse childhood experiences and severely traumatic childhood experiences can result in problematic emotion regulation strategies (Krause-Utz et al. 2022) and deficiencies in adaptive coping strategies and consciously volitional efforts to regulate emotion, cognition, physiological, and the environmental response to stress (Compas et al. 2001). In other words, the accumulation of aversive stressful experiences is associated with alteration of the course of adjustment with stress over time (Gruhn and Compas 2020). Emotion regulation refers to broad efforts to impact which emotions a person has and how the person experiences or expresses these emotions (Gross 1998a, b, 2013, 2015, 2019, 2024). Emotion regulation is defined as the process by which individuals impact the occurrence, duration, nature, experience, and expression of their emotion (Gross 2013). Traumatic life experiences raise the development of BPD, because early traumas take action as triggers for the formation of several BPD characteristics including affect instability, emotion dysregulation, and self-destructive behaviors (Herzog and Schmahl 2018). Children who experience different forms of adverse childhood experiences display problematic alterations in emotional expression and emotional awareness, as well as a strong tendency toward using various types of maladaptive emotion regulation strategies (McLaughlin et al. 2017; Reyes et al. 2019a, b, 2024) and impairment in the ability of mentalizing and symbolizing emotions (Gabbard 2017; Gunderson 2009) later in their life. Geselowitz et al. (2021) proposed that adverse childhood experiences encompassing child emotional and physical abuse, parental psychiatric disorders, and being exposed to poverty in childhood can be a significant predictor of BPD symptoms in 14–19-year-old participants, even after excluding the effects of parental mental illness and parental childhood poverty (Geselowitz et al. 2021). Based on experimental studies, an association between childhood emotional abuse and neglect and difficulties in emotion regulation impact the relationship between emotional abuse and acute symptomatology in BPD (Carvalho Fernando et al. 2014; Linehan 1993). It has been found that individuals with a history of childhood maltreatment tend to display high levels of emotional/affective lability and against law behaviors (Almeida et al. 2023). However, coping includes only controlled effortful processes which cover a wider array of goal-directed regulatory endeavors, whereas emotion regulation encompasses both controlled and automatic processes which concentrate on the purpose of altering individual's own emotional experience; adverse childhood experiences lead to insufficient coping and maladaptive emotion regulation efforts as well. As indicated by a meta-analytic review, it was indicated that maltreatment is widely related to poor emotion regulation as well as intensified avoidance, emotional suppression, and expression of negative emotions in response to stress (Gruhn and Compas 2020). Yuan et al. (2023) identified a significant association between emotional abuse and high BPD features. In addition, with data collected for a longitudinal study, they demonstrated that emotional abuse mediated the path from trauma to BPD characteristics (Yuan et al. 2023).

Emotional working memory (EWM) refers to the ability to apply working memory in emotional contexts such as during emotional distraction and is considered as a crucial component for coping with emotionally distressing information (Koch Koch and Jones 2018), cognitive emotion regulation (Krause-Utz et al. 2022), and shifting attention away from aversive material while concentrating on goal-directed tasks (Schweizer et al. 2019). Moreover, in previous empirical studies, it has been documented that high-frequency heart rate variability (HF-HRV) has an important role in the flexible adaptation to stressful environmental demands, comprising emotion regulation (Shaffer and Ginsberg 2017). Krause-Utz et al. (2022) studied reaction times (RTs) as well as HF-HRV during an emotional working memory task (EWMT) in association with the severity of childhood maltreatment and comorbid for PTSD in BPD among 53 BPD patients and 28 health controls. To compare with healthy control, the BPD patients demonstrated prolonged RTs across all distractor situations with social cues, regardless with emotional valence. In addition, the findings indicated that BPD patients, especially those comorbid with PTSD, revealed decreased HF-HRV both at rest and during EWMT. Finally, in compliance with the results, longer RTs and lower HF-HRV during the EWMT were predicted by the severity of childhood maltreatment (Krause-Utz et al. 2022). Consistent with documented studies, dissociative symptoms including depersonalization and derealization are common consequences of child sexual abuse (Vonderlin et al. 2018), leading to increasing vulnerability for sexual revictimization (Hébert et al. 2020) because of leading to impaired encoding and processing of threat-related information (Lanius et al. 2010; Spiegel et al. 2011). Through a cross-sectional anonymous online survey, Krause-Utz et al. (2021a, b) investigated whether BPD features, dissociation, and maladaptive cognitive emotion regulation can be considered as a mediator for the link between self-reported child sexual abuse (CSA) and sexual intimate partner violence (IPV) among 100 CSA participants and 345 cases with at least one incidence of sexual IPV. According to the results, more severe CSA, more severe BPD features, higher dissociation, and more maladaptive predicted adult sexual IPV. In the separated model, each mediator variable indicated a substantial influence, while in the overall model, only dissociation and maladaptive emotion regulation mediated the relationship between CSA and sexual IPV with no association with BPD features (Krause-Utz et al. 2021a, b). Temes et al. (2020) examined the overall severity of sexual abuse among 104 inpatients adolescents with BPD and 290 adult inpatients with BPD to explore specific parameters of abusive experiences. Higher scores on an index of sexual abuse severity were reported in adults compared to adolescents, as well as higher proportion of adults reported more severe rang. In addition, adults with BPD revealed higher reports of experiencing sexual abuse occurred at multiple developmental stages, frequently in a longer duration, and were more often perpetrated by a parent (Temes et al. 2020).

In line with empirical investigation about autobiographical memories, the subjective recollections of experienced events that make up the building blocks of our personal life-narratives (Bertolote and De Leo 2012) have demonstrated incoherent autobiographical narratives in patients diagnosed BPD because of insecure attachment (Soloff et al. 2002), while it has not been explored whether incoherent autobiographical narratives in individuals with BPD are coupled to experiences of childhood adversities. Bendstrup et al. (2021) examined whether written autobiographical memories among 26 females diagnosed with BPD and 28 health female control participants had decreased narrative coherence, as well as whether greater rate of incoherent narratives was related with childhood adversities. The findings indicated that the autobiographical memories were reduced among BPD participants, especially inadequate orientation about the narrative and lack of narrative structure. In addition, the results showed lower orientation among participants with a history of child abuse and lowered narrative structure related to child abuse in BPD group (Bendstrup et al. 2021). The majority of extant literature on BPD concentrated on the course, consequences, etiology, and psychopathology of this disorder among adult population, while the emergence of BPD features and pathology in childhood has been paid less attention (Gratz et al. 2011). During past decades, several studies have been focused on the development of BP pathology and related factors among children (e.g., Fonagy et al. 2015; Zanarini et al. 2010, 2006, 2008; Hawton et al. 2012; Muehlenkamp et al. 2012; Hessels et al. 2018, 2022; Seon You et al. 2022; Baptista et al. 2023). Childhood maltreatment contributes to the development of negative emotional reactivity in children which can be considered as a marker of vulnerability leading to increasing the risk for the development of BPD (Stepp et al. 2015). Pursuant to several studies, experiencing childhood maltreatment results in negative outcomes later in life (Cheng and Langevin 2023). These dysfunctional changes in emotional processing contribute to the development of an association between adverse childhood experiences and later internalizing psychopathologies (McLaughlin et al. 2009), besides a relationship between the development of psychiatric disorders in childhood, adolescence, and adulthood (McLaughlin et al. 2012; Green et al. 2010; Reyes et al. 2019a, b, 2024). Some children indicate short-term pathologic symptoms, while others suffer from severe emotional problems and maladaptive behaviors over time throughout their life course, for whom formal interventions are required (Swenson and Schaeffer 2018). Stagaki et al. (2022) indicated that childhood maltreatment was directly related to the development of nonsuicidal self-harm and suicidal behaviors. In their findings, insecure attachment and impaired mentalizing relatively can potentially explain the relations between childhood maltreatment, self-inflicted injury, and suicidality (Stagaki et al. 2022). Experiencing childhood maltreatment is identified to be a predominant risk factor for self-inflicted injuries (e.g., Ford and Gómez 2015; Gratz 2003; Hawton et al. 2012; Lang and Sharma-Patel 2011), as well as, a significant association between nonsuicidal self-harm and childhood sexual, physical, and emotional abuse and neglect has been revealed especially among adolescents (e.g., Madge et al. 2011; Muehlenkamp et al. 2010, 2017; Muehlenkamp and Tillotson 2023; Wan et al. 2015; Layne et al. 2014). In line with a body of studies, it has been demonstrated that emotion dysregulation can mediate the association between interpersonal issues (with family and peers) and adolescents' nonsuicidal self-harm (e.g., Adrian et al. 2011), while, according to empirical studies, distress intolerance, impulsivity, self-criticism, and alexithymia have been indicated to mediate the relation between adverse childhood exposure and NSSH (e.g., Arens et al. 2014; Swannell et al. 2012). Through a cross-sectional study, Xu Peh et al. (2017) investigated the mediator's role of emotion dysregulation as an underlying mechanism, examining it in the pathway from childhood maltreatment exposure to adolescence self-harm behaviors. In keeping with the results, exposure to adverse childhood experiences can be considered as a distal associative factor for nonsuicidal self-harm among adolescents. This study suggested that self-injurious behaviors can be assumed as maladaptive endeavors to deal with emotion dysregulation caused by experiencing childhood maltreatment (Xu Peh et al. 2017).

The role of adverse childhood experiences in the etiology and development of BPD has not been fully developed yet, because there are several putative and highly intercorrelated risk factors such as childhood maltreatment, parental bonding issues, and chaotic familial context, which may contribute to the development of BPD. Despite the significance of these intercorrelated risk factors in the development of BPD in adolescence, less attention has been paid in the literature to highly correlated ADEs with current relationships (Hessels et al. 2018, 2022). A growing number of clinical and experimental investigations have indicated the substantial role of childhood adversity in the development of BPD (e.g., Quenneville et al. 2020; Brakemeier et al. 2018; Carlson et al. 2009; Kleindienst et al. 2020; Poter et al. 2020; Scheffers et al. 2020; Krause-Utz et al. 2022). Various etiological risk factors may contribute to developing BPD, and these sets of risk factors can be highly intercorrelated (Hessels et al. 2018, 2022). Elliott et al. (2016) demonstrated that early biological and neurological stressors contribute to DNA methylation which leading to the damage of normal brain functioning, interpersonal skills, cognitive functions, and other crucial skills that can appear similar to BPD deficits (Elliot et al. 2016). Various prominent epigenetic and neuro-morphological alterations due to child trauma are observed with childhood maltreatment, leading to the development of BPD, along with the influence and severity on both sexes (Mainali et al. 2020). In spite of the prominent role of genetic vulnerability in BPD, it cannot be claimed that genetics are the only factors contributing to BPD; it has been documented that genetic factors have little impact on the development of BPD in an appropriate environment with no harmful and risk factors, which provide the importance of individually unique environmental factors (Skoglund et al. 2021; Herzog et al. 2022). A considerable experimental and clinical investigations have revealed that a large number of BPD patients have reports of experiencing childhood mistreatment across their life (Pietrek et al. 2013; Tyrka et al. 2009; Zanarini et al. 2015; Lobbestael and Arntz (2010); Zanarini 1997; Temes et al. 2017; Mainali et al. 2020), and it has been indicated that patients with BPD were over 13 times more likely to report childhood maltreatment than nonclinical controls and other psychiatric clinical populations (Kleindienst et al. 2020; Porter et al. 2020; Herzog et al. 2022). Wu et al. (2022) reported that patients with BPD indicate intense clinical profiles, such as the comorbidity of personality disorders, as well as they display greater levels of childhood maltreatment than other types of personality disorders. Furthermore, it was shown that the higher levels of emotional neglect and emotional abuse were significantly associated with BPD; it indicated that, consistent with previous studies, physical and emotional neglect are two factors which distinguished BPD from other types of personality disorders (Wu et al. 2022, 2023a, b). Gratz et al. (2012) studied the interrelation among two borderline personality-relevant traits including affective dysfunction and impulsivity, borderline personality-relevant environmental stressors (e.g., emotional abuse), and childhood features in a sample of 225 children aged 11 to 14 years. The findings showed both affective dysfunction and impulsivity were uniquely related to childhood borderline features, specifically, the results indicated that affective dysfunction and impulsivity may independently predict childhood borderline features. Moreover, it was revealed that affective dysfunction moderated the association between emotional abuse and childhood borderline features, with emotional abuse showing an association with borderline features just among children with high levels of affective dysfunction (Gratz et al. 2012). Investigations have also indicated that experiencing childhood adversity and being exposed to negative experiences due to childhood maltreatment are associated to BPD, in particular experiencing physical and sexual abuse (e.g., Carr et al. 2018; You et al. 2022; DeShong et al. 2019; Cramer 2016; Allen et al. 2013; Wu et al. 2022, 2023a, b; Robin et al. 2022; Ghinea et al. 2021; Reyes et al. 2019a, b, 2024; Herzog et al. 2022).

The impact of adverse childhood experiences is empirically documented in the pathogenesis of BPD: intense maltreatment and parental dysfunction are assumed dose-dependent risk factors in BPD, contributing to more severe and earlier disorder onset (Porter et al. 2020). Greater levels of emotional and sexual abuse and emotional and physical neglect contribute to aggravation of the risk for BPD (Zhang et al. 2022) and antisocial personality disorder (Zhang et al. 2021; Nederlof et al. 2010a, b). A substantial body of studies have revealed a significant association between childhood sexual abuse and the onset of BPD in early youth (Geselowitz et al. 2021; Infurna et al. 2016; Biskin et al. 2011; Goodman et al. 2010; Venta et al. 2012; Kaplan et al. 2016; Rajan et al. 2021); however, some duplicated studies did not document this association (Hecht et al. 2014). In a cohort study among adolescents with various psychiatrics, who had been victims of child sexual abuse, the results indicated that BPD was the only diagnosis in the first year (Rajan et al. 2021). These identical findings suggest that emotional maltreatment and emotional neglect can be considered as the strongest predictor of BPD and the severity of BPD symptoms (Pietrek et al. 2013; Carvalho Fernando et al. 2014; Porter et al. 2020). Although childhood adversity influences anger and impulsivity (Quenneville et al. 2020), it has been shown that emotion regulation issues alone can be considered as a mediator for the impact of childhood maltreatment on impulsivity in BPD (Krause-Utz et al. 2019). Furthermore, a body of studies has revealed several difficulties in emotion perception in BPD patients including impairments in detecting accurately their emotional environment and identifying vigilantly others' emotional states. Identified links between childhood adversity and facial affect recognition in referring metal states of others have been proposed, including the descriptions of lower, unchanged, or improved capabilities in BPD patients in comparison to healthy population (Robin et al. 2022; Frick 2012; Berenson et al. 2018; Vestergaard et al. 2020). Adverse childhood experiences are associated with the automatic or intraindividual functions of deliberate self-harm (Nock and Prinstein 2004), consisting of emotion regulation function, anti-dissociative function, and self-punishment function (Klonsky 2007; Kaess et al. 2013). Through a cross-sectional study between the months of March and August 2022 among 411 participants, Kanj et al. (2023) examined the mediating impact of emotion regulation difficulties in the association between childhood emotional abuse and BPD. The findings revealed that difficulties in emotion regulation had an indirect impact between emotional abuse and BPD features. The results showed that higher emotional maltreatment scores indicated significant association with higher scores on the *Difficulties in Emotion Regulation Scale* (DERS-16) (e.g., Bjureberg et al. 2016; Shahabi et al. 2020), while a significant association with higher score of *Borderline Personality Questionnaire* (BPQ) (e.g., Ceylan et al. 2017; van Alebeek et al. 2015) was found. They concluded that among the various types of childhood maltreatment, emotional abuse may lead to the development of BPD (Kanj et al. 2023).

Various studies indicated significant association between mood disorders and BPD and frequently high rates of borderline pathology among individuals suffering from mood disorders and depression (e.g., Zimmerman and Mattia 1999; Zimmerman et al. 2013; Bellino et al. 2005; Baryshnikov et al. 2015). Moreover, it has been demonstrated that physical and sexual abuse are strongly associated with the elevated risk of mood disorders and depression (Carr et al. 2018), and also, emotional trauma may precede psychotic symptoms in individuals suffering BPD as well as with somatization symptoms in major depression (MDD) (Gulec et al. 2013). Seon You et al. (2022) investigated the association between childhood trauma and BPD features in mood disorder patients. In accord with the findings among 488 MDD, Bipolar I (BD-I), and Bipolar II (BD-II) diagnoses, as well as control group, it was shown that BD-II patients demonstrated significantly higher BPD features. In addition, it was found that emotional abuse and neglect displayed notable association with BPD, while emotional instability and chaotic relationships were strongly associated with childhood trauma. Also, a positive relationship between childhood trauma and BPD was found in MDD, BD-I, and BD-II patients. They concluded that mood disorder patients with a history of severe childhood trauma exhibit greater features of BPD, as well as BPD features are more likely to be detected among patients with BD-I than BD-II or MDD (Seon You et al. 2022).

However, studies have identified potential childhood contributors for later adult BPD, such as high-risk behaviors, and examined potential processes and pathways of BPD diagnosis development. Rogosch and Cicchetti (2005) proposed a developmental psychopathology perspective focused on present identifiable aspects of functioning that could lead to the later emergence of borderline pathology. Rogosch and Cicchetti (2005) studied the potential precursors of BPD among 185 maltreated school-aged children to investigate developmental constructs conceptualized to represent later revealing BPD. A set of aspects was selected to be assessed consisting of personality features, representational models of self, parent-child interactions issues, peer relationships matter, interpersonal difficulties with peers and adults, suicidal behaviors, and NSSH, as well as the assessment of three attention networks. The findings indicated that children with a history of childhood maltreatment displayed higher mean scores on the BPD precursors; simultaneously children categorized as having great levels of precursors were more prevalent in the group with a history of maltreatment. Moreover, the maltreated children with high level of BPD precursors exhibited less efficient processing of the conflict attention network. To conclude, childhood maltreatment and efficiency of the conflict attention network independently anticipated scores on the BPD precursors composite (Rogosch and Cicchetti 2005). Nock et al. (2010) suggested that elevated emotional reactivity can be a contributory mechanism through which stress results in increasing problem-coping behavior, such as NSSI (Nock 2009). Some experimental supports for Nock's Model were proposed to show that stress exposed, especially exposure to early abuse and other aversive family experiences, significantly caused an increased risk for involving in NSSH in adolescence and early adulthood (Brown et al. 2018; Titelius et al. 2018; Ford and Gómez 2015; Tatnell et al. 2017; Hamza et al. 2021). Through a path analysis among 87 female inpatients with a history of childhood abuse and neglect, Franzke et al. 2015 found that NSSI group reported significantly higher emotional, physical, and sexual as well as physical neglect and a higher number of overall experienced trauma types and abuse subtypes compared with individuals without NSSI. Furthermore, dissociative symptoms intensify substantial and unique risk for maltreated females to be involved in NSSH (Franzke et al. 2015). In a clinical cohort study exploring categorical and dimensional assessment among a clinical sample of 152 adolescents involving nonsuicidal self-injury disorder, Hessels et al. (2018) investigated whether it is possible to differentiate who has BPD from adverse childhood experiences, or from the quality of current relationships. The results demonstrated a greater association between more adverse childhood experiences and more BPD symptoms and BPD diagnosis, without low quality of current social relationships. In accordance with categorical approach, among individuals reporting higher quality of current parent-child relationship, greater association between childhood adversity and meeting full criteria for BPD was displayed.

In sum, the results highlighted the role of adverse childhood experiences as a risk factor of BPD; however, the role of current relations is more complicated (Hessels et al. 2018, 2022). Glenn and Klonsky et al. (2013) found in the children in the community study that there was a greater association between the documented childhood maltreatment and amplified risk for BPD among young adulthood, controlled for symptoms of other personality disorders, age, parental education, and parental mental issues (Glenn and Klonsky 2013). Various empirical findings have indicated an association between childhood maltreatment and suicidal ideation and attempts (Zatti et al. 2017; Thompson et al. 2019; Pompili et al. 2014). In a recent meta-analysis of 68 studies, Angelakis et al. (2019) found a significant association between childhood maltreatment and heightened rates of suicidal ideation in adults, reporting a two-fold increased risk for suicidal ideation among cases with a history of sexual abuse and emotional abuse, 2.5-fold heightened risk for suicidal ideation in physical abused case, and also 1.5-fold elevated risk for suicide ideation in individuals with a history of emotional and physical neglect (Angelakis et al. 2019). Furthermore, Angelakis et al. (2020) in a meta-analysis of 79 studies with 337,185 participants found that sexual abuse showed a significant association with 4.0-fold elevated rates for suicide plans (Angelakis et al. 2020). Kaplan et al. (2016) examined the contributory role of childhood maltreatment in increasing the high-risk behaviors in 29 female youth aged 13–21 years diagnosed with BPD with a history of child abuse, and 29 control group without BPD. The findings showed BPD participants reported greater past NSSI, and also, the occurrence of childhood maltreatment showed association with a 5-fold rise in the rate of lifetime suicide attempts. In addition, exploratory analyses indicated significant association between the co-occurrence of physical and sexual abuse and greater past NSSI and suicidality compared with control group (Kaplan et al. 2016). Based on a structural equation analysis, Marques-Feixa et al. (2021) assessed the association between childhood maltreatment comprising severity and frequency of different forms of neglect abuse; suicidal behaviors, including NSSI, suicide threat, suicide ideation, suicide plan and suicide attempts; recent stressful life events; and BPD traits consisting of emotion dysregulation, intense anger and impulsivity in 187 children and adolescents aged 7 to 17 years. The findings showed that young participants with a history of more severe/ frequent childhood maltreatment reported more notable BPD traits and were more likely to being exposed to recent stressful life events. Also, BPD traits elevated the risk for experiencing stressful life events. According to results, only emotion dysregulation and recent stressful life events indicated correlation with suicidal behaviors (Marques-Feixa et al. 2021). In a meta-analytic review, Gruhn and Compas (2020) tried to synthesize findings from 35 studies to explain patterns between experiences of child abuse and neglect and subsequent controlled/volitional efforts to respond to stress. The results revealed that childhood maltreatment was significantly associated to declined emotion regulation and raised emotion dysregulation, as well as maltreatment was significantly related to elevated avoidance, emotional suppression, and emotional expression (Gruhn and Compas 2020).

In recent decades, some researchers have begun to recognize the role of spirituality as a protective factor for suicide (e.g., Koenig et al. 2004, 2009, 2010, 2012, 2014; Esposito and Clum 2002). Tae and Chae (2021) studied the role of childhood abuse as a risk factor and spirituality as a protective factor in suicide attempts among 737 participants from 18 to 65 years old in an outpatient clinic from September 2010 to November 2017. The findings demonstrated that young age, a history of childhood emotional and sexual abuse, depression, and lower levels of spirituality were prominent independent factors for elevating suicide attempts. Furthermore, the result showed a mediator role of depression in the association between childhood emotional and sexual abuse, spirituality, and suicide attempts (Tae and Chae 2021).

Wu et al. (2022) have demonstrated that individuals with BPD were more likely to have experienced emotional abuse and neglect in comparison with individuals who suffer from other types of personality disorders. Beside, based on their findings, female gender and sexual abuse are considerable predictors of nonsuicidal self-harm and suicidal behaviors risk in BPD (Wu et al. 2022, 2023a, b). Hecht et al. (2014) examined maltreatment subtype including physical abuse (PA), sexual abuse (SA), emotional maltreatment (EM), physical neglect (PN), developmental timing, and chronicity of child maltreatment as significant factors in the development of BPD features in childhood among 314 maltreated and 285 non-maltreated children. The findings indicated that maltreated children showed significantly higher scores on each subscale consisting of affective instability, identity problems, negative relationships, and self-harm, in comparison with non-maltreated children. However, physically abused children displayed considerably higher borderline feature scores compared to the control group, and emotionally and sexually abused children did not show any difference with respect to overall four subscales of borderline features. Moreover, assessing the influence of exposure to multiple types of maltreatment experiences on the development of BPD, significant differences were illustrated between 1–2 subtypes and 3–4 subtypes. In addition, the results showed that the greater chronicity significantly predicted higher features of BPD. It meant that the number of developmental periods in which maltreatment happened substantially predicted borderline feature scores. Based on the findings, it was revealed that for each additional developmental period occurring maltreatment, an individual is 1.28 times more likely to meet criteria for a high-risk group leading to elevating scores on 3 out of 4 subscales (Hecht et al. 2014).

Through a cross-sectional study, Xie et al. (2021) examined the mediating role of self-esteem and resilience in all three types of childhood maltreatment (emotional abuse, physical abuse, and sexual abuse) and the development of BPD among 4034 college students. The result illustrated that when each type was tested separately, resilience and self-esteem were shown to be mediators of all three types of childhood abuse. While all three types of childhood abuse were entered into the model simultaneously, neither the indirect effect nor direct effects of physical or sexual abuse were detected to be significant; however, the relation between emotional abuse and BPD features was somewhat mediated by resilience and self-esteem (Xie et al. 2021). Although self-esteem and resilience mediate the association between child abuse (physical abuse and sexual abuse) and the features of BPD, emotional abuse had not only a direct influence on the features of BPD, but also an indirect effect via self-esteem and resilience (Trull et al. 2008; Wang et al. 2020; Xie et al. 2021). A growing body of studies have revealed that awareness of and sense of connectedness to one's own body may play a significant role as a mediator for the found association between traumatic childhood experiences and emotion dysregulation in individuals with BPD (Back and Bertsch 2020; Löffler et al. 2018, 2022). Consistent with this notion, both psychoform and somatoform dissociation contribute to impaired connection with one's body in people with a history of traumatic childhood experiences (Henschel et al. 2019; Mueller-Pfeiffer et al. 2010). As a part of a large cohort study, Schmitz et al. (2021) investigated the potential mediating role of body connection and emotion regulation in the association between traumatic childhood experiences and BPD core symptoms among 112 adult female patients with BPD and 96 healthy female control (HC). The findings revealed female patients with BPD distinctly reported significantly lower body awareness and higher bodily dissociation compared to a healthy control group. A significantly positive association was reported between body dissociation, traumatic childhood experiences, and emotion regulation in female BPD patients (Schmitz et al. 2021).

The preliminary evidence has shown that one of the most substantial risk factors for adolescent mentalizing issues and uncertainty/ confusion about mental state, BPD, depression, and anxiety symptoms includes childhood emotional abuse (Quek et al. 2017; Belvederi Murri et al. 2021). Through a path analysis, Martin-Gagnon et al. (2023) investigated the relation between child emotional abuse, adolescent borderline personality features, depression, and anxiety symptoms. In addition, they explored a pathway model where Uncertainty/Confusion about mental state mediates the association between child emotional abuse and adolescent BP features, depression, and anxiety symptoms among an outpatient psychiatric sample consisting of 94 adolescents. The findings indicated that Uncertainty/ Confusion about mental states partly mediated the association between child emotional abuse, borderline traits, and anxiety symptoms. Furthermore, an indirect influence was found where child emotional abuse predicted Uncertainty/Confusion about mental states contributing to anticipating depression (Martin-Gagnon et al. 2023). As indicated in a latent class analysis (LCA), Lee and Choi (2023) identified the patterns of CPTSD and BPD symptoms with childhood abuse experiences. They adopted a three-step LCA in 499 South Korean early and midlife adults to compare types of childhood maltreatment and abuse, invalidating environments, attachment styles, and pathological personality traits among various classes. The findings of LCA revealed four classes. Class 1, named a "CPTSD and BPD comorbid" class, indicated the highest scores in all symptoms and risk factors, while class 2, "an externalizing PBD class", was differentiated from class 3, and "avoidant BPD class", based on the externalizing versus internalizing related to pathological personality traits. Class 3 demonstrated experiencing a high level of emotional neglect, as well as other types of abuse and additional avoidant attachment style. Class 4 "low symptom class" displayed low symptomatology in both disorders. They concluded childhood maltreatment and abuse may elevate the risk for strong comorbidity of CPTSD and BPD and externalizing-internalizing subgroups of BPD as well (Lee and Choi 2023). In well-established literature, it has been revealed that there is conjoint comorbidity between the impact of all types of childhood maltreatment and PTSD symptomatology (Carr et al. 2018). According to a survey study, Gama et al. (2021) explored whether people who have a history of childhood maltreatment, especially emotional abuse, were more prone to experience other traumatic events and their harmful consequences and present greater levels of PTSD symptoms in being exposed to another trauma in life among 433 volunteers. Through a bivariate model, all types of childhood maltreatment showed significant association with revictimization and PTSD symptom severity. Moreover, multivariate models indicated that emotional maltreatment had a great association with the highest incidence rates of revictimization and PTSD symptom severity (Gama et al. 2021).

A body of documented studies have shown a strong association between insecure attachment and lower perceived social support with adverse childhood experiences leading to the development of borderline features (Crow and Levy 2019; Frias et al. 2016; Minzenberg et al. 2008). In an online international study that recruited 1682 participants and took place between March 2016 and May 2020, Schulze et al. (2023) examined the interplay of BPD subdomains (emotional instability, identity disturbance, self-harming impulsivity, and relationship matters), all types of adverse childhood experience (emotional, physical, and sexual abuse and neglect), attachment, and perceived social support utilizing a graph-theoretical approach. The findings showed the most central node in both networks and a bridge between all types of adverse childhood experiences and BPD features. In addition, an association between emotional abuse and all domains of BPD except emotional instability was found. Furthermore, adverse childhood experience was partially associated with BPD features, yet not fully elucidated by attachment and social support (Schulze et al. 2023).

To conclude, adverse childhood experiences (ACEs) have been recognized as severe and traumatic experiences including experiencing various forms of violence, childhood maltreatment and neglect, and domestic violence which contribute to the numerous mental health problems and psychiatric disorders, as well as personality difficulties, especially BPD. As discussed earlier, remarkable associations have been reported between having a history of childhood maltreatment and BPD. Furthermore, traumatic life experiences increase the risk of development of BPD by triggering the formation of several BPD features comprising affect instability, emotion dysregulation, and self-destructive behaviors. In addition, experiencing adverse childhood experiences contributes to different types of maladaptive emotion regulation strategies and disturbed mentalizing and symbolizing emotions in adulthood. Being exposed to various types of child abuse is directly associated with the development of nonsuicidal self-harm, suicidal attempts, impulsive behaviors, and other self-destructive behaviors. Several significant epigenetic and neuromorphological changes related to childhood traumatic experiences are reported because of childhood maltreatment, leading to the development of BPD. Moreover, difficulties in emotion regulation strategies have been indicated because of experiencing childhood adversities, as well as various issues in emotion perception in BPD patients. It has been documented that physical and sexual abuse are significantly related to the increased risk of psychiatric disorders among individuals with BPD. Further, high risk behaviors, emotional reactivity, and low quality of interpersonal relationships have been highly reported among individuals with BPD who had a history of childhood maltreatment.

References

Abbott M, Slack KS. Exploring the relationship between childhood adversity and adult depression: a risk versus strengths-oriented approach. Child Abuse Negl. 2021;120:105207. https://doi.org/10.1016/j.chiabu.2021.105207. Epub 2021 Jul 13

Adrian M, Zeman J, Erdley C, Lisa L, Sim L. Emotional dysregulation and interpersonal difficulties as risk factors for nonsuicidal self-injury in adolescent girls. J Abnorm Child Psychol. 2011;39:389–400.

Afifi TO, MacMillan HL. Resilience following child maltreatment: a review of protective factors. Can J Psychiatry. 2011;56(5):266–72.

Agnew-Blais J, Danese A. Childhood maltreatment and unfavourable clinical outcomes in bipolar disorder: a systematic review and meta-analysis. Lancet Psychiatry. 2016;3(4):342–9.

Allen B, Cramer RJ, Harris PB, Rufino KA. Borderline personality symptomatology as a mediator of the link between child maltreatment and adult suicide potential. Arch Suicide Res. 2013;17(1):41–51.

Almeida TC, Fernandes RM, Cunha O. The role of positive childhood experiences in the link between childhood maltreatment and affective lability in a sample of incarcerated men and women. Child Abuse Negl. 2023;135:105969.

Alvarez-Tomás I, Soler J, Bados A, Martín-Blanco A, Elices M, Carmona C, Bauzà J, Pascual JC. Long-term course of borderline personality disorder: a prospective 10-year follow-up study. J Personal Disord. 2017;31(5):590–605.

Amédée LM, Hébert M. Latent class analysis of post-traumatic stress symptoms and complex PTSD in child victims of sexual abuse and their response to Trauma-Focused Cognitive Behavioural Therapy. Eur J Psychotraumatol. 2020;11(1):1807171.

American Psychiatric Association. Diagnostic and statistical manual of mental disorders. 5th ed Text Revised (DSM-5-TR); 2022.

American Psychiatric Association. Understanding mental disorders: your guide to DSM-5-TR®. American Psychiatric Pub; 2023.

Anderson F, Howard L, Dean K, Moran P, Khalifeh H. Childhood maltreatment and adulthood domestic and sexual violence victimisation among people with severe mental illness. Soc Psychiatry Psychiatr Epidemiol. 2016;51:961–70.

Angelakis I, Gillespie EL, Panagioti M. Childhood maltreatment and adult suicidality: a comprehensive systematic review with meta-analysis. Psychol Med. 2019;49(7):1057–78.

Angelakis I, Austin JL, Gooding P. Childhood maltreatment and suicide attempts in prisoners: a systematic meta-analytic review. Psychol Med. 2020;50(1):1–0.

Antoniou G, Lambourg E, Steele JD, Colvin LA. The effect of adverse childhood experiences on chronic pain and major depression in adulthood: a systematic review and meta-analysis. Br J Anaesth. 2023;130:729.

Aouidad A, Cohen D, Mirkovic B, Pellerin H, Garny de La Rivière S, Consoli A, et al. Borderline personality disorder and prior suicide attempts define a severity gradient among hospitalized adolescent suicide attempters. BMC Psychiatry. 2020;20(1):525.

Appleyard K, Egeland B, van Dulmen MH, Alan SL. When more is not better: the role of cumulative risk in child behavior outcomes. J Child Psychol Psychiatry. 2005;46(3):235–45.

Arens AM, Gaher RM, Simons JS, Dvorak RD. Child maltreatment and deliberate self-harm: a negative binomial hurdle model for explanatory constructs. Child Maltreat. 2014;19(3–4):168–77.

Back SN, Bertsch K. Interoceptive processing in borderline personality pathology: a review on neurophysiological mechanisms. Curr Behav Neurosci Rep. 2020;7:232–8.

Baetens I, Claes L, Hasking P, Smits D, Grietens H, Onghena P, Martin G. The relationship between parental expressed emotions and nonsuicidal self-injury: the mediating roles of self-criticism and depression. J Child Fam Stud. 2015;24:491–8.

Baker AJ, Brassard M. Predictors of variation in sate reported rates of psychological maltreatment: a survey of statutes and a call for change. Child Abuse Negl. 2019;96:104102.

Baker AJ, Brassard MR, Rosenzweig J. Psychological maltreatment: definition and reporting barriers among American professionals in the field of child abuse. Child Abuse Negl. 2021;114:104941.

Baldwin JR, Reuben A, Newbury JB, Danese A. Agreement between prospective and retrospective measures of childhood maltreatment: a systematic review and meta-analysis. JAMA Psychiatry. 2019;76(6):584–93.

Balençon M, Pierre M, Roussey M. Childhood deprivation and neglect. In: Child abuse: diagnostic and forensic considerations; 2018. p. 257–73.

Baptista A, Chambon V, Hoertel N, Olfson M, Blanco C, Cohen D, Jacquet PO. Associations between early life adversity, reproduction-oriented life strategy, and borderline personality disorder. JAMA Psychiatry. 2023;80(6):558–66.

Barnett D, Ganiban J, Cicchetti D. Maltreatment, negative expressivity, and the development of type D attachments from 12 to 24 months of age. Monogr Soc Res Child Dev. 1999;1:97–118.

Baryshnikov I, Aaltonen K, Koivisto M, Näätänen P, Karpov B, Melartin T, Heikkinen M, Ketokivi M, Joffe G, Isometsä E. Differences and overlap in self-reported symptoms of bipolar disorder and borderline personality disorder. Eur Psychiatry. 2015;30(8):914–9.

Bateman A, Rüfenacht E, Perroud N, Debbané M, Nolte T, Shaverin L, Fonagy P. Childhood maltreatment, dissociation and borderline personality disorder: preliminary data on the mediational role of mentalizing in complex post-traumatic stress disorder. Psychol Psychother Theory Res Pract. 2023.

Battle CL, Shea MT, Johnson DM, Yen S, Zlotnick C, Zanarini MC, Sanislow CA, Skodol AE, Gunderson JG, Grilo CM, McGlashan TH. Childhood maltreatment associated with adult personality disorders: findings from the Collaborative Longitudinal Personality Disorders Study. J Personal Disord. 2004;18(2):193–211.

Bateman A, Rüfenacht E, Perroud N, Debbané M, Nolte T, Shaverin L, Fonagy P. Childhood maltreatment, dissociation and borderline personality disorder: preliminary data on the mediational role of mentalizing in complex post-traumatic stress disorder. In: Psychology and psychotherapy: theory, research and practice; 2023a.

Bateman A, Rüfenacht E, Perroud N, Debbané M, Nolte T, Shaverin L, Fonagy P. Childhood maltreatment, dissociation and borderline personality disorder: preliminary data on the mediational role of mentalizing in complex post-traumatic stress disorder. Psychol Psychother Theory Res Pract. 2023b;97:58.

Beilharz JE, Paterson M, Fatt S, Wilson C, Burton A, Cvejic E, Lloyd A, Vollmer-Conna U. The impact of childhood trauma on psychosocial functioning and physical health in a non-clinical community sample of young adults. Aust NZ J Psych. 2020;54(2):185–94.

Bellino S, Patria L, Ziero S, Bogetto F. Clinical picture of obsessive-compulsive disorder with poor insight: a regression model. Psychiatry Res. 2005;136(2–3):223–31.

Bellis MA, Hughes K, Ford K, Rodriguez GR, Sethi D, Passmore J. Life course health consequences and associated annual costs of adverse childhood experiences across Europe and North America: a systematic review and meta-analysis. Lancet Public Health. 2019;4(10):e517–28.

Belsky DW, Caspi A, Arseneault L, Bleidorn W, Fonagy P, Goodman M, Houts R, Moffitt TE. Etiological features of borderline personality related characteristics in a birth cohort of 12-year-old children. Dev Psychopathol. 2012;24(1):251–65.

Belvederi Murri M, Folesani F, Costa S, Biancosino B, Zerbinati L, Ounalli H, Rossetto A, Caruso R, Nanni MG, Grassi L. The relationship between cognitive abilities and trait clinical features in patients with borderline personality disorder. J Personal Disord. 2021;35(5):730–49.

Bendstrup G, Simonsen E, Kongerslev MT, Jørgensen MS, Petersen LS, Thomsen MS, Vestergaard M. Narrative coherence of autobiographical memories in women with borderline personality disorder and associations with childhood adversity. Borderline Personal Disord Emot Dysregul. 2021;8(1):18.

Berardelli I, Sarubbi S, Rogante E, Hawkins M, Cocco G, Erbuto D, Lester D, Pompili M. The role of demoralization and hopelessness in suicide risk in schizophrenia: a review of the literature. Medicina. 2019;55(5):200.

Berenson KR, Dochat C, Martin CG, Yang X, Rafaeli E, Downey G. Identification of mental states and interpersonal functioning in borderline personality disorder. Personal Disord Theory Res Treat. 2018;9(2):172.

Bertolote JM, De Leo D. Global suicide mortality rates–a light at the end of the tunnel? Crisis. 2012;33:249.

Biskin RS, Paris J, Renaud J, Raz A, Zelkowitz P. Outcomes in women diagnosed with borderline personality disorder in adolescence. J Can Acad Child Adolesc Psychiatry. 2011;20(3):168.

Bjureberg J, Ljótsson B, Tull MT, Hedman E, Sahlin H, Lundh LG, Bjärehed J, DiLillo D, Messman-Moore T, Gumpert CH, Gratz KL. Development and validation of a brief version of the difficulties in emotion regulation scale: the DERS-16. J Psychopathol Behav Assess. 2016;38:284–96.

Bornovalova MA, Huibregtse BM, Hicks BM, Keyes M, McGue M, Iacono W. Tests of a direct effect of childhood abuse on adult borderline personality disorder traits: a longitudinal discordant twin design. J Abnorm Psychol. 2013;122(1):180.

Bozzatello P, Bellino S, Bosia M, Rocca P. Early detection and outcome in borderline personality disorder. Front Psych. 2019;10:710.

Bozzatello P, Garbarini C, Rocca P, Bellino S. Borderline personality disorder: risk factors and early detection. Diagnostics. 2021;11(11):2142.

Brakemeier EL, Dobias J, Hertel J, Bohus M, Limberger MF, Schramm E, Radtke M, Frank P, Padberg F, Sabass L, Jobst A. Childhood maltreatment in women with borderline personal-

ity disorder, chronic depression, and episodic depression, and in healthy controls. Psychother Psychosom. 2018;87(1):49–51.
Brewer-Smyth K. Adverse childhood experiences: the neuroscience of trauma, resilience and healing throughout the life course. Springer Nature; 2022.
Brown RC, Fischer T, Goldwich AD, Keller F, Young R, Plener PL. # cutting: nonsuicidal self-injury (NSSI) on Instagram. Psychol Med. 2018;48(2):337–46.
Brüne M, Jiaqing O, Schojai M, Decker C, Edel MA. Mating strategies and experience of early adversity in female patients with borderline personality disorder: insights from life history theory. Personal Individ Differ. 2017;113:147–54.
Bunting L, McCartan C, Davidson G, Grant A, Mulholland C, Schubotz D, Hamill R, McBride O, Murphy J, Nolan E, Shevlin M. The influence of adverse and positive childhood experiences on young people's mental health and experiences of self-harm and suicidal ideation. Child Abuse Negl. 2023;140:106159.
Burgin XD, Daniel MC. Social emotional learning. In: Perspectives on evidence-based policy in human services, vol. 29; 2024. p. 168.
Bürgin D, Clemens V, Witt A, Sachser C, Jud A, Brähler E, et al. Adverse childhood experiences increase the risk for low perceived social participation and health-related quality of life in a large-scale population-based study in Germany. Child Abuse Negl. 2023;144:106382. https://doi.org/10.1016/j.chiabu.2023.106382. Epub 2023 Jul 30
Burke NN, Finn DP, McGuire BE, Roche M. Psychological stress in early life as a predisposing factor for the development of chronic pain: clinical and preclinical evidence and neurobiological mechanisms. J Neurosci Res. 2017;95(6):1257–70.
Carr O, Saunders KE, Tsanas A, Bilderbeck AC, Palmius N, Geddes JR, Foster R, Goodwin GM, De Vos M. Variability in phase and amplitude of diurnal rhythms is related to variation of mood in bipolar and borderline personality disorder. Sci Rep. 2018;8(1):1649.
Carr A, Duff H, Craddock F. A systematic review of the outcome of child abuse in long-term care. Trauma Violence Abuse. 2020;21(4):660–77.
Carlson EA, Egeland B, Sroufe LA. A prospective investigation of the development of borderline personality symptoms. Dev Psychopathol. 2009;21(4):1311–34.
Carvalho Fernando S, Beblo T, Schlosser N, Terfehr K, Otte C, Löwe B, Wolf OT, Spitzer C, Driessen M, Wingenfeld K. The impact of self-reported childhood trauma on emotion regulation in borderline personality disorder and major depression. J Trauma Dissociation. 2014;15(4):384–401.
Center for Disease Control and Prevention, 2012.
Center for Disease Control and Prevention, 2021, USA.
Centers for Disease Control and Prevention, National Center fro Injury Prevention and Control (NCPIC), 2022.
Ceylan V, Kose S, Akin E, Turkcapar MH. Normative data and factorial structure of the Turkish version of the Borderline Personality Questionnaire (Turkish BPQ). Psych Clin Psychopharmacol. 2017;27(2):143–51.
Chamberlain C, Gee G, Harfield S, Campbell S, Brennan S, Clark Y, Mensah F, Arabena K, Herrman H, Brown S. 'Healing the Past by Nurturing the Future'group. Parenting after a history of childhood maltreatment: a scoping review and map of evidence in the perinatal period. PLoS One. 2019a;14(3):e0213460.
Chamberlain SR, Tiego J, Fontenelle LF, Hook R, Parkes L, Segrave R, Hauser TU, Dolan RJ, Goodyer IM, Bullmore E, Grant JE. Fractionation of impulsive and compulsive trans-diagnostic phenotypes and their longitudinal associations. Aust NZ J Psychiatr. 2019b;53(9):896–907.
Cheng P, Langevin R. Difficulties with emotion regulation moderate the relationship between child maltreatment and emotion recognition. Child Abuse Negl. 2023;139:106094.
Cheng P, Ju P, Xia Q, Chen Y, Li J, Gao J, Zhang L, Yan F, Cheng X, Pei W, Chen L. Childhood maltreatment increases the suicidal risk in Chinese schizophrenia patients. Front Psych. 2022;13:927540.

Cicchetti D. Socioemotional, personality, and biological development: illustrations from a multilevel developmental psychopathology perspective on child maltreatment. Annu Rev Psychol. 2016;67:187–211.

Cicchetti D, Toth SL. Child maltreatment and developmental psychopathology: a multilevel perspective. Dev Psychopathol. 2016;3:457–512.

Clayton K, Lee JB, Cheung K, Theule J, Henrikson B. Quantifying the relationship between attention-deficit/hyperactivity disorder and experiences of child maltreatment: a meta-analysis. Child Abuse Rev. 2018;27(5):361–77.

Clemens V, Beschoner P, Jarczok MN, Weimer K, Kempf M, Morawa E, Geiser F, Albus C, Steudte-Schmiedgen S, Gündel H, Fegert JM. The mediating role of COVID-19-related burden in the association between adverse childhood experiences and emotional exhaustion: results of the egePan–VOICE study. Eur J Psychotraumatol. 2021;12(1):1976441.

Cloitre M, Garvert DW, Weiss B, Carlson EB, Bryant RA. Distinguishing PTSD, complex PTSD, and borderline personality disorder: a latent class analysis. Eur J Psychotraumatol. 2014;5(1):25097.

Cloitre M, Brewin CR, Bisson JI, Hyland P, Karatzias T, Lueger-Schuster B, Maercker A, Roberts NP, Shevlin M. Evidence for the coherence and integrity of the complex PTSD (CPTSD) diagnosis: response to Achterhof et al.(2019) and Ford (2020). Eur J Psychotraumatol. 2020;11(1):1739873.

Cloninger CR, Svrakic DM, Przybeck TR. A psychobiological model of temperament and character. Arch Gen Psychiatry. 1993;50(12):975–90.

Compas BE, Connor-Smith JK, Saltzman H, Thomsen AH, Wadsworth ME. Coping with stress during childhood and adolescence: problems, progress, and potential in theory and research. Psychol Bull. 2001;127(1):87.

Compas BE, Jaser SS, Bettis AH, Watson KH, Gruhn MA, Dunbar JP, Williams E, Thigpen JC. Coping, emotion regulation, and psychopathology in childhood and adolescence: a meta-analysis and narrative review. Psychol Bull. 2017;143(9):939.

Congdon E et al. Measurement and reliability of response inhibition. Front Psychol. 2012;3:37.

Courtney EA, Johnson JG, Alloy LB. Associations of childhood maltreatment with hopelessness and depression among adolescent primary care patients. Int J Cogn Ther. 2008;1(1):4–17.

Cramer P. Childhood precursors of adult borderline personality disorder features: a longitudinal study. J Nerv Ment Dis. 2016;204(7):494–9.

CRC U. Convention on the Rights of the Child. CRC becomes incorporates in Swedish law, 1989.

Crouch E, Probst JC, Radcliff E, Bennett KJ, McKinney SH. Prevalence of adverse childhood experiences (ACEs) among US children. Child Abuse Negl. 2019;92:209–18.

Crow TM, Levy KN. Adult attachment anxiety moderates the relation between self-reported childhood maltreatment and borderline personality disorder features. Personal Ment Health. 2019;13(4):239–49.

Crowell SE, Beauchaine TP, Linehan MM. A biosocial developmental model of borderline personality: elaborating and extending Linehan's theory. Psychol Bull. 2009;135(3):495.

Crowell SE, Kaufman EA, Lenzenweger MF. The development of borderline personality and self-inflicted injury. In: Child and adolescent psychopathology. Wiley; 2013. p. 577–609.

Crowell SE, Kaliush PR, Vlisides-Henry RD. Borderline personality disorder (BPD) Compass is a promising complementary intervention to dialectical behavior therapy: comment on Sauer-Zavala, 2022.

Dadomo H, Grecucci A, Giardini I, Ugolini E, Carmelita A, Panzeri M. Schema therapy for emotional dysregulation: theoretical implication and clinical applications. Front Psychol. 2016;7:1987.

Dadomo H, Panzeri M, Caponcello D, Carmelita A, Grecucci A. Schema therapy for emotional dysregulation in personality disorders: a review. Curr Opin Psychiatry. 2018;31(1):43–9.

Dadomo H, Ponzi D, Nicolini Y, Volpi R, Palanza P, Pelosi A, Bartolomucci A, Parmigiani S. Loss of socioeconomic condition and psychogenic erectile dysfunction: the role of temperament and depression. Adapt Hum Behav Physiol. 2020;6:57–74.

Dadomo H, Salvato G, Lapomarda G, Ciftci Z, Messina I, Grecucci A. Structural features predict sexual trauma and interpersonal problems in borderline personality disorder but not in controls: a multi-voxel pattern analysis. Front Hum Neurosci. 2022;16:773593.

D'arcy-Bewick S, Terracciano A, Turiano N, Sutin AR, Long R, O'Súilleabháin PS. Childhood abuse and neglect, and mortality risk in adulthood: a systematic review and meta-analysis. Child Abuse Negl. 2022;134:105922.

De Panfilis C, Schito G, Generali I, Gozzi LA, Ossola P, Marchesi C, Grecucci A. Emotions at the border: increased punishment behavior during fair interpersonal exchanges in borderline personality disorder. J Abnorm Psychol. 2019;128(2):162.

DeShong HL, Grant DM, Mullins-Sweatt SN. Precursors of the emotional cascade model of borderline personality disorder: the role of neuroticism, childhood emotional vulnerability, and parental invalidation. Personal Disord Theory Res Treat. 2019;10(4):317.

Di Pierro R, Sarno I, Perego S, Gallucci M, Madeddu F. Adolescent nonsuicidal self-injury: the effects of personality traits, family relationships and maltreatment on the presence and severity of behaviours. Eur Child Adolesc Psychiatry. 2012;21:511–20.

Division of Violence Prevention National Center for Injury Prevention and Control, CDC, 2019, 2021.

Douglas KR, Chan G, Gelernter J, Arias AJ, Anton RF, Weiss RD, Brady K, Poling J, Farrer L, Kranzler HR. Adverse childhood events as risk factors for substance dependence: partial mediation by mood and anxiety disorders. Addict Behav. 2010;35(1):7–13.

Dube SR, Anda RF, Felitti VJ, Croft JB, Edwards VJ, Giles WH. Growing up with parental alcohol abuse: exposure to childhood abuse, neglect, and household dysfunction. Child Abuse Negl. 2001;25(12):1627–40.

Edwards VJ, Anda RF, Gu D, Dube SR, Felitti VJ. Adverse childhood experiences and smoking persistence in adults with smoking-related symptoms and illness. Perm J. 2007;11(2):5.

Ehrlich KB, Ross KM, Chen E, Miller GE. Testing the biological embedding hypothesis: is early life adversity associated with a later proinflammatory phenotype? Dev Psychopathol. 2016;28(4pt2):1273–83.

Elliott E, Manashirov S, Zwang R, Gil S, Tsoory M, Shemesh Y, Chen A. Dnmt3a in the medial prefrontal cortex regulates anxiety-like behavior in adult mice. J Neurosci. 2016;36(3):730–40.

Elovainio M, Pulkki-Råback L, Jokela M, Kivimäki M, Hintsanen M, Hintsa T, Viikari J, Raitakari OT, Keltikangas-Järvinen L. Socioeconomic status and the development of depressive symptoms from childhood to adulthood: a longitudinal analysis across 27 years of follow-up in the Young Finns study. Soc Sci Med. 2012;74(6):923–9.

Elzy M, Clark C, Dollard N, Hummer V. Adolescent girls' use of avoidant and approach coping as moderators between trauma exposure and trauma symptoms. J Fam Violence. 2013;28:763–70.

Esposito CL, Clum GA. Social support and problem-solving as moderators of the relationship between childhood abuse and suicidality: applications to a delinquent population. J Traum Stress. 2002;15(2):137–46.

Fayaz I. Child abuse: effects and preventive measures. Int J Indian Psychol. 2019;7(2):871–84.

Fletcher JM, Stuebing KK, Morris RD, Lyon GR. Classification and definition of learning disabilities: a hybrid model. 2014.

Fonagy P, Speranza M, Luyten P, Kaess M, Hessels C, Bohus M. ESCAP Expert Article: borderline personality disorder in adolescence: an expert research review with implications for clinical practice. Eur Child Adolesc Psychiatry. 2015;24:1307–20.

Ford JD, Courtois CA. Complex PTSD and borderline personality disorder. Borderline Personal Disord Emot Dysregul. 2021;8(1):16.

Ford JD, Gómez JM. The relationship of psychological trauma and dissociative and posttraumatic stress disorders to nonsuicidal self-injury and suicidality: a review. J Trauma Dissociation. 2015;16(3):232–71.

Forester J, McKibbon G. Beyond blame: leadership, collaboration and compassion in the time of COVID-19. Socio-Ecol Pract Res. 2020;2:205–16.

Franzke I, Wabnitz P, Catani C. Dissociation as a mediator of the relationship between childhood trauma and nonsuicidal self-injury in females: a path analytic approach. J Trauma Dissociation. 2015;16(3):286–302.

Franklin JC, Ribeiro JD, Fox KR, Bentley KH, Kleiman EM, Huang X, Musacchio KM, Jaroszewski AC, Chang BP, Nock MK. Risk factors for suicidal thoughts and behaviors: a meta-analysis of 50 years of research. Psychol Bull. 2017;143(2):187.

Franklin A, Smeaton E. Listening to young people with learning disabilities who have experienced, or are at risk of, child sexual exploitation in the UK. Child Soc. 2018;32(2):98–109.

Franklin L, Theodore K, Foulds D, Cooper M, Mallaghan L, Wilshaw P, Colborne A, Flower E, Dickinson D, Lee JN. "They don't think I can cope, because I have got a learning disability…": experiences of stigma in the lives of parents with learning disabilities. J Appl Res Intellect Disabil. 2022;35(4):935–47.

Frias A, Palma C, Farriols N, Gonzalez L, Horta A. Anxious adult attachment may mediate the relationship between childhood emotional abuse and borderline personality disorder. Personal Ment Health. 2016;10(4):274–84.

Frick PJ. Developmental pathways to conduct disorder: implications for future directions in research, assessment, and treatment. J Clin Child Adolesc Psychol. 2012;41(3):378–89.

Fruzzetti AE, Shenk C, Hoffman PD. Family interaction and the development of borderline personality disorder: a transactional model. Dev Psychopathol. 2005;17(4):1007–30.

Gabbard GO. Long-term psychodynamic psychotherapy: a basic text. American Psychiatric Pub; 2017.

Gama CM, Portugal LC, Gonçalves RM, de Souza JS, Vilete LM, Mendlowicz MV, Figueira I, Volchan E, David IA, de Oliveira L, Pereira MG. The invisible scars of emotional abuse: a common and highly harmful form of childhood maltreatment. BMC Psychiatry. 2021;21:1–4.

Gardner MJ, Thomas HJ, Erskine HE. The association between five forms of child maltreatment and depressive and anxiety disorders: a systematic review and meta-analysis. Child Abuse Negl. 2019;96:104082.

Geselowitz B, Whalen DJ, Tillman R, Barch DM, Luby JL, Vogel A. Preschool age predictors of adolescent borderline personality symptoms. J Am Acad Child Adolesc Psychiatry. 2021;60(5):612–22.

Ghinea D, Fuchs A, Parzer P, Koenig J, Resch F, Kaess M. Psychosocial functioning in adolescents with nonsuicidal self-injury: the roles of childhood maltreatment, borderline personality disorder and depression. Borderline Personal Disord Emot Dysregul. 2021;8:1–1.

Gibson K, Morgan M. Narrative research on child sexual abuse: addressing perennial problems in quantitative research. Qual Res Psychol. 2013;10(3):298–317.

Gill H, El-Halabi S, Majeed A, Gill B, et al. The association between adverse childhood experiences and inflammation in patients with major depressive disorder: a systematic review. J Affect Disord. 2020;272:1–7. https://doi.org/10.1016/j.jad.2020.03.145. Epub 2020 Apr 5

Glassman LH, Weierich MR, Hooley JM, Deliberto TL, Nock MK. Child maltreatment, nonsuicidal self-injury, and the mediating role of self-criticism. Behav Res Ther. 2007;45(10):2483–90.

Glenn CR, Klonsky ED. Nonsuicidal self-injury disorder: an empirical investigation in adolescent psychiatric patients. J Clin Child Adolesc Psychol. 2013;42(4):496–507.

Goodman GS, Quas JA, Ogle CM. Child maltreatment and memory. Annu Rev Psychol. 2010;61:325–51.

Gratz KL. Risk factors for and functions of deliberate self-harm: an empirical and conceptual review. Clin Psychol Sci Pract. 2003;10(2):192.

Gratz KL, Hepworth C, Tull MT, Paulson A, Clarke S, Remington B, Lejuez C. An experimental investigation of emotional willingness and physical pain tolerance in deliberate self-harm: the moderating role of interpersonal distress. Compr Psychiatry. 2011;52(1):63–74.

Gratz KL, Latzman RD, Young J, Heiden LJ, Damon J, Hight T, Tull MT. Deliberate self-harm among underserved adolescents: the moderating roles of gender, race, and school-level and association with borderline personality features. Personal Disord Theory Res Treat. 2012;3(1):39.

Gratz KL, Weiss NH, McDermott MJ, Dilillo D, Messman-Moore T, Tull MT. Emotion dysregulation mediates the relation between borderline personality disorder symptoms and later physical health symptoms. J Personal Disord. 2017;31(4):433–48.

Gratz KL, Richmond JR, Dixon-Gordon KL, Chapman AL, Tull MT. Multimodal assessment of emotional reactivity and regulation in response to social rejection among self-harming adults with and without borderline personality disorder. Personal Disord Theory Res Treat. 2019;10(5):395.

Gratz KL, Kiel EJ, Mann AJ, Tull MT. The prospective relation between borderline personality disorder symptoms and suicide risk: the mediating roles of emotion regulation difficulties and perceived burdensomeness. J Affect Disord. 2022;313:186–95.

Green JG, McLaughlin KA, Berglund PA, Gruber MJ, Sampson NA, Zaslavsky AM, Kessler RC. Childhood adversities and adult psychiatric disorders in the national comorbidity survey replication I: associations with first onset of DSM-IV disorders. Arch Gen Psychiatry. 2010;67(2):113–23.

Gross JJ. The emerging field of emotion regulation: an integrative review. Rev Gen Psychol. 1998a;2(3):271–99.

Gross JJ. Antecedent-and response-focused emotion regulation: divergent consequences for experience, expression, and physiology. J Pers Soc Psychol. 1998b;74(1):224.

Gross JJ. Conceptualizing emotional labor: an emotion regulation perspective. Routledge/Taylor & Francis Group; 2013.

Gross JJ, Jazaieri H. Emotion, emotion regulation, and psychopathology: an affective science perspective. Clin Psychol Sci. 2015;2(4):387–401.

Gross J, Ford B. Handbook of emotion regulation. 3rd ed; 2024.

Gross JT, Cassidy J. Expressive suppression of negative emotions in children and adolescents: theory, data, and a guide for future research. Dev Psychol. 2019;55(9):1938.

Grove JL, Crowell SE. The Oxford handbook of dialectical behaviour therapy. Oxford University Press; 2019.

Gruhn MA, Compas BE. Effects of maltreatment on coping and emotion regulation in childhood and adolescence: a meta-analytic review. Child Abuse Negl. 2020;103:104446.

Gulec M, Selvi Y, Boysan M, Aydin A, Oral E, Aydin EF. Chronotype effects on general well-being and psychopathology levels in healthy young adults. Biol Rhythm Res. 2013;44(3):457–68.

Gunderson JG. Borderline personality disorder: ontogeny of a diagnosis. Am J Psychiatry. 2009;166(5):530–9.

Gunderson JG, Herpertz SC, Skodol AE, Torgersen S, Zanarini MC. Borderline personality disorder. Nat Rev Dis Primers. 2018;4(1):1–20.

Haj-Yahia MM, Greenbaum CW, Lahoud-Shoufany L. Palestinian adolescents' prolonged exposure to political violence, self-esteem, and post-traumatic stress symptoms. J Interpers Violence. 2021;36(9–10):4137–64.

Hamza CA, Goldstein AL, Heath NL, Ewing L. Stressful experiences in university predict nonsuicidal self-injury through emotional reactivity. Front Psychol. 2021;12:610670.

Hargreaves MK, Mouton CP, Liu J, Zhou YE, Blot WJ. Adverse childhood experiences and health care utilization in a low-income population. J Health Care Poor Underserved. 2019;30(2):749.

Hart H, Lim L, Mehta MA, Chatzieffraimidou A, Curtis C, Xu X, Breen G, Simmons A, Mirza K, Rubia K. Reduced functional connectivity of fronto-parietal sustained attention networks in severe childhood abuse. PLoS One. 2017;12(11):e0188744.

Hawton K, Saunders KE, O'Connor RC. Self-harm and suicide in adolescents. Lancet. 2012;379(9834):2373–82.

Hébert M, Smith K, Brodeur G, Cénat JM, Derivois D. Child sexual abuse as a risk factor for dating victimization in adolescent girls and young adult women in France. Theol Sex. 2020;29(4):e111–9.

Heck S. Adverse childhood experiences: exploring the impact on students' overall well-being, 2024.

Hecht KF, Cicchetti D, Rogosch FA, Crick NR. Borderline personality features in childhood: the role of subtype, developmental timing, and chronicity of child maltreatment. Dev Psychopathol. 2014;26(3):805–15.

Henschel S, Doba K, Nandrino JL. Emotion regulation processes and psychoform and somatoform dissociation in adolescents and young adults with cumulative maltreatment. J Trauma Dissociation. 2019;20(2):197–211.

Herzog JI, Schmahl C. Adverse childhood experiences and the consequences on neurobiological, psychosocial, and somatic conditions across the lifespan. Front Psych. 2018;9:357654.
Herzog P, Kube T, Fassbinder E. How childhood maltreatment alters perception and cognition–the predictive processing account of borderline personality disorder. Psychol Med. 2022;52(14):2899–916.
Hessels CJ, Laceulle OM, van Aken MA, Resch F, Kaess M. Differentiating BPD in adolescents with NSSI disorder: the role of adverse childhood experiences and current social relationships. Borderline Personal Disord Emot Dysregul. 2018;5:1–1.
Hessels CJ, van den Berg T, Lucassen SA, Laceulle OM, van Aken MA. Borderline personality disorder in young people: associations with support and negative interactions in relationships with mothers and a best friend. Borderline Personal Disord Emot Dysregul. 2022;9:1–1.
Huang ZH, Hou CL, Huang YH, He XY, Wang QW, Chen X, Wang ZL, Wang SB, Jia FJ. Individuals at high risk for psychosis experience more childhood trauma, life events and social support deficit in comparison to healthy controls. Psychiatry Res. 2019;273:296–302.
Hughes K, Bellis MA, Sethi D, Andrew R, Yon Y, Wood S, Ford K, Baban A, Boderscova L, Kachaeva M, Makaruk K. Adverse childhood experiences, childhood relationships and associated substance use and mental health in young Europeans. Eur J Pub Health. 2020a;29(4):741–7.
Hughes K, Ford K, Bellis MA, Glendinning F, Harrison E, Passmore J. Health and financial costs of adverse childhood experiences in 28 European countries: a systematic review and meta-analysis. Lancet Public Health. 2020b;6(11):e848–57.
Hughes K, Bellis MA, Hardcastle KA, Sethi D, Butchart A, Mikton C, Jones L, Dunne MP. The effect of multiple adverse childhood experiences on health: a systematic review and meta-analysis. Lancet Public Health. 2017;2(8):e356–66.
Hughes K, Ford K, Bellis MA, Glendinning F, Harrison E, Passmore J. Health and financial costs of adverse childhood experiences in 28 European countries: a systematic review and meta-analysis. Lancet Public Health. 2021;6(11):e848–57.
Humphreys KL, Guyon-Harris KL, Tibu F, Wade M, Nelson CA III, Fox NA, Zeanah CH. Psychiatric outcomes following severe deprivation in early childhood: follow-up of a randomized controlled trial at age 16. J Consult Clin Psychol. 2020;88(12):1079.
Hyland P, Shevlin M, Cloitre M, Karatzias T, Vallières F, McGinty G, Fox R, Power JM. Quality not quantity: loneliness subtypes, psychological trauma, and mental health in the US adult population. Soc Psychiatry Psychiatr Epidemiol. 2019;54:1089–99.
Ibrahim J, Cosgrave N, Woolgar M. Childhood maltreatment and its link to borderline personality disorder features in children: a systematic review approach. Clin Child Psychol Psychiatry. 2018;23(1):57–76.
Infurna MR, Reichl C, Parzer P, Schimmenti A, Bifulco A, Kaess M. Associations between depression and specific childhood experiences of abuse and neglect: a meta-analysis. J Affect Disord. 2016;190:47–55.
Jaffee SR. Child maltreatment and risk for psychopathology in childhood and adulthood. Annu Rev Clin Psychol. 2017;13:525–51.
Janusek LW, Tell D, Gaylord-Harden N, Mathews HL. Relationship of childhood adversity and neighborhood violence to a proinflammatory phenotype in emerging adult African American men: an epigenetic link. Brain Behav Immun. 2017;60:126–35.
Jenny C. Child abuse and neglect: diagnosis, treatment and evidence-expert consult. Online and Print. Elsevier Health Sciences; 2010.
Johnson RM, Hill AV, Jones VC, Lorraine TWP, et al. Racial/ethnic inequities in adverse childhood experiences and selected health-related behaviors and problems among Maryland adolescents. Health Promot Pract. 2022;23(6):935–40. https://doi.org/10.1177/15248399211008238.
Jones B, Currin-Mcculloch J, Pelletier W, Sardi-Brown V, Brown P, Wiener L. Psychosocial standards of care for children with cancer and their families: a national survey of pediatric oncology social workers. Soc Work Health Care. 2018;57(4):221–49.
Kaess M, Parzer P, Mattern M, Plener PL, Bifulco A, Resch F, Brunner R. Adverse childhood experiences and their impact on frequency, severity, and the individual function of nonsuicidal self-injury in youth. Psychiatry Res. 2013;206(2–3):265–72.

Kanj G, Hallit S, Obeid S. The relationship between childhood emotional abuse and borderline personality disorder: the mediating role of difficulties in emotion regulation among Lebanese adults. Borderline Personal Disord Emot Dysregul. 2023;10(1):34.

Kaplan C, Tarlow N, Stewart JG, Aguirre B, Galen G, Auerbach RP. Borderline personality disorder in youth: the prospective impact of child abuse on nonsuicidal self-injury and suicidality. Compr Psychiatry. 2016;71:86–94.

Kaufman EA, Victor SE, Hipwell AE, Stepp SD. Reciprocal influences of parent and adolescent borderline personality symptoms over 3 years. J Personal Disord. 2020;34(Supplement B):130–45.

Kessler RC, Aguilar-Gaxiola S, Alonso J, Benjet C, Bromet EJ, Cardoso G, Degenhardt L, de Girolamo G, Dinolova RV, Ferry F, Florescu S. Trauma and PTSD in the WHO world mental health surveys. Eur J Psychotraumatol. 2017;8(sup5):1353383.

Kealy D, Laverdière O, Pincus AL. Pathological narcissism and symptoms of major depressive disorder among psychiatric outpatients: the mediating role of impaired emotional processing. J Nerv Ment Dis. 2020;208(2):161–4.

Kempe CH. The battered-child syndrome. JAMA. 1962;181:17–24. https://doi.org/10.1001/jama.1962.03050270019004.

Khoury JE, Ahtam B, Sisitsky M, Ou Y, Gagoski B, Enlow MB, Teicher MH, Grant PE, Lyons-Ruth K. Maternal childhood maltreatment is associated with lower infant gray matter volume and amygdala volume during the first two years of life. Biol Psych Global Open Sci. 2022;2(4):440–9.

Kleindienst N, Löffler A, Herzig M, Bertsch K, Bekrater-Bodmann R. Evaluation of the own body in women with current and remitted borderline personality disorder: evidence for long-lasting effects of childhood sexual abuse. Eur J Psychotraumatol. 2020;11(1):1764707.

Klonsky ED. The functions of deliberate self-injury: a review of the evidence. Clin Psychol Rev. 2007;27(2):226–39.

Klonsky ED, May AM, Glenn CR. The relationship between nonsuicidal self-injury and attempted suicide: converging evidence from four samples. J Abnorm Psychol. 2013;122(1):231.

Klumparendt A, Nelson J, Barenbrügge J, Ehring T. Associations between childhood maltreatment and adult depression: a mediation analysis. BMC Psychiatry. 2019;19:1–1.

Koch KD, Jones BL. Supporting parent caregivers of children with life-limiting illness. Children. 2018;5(7):85.

Koenig JL, Barry RA, Kochanska G. Rearing difficult children: Parents' personality and children's proneness to anger as predictors of future parenting. Parent Sci Pract. 2010;10(4):258–73.

Koenig K, De Los RA, Cicchetti D, Scahill L, Klin A. Group intervention to promote social skills in school-age children with pervasive developmental disorders: reconsidering efficacy. J Autism Dev Disord. 2009;39:1163–72.

Koenig M, Stephens E. Characterizing children's responsiveness to cues of speaker trustworthiness: two proposals. In: Trust and skepticism. Psychology Press; 2014. p. 13–27.

Koenig MA, Jaswal VK. Characterizing children's expectations about expertise and incompetence: Halo or pitchfork effects? Child Dev. 2012;82(5):1634–47.

Koenig AL, Cicchetti D, Rogosch FA. Moral development: the association between maltreatment and young children's prosocial behaviors and moral transgressions. Soc Dev. 2004;13(1):87–106.

Koenigsberg HW, Harvey PD, Mitropoulou V, Schmeidler J, New AS, Goodman M, Silverman JM, Serby M, Schopick F, Siever LJ. Characterizing affective instability in borderline personality disorder. Am J Psychiatry. 2002;159(5):784–8.

Kolthof KA, Voorendonk EM, Van Minnen A, De Jongh A. Effects of intensive trauma-focused treatment of individuals with both post-traumatic stress disorder and borderline personality disorder. Eur J Psychotraumatol. 2022;13(2):2143076.

Krause-Utz A, Erol E, Brousianou AV, Cackowski S, Paret C, Ende G, Elzinga B. Self-reported impulsivity in women with borderline personality disorder: the role of childhood maltreatment severity and emotion regulation difficulties. Borderline Personal Disord Emot Dysregul. 2019;6:1–4.

Krause-Utz A, Mertens LJ, Renn JB, Lucke P, Wöhlke AZ, van Schie CC, Mouthaan J. Childhood maltreatment, borderline personality features, and coping as predictors of intimate partner violence. J Interpers Violence. 2021a;36(13–14):6693–721.

Krause-Utz A, Frost R, Chatzaki E, Winter D, Schmahl C, Elzinga BM. Dissociation in borderline personality disorder: recent experimental, neurobiological studies, and implications for future research and treatment. Curr Psychiatry Rep. 2021b;23(6):37.

Krause-Utz A, Walther JC, Kyrgiou AI, Hoogenboom W, Alampanou M, Bohus M, Schmahl C, Lis S. Severity of childhood maltreatment predicts reaction times and heart rate variability during an emotional working memory task in borderline personality disorder. Eur J Psychotraumatol. 2022;13(1):2093037.

Kruger DJ, Carrothers J, Franzen SP, Miller AL, Reischl TM, Stoddard SA, Zimmerman MA. The role of present time perspective in predicting early adolescent violence. J Interpers Violence. 2018;33(12):1893–908.

Laajasalo T, Cowley LE, Otterman G, Lamela D, Rodrigues LB, Jud A, Kemp A, Naughton A, Hurt L, Soldino V, Ntinapogias A. Current issues and challenges in the definition and operationalization of child maltreatment: a scoping review. Child Abuse Negl. 2023;140:106187.

Lang CM, Sharma-Patel K. The relation between childhood maltreatment and self-injury: a review of the literature on conceptualization and intervention. Trauma Violence Abuse. 2011;12(1):23–37.

Lanius RA, Vermetten E, Loewenstein RJ, Brand B, Schmahl C, Bremner JD, Spiegel D. Emotion modulation in PTSD: clinical and neurobiological evidence for a dissociative subtype. Am J Psychiatry. 2010;167(6):640–7.

Lapomarda G, Grecucci A, Messina I, Pappaianni E, Dadomo H. Common and different gray and white matter alterations in bipolar and borderline personality disorder: a source-based morphometry study. Brain Res. 2021;1762:147401.

Layne CM, Greeson JK, Ostrowski SA, Kim S, Reading S, Vivrette RL, Briggs EC, Fairbank JA, Pynoos RS. Cumulative trauma exposure and high risk behavior in adolescence: findings from the National Child Traumatic Stress Network Core Data set. Psychol Trauma Theory Res Pract Policy. 2014;6(S1):S40.

Lee J, Choi H. ICD-11 complex posttraumatic stress disorder and subclasses of borderline personality disorder in a South Korean adult population with childhood abuse experiences: a latent class analysis. Borderline Personal Disord Emot Dysregul. 2023;10(1):36.

Leeb RT. Child maltreatment surveillance: uniform definitions for public health and recommended data elements. Centers for Disease Control and Prevention, National Center for Injury Prevention and Control; 2008.

Lieb K, Zanarini MC, Schmahl C, Linehan MM, Bohus M. Borderline personality disorder. Lancet. 2004;364(9432):453–61.

Linehan M. Cognitive–behavioral treatment of borderline personality disorder. New York: Guilford Press; 1993.

Liu J, Wang L, Sun J, Liu G, Yan W, Xi B, Xiong F, Ding W, Huang G, Heymsfield S, Mi J. Bone mineral density reference standards for Chinese children aged 3–18: cross-sectional results of the 2013–2015 China Child and Adolescent Cardiovascular Health (CCACH) study. BMJ Open. 2018;7(5):e014542.

Liu Y, Li B, Hao F, Wang B, Zhu J, Liu D, Zhai J, Chen M, Wang J. Associations between borderline personality disorder features and the risk of first onset major depressive disorder: findings from a 2-year longitudinal study in a sample of first-year university students in China. J Affect Disord. 2021;295:5–10.

Liu Z, Yang K, Xie Q, Zhang T, Ananiadou S. Emollms: a series of emotional large language models and annotation tools for comprehensive affective analysis. In: In proceedings of the 30th ACM SIGKDD conference on knowledge discovery and data mining; 2024. p. 5487–96.

Lobbestael J, Arntz A. Emotional, cognitive and physiological correlates of abuse-related stress in borderline and antisocial personality disorder. Behav Res Ther. 2010;48(2):116–24.

Löffler A, Foell J, Bekrater-Bodmann R. Interoception and its interaction with self, other, and emotion processing: implications for the understanding of psychosocial deficits in borderline personality disorder. Curr Psychiatry Rep. 2018;20:1–9.

Löffler A, Kleindienst N, Neukel C, Bekrater-Bodmann R, Flor H. Pleasant touch perception in borderline personality disorder and its relationship with disturbed body representation. Borderline Personal Disord Emot Dysregul. 2022;9(1):3.

Lovis-Schmidt A, Bilz L, Pahlke K, Rindermann H. Physical health complaints in adolescents. Eur J Health Psychol. 2022a;29:121.

Lovis-Schmidt A, Schilling J, Pudschun C, Rindermann H. Adverse childhood experiences and physical diseases in adulthood: a summary of meta-analyses. 2022b;30:164.

Low LA, Schweinhardt P. Early life adversity as a risk factor for fibromyalgia in later life. Pain Res Treat. 2012;2012(1):140832.

Madge N, Hawton K, McMahon EM, Corcoran P, De Leo D, De Wilde EJ, Fekete S, van Heeringen K, Ystgaard M, Arensman E. Psychological characteristics, stressful life events and deliberate self-harm: findings from the Child & Adolescent Self-harm in Europe (CASE) study. Eur Child Adolesc Psychiatry. 2011;20(10):499–508.

Mainali P, Rai T, Rutkofsky IH. From child abuse to developing borderline personality disorder into adulthood: exploring the neuromorphological and epigenetic pathway. Cureus. 2020;12(7):e9474.

Mansueto G, Cavallo C, Palmieri S, Ruggiero GM, Sassaroli S, Caselli G. Adverse childhood experiences and repetitive negative thinking in adulthood: a systematic review. Clin Psychol Psychother. 2021;28(3):557–68.

Marques-Feixa L, Moya-Higueras J, Romero S, Santamarina-Pérez P, Rapado-Castro M, Zorrilla I, Martín M, Anglada E, Lobato MJ, Ramírez M, Moreno N. Risk of suicidal behavior in children and adolescents exposed to maltreatment: the mediating role of borderline personality traits and recent stressful life events. J Clin Med. 2021;10(22):5293.

Marques-Feixa L, Moya-Higueras J, Romero S, Santamarina-Pérez P, San Martín-Gonzalez N, Mas A, Rapado-Castro M, Blasco-Fontecilla H, Zorrilla I, Forner-Puntonet M, Anglada E. Complex post-traumatic stress disorder (CPTSD) of ICD-11 in youths with childhood maltreatment: associations with age of exposure and clinical outcomes. J Affect Disord. 2023;332:92–104.

Marshall CA, Jomeen J, Huang C, Martin CR. The relationship between maternal personality disorder and early birth outcomes: a systematic review and meta-analysis. Int J Environ Res Public Health. 2020;17(16):5778.

Martín-Blanco A, Ancochea A, Soler J, Elices M, Carmona C, Pascual JC. Changes over the last 15 years in the psychopharmacological management of persons with borderline personality disorder. Acta Psychiatr Scand. 2017;136(3):323–31.

Martin-Gagnon G, Normandin L, Fonagy P, Ensink K. Adolescent mentalizing and childhood emotional abuse: implications for depression, anxiety, and borderline personality disorder features. Front Psychol. 2023;14:1237735.

Mathur A, Graham-Engeland JE, Slavish DC, Smyth JM, Lipton RB, Katz MJ, Sliwinski MJ. Recalled early life adversity and pain: the role of mood, sleep, optimism, and control. J Behav Med. 2018;41:504–15.

Matjasko JL, Herbst JH, Estefan LF. Preventing adverse childhood experiences: the role of etiological, evaluation, and implementation research. Am J Prev Med. 2022;62(6):S6–15.

McLaughlin KA, Hatzenbuehler ML, Hilt LM. Emotion dysregulation as a mechanism linking peer victimization to internalizing symptoms in adolescents. J Consult Clin Psychol. 2009;77(5):894.

McLaughlin KA, Green JG, Gruber MJ, Sampson NA, Zaslavsky AM, Kessler RC. Childhood adversities and first onset of psychiatric disorders in a national sample of US adolescents. Arch Gen Psychiatry. 2012;69(11):1151–60.

McLaughlin KA, Peverill M, Gold AL, Alves S, Sheridan MA. Child maltreatment and neural systems underlying emotion regulation. J Am Acad Child Adolesc Psychiatry. 2015;54(9):753–62.

McLaughlin KA, Sheridan MA, Nelson CA. Neglect as a violation of species-expectant experience: neurodevelopmental consequences. Biol Psychiatry. 2017;82(7):462–71.
Mehta D, Kelly AB, Laurens KR, Haslam D, Williams KE, Walsh K, Baker PR, Carter HE, Khawaja NG, Zelenko O, Mathews B. Child maltreatment and long-term physical and mental health outcomes: an exploration of biopsychosocial determinants and implications for prevention. Child Psychiatry Hum Dev. 2021;29:1–5.
Mello MF, Faria AA, Mello AF, Carpenter LL, Tyrka AR, Price LH. Childhood maltreatment and adult psychopathology: pathways to hypothalamic-pituitary-adrenal axis dysfunction. Braz J Psychiatry. 2009;31:S41–8.
Mersky JP, Janczewski CE, Topitzes J. Rethinking the measurement of adversity: moving toward second-generation research on adverse childhood experiences. Child Maltreat. 2017;22:58–68.
Merrick MT, Ford DC, Haegerich TM, Simon T. Adverse childhood experiences increase risk for prescription opioid misuse. J Prim Prev. 2020a;41(2):139–52.
Merrick JS, Narayan AJ, Atzl VM, Harris WW, Lieberman AF. Type versus timing of adverse and benevolent childhood experiences for pregnant women's psychological and reproductive health. Child Youth Serv Rev. 2020b;114:105056.
Metzler M, Merrick MT, Klevens J, Ports KA, Ford DC. Adverse childhood experiences and life opportunities: shifting the narrative. Child Youth Serv Rev. 2017;72:141–9.
Minzenberg MJ, Fan J, New AS, Tang CY, Siever LJ. Frontolimbic structural changes in borderline personality disorder. J Psychiatr Res. 2008;42(9):727–33.
Mortensen JA, Rasmussen LA, Håberg A. Trait impulsivity in female patients with borderline personality disorder and matched controls. Acta Neuropsych. 2010;22(3):139–49.
Morgan CH, Pu DF, Rodriguez CM. Parenting style history in predicting harsh parenting and child abuse risk across the transition to parenthood: role of gender. Child Abuse Negl. 2022;127:105587.
Muehlenkamp JJ, Tillotson V. Overview and Epidemiology of NSSI in Clinical Samples. 2023.
Muehlenkamp JJ, Brausch AM, Washburn JJ. How much is enough? Examining frequency criteria for NSSI disorder in adolescent inpatients. J Consult Clin Psychol. 2017;85(6):611.
Muehlenkamp JJ, Kerr PL, Bradley AR, Larsen MA. Abuse subtypes and nonsuicidal self-injury: preliminary evidence of complex emotion regulation patterns. J Nerv Ment Dis. 2010;198(4):258–63.
Muehlenkamp JJ, Claes L, Havertape L, Plener PL. International prevalence of adolescent nonsuicidal self-injury and deliberate self-harm. Child Adolesc Psychiatry Ment Health. 2012;6:1–9.
Mueller-Pfeiffer C, Schumacher S, Martin-Soelch C, Pazhenkottil AP, Wirtz G, Fuhrhans C, Hindermann E, Assaloni H, Briner DP, Rufer M. The validity and reliability of the German version of the Somatoform Dissociation Questionnaire (SDQ-20). J Trauma Dissociation. 2010;11(3):337–57.
Mueller-Pfeiffer C, Rufibach K, Wyss D, Perron N, Pitman RK, Rufer M. Screening for dissociative disorders in psychiatric out-and day care-patients. J Psychopathol Behav Assess. 2013;35:592–602.
Narita Z, Stickley A, DeVylder J. Loneliness and psychotic experiences in a general population sample. Schizophr Res. 2020;218:146–50.
Nederlof E, Van der Ham JM, Dingemans PM, Oei TI. The relation between dimensions of normal and pathological personality and childhood maltreatment in incarcerated boys. J Personal Disord. 2010a;24(6):746–62.
Nederlof E, van der Ham A, Dingemans P, Oei K. The relation between dimensions of personality and personality pathology and offence type and severity in juvenile delinquents. J Forensic Psychiatry Psychol. 2010b;21(5):711–20.
Nock MK. Why do people hurt themselves? New insights into the nature and functions of self-injury. Curr Dir Psychol Sci. 2009;18(2):78–83.
Nock MK, Prinstein MJ. A functional approach to the assessment of self-mutilative behavior. J Consult Clin Psychol. 2004;72(5):885.

Nock MK, Hwang I, Sampson NA, Kessler RC. Mental disorders, comorbidity and suicidal behavior: results from the National Comorbidity Survey Replication. Mol Psychiatry. 2010;15(8):868–76.

Norman TR. Pharmacotherapy for mood and anxiety disorders. In: Mental health and illness of the elderly. Springer Science + Business Media; 2017. p. 427.

Oswald SH, Heil K, Goldbeck L. History of maltreatment and mental health problems in foster children: a review of the literature. J Pediatr Psychol. 2010;35(5):462–72.

Oswald LM, Wand GS, Kuwabara H, Wong DF, Zhu S, Brasic JR. History of childhood adversity is positively associated with ventral striatal dopamine responses to amphetamine. Psychopharmacology. 2014;231:2417–33.

Palusci VJ. Fatal child abuse. J Pain Manag. 2022;15(1):41.

Peh CX, Shahwan S, Fauziana R, Mahesh MV, Sambasivam R, Zhang Y, Ong SH, Chong SA, Subramaniam M. Emotion dysregulation as a mechanism linking child maltreatment exposure and self-harm behaviors in adolescents. Child Abuse Negl. 2017;67:383–90.

Pietrek C, Elbert T, Weierstall R, Müller O, Rockstroh B. Childhood adversities in relation to psychiatric disorders. Psychiatry Res. 2013;206(1):103–10.

Pompili M, Innamorati M, Lamis DA, Erbuto D, Venturini P, Ricci F, Serafini G, Amore M, Girardi P. The associations among childhood maltreatment,"male depression" and suicide risk in psychiatric patients. Psychiatry Res. 2014;220(1–2):571–8.

Porter C, Palmier-Claus J, Branitsky A, Mansell W, Warwick H, Varese F. Childhood adversity and borderline personality disorder: a meta-analysis. Acta Psychiatr Scand. 2020;141(1):6–20.

Ports KA, Ford DC, Merrick MT. Adverse childhood experiences and sexual victimization in adulthood. Child Abuse Negl. 2016;51:313–22.

Prokopez CR, Vallejos M, Farinola R, Alberio G, Caporusso GB, Cozzarin LG, Chiapella LC, Fuentes P, Daray FM. The history of multiple adverse childhood experiences in patients with schizophrenia is associated with more severe symptomatology and suicidal behavior with gender-specific characteristics. Psychiatry Res. 2020;293:113411.

Quek J, Newman LK, Bennett C, Gordon MS, Saeedi N, Melvin GA. Reflective function mediates the relationship between emotional maltreatment and borderline pathology in adolescents: a preliminary investigation. Child Abuse Negl. 2017;72:215–26.

Quenneville AF, Kalogeropoulou E, Küng AL, Hasler R, Nicastro R, Prada P, Perroud N. Childhood maltreatment, anxiety disorders and outcome in borderline personality disorder. Psychiatry Res. 2020;284:112688.

Rajan G, Syding S, Ljunggren G, Wändell P, Wahlström L, Philips B, Svedin CG, Carlsson AC. Health care consumption and psychiatric diagnoses among adolescent girls 1 and 2 years after a first-time registered child sexual abuse experience: a cohort study in the Stockholm region. Eur Child Adolesc Psychiatry. 2021;30:1803–11.

Raposo SM, Mackenzie CS, Henriksen CA, Afifi TO. Time does not heal all wounds: older adults who experienced childhood adversities have higher odds of mood, anxiety, and personality disorders. Am J Geriatr Psychiatry. 2014;22(11):1241–50.

Redfield RR. CDC. Antibiotic resistant threats in the United States. Atlanta: US Department of Health and Human Services US Centers for Disease Control and Prevention; 2019.

Reyes ME, Davis RD, Rojales AM, Zamora CP, Germodo DF, Lanuza LR, Manahan AN. Adverse childhood experiences and nonsuicidal self-injury as mediated by pathological personality traits. Suicidol Online. 2019a;10:9.

Reyes NM, Pickard K, Reaven J. Emotion regulation: a treatment target for autism spectrum disorder. Bull Menn Clin. 2019b;83(3):205–34.

Reyes CB, Randell H. Household shocks and adolescent well-being in Peru. Popul Res Policy Rev. 2023;42(3):44.

Reyes DR, Jocson RM, Alampay LP, Mamauag BL, Reyes JC, Lachman JM. Evaluation of a brief online parenting training for community service providers in The Philippines. Child Youth Serv Rev. 2024;161:107664.

Rey-Salmon C, De Boissieu P, Teglas JP, Adamsbaum C. Abusive head trauma in day care centers. Pediatrics. 2020;146(6):e2020013771.

Robin M, Belbèze J, Pham-Scottez A, Speranza M, Shadili G, Silva J, Corcos M. Adversity, attachment and emotion recognition in BPD adolescents: the distinct roles of disengaged and controlling environment. BMC Psychol. 2022;10(1):89.
Ross N, Gilbert R, Torres S, Dugas K, Jefferies P, McDonald S, Savage S, Ungar M. Adverse childhood experiences: assessing the impact on physical and psychosocial health in adulthood and the mitigating role of resilience. Child Abuse Negl. 2020;103:104440.
Rogosch FA, Cicchetti D. Child maltreatment, attention networks, and potential precursors to borderline personality disorder. Dev Psychopathol. 2005;17(4):1071–89.
Sahle BW, Reavley NJ, Li W, Morgan AJ, Yap MB, Reupert A, Jorm AF. The association between adverse childhood experiences and common mental disorders and suicidality: an umbrella review of systematic reviews and meta-analyses. Eur Child Adolesc Psychiatry. 2021;27:1–1.
Sansone RA, Sansone LA. Gender patterns in borderline personality disorder. Innov Clin Neurosci. 2011;8(5):16.
Scheffers F, van Vugt E, Moonen X. Resilience in the face of adversity in adults with an intellectual disability: a literature review. J Appl Res Intellect Disabil. 2020;33(5):828–38.
Schneider FD, Loveland Cook CA, Salas J, Scherrer J, Cleveland IN, Burge SK, Residency Research Network of Texas Investigators. Childhood trauma, social networks, and the mental. 2020.
Schlensog-Schuster F, Keil J, Von Klitzing K, Gniewosz G, Schulz CC, Schlesier-Michel A, Mayer S, Stadelmann S, Döhnert M, Klein AM, Sierau S. From maltreatment to psychiatric disorders in childhood and adolescence: the relevance of emotional maltreatment. Child Maltreat. 2024;29(1):142–54.
Schmitz M, Bertsch K, Löffler A, Steinmann S, Herpertz SC, Bekrater-Bodmann R. Body connection mediates the relationship between traumatic childhood experiences and impaired emotion regulation in borderline personality disorder. Borderline Personal Disord Emot Dysregul. 2021;8(1):17.
Schulze A, Streit F, Zillich L, Awasthi S, Hall AS, Jungkunz M, Kleindienst N, Frank J, Schwarze CE, Dahmen N, Schott BH. Evidence for a shared genetic contribution to loneliness and borderline personality disorder. Transl Psychiatry. 2023;13(1):398.
Schweizer S, Satpute AB, Atzil S, Field AP, Hitchcock C, Black M, Barrett LF, Dalgleish T. The impact of affective information on working memory: a pair of meta-analytic reviews of behavioral and neuroimaging evidence. Psychol Bull. 2019;145(6):566.
Selby EA, Yen S. Six-month trajectory of suicidal ideation in adolescents with borderline personality disorder. Suicide Life Threat Behav. 2014;44(1):89–100.
Shaffer F, Ginsberg JP. An overview of heart rate variability metrics and norms. Front Public Health. 2017;5:290215.
Shahabi M, Hasani J, Bjureberg J. Psychometric properties of the brief persian version of the Difficulties in Emotion Regulation Scale (the DERS-16). Assess Eff Interv. 2020;45(2):135–43.
Shonkoff JP, Garner AS, Committee on Psychosocial Aspects of Child and Family Health, Committee on Early Childhood, Adoption, and Dependent Care, and Section on Developmental and Behavioral Pediatrics, Siegel BS, Dobbins MI, Earls MF, Garner AS, McGuinn L, Pascoe J, Wood DL. The lifelong effects of early childhood adversity and toxic stress. Pediatrics. 2012;129(1):e232–46.
Skoglund C, Tiger A, Rück C, Petrovic P, Asherson P, Hellner C, Mataix-Cols D, Kuja-Halkola R. Familial risk and heritability of diagnosed borderline personality disorder: a register study of the Swedish population. Mol Psychiatry. 2021;26(3):999–1008.
Soloff PH, Lynch KG, Kelly TM. Childhood abuse as a risk factor for suicidal behavior in borderline personality disorder. J Personal Disord. 2002;16(3):201–14.
Spiegel D, Loewenstein RJ, Lewis-Fernández R, Sar V, Simeon D, Vermetten E, Cardeña E, Dell PF. Dissociative disorders in DSM-5. Depress Anxiety. 2011;28(12):E17–45.
Stagaki M, Nolte T, Feigenbaum J, King-Casas B, Lohrenz T, Fonagy P, Montague PR, Personality and Mood Disorder Research Consortium. The mediating role of attachment and mentalising in the relationship between childhood maltreatment, self-harm and suicidality. Child Abuse Negl. 2022;128:105576.

Stapp EK, Mendelson T, Merikangas KR, Wilcox HC. Parental bipolar disorder, family environment, and offspring psychiatric disorders: a systematic review. J Affect Disord. 2020;268:69–81.
Steenkamp L, Weijers J, Gerrmann J, Eurelings-Bontekoe E, Selten JP. The relationship between childhood abuse and severity of psychosis is mediated by loneliness: an experience sampling study. Schizophr Res. 2022;241:306–11.
Stein DJ, Fernandes Medeiros L, Caumo W, Torres IL. Transcranial direct current stimulation in patients with anxiety: current perspectives. Neuropsychiatr Dis Treat. 2020;14:161–9.
Stepp SD, Lazarus SA, Byrd AL. A systematic review of risk factors prospectively associated with borderline personality disorder: taking stock and moving forward. Personal Disord Theory Res Treat. 2015;7(4):316.
Stepp SD, Scott LN, Jones NP, Whalen DJ, Hipwell AE. Negative emotional reactivity as a marker of vulnerability in the development of borderline personality disorder symptoms. Dev Psychopathol. 2016a;28(1):213–24.
Stepp SD, Lazarus SA, Byrd AL. A systematic review of risk factors prospectively associated with borderline personality disorder: taking stock and moving forward. Personal Disord Theory Res Treat. 2016b;7(4):316.
Stoltenborgh M, Van Ijzendoorn MH, Euser EM, Bakermans-Kranenburg MJ. A global perspective on child sexual abuse: meta-analysis of prevalence around the world. Child Maltreat. 2011;16(2):79–101.
Stoltenborgh M, Bakermans-Kranenburg MJ, Van Ijzendoorn MH. The neglect of child neglect: a meta-analytic review of the prevalence of neglect. Soc Psychiatry Psychiatr Epidemiol. 2013;48:345–55.
Stoltenborgh M, Bakermans-Kranenburg MJ, Alink LR, van IJzendoorn MH. The prevalence of child maltreatment across the globe: review of a series of meta-analyses. Child Abuse Rev. 2015;24(1):37–50.
Struck N, Krug A, Yuksel D, Stein F, Schmitt S, Meller T, Brosch K, Dannlowski U, Nenadić I, Kircher T, Brakemeier EL. Childhood maltreatment and adult mental disorders–the prevalence of different types of maltreatment and associations with age of onset and severity of symptoms. Psychiatry Res. 2020a;293:113398.
Struck N, Krug A, Feldmann M, Yuksel D, Stein F, Schmitt S, Meller T, Brosch K, Dannlowski U, Meinert S, Opel N. Attachment and social support mediate the association between childhood maltreatment and depressive symptoms. J Affect Disord. 2020b;273:310–7.
Swannell S, Martin G, Page A, Hasking P, Hazell P, Taylor A, Protani M. Child maltreatment, subsequent nonsuicidal self-injury and the mediating roles of dissociation, alexithymia and self-blame. Child Abuse Negl. 2012;36(7–8):572–84.
Swenson CC, Schaeffer CM. A multisystemic approach to the prevention and treatment of child abuse and neglect. Int J Child Maltreat: Res Policy Pract. 2018;1(1):97–120.
Tae H, Chae JH. Factors related to suicide attempts: the roles of childhood abuse and spirituality. Front Psych. 2021;12:565358.
Tanaka M, Georgiades K, Boyle MH, MacMillan HL. Child maltreatment and educational attainment in young adulthood: results from the Ontario Child Health Study. J Interpers Violence. 2015;30(2):195–214.
Tatnell R, Hasking P, Newman L, Taffe J, Martin G. Attachment, emotion regulation, childhood abuse and assault: examining predictors of NSSI among adolescents. Arch Suicide Res. 2017;21(4):610–20.
Temes CM, Magni LR, Fitzmaurice GM, Aguirre BA, Goodman M, Zanarini MC. Prevalence and severity of childhood adversity in adolescents with BPD, psychiatrically healthy adolescents, and adults with BPD. Personal Ment Health. 2017;11(3):171–8.
Temes CM, Magni LR, Aguirre BA, Goodman M, Ridolfi ME, Zanarini MC. Parameters of reported childhood sexual abuse and assault in adolescents and adults with borderline personality disorder. Personal Ment Health. 2020;14(3):254–62.
Thompson MP, Kingree JB, Lamis D. Associations of adverse childhood experiences and suicidal behaviors in adulthood in a US nationally representative sample. Child Care Health Dev. 2019;45(1):121–8.

Thornberry TP, Henry KL, Ireland TO, Smith CA. The causal impact of childhood-limited maltreatment and adolescent maltreatment on early adult adjustment. J Adolesc Health. 2010;46(4):359–65.
Titelius EN, Cook E, Spas J, Orchowski L, Kivisto K, O'Brien K, Frazier E, Wolff JC, Dickstein DP, Kim KL, Seymour KE. Emotion dysregulation mediates the relationship between child maltreatment and nonsuicidal self-injury. J Aggress Maltreat Trauma. 2018;27(3):323–31.
Tobin J, Cashmore J. Thirty years of the CRC: child protection progress, challenges and opportunities. Child Abuse Negl. 2020;110:104436.
Toth SL, Manly JT. Developmental consequences of child abuse and neglect: implications for intervention. Child Dev Perspect. 2019;13(1):59–64.
Trickett PK, Negriff S, Ji J, Peckins M. Child maltreatment and adolescent development. J Res Adolesc. 2011;21(1):3–20.
Trull TJ, Solhan MB, Tragesser SL, Jahng S, Wood PK, Piasecki TM, Watson D. Affective instability: measuring a core feature of borderline personality disorder with ecological momentary assessment. J Abnorm Psychol. 2008;117(3):647.
Turner S, Taillieu T, Carleton RN, Sareen J, Afifi TO. Association between a history of child abuse and suicidal ideation, plans and attempts among Canadian public safety personnel: a cross-sectional survey. Canadian Med Assoc Open Access J. 2018;6(4):E463–70.
Turner HA. Collecting child victimization information from youth and parents: ethical and methodological considerations. In: Handbook of interpersonal violence and abuse across the lifespan: a project of the National Partnership to End Interpersonal Violence across the lifespan (NPEIV); 2021. p. 1851–79.
Trygg NF, Månsdotter A, Gustafsson PE. Intersectional inequalities in mental health across multiple dimensions of inequality in the Swedish adult population. Soc Sci Med. 2021;283:114184.
Turecki G, Ota VK, Belangero SI, Jackowski A, Kaufman J. Early life adversity, genomic plasticity, and psychopathology. Lancet Psychiatry. 2014;1(6):461–6.
Turner S, Menzies C, Fortier J, Garces I, Struck S, Taillieu T, Georgiades K, Afifi TO. Child maltreatment and sleep problems among adolescents in Ontario: a cross sectional study. Child Abuse Negl. 2020;99:104309.
Turniansky H, Ben-Dor D, Krivoy A, Weizman A, Shoval G. A history of prolonged childhood sexual abuse is associated with more severe clinical presentation of borderline personality disorder in adolescent female inpatients–a naturalistic study. Child Abuse Negl. 2019;98:104222.
Tyrka AR, Wyche MC, Kelly MM, Price LH, Carpenter LL. Childhood maltreatment and adult personality disorder symptoms: influence of maltreatment type. Psychiatry Res. 2009;165(3):281–7.
Tzouvara V, Kupdere P, Wilson K, Matthews L, Simpson A, Foye U. Adverse childhood experiences, mental health, and social functioning: a scoping review of the literature. Child Abuse Negl. 2023;139:106092.
van Alebeek A, van der Heijden PT, Hessels C, Thong MS, van Aken M. Comparison of three questionnaires to screen for borderline personality disorder in adolescents and young adults. Eur J Psychol Assess. 2015;33:123.
Venta A, Sharp C, Hart J. The relation between anxiety disorder and experiential avoidance in inpatient adolescents. Psychol Assess. 2012;24(1):240.
Vestergaard M, Kongerslev MT, Thomsen MS, Mathiesen BB, Harmer CJ, Simonsen E, Miskowiak KW. Women with borderline personality disorder show reduced identification of emotional facial expressions and a heightened negativity bias. J Personal Disord. 2020;34(5):677–98.
Vial A, Assink M, Stams GJ, Van der Put C. Child safety assessment: do instrument-based decisions concur with decisions of expert panels? Soc Sci. 2021;10(5):167.
Vonderlin R, Kleindienst N, Alpers GW, Bohus M, Lyssenko L, Schmahl C. Dissociation in victims of childhood abuse or neglect: a meta-analytic review. Psychol Med. 2018;48(15):2467–76.
Walsh D, McCartney G, Smith M, Armour G. Relationship between childhood socioeconomic position and adverse childhood experiences (ACEs): a systematic review. J Epidemiol Community Health. 2019;73(12):1087–93.
Wan Y, Chen J, Sun Y, Tao F. Impact of childhood abuse on the risk of nonsuicidal self-injury in mainland Chinese adolescents. PLoS One. 2015;10(6):e0131239.

Wan G, Wang M, Chen S. Child abuse in ethnic regions: evidence from 2899 girls in Southwest China. Child Youth Serv Rev. 2019;105:104457.

Wang S, Xu H, Zhang S, Yang R, Li D, Sun Y, Wan Y, Tao F. Linking childhood maltreatment and psychological symptoms: the role of social support, coping styles, and self-esteem in adolescents. J Interpers Violence. 2022;37(1-2):NP620-50.

Wang G, Zhang Y, Zhao J, Zhang J, Jiang F. Mitigate the effects of home confinement on children during the COVID-19 outbreak. Lancet. 2020;395(10228):945–7.

Waxman R, Fenton MC, Skodol AE, Grant BF, Hasin D. Childhood maltreatment and personality disorders in the USA: specificity of effects and the impact of gender. Personal Ment Health. 2014;8(1):30–41.

White OG, Hindley N, Jones DP. Risk factors for child maltreatment recurrence: an updated systematic review. Med Sci Law. 2015;55(4):259–77.

Widom CS, Czaja SJ, Kozakowski SS, Chauhan P. Does adult attachment style mediate the relationship between childhood maltreatment and mental and physical health outcomes? Child Abuse Negl. 2018;76:533–45.

Winsper C, Zanarini M, Wolke D. Prospective study of family adversity and maladaptive parenting in childhood and borderline personality disorder symptoms in a non-clinical population at 11 years. Psychol Med. 2012;42(11):2405–20.

Winter SM, Dittrich K, Dörr P, Overfeld J, Moebus I, Murray E, Karaboycheva G, Zimmermann C, Knop A, Voelkle M, Entringer S. Immediate impact of child maltreatment on mental, developmental, and physical health trajectories. J Child Psychol Psychiatry. 2022;63(9):1027–45.

Wolf JP, Baiocchi A, Argüello T. Child maltreatment reporting in the general population: examining the roles of community, collective efficacy, and adverse childhood experiences. Child Abuse Negl. 2018;82:201–9.

Wolfe VV, Kelly BM. Child maltreatment, 2018.

Wolfe VV, Kelly BM. Child maltreatment, 2019.

Wong SY, Zhang D, Sit RW, Yip BH, Chung RY, Wong CK, Chan DC, Sun W, Kwok KO, Mercer SW. Impact of COVID-19 on loneliness, mental health, and health service utilisation: a prospective cohort study of older adults with multimorbidity in primary care. Br J Gen Pract. 2020;70(700):e817–24.

Wota AP, Byrne C, Murray I, Ofuafor T, Nisar Z, Neuner F, Hallahan BP. An examination of childhood trauma in individuals attending an adult mental health service. Ir J Psychol Med. 2014;31(4):259–70.

World Health Organization. Report of the consultation on child abuse prevention, 29–31 March 1999, WHO. Geneva: World Health Organization; 1999.

World Health Organization, 2012.

White K, Barnett J, Hill M. Religion medicine and deviance-child abuse and the social structure. Int Rev Sociol. 1993;4(3):144–66.

Wu Y, Zheng Y, Wang J, Zhang T. Specific type of childhood trauma and borderline personality disorder in Chinese patients. Front Psych. 2022;13:936739.

Wu J, Liu S, Luo J, Li X, You J. The effects of childhood abuse, depression, and self-compassion on adolescent nonsuicidal self-injury: a moderated mediation model. Child Abuse Negl. 2023a;136:105993.

Wu AD, Gao M, Aveyard P, Taylor G. Smoking cessation and changes in anxiety and depression in adults with and without psychiatric disorders. JAMA Netw Open. 2023b;6(5):e2316111.

Xie GD, Chang JJ, Yuan MY, Wang GF, He Y, Chen SS, Su PY. Childhood abuse and borderline personality disorder features in Chinese undergraduates: the role of self-esteem and resilience. BMC Psychiatry. 2021;21:1–9.

You JS, Lee CW, Park JY, Jang Y, Yu H, Yoon J, Kwon SS, Oh S, Park YS, Ryoo HA, Lee JH. Borderline personality pathology in major depressive disorder, bipolar I and II disorder, and its relationship with childhood trauma. Psychiatry Investig. 2022;19(11):909.

Yuan Y, Lee H, Newhill CE, Eack SM, Fusco R, Scott LN. Differential associations between childhood maltreatment types and borderline personality disorder from the perspective of emotion dysregulation. Borderline Personal Disord Emot Dysregul. 2023;10(1):1–4.
Zanarini MC. Role of sexual abuse in the etiology of borderline personality disorder. American Psychiatric Pub; 1997.
Zanarini MC, Frankenburg FR, Reich DB, Marino MF, Haynes MC, Gunderson JG. Violence in the lives of adult borderline patients. J Nerv Ment Dis. 1999;187(2):65–71.
Zanarini MC, Frankenburg FR, Hennen J, Reich DB, Silk KR. Prediction of the 10-year course of borderline personality disorder. Am J Psychiatry. 2006;163(5):827–32.
Zanarini MC, Reichman CA, Frankenburg FR, Reich DB, Fitzmaurice G. The course of eating disorders in patients with borderline personality disorder: a 10-year follow-up study. Int J Eat Disord. 2010;43(3):226–32.
Zanarini MC, Frankenburg FR, Reich DB, Fitzmaurice G, Weinberg I, Gunderson JG. The 10-year course of physically self-destructive acts reported by borderline patients and axis II comparison subjects. Acta Psychiatr Scand. 2008;117(3):177–84.
Zanarini MC, Wedig MM. Childhood adversity and the development of borderline personality disorder. In: Handbook of borderline personality disorder in children and adolescents. New York: Springer New York; 2014. p. 265–76.
Zanarini MC, Gunderson JG, Marino MF, Schwartz EO, Frankenburg FR. Childhood experiences of borderline patients. Compr Psychiatry. 1989;30(1):18–25.
Zanarini MC, Frankenburg FR, Reich DB, Conkey LC, Fitzmaurice GM. Treatment rates for patients with borderline personality disorder and other personality disorders: a 16-year study. Psychiatr Serv. 2015;66(1):15–20.
Zatti C, Rosa V, Barros A, Valdivia L, Calegaro VC, Freitas LH, Ceresér KM, da Rocha NS, Bastos AG, Schuch FB. Childhood trauma and suicide attempt: a meta-analysis of longitudinal studies from the last decade. Psychiatry Res. 2017;256:353–8.
Zhang L, Simmel C, Nepomnyaschy L. Income inequality and child maltreatment rates in US counties, 2009–2018. Child Abuse Negl. 2021;130:105328.
Zhang Z, Xu Y, Wang Y, Yao B, Ritchie D, Wu T, Yu M, Wang D, Li TJ. Storybuddy: a human-ai collaborative chatbot for parent-child interactive storytelling with flexible parental involvement. In: Proceedings of the 2022 CHI conference on human factors in computing systems; 2022, Apr 29. p. 1–21.
Zimmerman M, Mattia JI. Axis I diagnostic comorbidity and borderline personality disorder. Compr Psychiatry. 1999;40(4):245–52.
Zimmerman M, Chelminski I, Young D, Dalrymple K, Martinez J. Is dimensional scoring of borderline personality disorder important only for subthreshold levels of severity? J Personal Disord. 2013;27(2):244–51.

Chapter 5
Emotion Regulation and Dysregulation in Borderline Personality Disorder

Introduction

Borderline personality disorder (BPD) is a severely persistent impairing mental state characterized by intensely pervasive emotional dysregulation, as well as dysregulation of behavior and cognition, and considerably unstable interpersonal relationships (Crowell et al. 2009; O'Grady and Hinshaw 2023; Selby et al. 2009). Numerous theoretical perspectives have suggested that BPD is a pervasive personality disorder of different emotional issues (e.g., Selby and Joiner Jr 2009; Linehan 1993; Bradley et al. 2005). The core features of BPD are affective instability due to a marked reactivity of mood and inappropriate, intense anger or difficulty controlling anger (American Psychiatric Association 2022). Moreover, other BPD criteria, such as self-destructive behaviors and self-inflicted behaviors, seem to be the result of emotional difficulties, because in accordance with investigations, it has been demonstrated that suicidal behaviors and attempts and nonsuicidal self-injury (NSSI) are frequently performed to escape and provide relief from overwhelming negative emotions (e.g., Glenn and Klonsky 2009; 2012, 2013; Kaufman et al. 2020). Also, a central theory of BPD, especially Linehan's biosocial theory (Linehan 1993), has a great emphasize on the emotional difficulties and affective issues (Glenn and Klonsky 2009). A great body of investigations has depicted that affective instability and issues in emotion regulation are presented as the core problems in individuals with BPD (e.g., Dixon-Gordon et al. 2020; Skodol et al. 2002; Mirkovic et al. 2021; Carpenter and Trull 2013). The majority of those diagnosed with BPD generally express negative emotional states, such as anger and hopelessness, often before being involved in episodes of self-destructive behaviors (Sosic-Vasic et al. 2024). Several abnormalities in emotional functioning have been presented, such as emotional and affective instability, intense and inappropriate anger, and chronic feeling of emptiness in the *Diagnostic and Statistical Manual of*

E. A. Selby, M. Salavati, *Theories of Borderline Personality Disorder*,
https://doi.org/10.1007/978-3-031-75503-3_5

Mental Disorders, fifth Edition (American Psychiatric Association 2022; Glenn and Klonsky 2009; Dixon-Gordon et al. 2020).

The term *emotion* relegates to a various lineup of phenomena (Suri and Gross 2022), and can be subtle or intense; *brief* or *extended; partially simple* or *complex; and private* or *public* (Gross 2024). Therefore, issues in the process of emotional experience can contribute to the disturbance of adaptive psychological states. When emotional regulatory processes become no longer optimal and inappropriate with the current context, emotions can be maladaptive (Heller et al. 2018). Gross (2014) defined emotion as "an astonishing array of responses, from the mild to the intense, the brief to the extended, the simple to the complex, and the private to the public" (Gross 2014, p. 4). One of the most challenging points in the emotion literature is the terminology referred to emotion-related processes, comprising affect, emotion, stress, and mood. Gross (2014) pointed out that affect is such an umbrella term for states that consist partially quick good-bad dis-circumstances. In line with this view, affective states consist of (1) emotion such as anxiety; (2) stress response to situations that exceed a person's capability to cope; and (3) moods such as depression. *Affect* refers to the experiential element of emotion, and behavioral component of emotion; *Emotion* refers to both negative unspecified affective responses, and both negative and positive affective states; and *Moods* last more than emotion and more diffuse (Gross 2014). Emotions elicit due to individual-situation transactions (Moors 2017), and include coordinated but flexible multisystem responses that alter current individual-situation transactions (Gross 2024). Gross (2015) and Gross and Ford (2024) proposed that based on cybernetic theory, emotions may be provoked through a constellation of iterative cycles encompassing four components: (1) a *situation* which may be experienced or imagined; (2) *attention* that assigns aspects of situation are perceived; (3) *evaluation* or *appraisal* of the situation associated with active objectives; (4) a *response* to the situation, comprising alterations in experience, physiology, and/or facial or whole-body behavior (Gross 2024). In line with empirical investigations, emotions comprise an integrated function consisting of appraisal and response tendencies which are automated, rapid and dynamic contributing to appropriate responses in a specified contest (Hughes et al. 2012, 2020; Cole et al. 2008, 2009; Gross 1998, 2014, 2024). Emotions constitute two integrated processes: appraisal and action readiness, which include a type of psychological sonar and a readiness system to reply. Appraisal is a process by which we can appraise and evaluate the importance of circumstances surrounding us in association with our aims for well-being. On the other hand, action readiness a biological or learned predisposition to reply in a specific manner and style which can enable us to recover and maintain our well-being. Hence, emotions structure and organize responses to understand, perceive, and facilitate awareness of circumstances (Cole et al. 2017, 2020; Lazarus 1991; Frijda 1986). Based on Gross and Ford (2014, 2024), emotion has a set of three core features. The first core feature of emotion is related to the time of occurring, *"when it occurs."* It means that emotions arise whenever an individual enters into a situation and appraise that situation as being related to a specific kind of current activity and purposes that are relevant to the achievement of a meaningful personal purpose (see, Scherer et al. 2001; Gross

2014). The underlying goals in these evaluations maybe protracted or ephemeral; conscious and complex; unconscious and simple; and highly distributed or widely personal and idiosyncratic. The second core feature of emotion is related to its *"multifaceted nature."* It means that emotions are whole-body phenomena including alterations in the experiential, behavioral, and central and peripheral physiological domains, which commence specific action tendencies (e.g., Mauss et al. 2005; Gross 2014). The third core feature is the multisystem changes related to emotion are seldom mandatory. Suri and Gross (2022) elucidate emotions as a type of valuation. Based on the valuation perspective, "emotions are a particular type of valuation that (1) have a well-specified object, (2) unfold over seconds to minutes, and (3) involve coordinated changes in subjective experience, behavior and physiology" (Barret et al. 2017). Consistent with this perspective's core features, Gross (2008) conceptualized the Modal Model of emotion.

According to the Modal Model of emotion, "emotions involve person-situation transactions that compel attention, have meaning to an individual in light of currently active goals, and give rise to coordinated yet flexible multi-system responses that modify the ongoing person-situation transaction in crucial ways" (Gross 2014, p. 5). The Modal Model of emotion proposes one approach to specify a sequence of processes to generate an emotion: situation-attention-appraisal-response sequence. In line with this model, this sequence commences through entering a situation and being exposed to relevant stimuli, external or internal. These situations are then attended to in several ways, being evaluated by individual's appraisal system to generate emotional responses including changes in experiential, behavioral, and neurological response systems.

What Is Emotion Regulation?

There are several challenges in defining emotion regulation because of its role in the development of psychopathology and the judgment about how has adaptive function in an individual. In an attempt to encapsulate the complicated nature of emotion regulation, Cole et al. (2017) conceptualized emotion regulation as alterations in initial appraisal/action readiness responses to situations that can be modified and managed by a series of processes including attentional, cognitive, social, and behavioral (Cole et al. 2017, 2020). In line with a substantial body of investigations, emotional process modifies cognitive processes such as executive function contributing to the development of a goal-directed, flexible and adaptive behavior (Diamond 2013; Zelada et al. 2023; Genet and Siemer 2011; D'Aurizio et al. 2023). Furthermore, emotional responses can be secondarily exacerbated by cognitive appraisal of environmental stimulus (Bargh and Williams 2007), which would be associated with normal daily-life functioning (D'Aurizio et al. 2023). The emotion regulation process, identification and analysis of emotional stimuli, and the consequent provoked responses have a fundamental role in human behavior (Koziol and

Budding 2009; Gross 2008, 2014; D'Aurizio et al. 2023). Emotion regulation refers to processes in which individuals utilize top-down cortical mechanisms to identify, choose, implement, and monitor the way of experiencing and expressing emotions associated to their personal goals (Beauchaine 2015; Beauchaine et al. 2017; Gross 1998; Crowell et al. 2021; Sheppes et al. 2015). Emotion regulation is almost defined as an individual process (Hughes et al. 2012), and involves awareness, evaluation, maintenance, and modulation of an individual's emotional state to achieve goal-directed behaviors (Paley and Hajal 2022). According to reviewing current literature about emotion regulations definitions, some of them will propose here. Emotion regulation is conceptualized as encompassing the (a) awareness and understanding of emotions, (b) acceptance of emotions, (c) ability to control and manage impulsive behaviors and act based on desired purposes when experiencing intensely negative emotions, and (d) ability to recruit situationally suitable emotion regulation strategies flexibly to modify emotional responses as desired to meet individual objectives situational demands (Gratz and Roemer 2004). Gross (2014) state three core features of emotion regulation: first, main feature of emotion regulation is the activation of a goal to modulate the emotion-generative process (activation of a regulatory goal); and can be *intrinsic emotion regulation* which becomes activated in individual or *extrinsic emotion regulation* contributing to the activation of a goal in another; and second, the involving of the processes which are responsible for changing the emotion trajectory (the engagement of regulatory processes) (Gross 2014). Depending on the personal goals, there is an escalation or reduction in the dormancy, rise time, expansion, duration, or offset of the emotional response (Gross 2014).

Five families of the emotion process model of emotion can be distinguished according to where these prosses have their main influence on emotion generation, which is shown in Fig. 5.1 (Gross 2024).

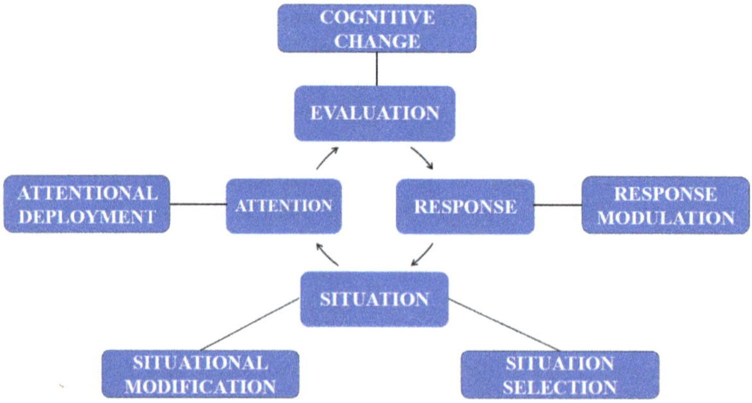

Fig. 5.1 Five families of emotion regulation strategies. (Adapted from Gross 2024)

According to the process model of emotion regulation, there are five groups of emotion regulation processes: situation selection, situation modification, attentional deployment, cognitive change, and response modulation (Gross 1998, 2014; Gross and Cassidy 2024; Tull et al. 2020; Fassbinder et al. 2016; Gross and Jazaieri 2014; Sheppes et al. 2015). *Situation selection* consists of conducting an action in a situation to raise the likelihood of an expected desire or undesirable emotions. *Situation modification* refers straightforward modification of a situation to change its emotional impact. *Attentional deployment* refers to influencing one's emotions via directing attention to a specific situation. *Cognitive change* refers to modifying the way an individual appraises a situation in order to change its emotional importance, either by altering the style of thinking about the situation or changing individual's capacity to manage the demands of situation. Response modulation happens at the end of emotion-generative process and refer to influencing experiential, behavioral, and physiological components of the emotional response (Gross 1998, 2014, 2015).

Recently, the Extended Process Model of Emotion Regulation has been introduced (Gross 2015; Sheppes et al. 2015). The new model considers emotion regulation as *meta-valuation*. According to this model, emotion regulation processes happen afterwards a generated emotion. In other words, "emotion can be thought of as a world, perception, valuation, action (W-PVA) sequence, emotion regulation may be also be conceptualized as a W-PVA sequence that takes as its input another W-PVA system, namely the one that is generating the underlying emotion". It means that the extended model has a great emphasis on subjective valuation processes, which escalate the following action processes. These actions recruited to overcome perceived inconsistencies between at the moment and desired state (Gross 2015; Sheppes et al. 2015).

Emotion regulation can be considered as skills and deficits. In their extended model of emotion regulation, Berking et al. (2008) posited that there are eight main emotion-regulation skill including the ability (1) consciously process emotions, (2) identify and label emotions, (3) interpret emotion-related sensations correctly, (4) understand the prompts of emotions, (5) accept emotions, (6) tolerate emotions, (7) confront emotionally distressing situations to attain important goals, and (8) actively modify negative emotions to feel better (e.g., Berking et al. 2008; Linehan et al. 2015; Eid et al. 2003; Mennin and Fresco 2014; Linehan et al. 2006; Berking et al. 2019). In line with the extended model of emotion regulation, Neacsiu et al. (2014) have developed a DBT extended model of emotion regulation which is adopted with Gross (2015). As mentioned in the extended model of emotion regulation, the basic emotion vulnerability factors include the effects of distal and proximal prior events, effect on situation selection, situation modification and attention deployment, and impact on the emotional responses consisting of biological/experiential, and expression/action. In other words, emotions initiate in a contextual situation, where stimuli catch an individual's attention. The stimuli are appraised and interpreted and contributed to trigger emotional responses. Then, the emotional responses are followed by aftereffects: secondary emotions (Neacsiu et al. 2014).

What Is Emotion Dysregulation?

As stated by Hofmann et al. (2014), emotional experiences are complex and may be varied according to their degree of intensity, valence, duration, complexity, controllability, and action tendency (Hofmann 2014; Barrett et al. 2001). Yet, the frequency and intensity of experiencing emotions concurrent with an inability to control and manage their occurrence can contribute to severely dysfunctional behaviors in individuals (Matusiewicz et al. 2014). When emotion dysregulation difficulties arise, an individual can feel emotionally "out of control" (e.g., Cole 2014), experience and express intense labile emotions (e.g., Crowell et al. 2021; Matusiewicz et al. 2014; Thompson 2019), have difficulty in tolerating and modulating emotional responses (e.g., Matusiewicz et al. 2014), and attempt to reduce undesirable emotions via conducting self-destructive behaviors such as self-inflicted behaviors and suicidal attempts (e.g., Gratz et al. 2014; McLaughlin et al. 2011; Wolff et al. 2019; Bookhout et al. 2017; Cavicchioli et al. 2021). According to Crowell et al. (2021), emotion dysregulation is a pattern of intense experience and expression of emotions that are severely labile and rigid, which are too prolonged and are interfered with adaptive and appropriate goal-directed behaviors and interpersonal relationships (Crowell et al. 2021; Beauchaine 2015). It has been emphasized that emotion dysregulation should not be considered only as a opposite to emotion regulation (Cole and Hall 2008; Cole and Deater-Deckard 2009; Cole et al. 2017, 2020). In line with Gross and Cassidy (2024), emotion dysregulation encompasses three ways in which emotion regulation may be deviated: emotion regulation failure, emotion mis-regulation, and emotion regulation mis-execution (Gross and Cassidy 2024). Substantial body of investigations have demonstrated that the emergence of emotion dysregulation is earlier than the starting of emotion regulation along life span (e.g., Crowell et al. 2021; Vohs and Baumeister 2016). As per Linehan (1993), the origins of issues in emotion regulation stem from the transactions and interactions between familial invalidating environment and a biological vulnerability to react emotionally (see, Linehan 1993; Yamaguchi et al. 2022). Consequently, these interactions between biological and environmental vulnerabilities might cause a heightened sensitivity to emotional stimuli and dramatical elevation in emotional intensity, and at the same time, a slow return to baseline (e.g., Glenn and Klonsky 2009; Yamaguchi et al. 2022; Linehan 1993; Crowell et al. 2009; Kuo and Linehan 2009; Dimeff et al. 2021). As mentioned, Gratz and Roemer (2004) proposed that emotion regulation includes a constellation of skills; therefore, it has been presented that emotion dysregulation involves any issues and difficulties in these mentioned emotional skills (Gratz and Roemer 2004). Emotion dysregulation implies a disintegration in the ability to employ emotion regulation strategies successfully (Daros et al. 2018, 2020). In line with a developmental viewpoint, emotion regulation is joined to emotion generation, especially early in life. Based on individuals' differences in neural functions of motivational systems, emotion dysregulation can be escalated into two pathways: (1) directly, because of temperamental variations in emotional intensity or duration, and/or (2) indirectly, as when in spite of attempts at self-regulation, distressful dates remain unchanged (Crowell et al. 2021). Cole et al. (2017)

attempted to distinguish between emotional competence, the ability to experience a full spectrum of emotions and being able to respond to other's emotional state, and emotion dysregulation (Cole et al. 2017; Thompson 2019), and accordingly, emotion dysregulation is a state of (1) any insufficient attempt to tolerate and regulate emotions; (2) disturbed appropriate behaviors due to interfering emotions; (3) inappropriate emotions based on context; and (4) sudden or blunted alterations in emotions (Cole et al. 2017).

Emotion Dysregulation and BPD

Despite numerous investigations into the features of emotion regulation and dysregulation across a wide range of mental disorders, some of the most intensive research has been done in people diagnosed with BPD (Fitzpatrick and Dixon-Gordon 2024). Numerous empirical investigations have exhibited higher levels of negative emotions in BPD in comparison to nonclinical controls and other personality disorders (Linehan 1993; Koerner and Linehan 1993; Koenigsberg et al. 2002, 2014; Reeve et al. 2010; Burton et al. 2022; Berghoff et al. 2022). The origin of studies in the field of emotion regulation and BPD is in 1947, when for the first time, Schmideberg (1947) proposed that a deteriorated affect regulation can be a core characteristic of "borderline" cases and suggested these patients suffer from emotional instability which disturb different aspects of their personality functioning (Schmideberg 1947; Putnam and Silk 2005). Difficulties in emotion regulation, inability to manage intense negative emotions, and behavioral instability are considered as core features underlying BPD (Scott et al. 2014; Carpenter and Trull 2013; Putnam and Silk 2005), and it has been frequently emphasized that there are fundamental emotion regulations problems among individuals with BPD (e.g., Linehan 1993). In many studies, BPD has been defined as an emotional disorder (e.g., Sauer-Zavala and Barlow 2014; Sauer-Zavala et al. 2019), in which frequent and intense negative emotions, extreme aversive reactions to emotional experiences, and effort to escape or avoid them (Barlow et al. 2017). According to DSM-5-TR, there are three of nine hallmark diagnostic criteria for BPD consist of "affective instability due to a marked reactivity of mood; Chronic feelings of emptiness; and, inappropriate, intense anger or difficulty controlling anger" (APA 2022, p. 753–754). Furthermore, in accordance with the *Psychodynamic Diagnostic Manual* (PDM-2, 2017), central influences of BPD encompass intense affects generally, especially rage, shame and fear in adults, and in the individual's clinical history several notably intense emotional reactivity to different environmental situations have been found (Del Corno and Plotkin 2017; Lingiardi and McWilliams 2018). This means that even psychoanalytic and psychodynamic perspective consider emotional issues as core features of BPD, consistent with the predominant cognitive behavioral view of BPD. Along these lines, affective instability was found to be a criterion to differentiate BPD patients from patients without BPD (Kröger et al. 2011). Although it has been accepted that emotion regulation/dysregulation has a key role in the development of BPD and emotion dysregulation is a core feature of BPD (e.g., Putnam and Silk 2005; Crowell et al. 2009; Glenn and Klonsky 2009; Dixon-Gordon et al. 2020, 2022), there remains a paucity of studies on the extent to which emotion dysregulation represents a general risk factor for mental health problems versus a predisposition for a specific type of psychopathology (McLaughlin et al. 2011).

In line with behavioral/biosocial models (Linehan 1993), emotion dysregulation has been considered as a core characteristic of BPD, and it has been emphasized that emotion dysregulation has a key role in the development of BPD and the severity of BPD symptoms. Biosocial theory (Linehan 1993) focuses on the deficient capacity to regulate emotion, which is due to a neurobiological predisposition that may contribute to excessively experiencing of intense and prolonged emotions. This biological predisposition and capacity deficiency can appear only when a BPD patient experiences an invalidating environment in childhood before meeting BPD diagnostic criteria. The dysregulated emotions trigger the BPD behavioral and interpersonal difficulties (e.g., Linehan 1993; Crowell et al. 2009, 2014; Matusiewicz et al. 2014; Kaufman et al. 2020; Dimeff et al. 2021; Gunderson et al. 2018; Fitzpatrick et al. 2024; Gratz et al. 2016). Linehan's biosocial theory (1993) proposes two features of emotion which are disturbed in BPD: (1) hyperintensity/reactivity and (2) poor regulation (Glenn and Klonsky 2009). Linehan (1993) focused on emotion vulnerability, which refers to the patient's experience of great vulnerability and reactivity to the environment. Moreover, it has a remarkable emphasize on self-invalidation which stems from the interaction between emotional vulnerable patients and invalidating environments. Consequently, Linehan (1993) proposes three common patterns in BPD which consist of (1) the inhibition of emotional experiences and expression; (2) a distorted sense of self as a hated disgusted self and being undeserved and disrespected; and (3) oversimplifying the current problems (Linehan 1993; McMain et al. 2001; Dixon-Gordon et al. 2017a, b, 2021, 2022). Crowell et al. (2009) suggest a developmental biosocial model to emphasize on the role of emotional dysregulation and impulsivity as core factors to the development of BPD (Crowell et al. 2009). An investigation done to support Linehan's biosocial theory in a nonclinical sample showed that emotional vulnerability and emotional dysregulation were uniquely associated with BPD symptoms, and emotion dysregulation mediated the relation between emotional vulnerability and BPD (Reeve et al. 2010).

Individuals with BPD recruit less effective emotion regulation strategies (Daros et al. 2018, 2020; Kuo et al. 2016). Emotional vulnerability in individuals with BPD is displayed by an escalated sensitivity to emotional stimuli, inappropriate emotional intensity, and a slow return to baseline. As well as, emotional identification, expression, and inhibition are problematic and disturbed in BPD patients (Linehan 1993; Svaldi et al. 2012; Eddie et al. 2018). Zanarini et al. (2004) found emotion dysregulation is a core feature in 90% of patients who meet BPD diagnostic criteria (Zanarini et al. 2004). Gratz and Roemer (2004) conceptualized a model of six elements of emotion regulation including emotional awareness, emotional clarity, acceptance of one's perceived as effective, impulse control experiencing negative affect, and the ability to perform goal-directed behavior when experiencing negative emotion (Gratz and Roemer 2004). Experimental and psychophysiological studies using ecological momentary paradigms showed mixed results (Fitzpatrick et al. 2024). Although it has been shown that BPD patients are inclined to apply more maladaptive emotion regulation strategies in daily life, such suppression, rumination, and avoidance, while using less cognitive reappraisal, problem solving and acceptance, the principal issue refers to an inflexible implementation of emotion regulation rather than the lack of it (Daros and Williams 2019). Various studies have demonstrated that individuals with BPD do not reveal deficiencies in the applying of emotion regulation strategies, and they exhibit some reduced self-reported, sympathetic, and parasympathetic markers of emotions and deficits in using cognitive reappraisal (Baczkowski et al. 2017; Schulze et al. 2011), suppress emotional expressions (Evans et al. 2016), and implementation mindfulness/acceptance (Fitzpatrick et al. 2024; Dixon-Gordon et al. 2017a, b, 2021, 2022). A body of findings have been achieved in the field of issues in emotion regulation strategies in individuals with BPD. Some of these findings suggest that BPD features are more related to positive emotions when applying avoidance (Turner et al. 2021), while another suggest that individuals with BPD indicate less improvements in self-reported emotions recruiting distraction rather than controls. Moreover, some findings have proposed that BPD patients do not display insufficiencies in the structure or in the implementation of emotion regulation strategies and report short-term benefits in disengaging from emotion, as well as increased emotional intensity at baseline in comparison to controls (Fitzpatrick et al. 2024; Kuo et al. 2016).

Several studies have been conducted to investigate a heightened sensitivity to emotional stimuli and the importance of emotional responses in BPD, especially self-destructive behaviors such as NSSI and suicidal behaviors (e.g., Tragesser et al. 2008; Sadikaj et al. 2010; Lobbestael and Arntz 2010; Gratz et al. 2010; Baskin-Sommers et al. 2012; Domes et al. 2011; Sharp et al. 2012; Lawrence et al. 2011; Burke 2016; Boylan et al. 2019; Bresin et al. 2013; Burton et al. 2022; Berghoff et al. 2022). Lynch et al. (2006) proposed that patients who meet BPD criteria reported heightened emotional sensitivity (see, Lynch et al. 2006; Glenn and Klonsky 2009). In addition, studies demonstrated that individuals with BPD indicated fluctuations between positive and negative emotions (Mneimne et al. 2018). Robin et al. (2012) found that in order to identify anger and happiness correctly, the BPD patient needs more intense facial expression (Robin et al. 2012). Moreover, various research has indicated that emotional dysfunction can anticipate BPD in both male and female adolescents, and also, interaction between affective dysfunction and disinhibition predict BPD features in female adolescents (Gratz et al. 2009). Koenigsberg et al. (2002) posited that individuals with BPD exhibited greater instability in anger and anxiety in comparison with patients with other personality disorders (Koenigsberg et al. 2002). One study indicated that BPD patients reported higher score in negative emotions and emotion dysregulation compared to controls (Conklin et al. 2006). Further, traditional laboratory-based cognitive tasks such as the emotional Stroop task demonstrated that individuals who are sensitive to emotionally charged stimuli have more difficulties in the suppression of their sentiment to read the words, slowing their reaction times (Carpenter and Trull 2013; Domes et al. 2006; Wingenfeld et al. 2009). Whereas, some investigations have revealed that individuals with BPD display slower reaction times on the emotional Stroop task (Sieswerda et al. 2007; Arntz et al. 2000). Wingenfeld et al. (2009) found that BPD patients may have a cognitive and attentional bias toward processing negative stimuli (Carpenter and Trull 2013; Wingenfeld et al. 2009). Many investigations have found that BPD individuals indicated a negativity bias in emotion recognition (e.g., Domes et al. 2009), and a bias toward identifying negative emotions in other people (e.g., Domes et al. 2008; Scott et al. 2011, 2017; Wagner and Linehan 1999; Koenigsberg et al. 2009, 2010, 2014). Moreover, a substantial number of studies have demonstrated that both intensity and reactivity of negative emotions are strongly associated with BPD (Carpenter and Trull 2013; Kuo and Linehan 2009; Trull et al. 2010). Research on ecological momentary assessment (EMA) revealed acute elevations in negative affect moment-to-moment, to assess the dynamics of mood states, extreme alterations of mood, and environmental triggers for mood changes, found greater instability and lability in negative emotion in BPD (Nica and Links 2009). Accordingly, Ebner-Priemer and Trull (2009) examined the affective states of 50 female with BPD and 50 female healthy controls (HC) during 24 h of their everyday life. The results showed that elevated affective instability for both emotional valence and distress was clearly displayed in the BPD group but not in the HC group. Moreover, a group-specific pattern of instability was recognized in the BPD group manifested by sudden large reduces from positive mood states. In addition, 48% of the declines from a very positive mood state in BPD were so large that they reached a negative mood state. Based on their findings, BPD patients, on average, take less time to fluctuate from a very positive mood state to a negative mood state (Ebner-Priemer and Trull 2009). Trull et al. (2008) found greater instability of negative affects over a long period of time in comparison with other clinical groups (Trull et al. 2008; Carpenter and Trull 2013).

As mentioned, one of the most crucial elements of emotion regulation is emotion regulation strategies, which are inadequate in that condition of emotion dysregulation (e.g., Dimeff et al. 2021; Crowell et al. 2009, 2014; Linehan 1993; Selby et al. 2014; Gratz et al. 2017, 2019, 2022; Kaufman et al. 2020; Palmer et al. 2018, 2021; Bookhout et al. 2017; Garofalo 2022; Garofalo et al. 2018; Fitzpatrick and Dixon-Gordon 2024). Several studies have indicated that individuals with BPD reveal lower emotional awareness and inability to distinguish among emotional states or emotional granularity. This research has suggested that BPD patients' scores in tasks measuring emotional clarity, mood labeling, and emotional labeling are lower than controls (see, Leible and Snell Jr 2004; Suvak et al. 2011). Other studies indicate that BPD symptoms have been related to lack of emotional clarity (Vine and Aldao 2014; Dixon-Gordon et al. 2022), toughness in identifying and naming specific emotional states (e.g., Wolf et al. 2007, 2018), experiencing over-arousal in the case of experiencing emotions (Suvak et al. 2011), and lower ability to distinguish different emotions in their daily life (Zaki and Williams 2013; Dixon-Gordon et al. 2020). Furthermore, several investigations have found that individuals with BPD have more difficulties recruiting emotion regulation strategies (e.g., Salsman and Linehan 2012; Bornovalova et al. 2008; Chapman et al. 2008; Gratz et al. 2017,

2019, 2022; Leyro et al. 2010). Mirkovic et al. (2021) assessed the role of emotion dysregulation in adolescent suicide attempts. The findings suggested that emotional dysregulation had a mediating role in suicide attempts among BPD adolescents (Mirkovic et al. 2021). Scott et al. (2014) tested unique prospective associations between BPD symptoms, trait impulsivity, difficulties in emotion regulation, and psychological and physical aggression in antisocial and borderline cases. The results showed that although there are associations between BPD and ASPD with aggressive behaviors, the relation between BPD symptoms and aggression is mediated by difficulties in emotion regulation. The authors suggested that most studies on BPD have been focused on internalizing emotional processes and self-inflicted behaviors, and more research should be conducted to assess externalizing behaviors, especially aggression and victimization (Scott et al. 2014). As stated by Reitz et al. (2012), self-inflicted injurious behaviors, suicidal attempts and other self-destructive behaviors, such as impulsive behaviors, are maladaptive problem-solving strategies (Reitz et al. 2012). Neacsiu et al. (2014) suggested that these difficulties can be due to biological and expressive components of emotions or toughness in other emotion regulation strategies especially selecting effective situation modification strategies (Neacsiu et al. 2014). Woods et al. (2021) examined interpersonal and emotional processes that are core elements for diagnostic BPD. The findings suggested that within the BPD subsample, BPD patients were heterogeneous and were better described by emotional dynamics and the associations between interpersonal and emotional domains (Woods et al. 2021). As will be discussed in more detail in a subsequent chapter, Selby et al. (2008) proposed an emotional cascade model to explain why behavior occurs instead of appropriate and adaptive emotion regulation strategies. In line with the emotional cascade model, individuals have a strong tendency to choose maladaptive behaviors rather than adaptive ones, while they experience extremely intensely negative affect. Because maladaptive behaviors often have a much more effective impact to reduce intense emotions, therefore, individuals with BPD have a marked tendency to utilize these insufficient behaviors instead of more adaptive or healthy ones. Unfortunately, impulsive behaviors are ultimately problematic and followed by negative consequences over the long-term (Selby et al. 2008; Selby and Joiner Jr 2009, 2013). Selby et al. (2009) found support for this model in BPD patients (Selby et al. 2009).

Familial studies propose that emotional instability and impulsivity are considered as two core heritable traits in BPD (e.g., Silverman et al. 1995; Beauchaine et al. 2009). To investigate emotional sensitivity in BPD, Gibb et al. (2001) studied the effects of 5-HTTLPR and maternal criticism on children's attentional biases toward emotional information. The results indicated a significant three-way interaction between child 5HTTLPR gene presence, maternal criticism, and facial expression. This means that children with a history of maternal criticism experiences demonstrated more attentional avoidance toward angry, with no facial expression of sadness and happiness (Gibb et al. 2011; Carpenter et al. 2013). The gene-environmental interaction theory concentrates on the role of interpersonal vulnerability factors in the development of BPD (Gunderson et al. 2018; Gunderson and Lyons-Ruth 2008). This theory emphasizes on biological-based interpersonal high sensitivity to emotional stimuli in combination with tendency for emotional vulnerability and impulsivity contribute to a strengthened emotional reactivity in interpersonal contexts, disrupting the development of a secured attachment in the relationship between the child and mother/caregiver. This unsecured attachment contributes to the development of psychopathology and causes increased more proneness to any distress and interpersonal sensitivity in children, which might elicit inappropriate caregiver's behaviors. Consequently, this reciprocal maladaptive interaction between child and caregiver leads to a disorganized/ambivalent attachment style which covers all child's life span (Dixon-Gordon et al. 2020). Crowell and Schmeichel (2016) posits that because of the hypersensitiveness in an individual which appears toward interpersonal signals, an individual tries to inhibit his/her interpersonal needs. Therefore, it contributes to interpersonal relationship issues which soar emotion dysregulation (Crowell et al. 2017).

Neuroimaging studies have demonstrated that BPD patients show reduction in amygdala, orbitofrontal, and hippocampal sizes and escalated amygdala function in response to emotional cues (see, Sauer-Zavala et al. 2019; Ruocco and Carcone 2016; Rosenthal et al. 2008). There is a great deal of evidence proving that individuals with BPD engage in maladaptive emotion regulation strategies to reduce their negative emotions (Carpenter and Trull 2013), such as rumination (e.g., Chapman et al. 2011), thought suppression (e.g., Cheavens et al. 2005; Rosenthal et al. 2005), thought avoidance (Rosenthal et al. 2005), self-criticism, emotional suppression, anger rumination (Dixon-Gordon et al. 2020, 2022; Aldao and Dixon-Gordon 2014; Baer and Sauer 2011), and emotional suppression (Beblo et al. 2013). Empirical investigations have demonstrated experiential avoidance (Hayes et al. 1996), and an escalation in the severity of BPD due to high frequency of negative emotions (Iverson et al. 2012). Based on several studies, it can be concluded that BPD symptoms are not merely a product of increased levels of negative emotions; rather, the combination of intense negative emotions and the style of the relations to these negative emotions are crucial for the development of BPD (Sauer-Zavala et al. 2019). After controlling for negative emotions such as depression, Glenn and Klonsky (2009) documented emotion dysregulation has a unique role in the development of BPD (Glenn and Klonsky 2009a; Kröger et al. 2011). BPD patients who experience strong levels of negative emotions try to find different coping strategies to escape or avoid from experiencing extremely negative emotions such as suppression, substance and alcohol use, and self-injury behaviors (e.g., Bentley et al. 2014; Baer and Sauer 2011; Selby et al. 2009; Nock and Prinstein 2004; Dimeff et al. 2021; Kaufman et al. 2020; Sauer-Zavala et al. 2019).

Consistent with the empirical findings in emotional sensitivity and emotional hyperactivity, a number of studies have attempted to demonstrate subjective emotional reactivity in BPD consists of "personally relevant emotional sounds (Rosenthal et al. 2016); social rejection stressors (Reichenberger et al. 2017), and an abused-themed film clip (Lobbestael and Arntz 2010)" (Dixon-Gordon et al. 2020, p. 365). In sum, investigations in these areas have illustrated that BPD patients reported less positive emotion reactivities to emotional stimuli (Reichenberger et al. 2017);

therefore, subjective emotional reactivity in BPD may be restricted to intense negative emotions (Dixon-Gordon et al. 2020).

Several laboratory investigations have exhibited that individuals with BPD indicate high reactivity to emotional cues (e.g., Dixon-Gordon et al. 2017a, b, 2021; Weinberg et al. 2009). In contrast, some studies have demonstrated despite higher negative emotion at baseline in BPD cases (Kuo and Linehan 2009; Reitz et al. 2012), no difference has been found in reactivity than control groups. This point can be associated with BPD's responses to social stressors and in interpersonal and self-conscious emotions (Dixon-Gordon et al. 2017a, b, 2021; Chapman 2019). Furthermore, Dixon-Gordon et al. (2017a, b) cited that there are several evidence of higher subjective reactivity in terms of shame (Gratz et al. 2010), anger (Kuo et al. 2014), and fear/anxiety (Dixon-Gordon et al. 2022). Deficits in emotion regulation strategies and emotional dysregulation may contribute to nonsuicidal self-injurious behaviors (Nock and Prinstein 2004; Haywood et al. 2022). Robin et al. (2021) proposed that individuals with BPD reveal paradoxical emotional reactions: no rise of hopelessness and emotional symptoms with a peak of parental dysfunction; meanwhile, a decline in emotional symptoms and hopelessness with cumulative stressful life events. These paradoxical emotional reactions may occur because of emotional dysregulation processes for child-parent interactions, and, independent of attachment versus dependent on early interactions, and involving alexithymia, as well (Robin et al. 2021). As reported by Dixon-Gordon et al. (2015), individuals who were categorized as high regulators, such as frequent use of all emotion regulation strategies, and maladaptive regulators such as frequent maladaptive emotion regulation strategies, indicated greater BPD symptoms in comparison with low regulated group (Dixon-Gordon et al. 2015). Correspondingly, Chapman et al. (2013) posited BPD patients reported higher rate of utilizing emotion regulation strategies, such as distraction and emotion suppression, and less spontaneous using emotional acceptance in response to laboratory-made stressors in comparison with controls (Chapman et al. 2013). Iverson et al. (2012) investigated three domains of emotional functioning, such as emotion dysregulation, distress tolerance, and experiential avoidance, and suggested that experiential avoidance may be a central process in BPD symptoms severity (Iverson et al. 2012). Individuals with BPD may shift to the most potentially effective behavioral strategies to regulate their intense emotions, such as more problematic ones, such as self-injury and eating disorder behaviors (Selby et al. 2009), which then perpetuate symptoms of emotion dysregulation over the long-term (Selby et al. 2009; Sansone et al. 2001). Mclachlan et al. (2021) measured BPD traits, beliefs about emotions, treatment preference, cognitive reappraisal, and rumination via modifying beliefs about emotions using virtual reality (VR) in adolescents. The findings showed that adolescents with higher levels of BPD traits supported fixed beliefs of emotion and indicated higher levels of rumination and lower levels of cognitive reappraisal (McLachlan et al. 2021). Consistent with the biosocial theory, Evans et al. (2016) demonstrated greater borderline severity associated with greater implementation of suppression and reduced emotional state and use of acceptance. They claim these data support the viewpoint that individuals with BPD have a strong tendency to adopt avoidant emotion regulation strategies at both state and trait levels (Evans et al. 2016). Dixon-Gordon et al. (2020) proposed that despite a great deal of work on emotion dysregulation in BPD which contribute to utilizing insufficient emotion regulation strategies, it is not clear whether BPD patients are using emotion regulation strategies ineffectively or they are recruiting emotion regulation strategies in a messy and disorganized war just to reduce distressing emotions (Dixon-Gordon et al. 2020). Based on growing literature, BPD individuals indicate under-recruit brain regions related to cognitive control while utilizing the emotion regulation strategy of reappraisal (Mauchnik and Schmahl 2010), and have less activation in brain sections associated with cognitive control, specifically prefrontal cortex region (Lang and Berglundh 2011). Furthermore, BPD patients demonstrated various neural dynamics in brain regions associated with cognitive control and regions associated with emotional responding. This research proposed that BPD individuals might utilize less cognitive control regions in recruiting emotion regulation strategies (Dixon-Gordon et al. 2020). Several studies have documented difficulties with cognitive flexibility (Ruocco 2005, 2010), cognitive change (Selby and Joiner Jr 2009, 2013), emotional awareness (Levine 1997), and aftereffects (Korfine and Hooley 2000).

Daros et al. (2018) found that BPD patients engage in potentially harmful behaviors more often, and the subthreshold of BPD symptoms can affect the rate and frequency of using emotion regulation strategy in comparison with other mental disorders (Daros et al. 2018). Kuo and Linehan (2009) demonstrated that individuals with BPD revealed heightened biological vulnerability compared with normal control group, and also displayed higher baseline emotional intensity, expanded skin conductance response, in spite of showing no heightened reactivity (Kuo and Linehan 2009). Adults with BPD have manifested evidence of a wide range of cognitive, physiological, and behavioral features of emotion dysregulation and development of psychopathology (Chapman 2019; Garofalo 2022; Garofalo et al. 2018; Ponzoni et al. 2021). Through a narrative review of literature, Paulus et al. (2021) proposed emotion dysregulation as a transdiagnostic construct and defined emotion dysregulation an inability to regulate the intensity and quality of emotions. They mentioned that the basic condition of emotion dysregulation includes a genetic disposition, a history of experiencing trauma, especially sexual and physical abuse, emotional neglect in childhood and adolescence, and experiencing several stressful life events. Furthermore, they stated that emotion dysregulation is a complicated structure and an expansive concept, which can be considered as a disposition for a large number of mental disorders (Paulus et al. 2021). Ebner-Priemer et al. (2015) elucidated the transdiagnostic nature of emotion dysregulation may assist individuals to illustrate the common and independent mechanisms that subordinate many of different mental disorders with affective dysregulation characteristics (Ebner-Priemer et al. 2015).

At present, a growing body of investigations and theories have been conducted to examine emotion dysregulation as core impairment in BPD and have been achieved a great deal of evidence to support this hypothesis (e.g., Dixon-Gordon et al. 2015, 2016, 2022; Crowell et al. 2009; Reichenberger et al. 2017; Glenn and Klonsky

2009a; Kaufman et al. 2020; Sauer-Zavala et al. 2019), there are some unanswered interrogations in this area, such as emotion regulation strategies recruited by BPD individuals. Moreover, several critical points have been proposed that in the field of assessing and doing psychotherapy in BPD individuals (Dixon-Gordon et al. 2020, 2022). Chapman (2019) cited that however the precursors to the development of BPD and emotion dysregulation have been documented, prevention and treatment attempts sustain great support for reducing the long-term suffering, functional disturbances, and noticeable societal consequences with BPD (Chapman 2019). Dixon-Gordon et al. (2020) gathered a few consistent themes appear from related literature and adapted them in a graphical deception of BPD. Based on Fig. 4, BPD patients seem to have an escalated biased tendency toward emotional stimuli. In addition, BPD patients significantly own baseline negative emotions, as well as, there are an expanded emotional reactivity to interpersonal cues and trauma/abandonment-themed stressors, especially anger, shame, and anxiety reactivity. Moreover, it seems an exaggerated emotional responding will appear later in the emotional response. Whether individuals with BPD utilize emotion regulation strategies more or less than other people, there are evidence to exhibit that BPD patients underrecruited emotional acceptance, underutilize cognitive control regions to regulate emotions, and so they recognize their own emotion regulation strategies less effective. Besides, several studies have been documented that negative emotional intensity may contribute to several difficulties in BPD, such as impulsive behaviors, problematic interpersonal relationships, and poor problem-solving strategies in various parts of their life. Ultimately, emotion dysregulation is a core component which should be altered in the treatment of BPD (See, Dixon-Gordon et al. 2020; Bateman and Fonagy 2005; Crowell et al. 2009; Gunderson and Lyons-Ruth 2008; Linehan 1993).

To conclude, as mentioned one of the most substantial core characteristics of BPD comprise emotional instability, remarkable reactivity of mood, intense anger with problems in management of anger, self-destructive behaviors which have been documented as the result of emotional issues. Affective instability and emotion dysregulation have been proposed as major issues in individuals with BPD. Moreover, issues in emotional regulation strategies, inability to manage emotions, and behavioral instability are found as major characteristics underlying BPD. Emotion dysregulation has been shown a key role in the development, severity, and maintenance of BPD symptoms. Furthermore, Linehan's biosocial theory suggested hyperintensity/reactivity, and poor regulation as two core characteristics of BPD, and emphasized on emotion vulnerability and emotional reactivity among individuals with BPD. Moreover, self-invalidation, stemmed from the interaction between emotional vulnerable patients and invalidating environments, has been shown common among BPD patients. Emotion dysregulation has documented as a core psychopathology in etiology of BPD which caused several features of BPD, including NSSI, suicidal thoughts and attempts, intense anger, mood fluctuations, impulsive behaviors, and highly emotional sensitivity and reactivity.

References

Aldao A, Dixon-Gordon KL. Broadening the scope of research on emotion regulation strategies and psychopathology. Cogn Behav Ther. 2014;43(1):22–33.

American Psychiatric Association. Diagnostic and statistical manual of mental disorders. 5th ed. Washington, DC: Author; 2022.

Arntz A, Appels C, Sieswerda S. Hypervigilance in borderline disorder: a test with the emotional Stroop paradigm. J Personal Disord. 2000;14(4):366–73.

Baczkowski BM, van Zutphen L, Siep N, Jacob GA, Domes G, Maier S, Sprenger A, Senft A, Willenborg B, Tüscher O, Arntz A. Deficient amygdala–prefrontal intrinsic connectivity after effortful emotion regulation in borderline personality disorder. Eur Arch Psychiatry Clin Neurosci. 2017;267:551–65.

Baer RA, Sauer SE. Relationships between depressive rumination, anger rumination, and borderline personality features. Personal Disord Theory Res Treat. 2011;2(2):142.

Bargh JA, Williams LE. The nonconscious regulation of emotion. Handbook of Emotion Regulation. 2007;1:429–45.

Barlow DH, Farchione TJ, Bullis JR, Gallagher MW, Murray-Latin H, Sauer-Zavala S, Bentley KH, Thompson-Hollands J, Conklin LR, Boswell JF, Ametaj A. The unified protocol for transdiagnostic treatment of emotional disorders compared with diagnosis-specific protocols for anxiety disorders: a randomized clinical trial. JAMA Psychiatry. 2017;74(9):875–84.

Barrett LF, Gross J, Christensen TC, Benvenuto M. Knowing what you're feeling and knowing what to do about it: mapping the relation between emotion differentiation and emotion regulation. Cognit Emot. 2001;15(6):713–24.

Barrett CE, Hennessey TM, Gordon KM, Ryan SJ, McNair ML, Ressler KJ, Rainnie DG. Developmental disruption of amygdala transcriptome and socioemotional behavior in rats exposed to valproic acid prenatally. Mol Autism. 2017;8:1–7.

Baskin-Sommers AR, Vitale JE, MacCoon D, Newman JP. Assessing emotion sensitivity in female offenders with borderline personality symptoms: results from a fear-potentiated startle paradigm. J Abnorm Psychol. 2012;121(2):477.

Bateman A, Fonagy P. Psychotherapy for borderline personality disorder. Psychol Med. 2005;35:163–74.

Bentley KH, Nock MK, Barlow DH. The four-function model of nonsuicidal self-injury: key directions for future research. Clin Psychol Sci. 2014;2(5):638–56.

Beauchaine TP. Future directions in emotion dysregulation and youth psychopathology. J Clin Child Adolesc Psychol. 2015;44(5):875–96.

Beauchaine TP, Klein DN, Crowell SE, Derbidge C, Gatzke-Kopp L. Multifinality in the development of personality disorders: a biology × sex × environment interaction model of antisocial and borderline traits. Dev Psychopathol. 2009;21(3):735–70.

Beauchaine TP, Zisner AR, Sauder CL. Trait impulsivity and the externalizing spectrum. Annu Rev Clin Psychol. 2017;13:343–68.

Beblo T, Fernando S, Kamper P, Griepenstroh J, Aschenbrenner S, Pastuszak A, Schlosser N, Driessen M. Increased attempts to suppress negative and positive emotions in borderline personality disorder. Psychiatry Res. 2013;210(2):505–9.

Berghoff CR, Dixon-Gordon KL, Chapman AL, Baer MM, Turner BJ, Tull MT, Gratz KL. Daily associations of interpersonal and emotional experiences following stressful events among young adults with and without nonsuicidal self-injury. J Clin Psychol. 2022;78(11):2329–40.

Berking M, Wupperman P, Reichardt A, Pejic T, Dippel A, Znoj H. Emotion-regulation skills as a treatment target in psychotherapy. Behav Res Ther. 2008;46(11):1230–7.

Berking M, Eichler E, Luhmann M, Diedrich A, Hiller W, Rief W. Affect regulation training reduces symptom severity in depression – a randomized controlled trial. PLoS One. 2019;14(8):e0220436.

Bookhout MK, Hubbard JA, Moore CC. Emotion regulation. In: The Wiley handbook of disruptive and impulse-control disorders; 2017. p. 221–36.

Bornovalova MA, Gratz KL, Daughters SB, Nick B, Delany-Brumsey A, Lynch TR, Kosson D, Lejuez CW. A multimodal assessment of the relationship between emotion dysregulation and borderline personality disorder among inner-city substance users in residential treatment. J Psychiatr Res. 2008;42(9):717–26.

Boylan K, Chahal J, Courtney DB, Sharp C, Bennett K. An evaluation of clinical practice guidelines for self-harm in adolescents: the role of borderline personality pathology. Personal Disord Theory Res Treat. 2019;10(6):500.

Bradley PJ, Ward C, Cheng SJ, Alexander DL, Coller S, Coombs GH, Dunn JD, Ferguson DJ, Sanderson SJ, Wastling JM, Boothroyd JC. Proteomic analysis of rhoptry organelles reveals many novel constituents for host-parasite interactions in Toxoplasma gondii. J Biol Chem. 2005;280(40):34245–58.

Bresin K, Finy MS, Verona E. Childhood emotional environment and self-injurious behaviors: the moderating role of the BDNF Val66Met polymorphism. J Affect Disord. 2013;150(2):594–600.

Brown SB, van Steenbergen H, Band GP, de Rover M, Nieuwenhuis S. Functional significance of the emotion-related late positive potential. Front Hum Neurosci. 2012;6:33.

Brown KW, Goodman RJ, Inzlicht M. Dispositional mindfulness and the attenuation of neural responses to emotional stimuli. Soc Cogn Affect Neurosci. 2013;8(1):93–9.

Brown BK, Murrell J, Karne H, Anand A. The effects of DAT1 genotype on fMRI activation in an emotional go/no-go task. Brain Imaging Behav. 2017;11:185–93.

Burton AL, Brown R, Abbott MJ. Overcoming difficulties in measuring emotional regulation: assessing and comparing the psychometric properties of the DERS long and short forms. Cogent Psychology. 2022;9(1):2060629.

Burke M. Affective forecasting ability: individual differences in emotional intelligence and prosocial behaviour. 2016.

Carpenter RW, Bagby-Stone S, Trull TJ. Emotional awareness. In: Handbook of cognition and emotion; 2013. p. 462.

Carpenter RW, Trull TJ. Components of emotion dysregulation in borderline personality disorder: a review. Curr Psychiatry Rep. 2013;15:1–8.

Cavicchioli M, Scalabrini A, Northoff G, Mucci C, Ogliari A, Maffei C. Dissociation and emotion regulation strategies: a meta-analytic review. J Psychiatr Res. 2021;143:370–87.

Chapman AL, Leung DW, Lynch TR. Impulsivity and emotion dysregulation in borderline personality disorder. J Personal Disord. 2008;22(2):148–64.

Chapman BP, Fiscella K, Kawachi I, Duberstein P, Muennig P. Emotion suppression and mortality risk over a 12-year follow-up. J Psychosom Res. 2013;75(4):381–5.

Chapman AL, Dixon-Gordon KL, Walters KN. Experiential avoidance and emotion regulation in borderline personality disorder. J Ration Emot Cogn Behav Ther. 2011;29:35–52.

Chapman AL. Borderline personality disorder and emotion dysregulation. Dev Psychopathol. 2019;31(3):1143–56.

Cheavens JS, Rosenthal MZ, Daughters SB, Nowak J, Kosson D, Lynch TR, Lejuez CW. An analogue investigation of the relationships among perceived parental criticism, negative affect, and borderline personality disorder features: the role of thought suppression. Behav Res Ther. 2005;43(2):257–68.

Conklin CZ, Bradley R, Westen D. Affect regulation in borderline personality disorder. J Nerv Ment Dis. 2006;194(2):69–77.

Cole PM, Deater-Deckard K. Emotion regulation, risk, and psychopathology. J Child Psychol Psychiatry. 2009;50(11):1327.

Cole PM, Hall SE. Emotion dysregulation as a risk factor for psychopathology. In: Child and adolescent psychopathology; 2008. p. 265–98.

Cole PM. Moving ahead in the study of the development of emotion regulation. Int J Behav Dev. 2014;38(2):203–7.

Cole PM, Hall SE, Hajal NJ. Emotion dysregulation as a vulnerability to psychopathology. In: Child and adolescent psychopathology. 3rd ed; 2017. p. 346–86.

Cole PM, Lougheed JP, Chow SM, Ram N. Development of emotion regulation dynamics across early childhood: a multiple time-scale approach. Affect Sci. 2020;1:28–41.

Crowell SE, Beauchaine TP, Linehan MM. A biosocial developmental model of borderline personality: elaborating and extending Linehan's theory. Psychol Bull. 2009;135(3):495.

Crowell SE, Butner JE, Wiltshire TJ, Munion AK, Yaptangco M, Beauchaine TP. Evaluating emotional and biological sensitivity to maternal behavior among self-injuring and depressed adolescent girls using nonlinear dynamics. Clin Psychol Sci. 2017;5(2):272–85.

Crowell SE, Baucom BR, Yaptangco M, Bride D, Hsiao R, McCauley E, Beauchaine TP. Emotion dysregulation and dyadic conflict in depressed and typical adolescents: evaluating concordance across psychophysiological and observational measures. Biol Psychol. 2014;98:50–8.

Crowell A, Schmeichel BJ. Approach motivation and cognitive resources combine to influence memory for positive emotional stimuli. Cognit Emot. 2016;30(2):389–97.

Crowell JA. Development of emotion regulation in typically developing children. Child Adolesc Psychiatric Clin. 2021;30(3):467–74.

D'Aurizio G, Di Stefano R, Socci V, Rossi A, Barlattani T, Pacitti F, Rossi R. The role of emotional instability in borderline personality disorder: a systematic review. Ann General Psychiatry. 2023;22(1):9.

Daros AR, Williams GE, Jung S, Turabi M, Uliaszek AA, Ruocco AC. More is not always better: strategies to regulate negative mood induction in women with borderline personality disorder and depressive and anxiety disorders. Personal Disord Theory Res Treat. 2018;9(6):530.

Daros AR, Williams GE. A meta-analysis and systematic review of emotion-regulation strategies in borderline personality disorder. Harv Rev Psychiatry. 2019;27(4):217–32.

Daros AR, Guevara MA, Uliaszek AA, McMain SF, Ruocco AC. Cognitive emotion regulation strategies in borderline personality disorder: diagnostic comparisons and associations with potentially harmful behaviors. Psychopathology. 2018;51(2):83–95.

Daros AR, Daniel KE, Boukhechba M, Chow PI, Barnes LE, Teachman BA. Relationships between trait emotion dysregulation and emotional experiences in daily life: an experience sampling study. Cognit Emot. 2020;34(4):743–55.

Del Corno F, Plotkin D. Personality patterns and syndromes in the elderly – PE Axis. 2017.

Diamond A. Executive functions. Annu Rev Psychol. 2013;64:135–68.

Dimeff LA, Jobes DA, Koerner K, Kako N, Jerome T, Kelley-Brimer A, Boudreaux ED, Beadnell B, Goering P, Witterholt S, Melin G. Using a tablet-based app to deliver evidence-based practices for suicidal patients in the emergency department: pilot randomized controlled trial. JMIR Mental Health. 2021;8(3):e23022.

Dixon-Gordon KL, Aldao A, De Los RA. Emotion regulation in context: examining the spontaneous use of strategies across emotional intensity and type of emotion. Personal Individ Differ. 2015;86:271–6.

Dixon-Gordon KL, Whalen DJ, Scott LN, Cummins ND, Stepp SD. The main and interactive effects of maternal interpersonal emotion regulation and negative affect on adolescent girls' borderline personality disorder symptoms. Cogn Ther Res. 2016;40:381–93.

Dixon-Gordon KL, Turner BJ, Rosenthal MZ, Chapman AL. Emotion regulation in borderline personality disorder: an experimental investigation of the effects of instructed acceptance and suppression. Behav Ther. 2017a;48(6):750–64.

Dixon-Gordon KL, Peters JR, Fertuck EA, Yen S. Emotional processes in borderline personality disorder: an update for clinical practice. J Psychother Integr. 2017b;27(4):425.

Dixon-Gordon KL, Marsh NP, Balda KE, McQuade JD. Parent emotion socialization and child emotional vulnerability as predictors of borderline personality features. Research on Child and Adolescent Psychopathology. 2020;48:135–47.

Dixon-Gordon KL, Fitzpatrick S, Haliczer LA. Emotion regulation and borderline personality features in daily life: the role of social context. J Affect Disord. 2021;282:677–85.

Dixon-Gordon KL, Turner BJ, Haliczer LA, Gratz KL, Tull MT, Chapman AL. Self-injury motives: a person-centered examination. Suicide Life Threat Behav. 2022;52(4):812–27.

Domes G, Winter B, Schnell K, Vohs K, Fast K, Herpertz SC. The influence of emotions on inhibitory functioning in borderline personality disorder. Psychol Med. 2006;36(8):1163–72.

Domes G, Czieschnek D, Weidler F, Berger C, Fast K, Herpertz SC. Recognition of facial affect in borderline personality disorder. J Personal Disord. 2008;22(2):135–47.

Domes G, Schulze L, Herpertz SC. Emotion recognition in borderline personality disorder—a review of the literature. J Personal Disord. 2009;23(1):6–19.

Domes G, Grabe HJ, Czieschnek D, Heinrichs M, Herpertz SC. Alexithymic traits and facial emotion recognition in borderline personality disorder. Psychother Psychosom. 2011;80(6):383–5.

Ebner-Priemer UW, Trull TJ. Ecological momentary assessment of mood disorders and mood dysregulation. Psychol Assess. 2009;21(4):463.

Ebner-Priemer UW, Houben M, Santangelo P, Kleindienst N, Tuerlinckx F, Oravecz Z, Verleysen G, Van Deun K, Bohus M, Kuppens P. Unraveling affective dysregulation in borderline personality disorder: a theoretical model and empirical evidence. J Abnorm Psychol. 2015;124(1):186.

Eddie D, Bates ME, Vaschillo EG, Lehrer PM, Retkwa M, Miuccio M. Rest, reactivity, and recovery: a psychophysiological assessment of borderline personality disorder. Front Psych. 2018;9:505.

Eid M, Lischetzke T, Nussbeck FW, Trierweiler LI. Separating trait effects from trait-specific method effects in multitrait-multimethod models: a multiple-indicator CT-C (M-1) model. Psychol Methods. 2003;8(1):38.

Evans SC, Blossom JB, Canter KS, Poppert-Cordts K, Kanine R, Garcia A, Roberts MC. Self-reported emotion reactivity among early-adolescent girls: evidence for convergent and discriminant validity in an urban community sample. Behav Ther. 2016;47(3):299–311.

Fassbinder E, Schweiger U, Martius D, Brand-de Wilde O, Arntz A. Emotion regulation in schema therapy and dialectical behavior therapy. Front Psychol. 2016;7:1373.

Fitzpatrick C, Pan PM, Lemieux A, Harvey E, de Andrade RF, Garon-Carrier G. Early-childhood tablet use and outbursts of anger. JAMA Pediatr. 2024;178(10):1035–40.

Fitzpatrick S, Dixon-Gordon KL. Emotion regulation in personality disorders 2024.

Frijda NH. The emotions. Cambridge University Press; 1986.

Garofalo C. Emotion and emotion regulation. Clinical forensic psychology: Introductory perspectives on offending; 2022. p. 87–107.

Garofalo C, Velotti P, Zavattini GC. Emotion regulation and aggression: the incremental contribution of alexithymia, impulsivity, and emotion dysregulation facets. Psychol Violence. 2018;8(4):470.

Genet JJ, Siemer M. Flexible control in processing affective and non-affective material predicts individual differences in trait resilience. Cognit Emot. 2011;25(2):380–8.

Gibb BE, Wheeler R, Alloy LB, Abramson LY. Emotional, physical, and sexual maltreatment in childhood versus adolescence and personality dysfunction in young adulthood. J Personal Disord. 2001;15(6):505–11.

Gibb BE, Johnson AL, Benas JS, Uhrlass DJ, Knopik VS, McGeary JE. Children's 5-HTTLPR genotype moderates the link between maternal criticism and attentional biases specifically for facial displays of anger. Cognit Emot. 2011;25(6):1104–20.

Glenn CR, Klonsky ED. Social context during nonsuicidal self-injury indicates suicide risk. Personal Individ Differ. 2009;46(1):25–9.

Glenn CR, Klonsky ED. Emotion dysregulation as a core feature of borderline personality disorder. J Personal Disord. 2009a;23(1):20–8.

Gratz KL, Roemer L. Multidimensional assessment of emotion regulation and dysregulation: development, factor structure, and initial validation of the difficulties in emotion regulation scale. J Psychopathol Behav Assess. 2004;26:41–54.

Gratz KL, Tull MT, Reynolds EK, Bagge CL, Latzman RD, Daughters SB, Lejuez CW. Extending extant models of the pathogenesis of borderline personality disorder to childhood borderline personality symptoms: the roles of affective dysfunction, disinhibition, and self-and emotion-regulation deficits. Dev Psychopathol. 2009;21(4):1263–91.

Gratz KL, Rosenthal MZ, Tull MT, Lejuez CW, Gunderson JG. An experimental investigation of emotional reactivity and delayed emotional recovery in borderline personality disorder: the role of shame. Compr Psychiatry. 2010;51(3):275–85.

Gratz KL, Tull MT, Levy RJ. Randomized controlled trial and uncontrolled 9-month follow-up of an adjunctive emotion regulation group therapy for deliberate self-harm among women with borderline personality disorder. Psychol Med. 2014;44(10):2099–112.

Gratz KL, Moore KE, Tull MT. The role of emotion dysregulation in the presence, associated difficulties, and treatment of borderline personality disorder. Personal Disord Theory Res Treat. 2016;7(4):344.

Gratz KL, Kiel EJ, Mann AJ, Tull MT. The prospective relation between borderline personality disorder symptoms and suicide risk: the mediating roles of emotion regulation difficulties and perceived burdensomeness. J Affect Disord. 2022;313:186–95.

Gratz KL, Richmond JR, Dixon-Gordon KL, Chapman AL, Tull MT. Multimodal assessment of emotional reactivity and regulation in response to social rejection among self-harming adults with and without borderline personality disorder. Personal Disord Theory Res Treat. 2019;10(5):395.

Gratz KL, Weiss NH, McDermott MJ, Dilillo D, Messman-Moore T, Tull MT. Emotion dysregulation mediates the relation between borderline personality disorder symptoms and later physical health symptoms. J Personal Disord. 2017;31(4):433–48.

Gross JT, Cassidy J. Hidden feelings: expressive suppression in middle childhood and links with physiology and negative emotion. Emotion. 2024;24(1):255.

Gross JJ. Emotion regulation. In: Handbook of emotions, vol. 3(3); 2008. p. 497–513.

Gross JJ. Emotion regulation: conceptual and empirical foundations. In: Handbook of emotion regulation, vol. 2; 2014. p. 3–20.

Gross JJ. Emotion regulation: current status and future prospects. Psychol Inq. 2015;26(1):1–26.

Gross JJ. The emerging field of emotion regulation: an integrative review. Rev Gen Psychol. 1998;2(3):271–99.

Gross JJ. Emotion regulation: conceptual and empirical foundations. Handbook of Emotion Regulation. 2014;2:3–20.

Gross F, Ford B. Handbook of emotion regulation. 3rd ed. Guilford Press; 2024.

Gross JJ, Jazaieri H. Emotion, emotion regulation, and psychopathology: an affective science perspective. Clin Psychol Sci. 2014;2(4):387–401.

Gunderson JG, Lyons-Ruth K. BPD's interpersonal hypersensitivity phenotype: a gene-environment-developmental model. J Personal Disord. 2008;22(1):22–41.

Gunderson JG, Fruzzetti A, Unruh B, Choi-Kain L. Competing theories of borderline personality disorder. J Personal Disord. 2018;32(2):148–67.

Hayes SC, Wilson KG, Gifford EV, Follette VM, Strosahl K. Experiential avoidance and behavioral disorders: a functional dimensional approach to diagnosis and treatment. J Consult Clin Psychol. 1996;64(6):1152.

Haywood SB, Hasking P, Boyes ME. We have so much in common: does shared variance between emotionrelated constructs account for relationships with self-injury? J Affect Disord Rep. 2022;8:100332.

Hayward M, Jones AM, Strawson WH, Quadt L, Larsson DE, Silva M, Davies G, Fielding-Smith S, Hazell CM, Critchley HD, Garfinkel SN. A cross-sectional study of auditory verbal hallucinations experienced by people with a diagnosis of borderline personality disorder. Clin Psychol Psychother. 2022;29(2):631–41.

Heller J, Mirzazade S, Romanzetti S, Habel U, Derntl B, Freitag NM, Schulz JB, Dogan I, Reetz K. Impact of gender and genetics on emotion processing in Parkinson's disease – a multimodal study. NeuroImage: Clinical. 2018;18:305–14.

Hofmann SG. Interpersonal emotion regulation model of mood and anxiety disorders. Cogn Ther Res. 2014;38:483–92.

Hofmann W, Luhmann M, Fisher RR, Vohs KD, Baumeister RF. Yes, but are they happy? Effects of trait self-control on affective Well-being and life satisfaction. J Pers. 2014;82(4):265–77.

Hughes AE, Crowell SE, Uyeji L, Coan JA. A developmental neuroscience of borderline pathology: emotion dysregulation and social baseline theory. J Abnorm Child Psychol. 2012;40:21–33.

Hughes DJ, Kratsiotis IK, Niven K, Holman D. Personality traits and emotion regulation: a targeted review and recommendations. Emotion. 2020;20(1):63.

Iverson KM, Follette VM, Pistorello J, Fruzzetti AE. An investigation of experiential avoidance, emotion dysregulation, and distress tolerance in young adult outpatients with borderline personality disorder symptoms. Personal Disord Theory Res Treat. 2012;3(4):415.

Kaufman EA, Puzia ME, Godfrey DA, Crowell SE. Physiological and behavioral effects of interpersonal validation: a multilevel approach to examining a core intervention strategy among self-injuring adolescents and their mothers. J Clin Psychol. 2020;76(3):559–80.

Koenigsberg HW, Fan J, Ochsner KN, Liu X, Guise K, Pizzarello S, Dorantes C, Tecuta L, Guerreri S, Goodman M, New A. Neural correlates of using distancing to regulate emotional responses to social situations. Neuropsychologia. 2010;48(6):1813–22.

Koenigsberg HW, Siever LJ, Lee H, Pizzarello S, New AS, Goodman M, Cheng H, Flory J, Prohovnik I. Neural correlates of emotion processing in borderline personality disorder. Psychiatry Res Neuroimaging. 2009;172(3):192–9.

Koenigsberg HW, Denny BT, Fan J, Liu X, Guerreri S, Mayson SJ, Rimsky L, New AS, Goodman M, Siever LJ. The neural correlates of anomalous habituation to negative emotional pictures in borderline and avoidant personality disorder patients. Am J Psychiatry. 2014;171(1):82–90.

Korfine L, Hooley JM. Directed forgetting of emotional stimuli in borderline personality disorder. J Abnorm Psychol. 2000;109(2):214.

Koenigsberg HW, Harvey PD, Mitropoulou V, Schmeidler J, New AS, Goodman M, Silverman JM, Serby M, Schopick F, Siever LJ. Characterizing affective instability in borderline personality disorder. Am J Psychiatry. 2002;159(5):784–8.

Koerner K, Linehan MM. Research on dialectical behavior therapy for patients with borderline personality disorder. Personality and Personality Disorders: The Science of Mental Health. 2013;7(1):315.

Koziol LF, Budding DE. Subcortical structures and cognition: implications for neuropsychological assessment. New York: Springer; 2009.

Kröger C, Vonau M, Kliem S, Kosfelder J. Emotion dysregulation as a core feature of borderline personality disorder: comparison of the discriminatory ability of two self-rating measures. Psychopathology. 2011;44(4):253–60.

Kuo JR, Fitzpatrick S, Metcalfe RK, McMain S. A multi-method laboratory investigation of emotional reactivity and emotion regulation abilities in borderline personality disorder. J Behav Ther Exp Psychiatry. 2016;50:52–60.

Kuo JR, Neacsiu AD, Fitzpatrick S, MacDonald DE. A methodological examination of emotion inductions in borderline personality disorder: a comparison of standardized versus idiographic stimuli. J Psychopathol Behav Assess. 2014;36:155–64.

Kuo JR, Linehan MM. Disentangling emotion processes in borderline personality disorder: physiological and self-reported assessment of biological vulnerability, baseline intensity, and reactivity to emotionally evocative stimuli. J Abnorm Psychol. 2009;118(3):531.

Lang NP, Berglundh T. Working group 4 of the seventh European workshop on periodontology. Periimplant diseases: where are we now? Consensus of the seventh European workshop on periodontology. J Clin Periodontol. 2011;38:178–81.

Lawrence KA, Allen JS, Chanen AM. A study of maladaptive schemas and borderline personality disorder in young people. Cogn Ther Res. 2011;35:30–9.

Lazarus RS. Progress on a cognitive-motivational-relational theory of emotion. Am Psychol. 1991;46(8):819.

Leible TL, Snell WE Jr. Borderline personality disorder and multiple aspects of emotional intelligence. Personal Individ Differ. 2004;37(2):393–404.

Levine LJ. Reconstructing memory for emotions. J Exp Psychol Gen. 1997;126(2):165.

Leyro TM, Zvolensky MJ, Bernstein A. Distress tolerance and psychopathological symptoms and disorders: a review of the empirical literature among adults. Psychol Bull. 2010;136(4):576.

Linehan MM. Cognitive-behavioral treatment of borderline personality disorder. New York: Guilford Press; 1993.

Linehan MM, Comtois KA, Murray AM, Brown MZ, Gallop RJ, Heard HL, Korslund KE, Tutek DA, Reynolds SK, Lindenboim N. Two-year randomized controlled trial and follow-up of dialectical behavior therapy vs therapy by experts for suicidal behaviors and borderline personality disorder. Arch Gen Psychiatry. 2006;63(7):757–66.

Linehan MM, Korslund KE, Harned MS, Gallop RJ, Lungu A, Neacsiu AD, McDavid J, Comtois KA, Murray-Gregory AM. Dialectical behavior therapy for high suicide risk in individuals with borderline personality disorder: a randomized clinical trial and component analysis. JAMA Psychiatry. 2015;72(5):475–82.

Lingiardi V, McWilliams N. Introduction to the special issue on the psychodynamic diagnostic manual, (PDM-2): the PDM: yesterday, today, tomorrow. Psychoanal Psychol. 2018;35(3):289.
Lobbestael J, Arntz A. Emotional, cognitive and physiological correlates of abuse-related stress in borderline and antisocial personality disorder. Behav Res Ther. 2010;48(2):116–24.
Lynch TR, Rosenthal MZ, Kosson DS, Cheavens JS, Lejuez CW, Blair RJ. Heightened sensitivity to facial expressions of emotion in borderline personality disorder. Emotion. 2006;6(4):647.
Matusiewicz A, Weaverling G, Lejuez CW. Emotion dysregulation among adolescents with borderline personality disorder. In: Handbook of borderline personality disorder in children and adolescents. New York: Springer; 2014. p. 177–94.
Mauchnik J, Schmahl C. The latest neuroimaging findings in borderline personality disorder. Curr Psychiatry Rep. 2010;12:46–55.
Mauss IB, Levenson RW, McCarter L, Wilhelm FH, Gross JJ. The tie that binds? Coherence among emotion experience, behavior, and physiology. Emotion. 2005;5(2):175.
McLachlan K, Mullally K, Ritter C, Mela M, Pei J. Fetal alcohol Spectrum disorder and neurodevelopmental disorders: an international practice survey of forensic mental health clinicians. Int J Forensic Ment Health. 2021;20(2):177–97.
McLaughlin KA, Hatzenbuehler ML, Mennin DS, Nolen-Hoeksema S. Emotion dysregulation and adolescent psychopathology: a prospective study. Behav Res Ther. 2011;49(9):544–54.
McMain S, Korman LM, Dimeff L. Dialectical behavior therapy and the treatment of emotion dysregulation. J Clin Psychol. 2001;57(2):183–96.
Mennin DS, Fresco DM. Emotion regulation therapy. Handbook of Emotion Regulation. 2014;2:469–90.
Mirkovic B, Delvenne V, Robin M, Pham-Scottez A, Corcos M, Speranza M. Borderline personality disorder and adolescent suicide attempt: the mediating role of emotional dysregulation. BMC Psychiatry. 2021;21:1.
Mneimne M, Fleeson W, Arnold EM, Furr RM. Differentiating the everyday emotion dynamics of borderline personality disorder from major depressive disorder and bipolar disorder. Personal Disord Theory Res Treat. 2018;9(2):192.
Moors A. The integrated theory of emotional behavior follows a radically goal-directed approach. Psychol Inq. 2017;28(1):68–75.
Neacsiu AD, Eberle JW, Kramer R, Wiesmann T, Linehan MM. Dialectical behavior therapy skills for transdiagnostic emotion dysregulation: a pilot randomized controlled trial. Behav Res Ther. 2014;59:40–51.
Nica EI, Links PS. Affective instability in borderline personality disorder: experience sampling findings. Curr Psychiatry Rep. 2009;11(1):74–81.
Nock MK, Prinstein MJ. A functional approach to the assessment of self-mutilative behavior. J Consult Clin Psychol. 2004;72(5):885.
O'Grady SM, Hinshaw SP. Developmental predictors of young adult borderline personality disorder: a prospective, longitudinal study of females with and without childhood ADHD. BMC Psychiatry. 2023;23(1):106.
Paley B, Hajal NJ. Conceptualizing emotion regulation and coregulation as family-level phenomena. Clin Child Fam Psychol Rev. 2022;25(1):19–43.
Palmer CA, Oosterhoff B, Bower JL, Kaplow JB, Alfano CA. Associations among adolescent sleep problems, emotion regulation, and affective disorders: findings from a nationally representative sample. J Psychiatr Res. 2018;96:1–8.
Palmer CA, Oosterhoff B, Gentzler AL. Don't worry, be happy: associations between worry and positive emotion regulation. Int J Cogn Ther. 2021;14:417–35.
Paulus DJ, Heggeness LF, Raines AM, Zvolensky MJ. Difficulties regulating positive and negative emotions in relation to coping motives for alcohol use and alcohol problems among hazardous drinkers. Addict Behav. 2021;115:106781.
Ponzoni S, Beomonte Zobel S, Rogier G, Velotti P. Emotion dysregulation acts in the relationship between vulnerable narcissism and suicidal ideation. Scand J Psychol. 2021;62(4):468–75.

Psychotherapy research and the Psychodynamic Diagnostic Manual (PDM–2). Psychoanalytic Psychology. 2018.

Putnam KM, Silk KR. Emotion dysregulation and the development of borderline personality disorder. Dev Psychopathol. 2005;17(4):899–925.

Reeve J, Lloyd-Williams M, Payne S, Dowrick C. Revisiting biographical disruption: exploring individual embodied illness experience in people with terminal cancer. Health. 2010;14(2):178–95.

Reichenberger J, Eibl JJ, Pfaltz M, Wilhelm FH, Voderholzer U, Hillert A, Blechert J. Don't praise me, don't chase me: emotional reactivity to positive and negative social-evaluative videos in patients with borderline personality disorder. J Personal Disord. 2017;31(1):75–89.

Reitz S, Krause-Utz A, Pogatzki-Zahn EM, Ebner-Priemer U, Bohus M, Schmahl C. Stress regulation and incision in borderline personality disorder – a pilot study modeling cutting behavior. J Personal Disord. 2012;26(4):605–15.

Robin M, Belbèze J, Pham-Scottez A, Shadili G, Peres V, Silva J, Corcos M, Speranza M. Paradoxes in borderline emotional dysregulation in adolescence: influence of parenting, stressful life events, and attachment. Front Psych. 2021;12:735615.

Robin M, Pham-Scottez A, Curt F, Dugre-Le Bigre C, Speranza M, Sapinho D, Corcos M, Berthoz S, Kedia G. Decreased sensitivity to facial emotions in adolescents with borderline personality disorder. Psychiatry Res. 2012;200(2–3):417–21.

Rosenthal MZ, Cheavens JS, Lejuez CW, Lynch TR. Thought suppression mediates the relationship between negative affect and borderline personality disorder symptoms. Behav Res Ther. 2005;43(9):1173–85.

Rosenthal MZ, Gratz KL, Kosson DS, Cheavens JS, Lejuez CW, Lynch TR. Borderline personality disorder and emotional responding: a review of the research literature. Clin Psychol Rev. 2008;28(1):75–91.

Rosenthal MZ, Neacsiu AD, Geiger PJ, Fang C, Ahn R, Larrauri J. Emotional reactivity to personally-relevant and standardized sounds in borderline personality disorder. Cogn Ther Res. 2016;40:314–27.

Ruocco AC, Medaglia JD, Ayaz H, Chute DL. Abnormal prefrontal cortical response during affective processing in borderline personality disorder. Psychiatry Res Neuroimaging. 2010;182(2):117–22.

Ruocco AC. The neuropsychology of borderline personality disorder: a meta-analysis and review. Psychiatry Res. 2005;137(3):191–202.

Ruocco AC, Carcone D. A neurobiological model of borderline personality disorder: systematic and integrative review. Harv Rev Psychiatry. 2016;24(5):311–29.

Sadikaj G, Russell JJ, Moskowitz DS, Paris J. Affect dysregulation in individuals with borderline personality disorder: persistence and interpersonal triggers. J Pers Assess. 2010;92(6):490–500.

Salsman NL, Linehan MM. An investigation of the relationships among negative affect, difficulties in emotion regulation, and features of borderline personality disorder. J Psychopathol Behav Assess. 2012;34:260–7.

Sansone RA, Whitecar P, Meier BP, Murry A. The prevalence of borderline personality among primary care patients with chronic pain. Gen Hosp Psychiatry. 2001;23(4):193–7.

Sauer-Zavala S, Barlow DH. The case for borderline personality disorder as an emotional disorder: implications for treatment. Clin Psychol Sci Pract. 2014;21(2):118.

Sauer-Zavala S, Wilner JG, Cassiello-Robbins C, Saraff P, Pagan D. Isolating the effect of opposite action in borderline personality disorder: a laboratory-based alternating treatment design. Behav Res Ther. 2019;117:79–86.

Scherer KR, Banse R, Wallbott HG. Emotion inferences from vocal expression correlate across languages and cultures. J Cross-Cult Psychol. 2001;32(1):76–92.

Schmideberg M. Learning to talk. The Psychoanalytic Review (1913–1957). 1947;34:296.

Scott LN, Levy KN, Adams RB Jr, Stevenson MT. Mental state decoding abilities in young adults with borderline personality disorder traits. Personal Disord Theory Res Treat. 2011;2(2):98.

Scott LN, Stepp SD, Pilkonis PA. Prospective associations between features of borderline personality disorder, emotion dysregulation, and aggression. Personal Disord Theory Res Treat. 2014;5(3):278.

Scott LN, Wright AG, Beeney JE, Lazarus SA, Pilkonis PA, Stepp SD. Borderline personality disorder symptoms and aggression: a within-person process model. J Abnorm Psychol. 2017;126(4):429.

Schulze L, Domes G, Krüger A, Berger C, Fleischer M, Prehn K, Schmahl C, Grossmann A, Hauenstein K, Herpertz SC. Neuronal correlates of cognitive reappraisal in borderline patients with affective instability. Biol Psychiatry. 2011;69(6):564–73.

Selby EA, Nock MK, Kranzler A. How does self-injury feel? Examining automatic positive reinforcement in adolescent self-injurers with experience sampling. Psychiatry Res. 2014;215(2):417–23.

Selby EA, Joiner TE Jr. Cascades of emotion: the emergence of borderline personality disorder from emotional and behavioral dysregulation. Rev Gen Psychol. 2009;13(3):219–29.

Selby EA, Joiner TE Jr. Emotional cascades as prospective predictors of dysregulated behaviors in borderline personality disorder. Personal Disord Theory Res Treat. 2013;4(2):168.

Selby EA, Braithwaite SR, Joiner TE Jr, Fincham FD. Features of borderline personality disorder, perceived childhood emotional invalidation, and dysfunction within current romantic relationships. J Fam Psychol. 2008;22(6):885.

Selby EA, Anestis MD, Bender TW, Joiner TE Jr. An exploration of the emotional cascade model in borderline personality disorder. J Abnorm Psychol. 2009;118(2):375.

Sharp C, Ha C, Michonski J, Venta A, Carbone C. Borderline personality disorder in adolescents: evidence in support of the childhood interview for DSM-IV borderline personality disorder in a sample of adolescent inpatients. Compr Psychiatry. 2012;53(6):765–74.

Sheppes G, Suri G, Gross JJ. Emotion regulation and psychopathology. Annu Rev Clin Psychol. 2015;11:379–405.

Sieswerda S, Arntz A, Mertens I, Vertommen S. Hypervigilance in patients with borderline personality disorder: specificity, automaticity, and predictors. Behav Res Ther. 2007;45(5):1011–24.

Silverman WK, La Greca AM, Wasserstein S. What do children worry about? Worries and their relation to anxiety. Child Dev. 1995;66(3):671–86.

Skodol AE, Gunderson JG, McGlashan TH, Dyck IR, Stout RL, Bender DS, Grilo CM, Shea MT, Zanarini MC, Morey LC, Sanislow CA. Functional impairment in patients with schizotypal, borderline, avoidant, or obsessive-compulsive personality disorder. Am J Psychiatry. 2002;159(2):276–83.

Sosic-Vasic Z, Schaitz C, Mayer B, Maier A, Connemann B, Kroener J. Treating emotion dysregulation in patients with borderline personality disorder using imagery rescripting: a two-session randomized controlled trial. Behav Res Ther. 2024;173:104454.

Suri G, Gross JJ. What is an emotion? A connectionist perspective. Emotion Review. 2022;14(2):99–110.

Suvak MK, Litz BT, Sloan DM, Zanarini MC, Barrett LF, Hofmann SG. Emotional granularity and borderline personality disorder. J Abnorm Psychol. 2011;120(2):414.

Svaldi J, Griepenstroh J, Tuschen-Caffier B, Ehring T. Emotion regulation deficits in eating disorders: a marker of eating pathology or general psychopathology? Psychiatry Res. 2012;197(1–2):103–11.

Trull TJ, Tomko RL, Brown WC, Scheiderer EM. Borderline personality disorder in 3-D: dimensions, symptoms, and measurement challenges. Soc Personal Psychol Compass. 2010;4(11):1057–69.

Trull TJ, Solhan MB, Tragesser SL, Jahng S, Wood PK, Piasecki TM, Watson D. Affective instability: measuring a core feature of borderline personality disorder with ecological momentary assessment. J Abnorm Psychol. 2008;117(3):647.

Tull MT, Barbano AC, Scamaldo KM, Richmond JR, Edmonds KA, Rose JP, Gratz KL. The prospective influence of COVID-19 affective risk assessments and intolerance of uncertainty on later dimensions of health anxiety. J Anxiety Disord. 2020;75:102290.

Thompson RA. Emotion dysregulation: a theme in search of definition. Dev Psychopathol. 2019;31(3):805–15.

Turner MJ, Wood AG, Boatwright D, Chadha N, Jones JK, Bennett R. Assessing beliefs about emotion generation and change: the conceptualisation, development, and validation of the Cognitive Mediation Beliefs Questionnaire (CMBQ). Psychother Res. 2021;31(7):932–49.

Tragesser SL, Lippman LG, Trull TJ, Barrett KC. Borderline personality disorder features and cognitive, emotional, and predicted behavioral reactions to teasing. J Res Pers. 2008;42(6):1512–23.

Vine V, Aldao A. Impaired emotional clarity and psychopathology: a transdiagnostic deficit with symptom-specific pathways through emotion regulation. J Soc Clin Psychol. 2014;33(4):319–42.

Vohs KD, Baumeister RF, editors. Handbook of self-regulation: research, theory, and applications. Guilford Publications; 2016.

Wagner AW, Linehan MM. Facial expression recognition ability among women with borderline personality disorder: implications for emotion regulation? J Personal Disord. 1999; 13(4):329–44.

Wolff JC, Thompson E, Thomas SA, Nesi J, Bettis AH, Ransford B, Scopelliti K, Frazier EA, Liu RT. Emotion dysregulation and nonsuicidal self-injury: a systematic review and meta-analysis. Eur Psychiatry. 2019;59:25–36.

Wolf D, Klasen M, Eisner P, Zepf FD, Zvyagintsev M, Palomero-Gallagher N, Weber R, Eisert A, Mathiak K. Central serotonin modulates neural responses to virtual violent actions in emotion regulation networks. Brain Struct Funct. 2018;223:3327–45.

Woods KE, Mazursky-Horowitz H, Thomas SR, Dougherty LR, Chronis-Tuscano A. The unique effects of maternal ADHD symptoms and emotion dysregulation on parenting behavior. J Atten Disord. 2021;25(5):672–84.

Weinberg A, Klonsky ED, Hajcak G. Autonomic impairment in borderline personality disorder: a laboratory investigation. Brain Cogn. 2009;71(3):279–86.

Wingenfeld K, Rullkoetter N, Mensebach C, Beblo T, Mertens M, Kreisel S, Toepper M, Driessen M, Woermann FG. Neural correlates of the individual emotional Stroop in borderline personality disorder. Psychoneuroendocrinology. 2009;34(4):571–86.

Wolff S, Stiglmayr C, Bretz HJ, Lammers CH, Auckenthaler A. Emotion identification and tension in female patients with borderline personality disorder. Br J Clin Psychol. 2007;46(3):347–60.

Yamaguchi S, Kawata Y, Murofushi Y, Ota T. The development and validation of an emotional vulnerability scale for university students. Front Psychol. 2022;13:941250.

Zanarini MC, Frankenburg FR, Hennen J, Reich DB, Silk KR. Axis I comorbidity in patients with borderline personality disorder: 6-year follow-up and prediction of time to remission. Am J Psychiatry. 2004;161(11):2108–14.

Zaki J, Williams WC. Interpersonal emotion regulation. Emotion. 2013;13(5):803.

Zelada MI, Garrido V, Liberona A, Jones N, Zúñiga K, Silva H, Nieto RR. Brain-derived neurotrophic factor (BDNF) as a predictor of treatment response in major depressive disorder (MDD): a systematic review. Int J Mol Sci. 2023;24(19):14810.

Chapter 6
Linehan's Biosocial Model and Borderline Personality Disorders

Introduction

The core features in the symptomology of borderline personality disorder (BPD) include emotional instability, impulsivity, identity disturbance, chaotic interpersonal relationships, and suicide/self-injurious behaviors (DSM-5-TR 2022). As stated by Kuo and Linehan (2009), over two decades, several studies have been conducted to identify various biological factors that contribute to the development of BPD. An expansive spectrum of biological factors has been assessed from neurotransmitter dysfunction through focus on the serotonergic system (e.g., Gurvits et al. 2000; Ni et al. 2006), to electrophysiological studies (e.g., Boutros et al. 2003; Battaglia et al. 1999; Williams et al. 2006). However, all of these investigations have been proposed to contribute to the impulsiveness and emotional instability associated with BPD (Kuo and Linehan 2009). Moreover, from two decades before, a series of structural imaging studies have been done to demonstrate anatomical and structural brain dysfunctions in BPD cases (e.g., Tebartz van Elst et al. 2003; Schmahl et al. 2003; Schmaling and Fales 2018). In addition, many reports have been proposed alterations in brain metabolisms in prefrontal regions in BPD (see Schmahl and Bremner 2006). Hughes et al. (2012) suggested the developmental neuroscience of borderline pathology through the aspects of emotion dysregulation and social baseline theory. That said, widespread studies have endeavored to explain BPD development through different lenses of psychological aspects such as cognitive components (Sperry and Sperry 2015; Beck et al. 2016), social cognitive theory (Bandura 1999), and emotion (Linehan 1993; Selby et al. 2008a, b, 2013; Gross 2014; Gross and Ford 2024; Glenn and Klonsky 2013). In addition, as mentioned emotion dysregulation is defined as highly sensitive to emotional stimuli, intense responses to emotional evocation, and slow return to baseline (see e.g., Kuo and Linehan 2009; Linehan 1993, 1995; Crowell et al. 2014a, b; Chapman and Hope 2020; Grove and Crowell 2019).

E. A. Selby, M. Salavati, *Theories of Borderline Personality Disorder*,
https://doi.org/10.1007/978-3-031-75503-3_6

According to Harris and McDade (2018), social and biological phenomena are widely recognized as determining factors to develop human healthiness and acquiring socioeconomic positions across life span. Based on Harris and McDade (2018), the term biosocial is a broad concept to refer to the dynamic, bidirectional interactions between biological components and social interaction and contextual elements, led to shaping the process of human development over the life course. The "biological" aspect is characterized as processes and structures in human beings contributing to growth, reproduction, in other words being alive. This aspect is organized across multiple levels, including the genome, molecular interactions, integrated physiological and neurological systems, organs and other issues, and cells and cellular processes. The "social" phenomena are complex and multidimensional interactions, transactions and relationships among individuals living in groups in different social contexts, who share norms, values, rules, and hierarchies that organize and structure them. Therefore, a biosocial perspective proposes a model and a method which is drawn from biological, medical, behavioral, and social sciences (Harris and McDade 2018). In accordance with findings in the field of BPD development, the presence of biological trajectories and markers which influence the development of BPD is undeniable. One of the most prominent and comprehensive theories that explain the trajectories of formation and development BPD from both biological and environment perspectives is biosocial theory established by Linehan (1993).

Referring to theoretical and empirical studies, Linehan's biosocial theory of BPD (1993) is among the most thoroughly delineated etiological models of borderline pathology and it is a marked theory to elucidate the pathway of developing BPD (e.g., Crowell et al. 2008, 2009; Gunderson et al. 2018; Gill et al. 2021; Dixon-Gordon et al. 2020). As per the biological theory, the primary problem of BPD is a pervasive disorder of the emotion regulation system. This pervasive dysregulation is hypothesized to be developed and maintained by both biological and environmental factors. Linehan (1993) suggests that the fundamental and basic predilection of BPD is a pervasive difficulty in regulation of one's emotions. In other words, she posited that BPD individuals have a biological preparedness toward emotional dysregulation (Linehan 1993). A biosocial model formulates a specific identification of characteristics and manifestations of individuals who are in upward vulnerability trends to BPD psychopathology (Crowell et al. 2022). According to Evans et al. (2013), it has been claimed that the crucial component in the development of BPD is difficulties and deficits in emotion regulation, one of the most significant elements in Linehan' biosocial theory (1993). Pursuant to Evans et al. (2013), "emotion regulation has been defined as the automatic and intentional ways in which people influence their emotions and when and how they are experienced and expressed" (Evans et al. 2013; Dunn et al. 2009). Linehan (1993, 1997) posited that individuals with BPD have a biologically inherent predisposition toward emotional dysregulation. In other words, emotion dysregulation is considered an essential vulnerability which leads directly to the development and maintenance of BPD and other related cognitive, behavioral, interpersonal, and identity difficulties and dysregulations (see, Linehan 1993; Chapman and Hope 2020; Dixon-Gordon et al.

2020; Beauchaine and Crowell 2020; King et al. 2019). Per Niedtfeld and Bohus (2018), "emotion processing involves automatic and intentional processes influencing to occurrence, intensity, duration and expression of emotion." It should be noticed that from a psychological point of view, emotions crucially are complex and complicated and can be considered as a gradual evolutionary pattern of responses to both internal and external stimuli, providing a situation-based rapid interpretation along with a corresponding action tendency.

The core assumption of Linehan's (1993) theory is a transaction between emotional vulnerability and invalidated environment. According to this theory, the severe difficulties in emotion regulatory system, which lead to emotional dysregulation, is a consequence of interaction between innate biological vulnerability in the system of emotional regulation and an erratic environment, which is labeled as invalidated environment (e.g., Ritschel et al. 2018; Neacsiu et al. 2014a, b, Linehan and Schmidt 1995; Crowell et al. 2008, 2022; Kuo and Linehan 2009). Biosocial theory assumed that the interaction between *emotional vulnerability* (an innate biological deficiency of experiencing frequent and intense emotional state and a strong tendency toward emotional reactions to stimuli) and *invalidated environments* (series of specific negative traumatic environmental stressors) contribute to the development of psychological disorders especially characterological disturbances such as BPD (Linehan 1993; Linehan et al. 2006). According to biosocial theory (Linehan 1993), emotional vulnerability and emotion dysregulation in transaction with invalidated environment. To clarify, it should be noted that Linehan (1993) believes in a transactional mode of the individual-environment system. In other words, transactional processes between individual's emotional vulnerabilities especially in childhood and an invalid familial environment, which invalidate all psychological and behavioral aspects of a child during rearing, can contribute to the development of BPD. Linehan (1993) asserts that many of current psychopathological theories are based on interaction models, which emphasize the interaction between individual vulnerabilities and problematic characters and environment to produce different psychological disorders. In particular, she makes a reference to the "diathesis-stress model" to clarify this concept. As has been mentioned by Linehan (1993), diathesis refers to constitutional and biological predispositions, which can be considered as a heightened chance for shaping a psychopathology in individuals. As well, stress is assumed as any kind of notorious and unpleasant environmental stimuli and events, which can be noxious and aversive for a vulnerable person. As a consequence, an interaction between these both sides can contribute to develop mental disorders. On the contrary, in Linehan's view, the "transactional model assumes that individual functioning and environmental conditions are mutually and continuously interactive, reciprocal, and interdependent. Within social learning theory, this the principle of "reciprocal determinism: the environment and the individual adapt to and influence each other. Although the individual is surely affected by the environment, the environment is also affected by the individual." (Linehan 1993, p. 39).

According to biosocial theory, BPD diagnosis is assumed to appear from these biological changes, interacting with insufficient knowledge about emotion regulation, which is named *emotion dysregulation*. Neacsiu et al. (2014a, b) suggested that emotion dysregulation is the inability, even when individual efforts are applied to alter emotional cues, experiences, actions, verbal responses, and/or nonverbal expressions under normative conditions, in a desired way (Neacsiu et al. 2014a, b).

In line with biosocial theory, Linehan (1993) proposed that BPD is a serious psychological disorder with severe dysregulation of emotion system at its components. Linehan's (1993) biosocial theory of BPD is based on a transactional model of development which proposes a bidirectional relationship between the person and environment. Keeping with Linehan (1993), BPD is the outcome of a transaction between an individual with a constitutional and innate vulnerability to emotion regulation and an environment that is prone to invalidate the expression of private experiences, beliefs, and action (Linehan 1993; Chapman and Hope 2020). From this perspective, an individual's behavior is influenced and—under the effect of ongoing and constant interactions between personal factors (e.g., temperament) and the social environment—the environment and the individual adapt to and influence each other. It means that biosocial theory presents that an invalidating environment reinforces biological vulnerability to emotional sensitivity and emotional reactivity can contribute to the development of emotion dysregulation (see, Wagner and Linehan 2006; Sweezy 2011a, b; Chapman and Hope 2020). This model documented that a pervasive emotion dysregulation in BPD is generated as a result of interaction between biological (e.g., genetic, intrauterine factors, trauma to the biological system) vulnerability and aversive socio-biographical experiences (Neacsiu et al. 2014a, b). Stated by Crowell et al. (2022), the core assumption in biosocial theory is the emotional biological vulnerability in a child which is worsened in an invalidate environment; therefore, a severe emotion dysregulation appears which can be considered as a base for the development of BPD (Crowell et al. 2022). Linehan (1993) emphasizes that psychopathologies theories such as the stress-diathesis model claims that an inherent and constitutional disabling factor resides within the person, standing by being activated when some emotional-evoked events occur in environment; whereas, biosocial theory proposes that the individual and the environment are developmentally collaborative and co-active in providing conditions for the development of dysfunction in a wide aspects, especially emotional and behavioral areas. In accordance with this model, on one side, an individual evokes the environment that generates dysfunction, and on the other side, the environment embitters and intensifies vulnerabilities; in a more secure and benign environment, this dysfunction might not have developed (see, Linehan 1993, 1997; Linehan and Schmidt 1995; Crowell et al. 2008; Chapman and Hope 2020).

Linehan (1993) states that individuals who are at the risk BPD are born with a temperament and neurobiological alterations in the emotional circuity characterized by: (1) a low threshold for recognition of/arousal/response to emotional stimuli (heightened emotional sensitivity); this means that these difficulties with emotion regulation in turn are originated from a biological predisposition toward emotional hypersensitivity (Linehan 1993), in other words, higher emotional sensitivity (a low threshold to evoke and emotional reaction) (Dixon-Gordon et al. 2020; Chapman and Hope 2020) in interaction with an invalidating childhood environment; (2) a rapidly intense affective response, or heightened reactivity (inability to regulate intense emotional response; high amplitude of emotional responses) (Linehan 1993); meant that emotional responses and reactions to environmental stimuli happen more rapidly, are more intense and vigorous (Dixon-Gordon et al. 2020); (3) a slow return to emotional baseline following exposure to salient and emotional events and emotion induction (Linehan 1993), refer to a slower return to baseline in comparison with non-BPD individuals (Dixon-Gordon et al. 2020). These issues contribute to a heightened proneness in an individual which leads to not only replying forcefully and strongly, but also an increased tendency to show increasingly and drastically upward levels of responding ascribable to uninterrupted environmental input before throwback to baseline occurring, causing a vicious and perverse feedback cycle. In other words, the term which was mentioned by Linehan (1993) makes reference to the extreme sensitivity to emotional arousal and susceptibility to negative unpleasant emotions, along with the individual's awareness or experience of this vulnerability (Linehan 1993; Linehan and Schmidt 1995; Chapman and Hope 2020). "*High sensitivity*" means that the person reacts quickly and rapidly and has a low threshold for an emotional reaction; that is, it does not take much to provoke an emotional reaction. This means that events that do not annoy many people can be bothersome for emotionally vulnerable people. *"Emotional intensity"* refers to emotional reactions and responses which are significantly extreme. These individuals' response to emotional stimuli very dramatically, and their reactions are horribly exaggerated in some cases in the case of experiencing negative emotions, hastening really intense and painful grief, embarrassment, shame, guilt, anger, and other aversive emotions, even escalating to panic or outburst of negative emotions. On the positive side of emotions, again they experience severe and intense emotion such as falling in love and idealizing love object. Also, other positive and pleasant emotions can be intensified even to spiritual experiences (Linehan 1993). One of the most awful land disastrous drawbacks of these problems is difficulties in cognitive processes, especially attention ability and attention issues (Lewis et al. 1984; Neacsiu et al. 2014a, b; Niedtfeld and Bohus 2018; Crowell et al. 2008; Chapman and Hope 2020). *"Slow return to baseline"* refers to that individual's reactions which are long-lasting, continuous, and long-term. According to Linehan (1993), although all emotions are partly brief and short-term, and lasting from seconds to minutes, emotional arousal, or mood, have a great tendency to have a pervasive influences on a huge amount cognitive processes, especially attention, which in turn are associated with the activation and reactivation of emotional state (Linehan 1993; Crowell et al. 2008, 2009; Schulze et al. 2016; Dimeff et al. 2021a, b; Niedtfeld and Bohus 2018; Chapman and Hope 2020).

A substantial body of research has been conducted to test core elements of biosocial theory and to examine the roles of these components in the development of BPD via evidence-based studies and experiments (Ritschel et al. 2018). Based on these investigations, a great body of individuals with BPD reported elevated emotional intensity (e.g., Bland and Rossen 2005; Yen et al. 2002), more frequent and more severity in their experiences of their intensive negative emotions rather positive emotions (Ebner-Priemer et al. 2007), more difficulties in controlling their negative emotions and deficiencies in emotion regulation skills (Yen et al. 2002).

One of the most important research projects that Linehan referred to it as evidence to indicate emotional states is research conducted by Gilligan and Brower (1984). In these studies, they claimed that emotional states (1) selectively bias the recall of emotional toned material, which resulted in superior memory when emotional state at recall matches the learning state; (2) enhance the learning of mood-congruent material; and (3) can bias interpretations, fantasies, projections, free associations, personal forecasts, and social judgment in a fashion congruent with current mood (Linehan 1993). Conforming to Linehan (1993), since individuals with BPD have a significant tendency toward a severe intensity in their emotional response, it can be mentioned that emotions are more self-perpetuate among this group of patients. Linehan (1993) proposed that in a very high emotional arousal, the environment, even the therapist's behavior, can be selectively attended to, therefore, merely the actions and events which are compatible with the current mood state will be considered and the other might be missed. This problem can impact the cognitive processes, indicating that the emotions are full-system responses (Linehan 1993).

One of the most important concepts that have been proposed by Linehan (1993) to clarify the emotional problems in borderline personality disorder is that of *emotion modulation*. In describing this new concept, "emotion regulation requires two different and even paradoxical strategies". "First of all, the person should learn to experience and label the significant and specified emotion which are hard-weird into the neuro-physiological, behavioral-expressive, and sensory-feeling systems". Then, in the next stage, the person should learn to decrease emotionally related stimuli which provide the opportunity to react emotionally and experience ongoing negative emotions or deviate toward dysfunctional emotional responses. Linehan (1993) emphasized that as soon as an intense emotion being triggered and active, the person must be able to inhibit any kind of activation and behavior based on that intense emotion especially self-destructive behaviors, which are generated due to experiencing severe emotions (Linehan 1993). In other words, features of emotion dysregulation include an excess of negative aversive emotional experiences, an inability to regulate severely intensive physiological arousal, toughness in distracting attention away from emotional stimuli, cognitive distortions and failure in information processing, insufficient self-control of impulsive behaviors due to strong emotions, problems in organizing and coordinating activities to gain and achieve non-mood-dependent goals in the case of emotionally hyper-arousal, and a tendency to "freeze" or dissociate under really severe and high stressful situation (Linehan 1993; Crowell et al. 2008, 2009, 2014a, b; Neacsiu et al. 2014a, b; Ray et al. 2006; Linehan and Schmidt 1995). In line with Neacsiu et al. (2014a, b), psychological alterations include maladaptive, maladjusted, and insufficient learning in how to understand, label, regulate, or tolerate emotional responses effectively (e.g., Neacsiu et al. 2014a, b; Hernandez et al. 2012; Bornovalova et al. 2013; Crowell et al. 2008).

According to biosocial theory, the heightened biological sensitivity to emotional cues are innate and constitutional which encounters emotionally aversive experiences, such as interpersonal violence, social rejection, emotional neglect, and invalidation, and consequently developed biological and psychological alterations of the emotion regulation system (Linehan 1993; Distel et al. 2011; Neacsiu et al. 2014a, b; Linehan and Schmidt 1995; Crowell et al. 2008; Chapman and Hope 2020). Although the actual emotional response may be brief, the associated emotional arousal persists and has the potential influence on cognitive processes (e.g., attentional). As a result, the individual would be susceptible to the activation and reactivation of similar emotional states. Moreover, from Linehan's perspective, the construct of emotion (and thus of emotion dysregulation) is quite broad and includes emotion-linked cognitive processes, biochemistry and physiology, facial and muscle reaction, action urges, and emotion-linked actions (e.g., Crowell et al. 2009, 2013).

Although Linehan believed both DBT and modal model include the importance of attending to a cue within a relevant context, highlighted appraisals as potentially influencing the course of the emotion and present how emotions directly affect context. Nevertheless, dialectical behavior therapy (DBT) places more emphasis on issues in regulating the emotional response after it has already been initiated, especially when it is it could be suppressed. As stated by Linehan et al. (2014), the emotional response is broken into experiential and expressive responses. An additional difference is the inclusion of emotion vulnerability factors. The structure of *emotion vulnerability* refers to the effects of distal and proximal prior events on the initiation, course, and intensity of emotion responses, which would be occurred in BPD (Neacsiu et al. 2014a, b). To elaborate the concept of emotion vulnerability, Neacsiu et al. (2014a, b) have referred to this point that individuals diagnosed with BPD who meet diagnostic criteria for co-occurring posttraumatic stress disorder (PTSD; a distal vulnerability factor) report significantly higher emotion regulation (Harned et al. 2010), highly sufficient sleep (a proximal vulnerability factor) which lead to less emotional intensity when compared to lack of sleep (Gujar et al. 2011). As mentioned by Linehan (1993), the same patterns of emotion dysregulation and emotion vulnerability cause further dysregulation.

Referring to the previous argument, BPD is primarily a disorder of emotion dysregulation and emerges from transactions between individuals with biological vulnerabilities and specific environment influences. The dysfunction proposed by Linehan (1993) is one of the broad dysregulations across all aspects of emotional responding. In other words, the negative malignant consequences of transaction between emotion dysregulation and invalidated environment are cognitive, behavioral, interpersonal, and identity dysregulation. These concepts can explain and clarify BPD criteria in DSM. In sum, the best way to make a comparison between BPD criteria and parasuicidal characteristics of BPD case, which was proposed by Linehan (1993) can, has been shown in Table 6.1 (Linehan 1993, p. 13; Chapman and Hope 2020).

As mentioned by Crowell et al. (2022) biosocial theory is based on this assumption that since biological vulnerable children involve a contentious daily transaction

Table 6.1 Key facets of biopsychosocial theory

DSM BPD Symptom	Biopsychosocial Model Facet
Emotional dysregulation	
1. Emotional instability *2. Problems with anger*	*1. Chronis, aversive affect* *2. Anger, hostility, irritability*
Interpersonal dysregulation	
3. Unstable relationships *4. Efforts to avoid loss*	*3. Conflictual relationship* *4. Weak social support* *5. Interpersonal problems paramount* *6. Passive interpersonal problem solving*
Behavioral dysregulation	
5. Suicide threats, parasuicide *6. Self-damaging, impulsive behaviors, including alcohol and drug abuse*	*7. Suicide threats, parasuicide* *8. Alcohol, drug abuse, promiscuity*
Cognitive dysregulation	
7. Cognitive disturbances	*9. Cognitive rigidity, dichotomous thinking*
Self-dysregulation	
8. Unstable self, self-image *9. Chronic emptiness*	*10. Low self-esteem*

with their parents, caregivers, and different social-environmental pressures, they could be reinforced to develop ineffective and self-destructive behaviors while at the same time punishing effective strategies. Therefore, neither parents nor children can meet their core emotional-psychological needs. Subsequently, the children will fail to get effective and crucial skillful strategies for regulating emotions, managing distress, solving interpersonal conflicts, and being mindful (Crowell et al. 2022). As per Crowell et al. (2014a, b), the trajectory and markers of BPD development have existed from early childhood and include heritable biological vulnerabilities that are strengthened and potentiated by environmental and contextual risk factors. In line with Crowell et al. (2014a, b), BPD is the production of complicated transaction between individual-level vulnerabilities and environmental risk factor especially erratic and invalidating family environment, which if full of intermittent reinforcement of negative affect. BPD is manifested by constant and pervasive cognitive, emotional and behavioral dysregulation, and is one of the most severely notorious and perplexing behavioral disorders. In keeping with Crowell et al. (2009) "BPD is a heterogeneous phenotype and results from a polythetic criterion set of which only five of nine behavioral features are required for a diagnosis. Thus, two individuals receiving a diagnosis of BPD could potentially overlap on only one diagnosis criterion" (Crowell et al. 2008, 2009). This point can be seen in many clinical settings and psychotherapeutic experiences, in which a psychotherapist faces two BPD cases but with different signs and symptoms, although both of them meet DSM criteria for BPD. In other words, many clinicians have experienced the situation in which they visit some cases and they would be suspicious about the BPD criteria, and after assessing these cases via specific assessment methods, they find out that all of them meet BPD criteria based on DSM, but the most surprisingly point is although these cases have some shared and similar signs and symptoms, they are experiencing a group of problems which are completely specified to them, even in some cases, their features are profoundly controversial.

Pursuant to the perspective presented by Gunderson et al. (2018), Linehan's biosocial theory identifies a deficient capacity to regulate emotion. This deficiency is thought to be a neurobiological disposition that is evident in excessively intense and prolonged emotions, this deficit becomes manifest only when the pre-borderline child's experiences are not validated. The dysregulated emotions trigger the borderline patient's behavioral and interpersonal problems (Gunderson et al. 2018). According to Linehan (1993), these difficulties with the experience and management of emotion (e.g., intensity of affect activation and the lack of affect control) underlie the instability in identity, relationships, and behavior that define BPD. Specifically, the potentially destructive behaviors observed in cases with BPD are considered as a series of attempts to self-regulate intense and severe emotional experiences (e.g., Gratz et al. 2006; Linehan et al. 2006; Crowell et al. 2008). Therefore, the impulsive and self-destructive behaviors are considered as a reflection of the interference of intense emotion with cognitive functioning and effective problem-solving and self-regulation (e.g., Wagner and Linehan 1999).

Crowell et al. (2009) added to this discourse in highlighting the developmental course or trajectories that cause BPD in adulthood, a topic of investigation that remain ambiguous on many developmental fronts; thus, we are exposed to a series of unresolved questions (Crowell et al. 2009). Despite continuous progress in studies concerning the etiology and psychopathology of BPD, longitudinal studies are absolutely necessary to identify biological vulnerabilities, environmental risk and protective factors, and patterns of homotypic continuity that associated with the diagnosis of BPD (see Crowell et al. 2008, 2009; Lenzenweger and Cicchetti 2005; Chapman and Hope 2020). These ambiguous questions will be discussed in this chapter later as elaborated biosocial theory (Crowell et al. 2009).

Based on Linehan biosocial theory (1993), BPD is developed through the transaction of emotional vulnerability and invalidating environment. Up to this part of this chapter, the emotional vulnerability or emotional dysregulation has been explained as a biological aspect of biosocial theory. Linehan (1993) suggested in the case that the individual eliciting the invalidating environment, the theory is similar to Millon's (Millon et al. 2012) biosocial learning theory of personality disorders, wherein childhood biological substrates lead to behaviors that provoke particular groups of responses and reactions from caretakers and start to establish patterns of interaction that later "crystallize" into personality. Linehan (1993, 1995) posited that the most critical characteristic in familial environment which in transaction with emotional vulnerability contribute to produce BPD is invalidation. The body of work has demonstrated this crucial concept in familial environment of BPD individuals (e.g., Elzy 2013; Whalen 2014; Reeves et al. 2010, 2018; Lee et al. 2022; Crowell et al. 2008; Gill et al. 2018; Sauer and Baer 2010; Lyons-Ruth 2008; Beauchaine et al. 2009). Likewise, according to Lynch et al. (2006) in biosocial theory, invalidation is the crucial concept which can explain the critical role of context and environment where a child is raised (Lyons et al. 2006). Linehan (1993) suggests that the temperamental sensitivity is not a risk factor in and of itself. Rather, she proposes that emotional dysregulation occurs when the primary caregivers fail to support the adaptive expression of emotion in the vulnerable child, impeding the acquisition of skills required for successful emotional modulation.

Linehan (1993) proposed that invalidation has two core characteristics. First of all, its general message is that individual is wrong in describing and analyzing their own experiences and views about the casual factors of their emotions, thoughts, and actions. Second, invalidation leads individuals to attribute and relate all emotional experiences, beliefs, and behaviors to their individual personality traits and character. In other words, invalidation does not permit to individual analyze and make synthesis of their thoughts and accept their emotional experiences as valid, especially negative emotions. Linehan (1993) stated "negative emotional expressions may be attributed to traits such as overactivity, oversensitivity, paranoia, a distorted view of events, or failure to adopt a positive attitude. Behaviors that have unintended negative or painful consequences for others may be attributed to hostile or manipulative motives. Failure, or any deviation from socially defined success, is labeled as resulting from lack of motivation, lack of discipline, or not trying hard enough, or the like. Positive emotional expressions, beliefs, and action plans may be similarly invalidated of being attributed to lack of discrimination, naivete, overidealization, or immaturity. In any case, the individual's private experiences and emotional expressions are not viewed as valid responses to events" (Linehan 1993, p. 50). In an invalidating environment, the child's experiences are devalued and the communication of these experiences is met with erratic or extreme inappropriate responses (Fruzzetti et al. 2005; Linehan 1993). For instance, the child's display of emotion may be punished at times, which discourages expression of feelings. In this situation, the individual receives the message that their response to the environment is inaccurate or invalid and may start to doubt the veracity of their own thoughts and feelings. Consequently, labeling internal experiences becomes difficult (McMain et al. 2001) and the individual begins to base their emotional reactions in response to cues in their social environment. At other times, extreme displays of emotion may be reinforced, thereby strengthening emotional reactivity. Consequently, an invalidating environment may contribute to affective lability; the individual switches between strong inhibition of emotion and extreme displays of emotion. According to Linehan (1993), these difficulties with the experience and management of emotion (e.g., intensity of affect activation and the lack of affect control) underlie the instability in identity, interpersonal relationships, and behavior that define BPD. Specifically, the potentially harmful behaviors observed in patients with BPD are viewed as attempts to self-regulate intense emotional experience (e.g., Gratz et al. 2006; Linehan et al. 2006). From this perspective, the behavior of the individual is a reflection of the interference of intense emotion with cognitive functioning and effective problem solving (e.g., Wagner and Linehan 1999).

Based on Linehan (1997), the act of validating is "to attest to the truth or validity of something," "to communicate that a response is valid is to say that it is well-organized or justifiable: being at once relevant and meaningful.....logically correct.....appropriate to the end in view or effective", "having such force as to compel serous attention and usually accepted", "being well-founded on fact, or established on sound principles, and thoroughly applicable to the case or circumstances; soundness and strength" (Linehan 1997, p. 355). Although, a crucial point made by Linehan (1997) is that validation means the acknowledgment of that which is valid, validation does not involve "making" something valid. Nor does it mean validating that which invalid (Linehan 1997). In fact, through reviewing different definitions of validation, it can be inferred that validation is not an agreement with all individual's thoughts and emotions, ignoring limitations, allowing to any kind of expectation and letting go contingencies, and offering compliments to any kind of behaviors and action. Indeed, as mentioned in this chapter, based on biosocial theory and numerous studies associated with this model, it has been derived those individuals with BPD experience emotions especially negative emotions more intensive and unpleasant, extreme reactions to environment stimuli and slow return to baseline, which demonstrate the constitutional and biological parts of their problems. But, since they have been raised in an invalidating environment where their emotions, thoughts and behaviors will be replied with a series of notorious and unpredictable responses, they have serious problems in identifying their inner experiences. This is the environmental part of their life. Likewise, in an invalidating environment, individual's private emotional experiences will be dismissed, any type of displaying emotions are punished and there are significant punishing responses, instead of rewarding, toward child's behavior. Moreover, since no problem-solving strategies have been thought in these environment, oversimplifications of problems will have occurred in which can lead to even a series of traumatic experiences (e.g., Linehan 1993, 1995, 1997; Crowell et al. 2008, 2009, 2014a, b; Lee et al. 2022; Ramos-Luna and Oliver 2024; Dimeff et al. 2021a, b; Grove 2023). Linehan and Schmidt (1995) presented a description of invalidating environment as one in which all of the actions, communications, and private individual experiences such as feelings and attitudes are met by erratic, extreme, enmeshed, and in appropriate answers. Accordingly, Lynch et al. (2006) describe the biosocial theory of BPD as dialectical, in that the theory proposes that the transaction between a biological tendency toward emotional vulnerability and an invalidating rearing environment produces a dysregulation of the patient's emotional system (Lynch et al. 2006). Indeed, validation is like a gateway to help individuals to help and understand their own cognitive and emotional experiences to make them sense, to improve and expand their interpersonal relationships, to communicate with themselves and accept their emotions and beliefs as a valid phenomenon, to express their feelings and attitudes, and to elaborate their emotion regulation skills. In addition, Linehan (1993) proposed that invalidating environments during childhood contribute to the development of emotion dysregulation; they also fail to teach the child how to label and regulate arousal, how to tolerate emotional distress, and when to trust her own emotional responses as reflection of valid interpretations of events. Therefore, as adults, they tend to invalidate their own emotional experiences, look to others for accurate reflections of external reality, and oversimplify the ease of solving life's problems. In other words, invalidation can escalate emotional dysregulation and make difficulties for emotion regulation skill;

hence, any emotional experiences will be painful for BPD case and lead to the majority of intrapsychic and interpsychic problems for them (Linehan 1993).

Based on Linehan and Schmidt (1995), the core message of an invalidating environment that is delivered to individual is: "your typical responses to events and situations are invalid, wrong, inconsistent, meaningless, inaccurate and irrelevant." The invalidate environment is characterized by ignoring, punishing, dismissing, trivializing, disregarding the individual's communication of thoughts, beliefs, attitudes, emotions, and feelings as well as self-initiated behaviors and may involve traumatic experiences such as sexual abuse, molestation, physical maltreatment, and emotional-psychological abuse (Linehan 1993; Linehan and Schmidt 1995; Lycnh et al. 2006; Wagner and Linehan 1999; Sweezy 2011a, b; Crowell et al. 2009, 2014a, b; Gratz and Tull 2010; Bohus et al. 2020; Evans et al. 2015; Grove 2023). Dimeff et al. (2021a, b) have highlighted that issues appeared when a biologically vulnerable individual is in a pervasively invalidating environment. Invalidating environments communicate and provide a kind of relationship that the individual's characteristic and traits response to events (particularly their emotional responses) are incorrect, inappropriate, pathological, and problematic or not to be taken seriously. Not understanding how debilitating it is to struggle with emotion regulation, those in the environment oversimplify the ease of solving problems and fail to relate distress or to set realistic goals and expectations. By punishing and castigated communication of negative notorious experiences and only responding to negatively emotional displays when they are escalated, the individual would be thought by the environment to oscillate between emotional inhibition and extreme emotional communication (Dimeff et al. 2021a, b, p. 5).

Based on Crowell et al. (2009, 2013, 2014a, b) and Grove et al. (2017), there are three fundamental components of invalidating environment. First, in invalidating environment children's core psychological and emotional needs are chronically disregarded, ignored, dismissed, and rejected. It means that child's emotional expressions will be invalidated rather being accepted. In other words, the quality of caregiver-child relationship is overwhelmed by justification, punishment, and inappropriate responses. This pathological and conflictual communication can be overt such as blaming, discounting child's experience, and physically and emotionally abuse, or it can be covert such as making decisions for them before knowing what the problem is, body language and facial expressions. A growing body of work has shown that invalidating parent-child interaction can be contributed to the development of BPD (Linehan 1993, 1995; Dixon-Gordon et al. 2016; Selby et al. 2008a, b, 2014; Stepp et al. 2013). Grove et al. (2017) proposed that the biosocial theory identifies that invalidating environments are not merely due to either the caregiver or the sensitive child. Rather, it debates that both child and the contextual variables interact to generate an invalidating context, which can be further compounded by external forces such as poverty and environmental stressors (Grove et al. 2017).

The second component of the invalidating environmental theory cites that during parent-child interaction, parents or caregiver reinforce sporadically and intermittently child's extreme and intensive emotional expressions through conflictual, paradoxical, and problematic patterns (Grove 2023). Moreover, this kind of invalidating environment overwhelmed by intermittent reinforcement of a child's emotional response imposes the message on children that all of their emotional experiences are without good reason or are annoying, and that the child should deal with intense emotions without parents or caregivers' support and attention (Crowell et al. 2009). Linehan (1993) insisted that in invalidating environment, child's emotional experiences are ignored and dismissed. Consequently, the children learn all negative and positive emotions will not be addressed, even these experiences are unwarranted, so they learn to avoid, suppress, and invalidate their emotional experiences. Finally, the third component of invalidating environment theory includes the consequence of this conflictual and problematic parent-child interactions, or in other words, this invalidating environment is emotion dysregulation over time, which contribute to severe psychopathology, especially BPD.

In order to show the adverse consequences of problematic child-parent interaction which can be contributed to emotion dysregulation, Crowell et al. (2009) studied the respiratory sinus arrhythmia (RSA). RSA was defined as peripheral biomarker of emotion regulation capacity (Beauchaine 2012; Beauchaine et al. 2007). Crowell et al. (2013) found that high-high dyads adolescent-parent interaction showed the lowest RSA, which indicates poor self-regulatory capacity. In other words, these findings demonstrate that conflict upward the development of emotional instability and emotion dysregulation, which lead to self-destructive behaviors (Crowell et al. 2013). Subsequently, children cannot be able to identify, label, accept, tolerate, make their intense emotional responses valid as they are experiencing them, rather they began to oscillate between inhibition and extreme emotional lability (e.g., Linehan 1993; Crowell et al. 2009, 2014a, b, 2022; Grove and Crowell 2019; Chapman and Hope 2020). In keeping with coercive family dynamics, coercive, harsh, and conflictual parenting styles are related to the development of early conduct problems and different forms of antisocial behaviors (Waller et al. 2013; Odgers et al. 2008; Smith et al. 2014). Coercion theory describes a process of mutual reinforcement during which caregivers inadvertently reinforce children' difficult behaviors, which in turn elicits caregiver negativity, and so on, until the interaction is discounted when one of the participants "wins." These cycles may begin when the child reacts with anger or resistance to a caregiver's directive or request, evoking anger, and hostility from the caregiver, which is often intensified as the coercive escalates (Snyder and Ammons 1993). Thus, children learn a pattern of relating within the family that then carries over into interaction with others outside the family, such as peers and teachers in the school setting. When coercive interactions dominate within the family, child conduct problems emerge and then stabilize throughout development (Smith et al. 2014). Crowell et al. 2014a, b; Crowell and Kaufman 2016 make reference to coercive theory (Patterson and Capaldi 2013) to clarify the role of problematic dyadic interactions with parents which produce and maintain psychopathology, emotion dysregulation, and disturbed interpersonal relationships. Based on Crowell et al., (Crowell et al. 2014a, b), it can be deduced that there is an obvious similarity between coercive theory and biosocial. In other words, both these two theories emphasize on the erratic and intermittent confinement and inappropriate responses to child's negative intense emotional experiences (e.g., Crowell et al. 2014a, b). Crowell et al. (2013) demonstrated that the adolescents who had conflictual mutual relationships with problematic mothers and experienced several aversive responses in those erratic and inappropriate environments demonstrated dyads self-inflicted behaviors. According to coercion theory (Dodge et al. 2008) through the lens of developmental psychopathology, due to harsh, inconsistent parenting styles which overwhelmed by negative reinforcement patterns, maladaptive behaviors will be generated in parent-child interactions (Crowell and Kaufman 2016). Along these lines, Patterson et al. (2018) states, "family members' aversive behavior may be shaped by either positive or negative reinforcement. However, the negative reinforcement produces significant behavior change in fewer instances than does positive reinforcement" (Patterson et al. 2018; Dishion and Snyder 2016).

In the context of invalidating environments, children with biological emotional vulnerability are prone to get malicious and erratic messages from their caregivers that their cognitive and emotional reactions and behaviors are too unjustified and invalid. As a result, over time, they will be unable to trust to their emotions and even all the phenomena in their psychological atmosphere, which can contribute to the lack of self-regulation strategies, especially emotion regulation skills. Consequently, through these harmful transactions between temperamental vulnerabilities and invalidating environments, where one is surrounded by different risk factors, emotion dysregulation will be strengthened and intensified and invade to all parts of individual's life (Dixon-Gordon et al. 2020). Subsequently, the frequency, intensity, and duration of emotional experiences will be exacerbated, and BPD individuals cannot be able to clarify, identify, label and accept their intense negatively emotional experiences, and tolerate them as normal problems due to their vulnerabilities. Therefore, their emotion-dependent information processing deficits emerge (Dicxon-Gordon et al. 2020). Because there are lack of emotion regulation and distress tolerance skills, individuals with BPD began to attempt and being involved in maladaptive ways self-destructive behaviors to avoid from their dysregulated psychological states such as nonsuicidal self-injury (NSSI) (Gratz and Roemer 2004; Gratz and Tull 2010; Nock et al. 2006; Matera et al. 2021; Kaufman et al. 2017, 2023), suicidal behaviors (Linehan 1993, 1995; Crowell et al. 2009, 2014a, b; Grove 2023; Dimeff et al. 2021a, b; Kaufman et al. 2017, 2023; Neece 2014), binge eating (Selby et al. 2014; Mitchell et al. 1999). In line with Dimeff et al. (2021a, b), "On the biological side, individuals are thought to be more vulnerable to difficulties regulating their emotions due to differences in the central nervous system (e.g., due to genetics, events during fatal development, or early life trauma)" (Dimeff et al. 2021a, b). From this perspective, BPD criterion behaviors function to regulate emotions (e.g., suicidal behavior) or are a consequence of failed emotion regulation (e.g., dissociative symptoms or transient psychotic symptoms) (Dimeff and Koerner 2007).

According to Linehan (1993), there are three types of invalidating families that can lead to the development of BPD in children and adolescents: the "chaotic" family, the "perfect" family, and, the "typical" family. As mentioned, a body of work have shown that maltreatment and child abuse can predate the onset of psychopathology, escalate the risk of psychopathology, and maintain severe psychopathology (Zanarini and Wedig 2014). In a *Chaotic family*, Linehan (1993) posited that in the chaotic family, there may be several problems such as parental substance use disorder or poverty due to financial issues. In this type of family, due multiple challenges parents are exposed, generally children's core physical and psychological needs are not met, and the significant number of these needs are ignored, disregarded and dismissed. Therefore, different types of self-destructive behaviors will emerge due to the development emotion dysregulation. In these chaotic kinds of family, children are exposed to several painful, aversive, and negatives experiences, which can lead to the development of BPD (Linehan 1993; Fruzzetti et al. 2005, 2008). In a *Perfect family*, children are persuaded to suppress and inhibit their emotional experiences because their family has taught them that any kind of emotion is wrong. In other words, any emotional experiences and emotional expressions are not acceptable, so these children attempt to not tolerate any emotions because they believe that the control of emotion is impossible (Linehan 1993; Elzy 2013). Linehan (1993) proposed that these parents have an invalidating attitude toward emotions, such as "if they express their emotions, they cannot control their feeling" (Linehan 1993). In *Typical families,* the most emphasis is concentrated on the ability to cognitively control one's emotions (Elzy 2013), and the competence of self-control described as an individual's capability to control their own behavior through employing internal cues and resources (Linehan 1993). The most problematic aspect in these families is failing in identifying the child's capacity and ability to regulate and express their emotions. Therefore, it seems that there is a continuous battle in these families, in which there is a lack of internal capacity to manage intense emotions and a high parent's demanding for utilizing internal cognitive ability to regulate emotions without considering the real competency of the child's competency (e.g., Elzy 2013; Linehan 1993).

Dialectical Behavior Therapy in BPD

As mentioned, Linehan (1993) elucidated the etiology and maintenance of BPD through the perspective of a biosocial theory of emotional dysregulation. Biosocial theory explains that pervasive emotion dysregulation is generated from the combination of vulnerable biology and invalidating social environments (Koerner 2012; Koerner et al. 2021). DBT was initially developed to treat BPD individuals with chronic suicidality (Azevedo et al. 2024). During the treatment of highly suicidal complicated cases, Linehan explored some of the obstacles in the process of change-oriented treatment paradigm, especially several difficulties in acceptance of the necessity of change in thoughts and behaviors. To consider these limitations, Linehan (1993) incorporated perspectives comprising dialectical theory, and practices including mindfulness, Zen practice and acceptance. Furthermore, a substantial effective emphasis on the balance and synthesis of acceptance and change appeared (Chapman 2019; Swales 2018). Dialectical behavior therapy has been developed by Marsha Linehan (1993), which is considered as a psychotherapy approach for chronically suicidal individuals. Originally, it has been rooted from cognitive-behavior therapy and was adapted for suicidal women who met criteria for BPD (Koerner et al. 2021; Dimeff et al. 2021a, b; Chapman 2019; Linehan 1993; Zeyrek Rios 2020). DBT is a multicomponent and integrative psychotherapeutic approach which synthesized principles of Zen practice, behavioral theory, and dialectics (Azevedo et al. 2024; Linehan 1993). Theoretically, DBT has roots in the biosocial theory (Zeyrek Rios 2020; Linehan 1993), which consider BPD as a disorder of emotion regulation system that contributes to the activation of a behavioral pattern of instability as a coping mechanism (Gillespie et al. 2022). DBT helps these clients to find a way to establish lives that are worth living.

Moreover, Linehan presented dialectic dilemmas including secondary behavioral patterns. Due to issues in managing emotion vulnerability and ongoing invalidation, often clients are experiencing a dilemma between over-regulating under-regulating emotional experience and expression, named "dialectic dilemmas." These dialectic dilemmas cause failures in regulation of emotions leading to elevated invalidation that contribute to redoubled efforts to self-regulate in order to avoid fallowing invalidation. On the other side, individuals might increase expression as they endeavor to communicate why their responses are valid (Linehan 1993; Koerner 2012). In line with Linehan (1993), there are three dialectical dimensions in borderline behavioral patterns, comprising emotion vulnerability and self-invalidation; active passivity and apparent competence; and unrelenting crisis and inhibited grieving (Linehan 1993; Koerner 2012).

DBT concentrates on (1) the balancing between acceptance and validation of behavior as it is in the moment; (2) treating therapy interference behaviors which is similar to transference in psychodynamic approach; (3) the therapeutic relationship as a crucial element of psychotherapy, especially in working with suicidal patients; and (4) dialectical processes (Linehan 1993). DBT is addressed as a comprehensive treatment, as well as, is referred as a full-programmed psychotherapeutic approach, comprising four modes of treatment: individual psychotherapy, skills training, phone coaching, and consultation for therapists (Linehan 1993; Azevedo et al. 2024; Koerner et al. 2021; Swales and Heard 2016; Koerner 2012). DBT includes a complex of basic treatment strategies (Linehan 1993):

- **Dialectical treatment strategies:**
  - Balancing treatment strategies
  - Teaching dialectical behavior patterns
  - Specific dialectical strategies
- **Core strategies:**
  - Validation:

    Emotional validation strategies
    Behavioral validation strategies

Cognitive validation strategies
Cheerleading strategies

- Problem solving:

  Behavioral analysis strategies
  Insight strategies
  Didactic strategies
  Solution analysis strategies
  Orientation strategies
  Commitment strategies

- **Change procedures:**

  - Contingency procedures:

    Contingency management procedures
    Observing limit procedures

  - Skills training procedures:

    Mindfulness skills, emotion regulation skills, distress tolerance skills, and interpersonal effectiveness skills

  - Exposure
  - Cognitive modification

- **Stylistic strategies:**

  - Balancing communication:

    Reciprocal communication strategies
    Irreverent communication strategies

- **Case management strategies:**

  - Increasing with the community

The therapeutic benefits and effectiveness of DBT are supported by experimental investigations and empirical evidence. A large body of studies have shown the efficacy of DBT in diminishing self-injurious behaviors, self-harm attempts, suicidal thoughts, and suicidal behaviors among individuals with BPD, and other psychiatric disorders as well (e.g., May et al. 2016; Barnicot et al. 2022; Lakeman and Crighton 2021; Stiglmayr et al. 2014; Linehan et al. 2015; Kramer et al. 2016). Through applying a weekly skills training group among 82 outpatients with BPD, Lin et al. (2019) indicated significant improvements in suicidality, depression and suppression symptoms. In weekly individual therapy and skills training among 162 outpatients with BPD, Walton et al. (2020) found substantially improvements in reducing suicidal thoughts and behaviors and depressive symptoms. Through a 20 weekly 90-min group sessions among 31 outpatients with BPD, Euler et al. (2019) reported highly significant promotions in overall defense function. Bohus et al. (2020) demonstrated substantial improvements in BPD symptoms in 193 outpatients with BPD in one-on-one outpatients' treatment. In weekly group and individual sessions among 156 patients with BPD, Keefe et al. (2021) pointed out considerably significant improvements in suicidality and BPD symptoms after DBT treatment and at follow-ups. McMain et al. (2022) reported after 6 months applying four modes of DBT among 240 outpatients with BPD, significant improvements were found in suicidality, general psychopathology, and BPD symptoms. Through four modes of DBT, Soler et al. (2009) indicated prominent improvements in depression, irritability, anger, anxiety, mood instability and general psychiatric symptoms in 30outpatients with BPD. Linehan et al. (2015) applied four modes of DBT among 99 patients with BPD and showed that all treatment conditions contributed to similar improvements in the frequency and severity of suicide attempts, suicide ideation, use crisis services due to suicidality, and reason for living. Through a weekly individual and skills training groups among 58 outpatients, Van den Bosch et al. (2005) reported remarkably significant improvements in suicidal ideation and attempts, and impulsive behaviors in postintervention and at follow-up.

References

American Psychiatric Association. Diagnostic and statistical manual of mental disorders. 5th ed. Text Revised (DSM-5-TR); 2022.

Azevedo J, Carreiras D, Hibbs C, Guiomar R, Osborne J, Hibbs R, Swales M. Benchmarks for dialectical behavioural therapy intervention in adults and adolescents with borderline personality symptoms. Int J Clin Health Psychol. 2024;24(2):100446.

Bandura A. Social cognitive theory: an agentic perspective. Asian J Soc Psychol. 1999;2(1):21–41.

Barnicot K, Redknap C, Coath F, Hommel J, Couldrey L, Crawford M. Patient experiences of therapy for borderline personality disorder: commonalities and differences between dialectical behaviour therapy and mentalization-based therapy and relation to outcomes. Psychol Psychother Theory Res Pract. 2022;95(1):212–33.

Battaglia M, Strambi LF, Bertella S, Bajo S, Bellodi L. First-cycle REM density in never-depressed subjects with borderline personality disorder. Biol Psychiatry. 1999;45(8):1056–8.

Beauchaine TP, Klein DN, Crowell SE, Derbidge C, Gatzke-Kopp L. Multifinality in the development of personality disorders: a Biology× Sex× Environment interaction model of antisocial and borderline traits. Dev Psychopathol. 2009;21(3):735–70.

Beauchaine TP. Physiological markers of emotional and behavioral dysregulation in externalizing psychopathology. Monogr Soc Res Child Dev. 2012;77(2):79.

Beauchaine TP, Crowell SE, editors. The Oxford handbook of emotion dysregulation. Oxford University Press; 2020.

Beauchaine TP, Gatzke-Kopp L, Mead HK. Polyvagal theory and developmental psychopathology: emotion dysregulation and conduct problems from preschool to adolescence. Biol Psychol. 2007;74(2):174–84.

Beck E, Bo S, Gondan M, Poulsen S, Pedersen L, Pedersen J, Simonsen E. Mentalization-based treatment in groups for adolescents with borderline personality disorder (BPD) or subthreshold BPD versus treatment as usual (M-GAB): study protocol for a randomized controlled trial. Trials. 2016;17:1–3.

Bland AR, Rossen EK. Clinical supervision of nurses working with patients with borderline personality disorder. Issues Ment Health Nurs. 2005;26(5):507–17.

Bohus M, Kleindienst N, Hahn C, MüllerEngelmann M, Ludäscher P, Steil R, et al. Dialectical behavior therapy for posttraumatic stress disorder (DBT-PTSD) compared with Cognitive

Processing Therapy (CPT) in complex presentations of PTSD in women survivors of childhood abuse: a randomized clinical trial. JAMA Psychiatry. 2020;77(12):1235–45.

Bornovalova MA, Huibregtse BM, Hicks BM, Keyes M, McGue M, Iacono W. Tests of a direct effect of childhood abuse on adult borderline personality disorder traits: a longitudinal discordant twin design. J Abnorm Psychol. 2013;122(1):180.

Boutros NN, Torello M, McGlashan TH. Electrophysiological aberrations in borderline personality disorder: state of the evidence. J Neuropsychiatry Clin Neurosci. 2003;15(2):145–54.

Chapman AL. Borderline personality disorder and emotion dysregulation. Dev Psychopathol. 2019;31(3):1143–56.

Chapman AL, Hope NH. Dialectical behavior therapy and treatment of emotion dysregulation. In: The Oxford handbook of emotion dysregulation. New York: Oxford University Press; 2020. p. 463.

Crowell SE, Beauchaine TP, Lenzenweger MF, Beauchaine T, Hinshaw S. The development of borderline personality disorder and self-injurious behavior. In: Child and adolescent psychopathology. Wiley; 2008. p. 510–39.

Crowell SE, Beauchaine TP, Linehan MM. A biosocial developmental model of borderline personality: elaborating and extending Linehan's theory. Psychol Bull. 2009;135(3):495.

Crowell SE, Kaufman EA, Lenzenweger MF. The development of borderline personality and self-inflicted injury. Child Adolesc Psychol. 2013:577–609.

Crowell SE, Baucom BR, Yaptangco M, Bride D, Hsiao R, McCauley E, Beauchaine TP. Emotion dysregulation and dyadic conflict in depressed and typical adolescents: evaluating concordance across psychophysiological and observational measures. Biol Psychol. 2014a;98:50–8.

Crowell SE, Kaufman EA, Beauchaine TP. A biosocial model of BPD: theory and empirical evidence. In: Handbook of borderline personality disorder in children and adolescents. New York: Springer New York; 2014b. p. 143–57.

Crowell SE, Kaufman EA. Borderline personality disorder and the emerging field of developmental neuroscience. Personal Disord Theory Res Treat. 2016;7(4):324.

Crowell SE, Baucom BR, McCauley E, Potapova NV, Fitelson M, Barth H, Smith CJ, Beauchaine TP. Mechanisms of contextual risk for adolescent self-injury: invalidation and conflict escalation in mother–child interactions. J Clin Child Adolesc Psychol. 2013a;42(4):467–80.

Crowell SE, Kaliush PR, Vlisides-Henry RD. Borderline personality disorder (BPD) Compass is a promising complementary intervention to dialectical behavior therapy: comment on Sauer-Zavala, 2022.

Dimeff LA, Koerner K. Overview of dialectical behavior therapy. 2007.

Dimeff LA, Rizvi LS, Koerner K. Dialectical behavior therapy in clinical practice. 2nd ed. The Guilford Press; 2021a.

Dimeff LA, Jobes DA, Koerner K, Kako N, Jerome T, Kelley-Brimer A, Boudreaux ED, Beadnell B, Goering P, Witterholt S, Melin G. Using a tablet-based app to deliver evidence-based practices for suicidal patients in the emergency department: pilot randomized controlled trial. JMIR Ment Health. 2021b;8(3):e23022.

Dishion TJ, Snyder JJ. Coercion dynamics: past, present. In: The Oxford handbook of coercive relationship dynamics. Oxford: Oxford University Press; 2016. p. 396.

Distel MA, Carlier A, Middeldorp CM, Derom CA, Lubke GH, Boomsma DI. Borderline personality traits and adult attention-deficit hyperactivity disorder symptoms: a genetic analysis of comorbidity. Am J Med Genet B Neuropsychiatr Genet. 2011;156(7):817–25.

Dixon-Gordon KL, Whalen DJ, Scott LN, Cummins ND, Stepp SD. The main and interactive effects of maternal interpersonal emotion regulation and negative affect on adolescent girls' borderline personality disorder symptoms. Cogn Ther Res. 2016;40:381–93.

Dixon-Gordon KL, Haliczer LA, Conkey LC. Emotion dysregulation and borderline personality disorder. In: The Oxford handbook of emotion dysregulation. New York: Oxford University Press; 2020. p. 360–76.

Dodge KA, Greenberg MT, Malone PS. Conduct problems prevention research group. Testing an idealized dynamic cascade model of the development of serious violence in adolescence. Child Dev. 2008;79(6):1907–27.

Dunn R, Dunn K, Price GE. Learning style. J Educ Strateg. 2009:82.
Ebner-Priemer UW, Kuo J, Kleindienst N, Welch SS, Reisch T, Reinhard I, Lieb K, Linehan MM, Bohus M. State affective instability in borderline personality disorder assessed by ambulatory monitoring. Psychol Med. 2007;37(7):961–70.
Elzy MB. Emotional invalidation: an investigation into its definition, measurement, and effects; 2013.
Euler S, Stalujanis E, Allenbach G, Kolly S, de Roten Y, Despland JN, Kramer U. Dialectical behavior therapy skills training affects defense mechanisms in borderline personality disorder: an integrative approach of mechanisms in psychotherapy. Psychother Res. 2019;29(8):1074–85.
Evans K. Negotiating the self: identity, sexuality, and emotion in learning to teach. Routledge; 2013.
Evans D, Dalgleish T, Dudas RB, Denman C, Howard M, Dunn BD. Examining the shared and unique features of self-concept content and structure in borderline personality disorder and depression. Cogn Ther Res. 2015;39:613–26.
Fruzzetti AE, Shenk C, Hoffman PD. Family interaction and the development of borderline personality disorder: a transactional model. Dev Psychopathol. 2005;17(4):1007–30.
Fruzzetti AE, Crook W, Erikson KM, Lee JE, Worrall JM. 24 EMOTION REGULATION. Cognitive behavior therapy: Applying empirically supported techniques in your practice. 2008;23:174.
Gill D, Warburton W, Beath K. The specificity of the biosocial model to borderline traits. Clin Psychol. 2018;22(1):27–36.
Gill D, Warburton W, Sweller N, Beath K, Humburg P. The emotional dysregulation questionnaire: development and comparative analysis. Psychol Psychother Theory Res Pract. 2021;94:426–63.
Gillespie C, Murphy M, Joyce M. Dialectical behavior therapy for individuals with borderline personality disorder: a systematic review of outcomes after one year of follow-up. J Personal Disord. 2022;36(4):431–54.
Gilligan SG, Brower GH. Cognitive consequences of emotional arousal. In: Izard CE, Kagan J, Zajonc RB, editors. Emotions, cognitions, and behavior. Cambridge University Press; 1984. p. 547–88.
Glenn CR, Klonsky ED. Nonsuicidal self-injury disorder: an empirical investigation in adolescent psychiatric patients. J Clin Child Adolesc Psychol. 2013;42(4):496–507.
Gratz KL, Roemer L. Multidimensional assessment of emotion regulation and dysregulation: development, factor structure, and initial validation of the difficulties in emotion regulation scale. J Psychopathol Behav Assess. 2004;26:41–54.
Gratz KL, Tull MT. The relationship between emotion dysregulation and deliberate self-harm among inpatients with substance use disorders. Cogn Ther Res. 2010;34:544–53.
Gratz KL, Rosenthal MZ, Tull MT, Lejuez CW, Gunderson JG. An experimental investigation of emotion dysregulation in borderline personality disorder. J Abnorm Psychol. 2006;115(4):850.
Gross JJ. Emotion regulation: conceptual and empirical foundations. In: Handbook of emotion regulation, vol. 2. New York: The Guilford Press; 2014. p. 3–20.
Gross J, Ford B. Handbook of emotion regulation. 3rd ed; 2024.
Grove JL, Crowell SE. The Oxford handbook of dialectical behaviour therapy. Oxford: Oxford University Press; 2019.
Grove JL, Smith TW, Crowell SE, Ellis JH. Preliminary evidence for emotion dysregulation as a mechanism underlying poor sleep quality in borderline personality disorder. J Personal Disord. 2017;31(4):542–52.
Grove NS. Receding resilience: on the planetary moods of disruption. Rev Int Stud. 2023;49(1):3–19.
Gujar N, Yoo SS, Hu P, Walker MP. Sleep deprivation amplifies reactivity of brain reward networks, biasing the appraisal of positive emotional experiences. J Neurosci. 2011;31(12):4466–74.
Gunderson JG, Fruzzetti A, Unruh B, Choi-Kain L. Competing theories of borderline personality disorder. J Personal Disord. 2018;32(2):148–67.
Gurvits IG, Koenigsberg HW, Siever LJ. Neurotransmitter dysfunction in patients with borderline personality disorder. Psychiatr Clin N Am. 2000;23(1):27–40.
Harned MS, Rizvi SL, Linehan MM. Impact of co-occurring posttraumatic stress disorder on suicidal women with borderline personality disorder. Am J Psychiatry. 2010;167(10):1210–7.

Harris KM, McDade TW. The biosocial approach to human development, behavior, and health across the life course. RSF-Rus Sage J Soc S. 2018;4(4):2–6.

Hernandez A, Arntz A, Gaviria AM, Labad A, Gutiérrez-Zotes JA. Relationships between childhood maltreatment, parenting style, and borderline personality disorder criteria. J Personal Disord. 2012;26(5):727–36.

Hughes AE, Crowell SE, Uyeji L, Coan JA. A developmental neuroscience of borderline pathology: emotion dysregulation and social baseline theory. J Abnorm Child Psychol. 2012;40:21–33.

Kaufman EA, Crowell SE, Lenzenweger MF. The development of borderline personality and self-inflicted injury. In: Child and adolescent psychopathology. 3rd ed; 2017. p. 642–79.

Kaufman JR, Armstrong M, Maciarz J, Palekar N, Kim J, Koppelmans V, Welsh RC, Langenecker SA, Weisenbach SL. 31 sex differences in emotion regulation and emotional awareness in middle aged and older adults. J Int Neuropsychol Soc. 2023;29(s1):820–1.

Keefe JR, Kim TT, DeRubeis RJ, Streiner DL, Links PS, McMain SF. Treatment selection in borderline personality disorder between dialectical behavior therapy and psychodynamic psychiatric management. Psychol Med. 2021;51(11):1829–37.

King AC, Whitt-Glover MC, Marquez DX, Buman MP, Napolitano MA, Jakicic J, Fulton JE, Tennant BL. Physical activity promotion: highlights from the 2018 physical activity guidelines advisory committee systematic review. Med Sci Sports Exerc. 2019;51(6):1340–53.

Koerner K. Doing dialectical behavior therapy: a practical guide. The Gilford Press; 2012.

Koerner K, Dimeff LA, Rizvi SL. Overview of DBT. In: Dialectical behavior therapy in clinical practice. 2nd ed; 2021.

Kramer U, Pascual-Leone A, Berthoud L, de Roten Y, Marquet P, Kolly S, et al. Assertive anger mediates effects of dialectical behaviour-informed skills training for borderline personality disorder: a randomized controlled trial. Clin Psychol Psychother. 2016;23(3):189–202.

Kuo JR, Linehan MM. Disentangling emotion processes in borderline personality disorder: physiological and self-reported assessment of biological vulnerability, baseline intensity, and reactivity to emotionally evocative stimuli. J Abnorm Psychol. 2009;118(3):531.

Lakeman R, Crighton J. The impact of social distancing on people with borderline personality disorder: the views of dialectical behavioural therapists. Issues Ment Health Nurs. 2021;42(5):410–6.

Lee SS, Keng SL, Yeo GC, Hong RY. Parental invalidation and its associations with borderline personality disorder symptoms: a multivariate meta-analysis. Personal Disord Theory Res Treat. 2022;13(6):572.

Lenzenweger MF, Cicchetti D. Toward a developmental psychopathology approach to borderline personality disorder. Dev Psychopathol. 2005;17(4):893–8.

Lewis M, Sullivan MW, Michalson L. The cognitive-emotional fugue. Emot Cogn Behav. 1984:264.

Lin TJ, Ko HC, Wu JY, Oei TP, Lane HY, Chen CH. The effectiveness of dialectical behavior therapy skills training group vs. cognitive therapy group on reducing depression and suicide attempts for borderline personality disorder in Taiwan. Arch Suicide Res. 2019;23(1):82–99.

Linehan MM. Diagnosis and treatment of mental disorders: cognitive-behavioral treatment of borderline personality disorder. Guilford Press; 1993.

Linehan MM. Combining pharmacotherapy with psychotherapy for substance abusers with borderline personality disorder: strategies for enhancing compliance. NIDA Res Monogr. 1995;150:129–42.

Linehan MM. Behavioral treatments of suicidal behaviors. Definitional obfuscation and treatment outcomes a. Ann N Y Acad Sci. 1997;836(1):302–28.

Linehan MM, Schmidt III H. The dialectics of effective treatment of borderline personality disorder. 1995.

Linehan MM, Comtois KA, Murray AM, Brown MZ, Gallop RJ, Heard HL, Korslund KE, Tutek DA, Reynolds SK, Lindenboim N. Two-year randomized controlled trial and follow-up of dialectical behavior therapy vs therapy by experts for suicidal behaviors and borderline personality disorder. Arch Gen Psychiatry. 2006;63(7):757–66.

Linehan MM, Korslund KE, Harned MS, Gallop RJ, Lungu A, Neacsiu AD, McDavid J, Comtois KA, Murray-Gregory AM. Dialectical behavior therapy for high suicide risk in individuals with borderline personality disorder: a randomized clinical trial and component analysis. JAMA Psychiatry. 2014;72(5):475–82.

Linehan MM, Korslund KE, Harned MS, Gallop RJ, Lungu A, Neacsiu AD, et al. Dialectical behavior therapy for high suicide risk in individuals with borderline personality disorder: a randomized clinical trial and component analysis. JAMA Psychiatry. 2015;72(5):475–82.

Lynch TR, Rosenthal MZ, Kosson DS, Cheavens JS, Lejuez CW, Blair RJ. Heightened sensitivity to facial expressions of emotion in borderline personality disorder. Emotion. 2006;6(4):647.

Lyons EJ, Mehl MR, Pennebaker JW. Pro-anorexics and recovering anorexics differ in their linguistic internet self-presentation. J Psychosom Res. 2006;60(3):253–6.

Lyons-Ruth K. Contributions of the mother–infant relationship to dissociative, borderline, and conduct symptoms in young adulthood. Infant Ment Health J. 2008;29(3):203–18.

Matera E, Margari M, Serra M, Petruzzelli MG, Gabellone A, Piarulli FM, Pugliese A, Tassiello AR, Croce F, Renna C, Margari A. Nonsuicidal self-injury: an observational study in a sample of adolescents and young adults. Brain Sci. 2021;11(8):974.

May JM, Richardi TM, Barth KS. Dialectical behavior therapy as treatment for borderline personality disorder. Ment Health Clin. 2016;6(2):62–7.

McMain S, Korman LM, Dimeff L. Dialectical behavior therapy and the treatment of emotion dysregulation. J Clin Psychol. 2001;57(2):183–96.

McMain SF, Chapman AL, Kuo JR, DixonGordon KL, Guimond TH, Labrish C, et al. The effectiveness of 6 versus 12 months of dialectical behavior therapy for borderline personality disorder: a noninferiority randomized clinical trial. Psychother Psychosom. 2022;91(6):382–97.

Millon T, Millon CM, Meagher SE, Grossman SD, Ramnath R. Personality disorders in modern life. John Wiley & Sons; 2012.

Mitchell JE, Mussell MP, Peterson CB, Crow S, Wonderlich SA, Crosby RD, Davis T, Weller C. Hedonics of binge eating in women with bulimia nervosa and binge eating disorder. Int J Eat Disord. 1999;26(2):165–70.

Neacsiu AD, Bohus M, Linehan MM. Dialectical behavior therapy: an intervention for emotion dysregulation. In: Handbook of emotion regulation, vol. 2. New York: The Guilford Press; 2014a. p. 491–507.

Neacsiu AD, Eberle JW, Kramer R, Wiesmann T, Linehan MM. Dialectical behavior therapy skills for transdiagnostic emotion dysregulation: a pilot randomized controlled trial. Behav Res Ther. 2014b;59:40–51.

Neece CL. Mindfulness-based stress reduction for parents of young children with developmental delays: implications for parental mental health and child behavior problems. J Appl Res Intellect Disabil. 2014;27(2):174–86.

Ni X, Chan K, Bulgin N, Sicard T, Bismil R, McMain S, Kennedy JL. Association between serotonin transporter gene and borderline personality disorder. J Psychiatr Res. 2006;40(5):448–53.

Niedtfeld I, Bohus M. Understanding the bio in the biosocial theory of BPD. In: The Oxford handbook of dialectical behaviour therapy. Oxford University Press; 2018. p. 23.

Nock MK, Joiner TE Jr, Gordon KH, Lloyd-Richardson E, Prinstein MJ. Nonsuicidal self-injury among adolescents: diagnostic correlates and relation to suicide attempts. Psychiatry Res. 2006;144(1):65–72.

Odgers CL, Moffitt TE, Broadbent JM, Dickson N, Hancox RJ, Harrington H, Poulton R, Sears MR, Thomson WM, Caspi A. Female and male antisocial trajectories: from childhood origins to adult outcomes. Dev Psychopathol. 2008;20(2):673–716.

Patterson GR, Capaldi DM. Antisocial parents: unskilled and vulnerable. In: Family transitions. Routledge; 2013. p. 195–218.

Patterson CJ, Tate DP, Sumontha J, Xu R. Sleep difficulties among sexual minority adults: associations with family relationship problems. Psychol Sex Orientat Gend Divers. 2018;5(1):109.

Ramos-Luna ME, Oliver J. Relationship between differentiation of self, emotional intelligence and self-esteem in a Spanish sample. Curr Psychol. 2024;43(8):6797–806.

Reeves A. Auto-ethnography and the study of affect and emotion in world politics: investigating security discourses at London's Imperial War Museum. In: Researching emotions in international relations: methodological perspectives on the emotional turn; 2018. p. 103–27.

Reeves M, James LM, Pizzarello SM, Taylor JE. Support for Linehan's biosocial theory from a nonclinical sample. J Personal Disord. 2010;24(3):312–26.

Ritschel T, Schlüter S, Köhne JM, Vogel HJ, Totsche KU. Efficient prediction of multidomain flow and transport in hierarchically structured porous media. Water Resour Res. 2018;54(11):9033–44.

Sauer SE, Baer RA. Validation of measures of biosocial precursors to borderline personality disorder: childhood emotional vulnerability and environmental invalidation. Assessment. 2010;17(4):454–66.

Schmahl C, Bremner JD. Neuroimaging in borderline personality disorder. J Psychiatr Res. 2006;40(5):419–27.

Schmahl CG, Vermetten E, Elzinga BM, Bremner JD. Magnetic resonance imaging of hippocampal and amygdala volume in women with childhood abuse and borderline personality disorder. Psychiatry Res Neuroimaging. 2003;122(3):193–8.

Schmaling KB, Fales JL. The association between borderline personality disorder and somatoform disorders: a systematic review and meta-analysis. Clin Psychol Sci Pract. 2018;25(2):e12244.

Schulze L, Schmahl C, Niedtfeld I. Neural correlates of disturbed emotion processing in borderline personality disorder: a multimodal meta-analysis. Biol Psychiatry. 2016;79(2):97–106.

Selby EA, Anestis MD, Joiner TE. Understanding the relationship between emotional and behavioral dysregulation: emotional cascades. Behav Res Ther. 2008a;46(5):593–611.

Selby EA, Braithwaite SR, Joiner TE Jr, Fincham FD. Features of borderline personality disorder, perceived childhood emotional invalidation, and dysfunction within current romantic relationships. J Fam Psychol. 2008b;22(6):885.

Selby EA, Franklin J, Carson-Wong A, Rizvi SL. Emotional cascades and self-injury: investigating instability of rumination and negative emotion. J Clin Psychol. 2013;69(12):1213–27.

Selby EA, Kranzler A, Panza E. Development of emotional cascades in borderline personality disorder. In: Handbook of borderline personality disorder in children and adolescents. New York: Springer New York; 2014. p. 159–76.

Smith JD, Dishion TJ, Shaw DS, Wilson MN, Winter CC, Patterson GR. Coercive family process and early-onset conduct problems from age 2 to school entry. Dev Psychopathol. 2014;26(4pt1):917–32.

Soler J, Pascual JC, Tiana T, Cebrià A, Barrachina J, Campins MJ, et al. Dialectical behaviour therapy skills training compared to standard group therapy in borderline personality disorder: a 3-month randomised controlled clinical trial. Behav Res Ther. 2009;47(5):353–8.

Sperry L, Sperry J. Cognitive behavior therapy of DSM-5 personality disorders: assessment, case conceptualization, and treatment. Routledge; 2015.

Stiglmayr C, Stecher-Mohr J, Wagner T, Meiβner J, Spretz D, Steffens C, Roepke S, Fydrich T, Salbach-Andrae H, Schulze J, Renneberg B. Effectiveness of dialectic behavioral therapy in routine outpatient care: the Berlin borderline study. Bord Personal Disord Emot Dysregul. 2014;1:1–1.

Stepp SD, Olino TM, Klein DN, Seeley JR, Lewinsohn PM. Unique influences of adolescent antecedents on adult borderline personality disorder features. Personal Disord Theory Res Treat. 2013;4(3):223.

Snyder EE, Ammons R. Baseball's emotion work: getting psyched to play. Qual Sociol. 1993;16(2):111–32.

Swales MA. The Oxford handbook of dialectical behavior therapy. Oxford University Press; 2018.

Swales MA, Heard HL. Dialectical behaviour therapy: distinctive features. Routledge; 2016.

Sweezy M. Treating trauma after dialectical behavioral therapy. J Psychother Integr. 2011a;21(1):90.

Sweezy M. The teenager's confession: regulating shame in internal family systems therapy. Am J Psychother. 2011b;65(2):179–88.

van den Bosch LM, Koeter MW, Stijnen T, Verheul R, van den Brink W. Sustained efficacy of dialectical behaviour therapy for borderline personality disorder. Behav Res Ther. 2005;43(9):1231–41.

van Elst LT, Hesslinger B, Thiel T, Geiger E, Haegele K, Lemieux L, Lieb K, Bohus M, Hennig J, Ebert D. Frontolimbic brain abnormalities in patients with borderline personality disorder: a volumetric magnetic resonance imaging study. Biol Psychiatry. 2003;54(2):163–71.

Wagner AW, Linehan MM. Facial expression recognition ability among women with borderline personality disorder: implications for emotion regulation? J Personal Disord. 1999;13(4):329–44.

Wagner AW, Linehan MM. Applications of dialectical behavior therapy to posttraumatic stress disorder and related problems. Cogn Behav Ther Trauma. 2006;2:117–45.

Waller R, Gardner F, Hyde LW. What are the associations between parenting, callous–unemotional traits, and antisocial behavior in youth? A systematic review of evidence. Clin Psychol Rev. 2013;33(4):593–608.

Walton CJ, Bendit N, Baker AL, Carter GL, Lewin TJ. A randomised trial of dialectical behaviour therapy and the conversational model for the treatment of borderline personality disorder with recent suicidal and/or non-suicidal self-injury: an effectiveness study in an Australian public mental health service. Aust N Z J Psychiatry. 2020;54(10):1020–34.

Whalen D. The role of maternal invalidation in the development of BPD symptoms in adolescent girls (Doctoral dissertation, University of Pittsburgh), 2014.

Williams LM, Sidis A, Gordon E, Meares RA. "Missing links" in borderline personality disorder: loss of neural synchrony relates to lack of emotion regulation and impulse control. J Psychiatry Neurosci. 2006;31(3):181–8.

Yen S, Zlotnick C, Costello E. Affect regulation in women with borderline personality disorder traits. J Nerv Ment Dis. 2002;190(10):693–6.

Zanarini MC, Wedig MM. Childhood adversity and the development of borderline personality disorder. In: Handbook of borderline personality disorder in children and adolescents. New York: Springer New York; 2014. p. 265–76.

Zeyrek Rios EY. Dialectical behavior therapy in the treatment of borderline personality disorder. J Cogn Behav Psychother Res. 2020;9(2):148.

Chapter 7
A Developmental Biospecial Model of Borderline Personality Disorder

Introduction

In considering the developmental context of BPD, the following chapter focuses especially on a large body of foundational work generated by the following authors: Crowell et al. (2009, 2008, 2014), and Kaufman et al. (2017a). In considering the implications of Linehan's (1993) Biosocial Model of BPD, Crowell et al. (2014) described a complex, heterotypic trajectory from childhood vulnerabilities to adult BPD. They pointed out the significant role of trait impulsivity in the interaction with family-level risk factors which might contribute to the escalation of the risk of the development of BPD. In addition, they hypothesized that self-inflicted injurious behaviors and other features of self-destructive behaviors in adolescence can be considered a reliable predictor for later BPD in adulthood.

The extended developmental biosocial model (Crowell et al. 2009) is a developmental viewpoint to the BPD psychopathology. Crowell et al. (2014) mentioned that developmental psychopathology seeks an explanation for both equifinality and multifinality across development (Cicchetti 1989, 2016). *Equifinality* refers to multiple developmental trajectories converging on a phenotypically singular behavioral or diagnostic outcome. In contrast, *multifinality* occurs when one vulnerability or risk factor prompts many diverse outcomes in problematic behavior or diagnosis (Crowell et al. 2009). The extended biosocial model has emphasized the importance of equifinality and multifinality when considering the come out of BPD across development (Beauchaine et al. 2009). Based on Crowell et al. (2014), adults with BPD move across varied developmental pathways to shape BPD (equifinality), whereas many youths with early borderline features do not develop BPD (multifinality) (Crowell et al. 2014). Beauchaine and McNulty (2013) proposed that according to *heterotypic continuity* refer to any alterations in the obvious form of psychopathology, despite a common underlying vulnerability. Therefore, expression of inherent impulsive traits alters across development, so it can contribute to a

E. A. Selby, M. Salavati, *Theories of Borderline Personality Disorder*,
https://doi.org/10.1007/978-3-031-75503-3_7

variety of different diagnoses in different stages of development (Beauchaine and McNulty 2013).

Crowell et al. (2005) assumed that there are etiological trajectories toward BPD that are illuminated by the developmental psychopathology perspective. Therefore, Crowell et al. (2009) elaborated probable mechanisms underlying the development of BPD and tried to expand Linehan's model etiological concepts, including impulsivity, independent of emotion dysregulation as precursors to BPD. According to the basic and applied literature in the field of BPD, Crowell et al. (2009) established insight into the biological correlates and substrates of BPD formation. Likewise, the body of work on family interactive and transactive patterns contributes to the development of different psychological dysfunctions especially emotion dysregulation has been conducted (Granic and Patterson 2006). BPD is considered as a persistent pervasive and relatively intransigent condition that emerges in late adolescence and early adulthood like other personality disorders (APA 2022). A substantially long history of research has been investigated to follow these core assumptions (e.g., Crick et al. 2005), in which they believe that BPD is an enduring and stable diagnosis, a series of pathological traits such as neuroticism are underlying this disorder, BPD is a disorder which is resistant to treatment and emerges in late adolescent. On the other hand, over the three past decades, many investigations have attempted to look for more details and trajectories of personality disorders, especially BPD (Lenzenweger et al. 2012; Zanarini et al. 2003). In other words, a great attention has been emerged in investigating to challenge this assumption that BPD is just a disorder that can be diagnosed after age 18.

Following the postulates of Biosocial theory, Grove and Crowell (2018) and Crowell et al. (2022) emphasized the caregiver-child relationship. This means that complicated longitudinal transactions between a biologically vulnerable child and their invalidating environments contribute to a mismatch in the child and environment. Thus, psychopathology can come out in any familial context, even when there is no evidence of distress in any of family members. This generates an inherited base for the development of BPD, which will be getting worse in an invalidating environment (Grove et al. 2023; Crowell et al. 2022). Crowell et al. (2009) cited that Linehan (1993) emphasized on early emotional development and emotional vulnerability, without any focus on impulsivity as trait independent of emotion, and since Linehan's model has been developed as a therapeutic model to establish Dialectical behavior therapy (DBT), in which the therapeutic strategies are based on modifying any aspects of emotional experiences across the life that are associated with problematic feeling states and destructive behaviors. Linehan's model focused on mood-dependent behaviors (Crowell et al. 2009) and impulsive or self-destructive behaviors such as self-injury and suicidal attempts, which may occur directly to dysregulation in emotional response (Lynch et al. 2006). According to the elaborated biosocial model, behavioral component of emotion may be influenced by trait impulsivity, independent of emotion (Crowell et al. 2009). These risks are most likely to arise among individuals with inherited trait impulsivity from their parents, and consequently contribute to a failure to achieve skillful strategies to regulate severe emotions (Crowell et al. 2014; Kaufman et al. 2020). Crowell et al. (2009)

assert that "early impulsivity is a predisposing vulnerability for a marked subset of those who eventually meet criteria for BPD. This subset comprises those who continue as adults to manifest impulsive behaviors, encompassing suicidal and nonsuicidal, self-injurious behaviors" (Crowell et al. 2009). In sum, an elaborated biosocial model proposes that predisposing biological vulnerability to develop BPD consist of not only temperamental emotional vulnerability but also a propensity for impulsivity (Dixon-Gordon et al. 2020). Moreover, although impulsivity and emotion dysregulation are in almost unchangeable association with the development of BPD, impulsivity and emotion dysregulation may also emerge independently and sequentially during development of BPD; therefore, contributing to various difficulties in emotional, cognitive, behavioral, and identity functioning among individual with BPD. However, BPD is almost distinct from other impulse control disorders because of emotional instability dominance in BPD, a review of etiological factors and mechanisms has demonstrated a considerable level of biological correlates which have similarity between BPD and other impulse control disorders. This point can be useful for a richer and broader perspective of possible pathways to BPD (Crowell et al. 2009).

In reviewing Crowell et al. (2009) model, it is implicated that there is a reciprocal transaction between predisposing biological vulnerabilities and invalidating environment and environmental risk factors contribute to the development of BPD among high-risk individuals. This model emphasized that impulsive and emotionally sensitive children and adolescents are prone to be faced with a series of maltreatment in the context of invalidating environment, especially by their parents such as inappropriate punishment, and high level of aggressive interactions, because these children and adolescents have numerous difficulties in inhibiting extremely intense emotions (Crowell et al. 2009, 2022). Developmental approaches to the study of psychopathology have been become broadly expanded and pervasive over the past few decades. These approaches provide a more expansive window to elaborate our understanding of maladaptive functioning in childhood and adolescence. In addition, they help us to investigate and design therapeutic plans for psychological disorders (Achenbach et al. 2016; Cicchetti 2016). Through utilizing a developmental psychopathology framework to study emotion regulation, Calkins et al. (2016) presented a more elaborated understanding of multiple contributors consisting of familial, contextual, and individual differences, which may interact in various ways in different individuals to develop emotional problems, especially emotion dysregulation (Calkins et al. 2016; Cicchetti 2016). Based on Crowell's developmental psychopathology viewpoint, the development of BPD is influenced by traits and characters of child, caregiver, parents, the context of environment, and the dynamic of transactions among these traits and characteristics (Crowell et al. 2009). Hughes et al. (2012) cited that during childhood, a secure attachment bond between child and caregiver lead to an accepted assumptions of co-regulation and a strong sense of "the self" due to attachment figures (Hughes et al. 2012).

In line with Geselowitz et al. (2021), a growing body of studies in the field of BPD endorse the interaction between psychological variables, such as impulsivity (e.g., Crowell et al. 2009; Beauchaine and McNulty 2013; Neuhaus and Beauchaine

2017), emotional sensitivity and overreactivity (e.g., Linehan 2020; Crowell et al. 2009, 2014; Selby and Joiner Jr 2009), and social-environmental risk factors, including invalidating parenting (e.g., Crowell et al. 2009, 2014; Schaich et al. 2021a, b; De La Garza et al. 2021), disturbed attachment (e.g., Fonagy et al. 2018; Cicchetti 2016), and childhood trauma (e.g., De La Garza et al. 2021; Schaich et al. 2021a, b; Pohl et al. 2021).

Accordingly, Crowell et al. (2009, 2014) propose five suggestions according to the biosocial developmental model of borderline personality disorder: (these parts are not direct quotes and all of them are paraphrased).

1. Impaired impulse control likely appears in the development of borderline pathology, which can elucidate the overlapping biological vulnerabilities for BPD and other impulse control issues (Crowell et al. 2009) **or** Trait impulsivity—a marked inheritable biological predisposition—generates risk for BPD and other disorders of behavioral dyscontrol (Crowell et al. 2014,) **or** Trait impulsivity and emotional sensitivity are emerged in early stages of life, biologically are based on vulnerabilities that provide notable risk for self-inflicted injurious behaviors (SII), BPD, and other disorders manifested by disturbed behavioral control, such as issues on the externalizing spectrum (Kaufman et al. 2017a).
2. The development of severe emotional instability features of BPD is developed and maintained by the caregiving environment and is based on characteristics of the child (e.g., baseline emotional sensitivity) and the developmental context (Crowell et al. 2009) **or** affective instability is developed and maintained within high-risk familial contexts, which are manifested by intermittent reinforcement of adverse behavior and chronic invalidation of emotional expression (Crowell et al. 2014) **or** emotional lability is developed and perpetuated within high-risk contexts featured by emotional invalidation and intermittent reinforcement of intensely severe emotional expressions (Kaufman et al. 2017a).
3. Reciprocal reinforcement interactions between biological predispositions and environmental risk processes endorse emotion dysregulation and more severe behavioral control issues and therefore lead to negative cognitive and social consequences (Crowell et al. 2009) **or** inheritable impulsivity interacts across development with other environmental risk factors to reinforce more extremely severe behavior and emotion dysregulation, disturb peer relationships, and influence academic functioning (Crowell et al. 2014) **or** biological proneness transact with environmental risks over time to endorse internalizing and externalizing psychopathology manifested by increasingly extreme behavior and emotion dysregulation (Kaufman et al. 2017a).
4. By mid-to-late adolescence, there is a set of identifiable characteristics and maladaptive coping strategies that demonstrate elevated risk factor for following BPD (Crowell et al. 2009) **or** by adolescent, these Biology × Environment interactions improve a complex of identifiable issues and maladaptive coping strategies—comprising early borderline manifestations and repetitive self-injurious behaviors, which fall along a heterotypically continuous trajectory to BPD (Crowell et al. 2014) **or** by adolescence, these biology × environment interac-

tions provoke a constellation of identifiable difficulties and maladaptive coping strategies characteristic of BPD, such as self-injurious behaviors (Kaufman et al. 2017a).

5. These traits and behaviors may heighten the risk for BPD across developmental stages of life, because of evocative influences on interpersonal relationships and social performance and through interference with healthy emotional development (Crowell et al. 2009) **or** adolescent borderline pathology may further increase the risk for BPD in adulthood by interfering with normal processes of development, the capability to shape accepted interpersonal relationships, and development of adaptive coping strategies (Crowell et al. 2014) **or** early representations of borderline pathology such as self-injurious behaviors may further exacerbate risk for BPD by disturbing individual's abilities to navigate stage-salient developmental tasks, form supportive social associations, and shape healthy coping strategies (Kaufman et al. 2017a).

These hypotheses will be discussed in the following:

1. *Impaired impulse control likely appears in the development of borderline pathology, which can elucidate the overlapping biological vulnerabilities for BPD and other impulse control issues (Crowell et al.* 2009*)* ***or*** *Trait impulsivity—a marked inheritable biological predisposition—generates risk for BPD and other disorders of behavioral dyscontrol (Crowell et al.* 2014*)* ***or*** *Trait impulsivity and emotional sensitivity are emerged in early stages of life, biologically are based on vulnerabilities that provide notable risk for self-inflicted injurious behaviors (SII), BPD, and other disorders manifested by disturbed behavioral control, such as issues on the externalizing spectrum (Kaufman et al.* 2017a*).* Consistent with the first hypothesis postulated by Crowell et al. (2009), a large body of work has been conducted to date that proposes that BPD is a disorder with deficits in both impulse control and emotion regulation. A remarkable number of these studies have exhibited significant familial aggression, finding in both impulse control disorders and mood disorders frequently in BPD. This feature makes BPD unique in comparison to other externalizing disorders, which has been proposed a strong viewpoint about heritable biological vulnerabilities in BPD (see, White et al. 2003; Beauchaine 2012). Impulsivity is defined as a disinhibition of urges and drive impulse, with low levels of conscientiousness (Jacob et al. 2010). Impulsivity plays a major role in a broad range of disorders, including BPD, and is a clinical dimension associated with symptomatology and treatment issues (Martin et al. 2019). Impulsivity issues lead BPD individuals to become prone to rash actions and reckless reactions without forethought (Martin et al. 2019). The association between impulsivity and BPD is thoroughly documented in numerous studies (e.g., Kulacaoglu et al. 2017). Paris (2005) reported that BPD expresses a wide range of impulsive behaviors comprising repeated suicide attempts, self-mutilation, substance abuse, sexual promiscuity, and reckless driving or eating behavior (Martin et al. 2019). Kaufman et al. (2019) proposed that several investigations have pointed out impulsivity/behavioral undercontrol and emotional instability and negative affectivity as core features contributing to

BPD (Stevens et al. 2019; Littlefield et al. 2010; Dillahunt et al. 2022). Ecological models have highlighted the combination of trait-level vulnerabilities consisting of impulsivity and negative affectivity as genetically predisposing factors for BPD and other internalizing issues, such as alcohol drinking (Kaufman et al. 2020; Crowell et al. 2009). Neuhaus and Beauchaine (2017) stated that "according to developmental psychopathology models of externalizing behavior, extreme impulsivity expressed in the preschool years may represent the first stage in a trajectory that can progress via endorsing and mediating variables to early onset delinquency and other antisocial behaviors" (Neuhaus and Beauchaine 2017). Neuhaus and Beauchaine (2017) added that trait impulsivity underlies a broad range of disorders with externalizing problems falling along the externalizing spectrum, such as attention deficit/hyperactivity disorder (ADHD) and antisocial personality disorder (ASPD) (Beauchaine et al. 2009).

Moreover, temperamental disinhibition is a marker of early stages of development of a wide forms of internalizing problems such as self-harm and depression (e.g., Beauchaine et al. 2009). The observed impulsivity in the early stages of life may be a considerable marker for substantial risks for a wide range of destructive consequences (Neuhaus and Beauchaine 2017; Beauchaine et al. 2017). As mentioned by Neuhaus and Beauchaine (2017), many studies have tried to define impulsivity via behavioral symptoms, although some researchers have attempted a definition of impulsivity according to the result of neuropsychological tests, operational defined as poor attention to details, carelessness and lack of planning in maze solving (Porteus and Johnson 1965), difficulties in set-shifting tasks in Wisconsin Card Sorting Test (Avila et al. 2004), drawing tasks in Bender Gestalt (Bender 1950), and the Draw-A-Person test (Koppitz and De Moreau 1968). All such tests have been applied to the measurement of impulsivity through various tasks offered based on completion time, overall quality, omissions, asymmetry, detailing, and shading (Oas 1984; Neuhaus and Beauchaine 2017). To discuss this hypothesis, Crowell et al. (2014) concentrated on two interrelated forms of impulsivity: *behavioral impulsivity* and *trait impulsivity*. Behavioral impulsivity refers to actions which are emitted swiftly with no forethought (Oas 1985). Versus, trait impulsivity can be considered as an inheritable biological predisposition, developing behavioral impulsivity. Yet, it should be crucially addressed that trait impulsivity is a strong vulnerability for diverse forms of psychopathology in the externalizing continuum (Neuhaus and Beauchaine 2017). Heritable biological mechanisms of vulnerability cause impulsivity among children who were reared by impulsive parents (Crowell and Kaufman 2016; Beauchaine et al. 2009; Neuhaus and Beauchaine 2017). Crowell et al. (2014) demonstrated that trait impulsivity—primarily inheritable yet perhaps acquired through other mechanisms—has been indicated as a major predisposing vulnerability to BPD (Crowell et al. 2014). Based on this assumption, BPD is a disorder manifested first by trait impulsivity, with emotion dysregulation embarking later through complex interactions between impulsive individuals and high-risk environments (Crowell et al. 2014).

Impulsive-aggression and emotion dysregulation are in the center of the body of research of biological studies (Fruzzetti et al. 2005; Beauchaine et al. 2017; Shadara et al. 2021; Dillahunt et al. 2022). Furthermore, environmental risk factors can amplify and activate potential biological vulnerability, leading to more destructive and serious externalizing behaviors (Cicchetti 2016; Meier et al. 2008; Briscoe-Smith and Hinshaw 2006; Beauchaine et al. 2009). Moreover, there are significant correlations between genes, environment, and Gene × Environment interactions in the expression and the development of externalizing behaviors among impulsive and, therefore vulnerable children (Neuhaus and Beauchaine 2017; Beauchaine et al. 2009; Beauchaine 2012). However, according to externalizing psychopathology, impulsivity is a heritable vulnerability, its specific representation is associated with environmental factors (Neuhaus and Beauchaine 2017; Beauchaine and Neuhaus 2008; Beauchaine 2012). Indeed, the most seriously severe emotion and behavioral dysregulation among impulsive children emerge dependent on environmental risk (see, Jaffee 2017). Krause-utz et al. (2016) found that behavioral deficits in action withholding (but not in action cancellation) appear to be influenced by acute experimental stress in individuals with BPD. Delay discounting seems to be a general feature of BPD, independent of comorbid ADHD and acute stress, possibly underlying typical expressions of behavioral impulsivity in the disorder (Krause-Utz et al. 2016). Beauchaine (2012) proposed that in contrast to trait impulsivity emotion regulation encompasses the processes through which emotional experience and expression are developed—whether volitionally or automatically—in the service of adaptive behavior (Beauchaine 2012). Referring to this definition, emotion dysregulation is recognized as a pattern of emotional experiences and expression which has a destructive role in accessing to goal-directed behaviors. These negative emotions can be experienced in severely intense and maladaptive forms (Beauchaine 2012).

Crowell et al. (2009) proposed that dysregulated emotions and emotionally unstable anger become dramatically sensitive to environmental experiences and may even be covered by temperamental impulsivity as a downward consequence of repeated negative reinforcement in the familial context. In addition, various stressors that occur in the early stages of development can contribute to any kind of structural and neurotransmitter destructive changes (King-Casas et al. 2008). Therefore, elevated and amplified sensitivity to environmental stressors can mediate the relation between biological vulnerabilities and development of BPD (Crowell et al. 2009). Consistent with Linehan biosocial theory of BPD, Lynch et al. (2006) posited that individuals BPD demonstrate heightened emotion sensitivity. Selby and Joiner Jr (2009) suggested that individuals with BPD may demonstrate higher morning-to-evening mood variability and a more random distribution of morning moods than depressed patients and controls, as well as, mood instability related to anger, anxiety and fluctuation between depression and anxiety, which may be stronger than those experienced in depression, cyclothymia, and bipolar II disorder (Selby and Joiner Jr 2009). Another study found that extreme mood oscillation in hostile, fearful, and sad affects occurs in BPD individuals more frequently than in comparison to cases of depression (Trull et al. 2008). Dixon-Gordon et al. (2017) pointed out that issues with emotion regulation are core difficulties in BPD. Recent research has suggested that avoidance of emotions in general, and emotion suppression specifically, may be commonly used among BPD patients (Dixon-Gordon et al. 2017). An alternative approach to understanding borderline psychopathology may be concentrated on the core features of BPD rather the specific DSM criteria, specifically emotion dysregulation (Rufino et al. 2017; Sauer-Zavala and Barlow 2014). Along these lines, Selby and Joiner Jr (2009) presented the Emotional Cascade Model, which will be discussed in more detail in the next chapter, in which the model claims that individuals with BPD experience extreme vacillations in negative emotion induced by rumination on negative affect, progressively worsening the emotional state. This "emotional cascade" then results an intolerable emotional state that leads to dysregulated behaviors which are utilized to distract attention from the negative thoughts to the physical sensations of the dysregulated behaviors (Selby and Joiner Jr 2009). Recent research exploring the model revealed a three-way interaction between elevated BPD symptoms, elevated rumination, and negative emotions, which prospectively predicted dysregulated behavior within the next 2–3 h. Examples of dysregulated behaviors included nonsuicidal self-injury, alcohol use, physical fights, binge eating, and reckless driving (Selby and Joiner Jr 2013; Rufino et al. 2017).

2. *The development of severe emotional instability features of BPD is developed and maintained by the caregiving environment and is based on characteristics of the child* (e.g., *baseline emotional sensitivity) and the developmental context (Crowell et al.* 2009*)* ***or*** *affective instability is developed and maintained within high-risk familial contexts, which are manifested by intermittent reinforcement of adverse behavior and chronic invalidation of emotional expression (Crowell et al.* 2014*)* ***or*** *emotional lability is developed and perpetuated within high-risk contexts featured by emotional invalidation and intermittent reinforcement of intensely severe emotional expressions (Kaufman et al.* 2017a*).* In accordance with this hypothesis, Crowell et al. (2009) emphasized the considerable role of invalidating family contexts. As mentioned, the social part of biosocial theory refers to an invalidating social contextual environment, especially the role of caregivers. The ability to regulate emotion is a crucial part for developing a healthy and adaptive personality structure to adjust and having function in real life (Paley and Hajal 2022; Blair and Raver 2015; Panlilio et al. 2018). Dysfunctional relationships are a substantial feature of BPD (Whalen et al. 2015), and the quality of caregiver-child relationship has been pointed as a core factor in childhood and adolescence stages (Stepp et al. 2014). The environment may communicate that individual's emotions are wrong, weird, or bad. It can ignore emotional reactions and does nothing to help with appropriate emotional expression. Children who are raised in invalidating environments learn that they cannot trust their behaviors, emotions, thoughts, and perspectives. Parental criticism (Whalen et al. 2015; Hughes et al. 2012, 2020), family members criticism, hostility, and emotional over-involvement toward an individual (Hooley 2007; 2017), emotional invalidation (Elzy 2013), misattributing children's expressed emotions to undesirable personal characteristics and traits which contribute to exacerbated emotion dysregulation (Fruzzetti et al. 2005), discouraging or pun-

ishing adaptive attempts at socializing, problem solving or assertive communication; meanwhile, inconsistent and inappropriate response to self-harm and impulsive behaviors, and child abuse and maltreatment are core features of invalidating environments (Fruzzetti et al. 2005; Linehan 1993a).

Crowell et al. (2013) proposed that the invalidating environment theory posits that caregiver invalidation and conflict play a role in the development of emotion dysregulation, psychopathology, and self-injurious behaviors (Crowell et al. 2013). According to Linehan's biosocial model, though the child's emotional sensitivity makes child prone to the development of BPD, this vulnerability is greatly amplified within a negative invalidating familial environment (Linehan 1993a). Within this context, children's emotional expressions are rejected by caregivers and different life issues could be oversimplified. Therefore, several crucial skills cannot be taught, especially skills to modulate emotional arousal or distress tolerance skills (Crowell et al. 2009). Due to impaired toleration of emotional experiences in caregivers within invalidating environment, the child will experience difficulties to identify, label, and understand the momentary emotion experienced, as well as emotional components of interpersonal interactions and communications. Consequently, this process may contribute to emotion dysregulation followed by behavioral dysregulation such as impulsivity (e.g. Crowell et al. 2009, 2014; Linehan 1993a, 2016; Krause-Utz et al. 2021; Wilson and Durbin 2012; Sansone et al. 2018; Dixon-Gordon et al. 2020, 2022; Hughes et al. 2012). These outcomes can be observed in adolescents with self-injury behaviors, who suffer from externalizing psychopathology, borderline personality traits, and psychophysiological biomarkers of trait impulsivity (Crowell et al. 2012). For instance, Dixon-Gordon et al. (2016) found a powerful relation between a girl's negative emotional reactivity and borderline symptoms. The findings indicated that in conflict discussion task, there was an association between maternal problem-solving task and maternal support/validation level. In other words, they found in the case of high maternal support/validation during this task, the relationship between a girl's negative reactivity and borderline symptoms was significantly decreased and, in opposite, the relationship between girl's negative reactivity and borderline symptoms was dramatically elevated when there is low maternal support/validation (Macfie et al. 2020).

Within the context of the Coercion Model, the child's problematic behavior emerges such as impulsivity within family contexts in which parents tremendously treat harsh and inconsistent discipline strategies (Capaldi et al. 1997; Patterson and Capaldi 2013). This model is similar to Linehan's biosocial model in developing BPD (Crowell et al. 2014) and proposes that children's negative behavior may be neglected or may be met with equally negative or even severely negative behavior from the parent. Due to the inconsistency with which parenting strategies are applied in these families, children may have issues predicting what type of response is likely to happen from their own negative behavior. These negative discipline strategies tend to cooccur with lower rates of positive reinforcement for child's positive behavior (Fisher et al. 2019). The most considerable aspect of coercive process is a pattern in which aversive tactics escalate over time because they are effective in declining similarly aversive behaviors of interaction partner. In other words, via increasing conflict, a disagreement will be over. But these notorious negative reinforcement processes contribute to extreme emotional behaviors from both sides of children and their parents (Crowell et al. 2014).

Long-lasting, invasive, and originally interpersonal events such as severe child abuse and neglect by caregivers, domestic violence, sexual abuse and rape can be found in invalidating environment during childhood and adolescence contribute to the development of BPD (e.g., Krause-Utz et al. 2021). Chapman et al. (2020) indicated that having a history of psychopathology likely escalates both environmental and biological risks to the development of BPD (Chapman et al. 2020). Lobo and Lunkenheimer (2020) emphasized on the importance of considerable parent-child interactions as dynamic system to offer an enhanced understanding of how the parent-child transactions is associated with adaptive outcomes and maladaptive consequences in early childhood (Lobo and Lunkenheimer 2020). Mendez et al. (2022) suggested that adolescents with low perceived social support (PSS) are specifically more vulnerable for developing NSSI associated with exacerbated BPD characteristics and traits (Mendez et al. 2022). There are several predisposing factors of early BPD onset which can be considered as a precocious detection of high-risk individuals, such as positive history of traumatic experiences and precocious emotional or/and physical abuse and neglect by caregivers (Bornovalova et al. 2013; Bozzatello et al. 2019, 2021), maltreatment by peers (Crowell et al. 2009; Antila et al. 2017), invalidating familial environment and disturbed child-parent interaction (Vanwoerden et al. 2017, 2022, 2023), severe maternal psychopathology (Stepp et al. 2016; Mahan 2020). When individuals with specific temperamental trait (negative affectivity, impulsive behaviors, aggression, and anger in interpersonal relationships, or neurobiological characteristics) experience traumatic events, the risk of BPD will rise in young age (Bozzatello et al. 2019, 2021).

3. *Reciprocal reinforcement interactions between biological predispositions and environmental risk processes endorse emotion dysregulation and more severe behavioral control issues and therefore lead to negative cognitive and social consequences (Crowell et al.* 2009*)* ***or*** *inheritable impulsivity interacts across development with other environmental risk factors to reinforce more extremely severe behavior and emotion dysregulation, disturb peer relationships, and influence academic functioning (Crowell et al.* 2014*)* ***or*** *biological proneness transact with environmental risks over time to endorse internalizing and externalizing psychopathology manifested by increasingly extreme behavior and emotion dysregulation (Kaufman et al.* 2017a*).* In evaluating this postulate suggested by Crowell et al. (2009, 2013, 2014), impulsivity is one of the most substantial child's characteristics biologically driven presented in early child development (Crowell et al. 2009, 2013, 2014). Impulsivity, along with emotional dysregulation, is considered as a main feature of BPD (Jacob et al. 2010; Skodol et al. 2002). Further, impulsivity is one of the core diagnostic criteria according to APA (2022) and is related to the severity of BPD (e.g., Jacob et al. 2013; Neuhaus and Beauchaine 2017), especially self-destructive behaviors such as suicidal behavior (Paris 2005; Crowell et al. 2014). Based on Jacob et al.

(2013), typical manifestations of impulsivity in BPD can be observed in the form of behaviors like outbursts of anger and aggression, uncontrolled buying and money expenses, disinhibited sexual behaviors, eating issues like binges and substance use (Jacob et al. 2013). BPD is presented as a disorder which trait impulsivity is the main predisposing vulnerability. Trait impulsivity originates primarily from inheritable compromises in central dopaminergic and serotonergic function. Impulsivity is potentiated by high-risk family environments in which affective instability is developed and maintained by operant reinforcement contingencies. Over time, these endorsement contingencies cause long-lasting patterns of emotion dysregulation—contributing to antisocial and borderline personality disorder (ASPD & BPD) in vulnerable individuals. Sex effects modulate the behavioral expression of Biology × environment interactions to produce ASPD disproportionately in males, and BPD disproportionately in females (Beauchaine et al. 2009). Gene-Environment interaction (G × E) investigations have been widespread in the literature on psychopathology research (Dick 2011; Cicchetti 2016; Luyten and Fonagy 2016). In spite of growing research about the role of genetic and environmental factors in the development of BPD, studies on Gene-Environment interaction (G × E) are limited. Several studies have attempted to study impulsivity as a heritable-genetic factor and its transaction with environmental correlations to develop BPD (Crowell et al. 2014). Wilson et al. (2012) found a polymorphism in the tryptophan hydroxylase gene (TPH1) interacted with childhood abuse and could predict BPD in adulthood (Wilson et al. 2012). Respiratory sinus arrhythmia (RSA), which is utilized to mark the ability to adaptively regulate emotions, is measured by frequency of change in magnitude between rises and declines in heart rate across the respiratory cycle (Beauchaine et al. 2017). Beauchaine (2012) highlighted that low baseline RSA and/or excessive RSA withdrawal in response to emotionally evocative stimuli have been associated with conduct issues, trait hostility, eating disorders, anxiety disorders, depression, and panic disorder among other adverse consequences (Beauchaine 2012). Research about RSA greatly clarified that specific biological predispositions interact with contextual risk to stouten psychopathology. Besides psychophysiological markers of vulnerability, a number of Gene-Environment interactions (G × E) have been pointed out in the etiology of externalizing behavior disorders (Beauchaine 2012). According to Crowell et al. (2008), there is a synergistic association between biological vulnerabilities and environmental risk factors (Crowell et al. 2008).

4. *By mid-to-late adolescence there is a set of identifiable characteristics and maladaptive coping strategies that demonstrate elevated risk factor for following BPD (Crowell et al.* 2009*)* ***or*** *by adolescent, these Biology × Environment interactions improve a complex of identifiable issues and maladaptive coping strategies—comprising early borderline manifestations and repetitive self-injurious behaviors, which fall along a heterotypically continuous trajectory to BPD (Crowell et al.* 2014*)* ***or*** *by adolescence, these biology × environment interactions provoke a constellation of identifiable difficulties and maladaptive coping*

strategies characteristic of BPD, such as self-injurious behaviors (Kaufman et al. 2017a*)*. In this hypothesis, the main focus is on the trajectories of BPD in adolescence which can anticipate the later BPD in adults. Consistent with this, Crowell et al. (2014) postulated a series of specific BPD precursors that emerge by adolescence among people who are on a BPD trajectory, encompassing emotional instability and fluctuation, deregulated behaviors and impulsivity, outburst of anger, disturbed interpersonal relationships, lack of sense of self, feeling if emptiness, self-destructive behaviors and self-inflicted injuries (SII) (Crowell et al. 2014). Adolescence is a critical developmental stage of human life, when a majority of identifiable psychological and biological changes begin to emerge. Based on Crowell et al. (2009, 2014), a constellation of emotional and behavioral can appear in this stage which will not be labeled reliably as borderline pathology because they may be considered as normal signs in adolescence (Crowell et al. 2009, 2012, 2014; Miller and Resick 2007). Moreover, there are several overlaps among BPD symptoms and other psychological issues and psychiatric disorders, such as depression and conduct disorders (Crowell et al. 2014), and PTSD (Harned et al. 2014a, b, 2018, 2022), contributing to achieving a distinguished diagnosis of BPD harder (Crowell et al. 2014). By late adolescence, many youths with BPD can be diagnosed reliably (Hughes and Devine 2017, 2020; Miller et al. 2008). In addition, emotion-driven, impulsive behaviors such as self-inflicted injury, suicidal behaviors, substance use, often appear during adolescence (Crowell et al. 2008; Hughes et al. 2012). Repetitive self-inflicted injurious behaviors in adolescence may represent a precursor of adult BPD (Hughes et al. 2012; Crowell et al. 2009, 2014; Beauchaine et al. 2009), for example, studies have shown that self-injurious behaviors followed by interpersonal stressors such as conflict with parents, and these conflicts precipitate SII (Hughes et al. 2012; Berman et al. 2009). Like all developmental stages, during the adolescent stage, an individual actively attempts to shape specific strategies to solve age-dependent tasks via behavioral response patterns (Cicchetti 2006). Parental availability and support (Hughes et al. 2012), child temperament, and temperament × parenting interactions (Rothbart et al. 2000) are significant factors in the development of the emerging adult personality (Hughes et al. 2012, 2020). Crowell et al. (2012) proposed that self-inflicted injury (SII) and suicide are both manifested by severe emotion dysregulation (Crowell et al. 2014), and it has been indicated that 90% of BPD cases meet the criteria of self-inflicted injury (Zanarini et al. 2003), which is one of the most crucial functions of SII is to dampen escalated negative emotions (Crowell et al. 2005, 2014), and also, in more than two-thirds of BPD case, SII initiate before 18 (see., Zanarini et al. 2006). According to these findings, Crowell et al. (2014) stated that self-injuring adolescents are at heightened predisposition for later BPD (Crowell et al. 2014). Moreover, it has been demonstrated that reporting self-damaging impulsivity and frantic attempts to avoid abandonment were significantly higher than depressed adolescents (Crowell et al. 2012). BPD symptoms elevate in late adolescence, around 14–17 years of age (Courtney-Seidler et al. 2013). Through cross-sectional studies with adolescents, Stead et al. (2019) pointed out that there are remarkable associations between BPD and nonsuicidal self-injury in both clinical and community settings (Selby and Joiner Jr 2013; Cerutti et al. 2011; Klonsky and Olino 2008). Moreover, studies have shown that BPD symptoms are associated with earlier age of onset (Klonsky and Olino 2008), more frequent suicide attempts (Jacobson et al. 2008), and greater rate of repeated NSSI (Muehlenkamp et al. 2011). NSSI has been presented as a developmental trajectory of BPD pathology according to the biosocial developmental model (Stead et al. 2019; Gratz et al. 2017, 2019, 2022; Crowell et al. 2009, 2012; Homan et al. 2017). Stead et al. (2019) found significant longitudinal associations between NSSI and later BPD (Stead et al. 2019).

5. *These traits and behaviors may heighten the risk for BPD across developmental stages of life, because of evocative influences on interpersonal relationships and social performance and through interference with healthy emotional development (Crowell et al.* 2009*)* ***or*** *adolescent borderline pathology may further increase the risk for BPD in adulthood by interfering with normal processes of development, the capability to shape accepted interpersonal relationships, and development of adaptive coping strategies (Crowell et al.* 2014*)* ***or*** *early representations of borderline pathology such as self-injurious behaviors may further exacerbate risk for BPD by disturbing individual's abilities to navigate stage-salient developmental tasks, form supportive social associations, and shape healthy coping strategies (Kaufman et al.* 2017a*).* In this final hypothesis, the main focus is on a shared etiology between SII and BPD and suggests that SII exacerbates risk of adult BPD. Conceptualization of childhood borderline pathology is derived from studies on heterogeneous populations; therefore, it is unclear to what extend childhood borderline personality can predict the emergence of adult BPD (Petti and Vela 1990; Gratz et al. 2009). In order to test a full range of borderline personality symptom severity and dose-response relationships, a dimensional assessment of childhood borderline pathology should be addressed (Gratz et al. 2009; Bornovalova et al. 2010; Kaufman et al. 2017a, b). Through considering dimensional perspectives, we are able to evaluate the ways in which different factors, comprising biological, psychological, and socio-contextual, interact to predict normal and abnormal development across the life span (Cicchetti 2016), as well as, categorizing BPD symptoms in two subgroups comprising primarily internalizing and externalizing symptoms (Ramos-Loyo et al. 2012; Kaufman et al. 2020), and also, assessing the possibilities of various pathways to adaptive and maladaptive outcomes (Gratz et al. 2009). This constellation of symptoms in childhood may contribute to a wide range of different outcomes (multifinality) or one unique outcome as a result of several risk factors or developmental processes (equifinality) (Crowell et al. 2014; Gratz et al. 2009). Kaufman et al. (2017a, b) indicated that a developmental psychopathology approach in which BPD and self-injurious behaviors be conceptualized as consequences of several transactional processes, interacting risk factors, and casual events. This framework is especially beneficial for understanding the origins and different representations of psychopathology across development (Kaufman et al. 2017a, b). In sum, Crowell et al. (2009, 2014) and Kaufman et al. (2017a,

b) asserted that problematic behaviors propose a ground for the development of emotion regulation/avoidance strategy, these behaviors accelerate risk for BPD via influence not only interpersonal relationships, but also, on the development of healthy emotions (Crowell et al. 2009).

References

Achenbach TM, Ivanova MY, Rescorla LA, Turner LV, Althoff RR. Internalizing/externalizing problems: review and recommendations for clinical and research applications. J Am Acad Child Adolesc Psychiatry. 2016;55(8):647–56.
American Psychiatric Association. Diagnostic and statistical manual of mental disorders. 5th ed. Text Revised (DSM-5-TR); 2022.
Antila H, Arola R, Hakko H, Riala K, Riipinen P, Kantojärvi L. Bullying involvement in relation to personality disorders: a prospective follow-up of 508 inpatient adolescents. Eur Child Adolesc Psychiatry. 2017;26:779–89.
Avila C, Cuenca I, Félix V, Parcet MA, Miranda A. Measuring impulsivity in school-aged boys and examining its relationship with ADHD and ODD ratings. J Abnorm Child Psychol. 2004;32:295–304.
Beauchaine TP. Physiological markers of emotional and behavioral dysregulation in externalizing psychopathology. Monogr Soc Res Child Dev. 2012;77(2):79.
Beauchaine TP, McNulty T. Comorbidities and continuities as ontogenic processes: toward a developmental spectrum model of externalizing psychopathology. Dev Psychopathol. 2013;25(4pt2):1505–28.
Beauchaine TP, Neuhaus E. Impulsivity and vulnerability to psychopathology. In: Child and adolescent psychopathology. Hoboken: John Wiley & Sons; 2008. p. 129–56.
Beauchaine TP, Klein DN, Crowell SE, Derbidge C, Nehause-Kopp L. Multifinality in the development of personality disorders: a biology× sex× environment interaction model of antisocial and borderline traits. Dev Psychopathol. 2009;21(3):735–70.
Beauchaine TP, Gatzke-Kopp L, Gizer IR. Genetic, environmental, and epigenetic influences on behavior. In: Child and adolescent psychopathology. 3rd ed; 2017. p. 68–109.
Berman ME, Bradley TP, Fanning JR, Mccloskey MS. Self-focused attention reduces self-injurious behavior in alcohol-intoxicated men. Subst Use Misuse. 2009;44(9–10):1280–97.
Bender L. Anxiety in disturbed children. In: Annual meeting of the American Psychopathological Association, 39th, Jun, 1949, New York City, NY, US. Grune & Stratton; 1950.
Blair C, Raver CC. School readiness and self-regulation: a developmental psychobiological approach. Annu Rev Psychol. 2015;66:711–31.
Bornovalova MA, Levy R, Gratz KL, Lejuez CW. Understanding the heterogeneity of BPD symptoms through latent class analysis: initial results and clinical correlates among inner-city substance users. Psychol Assess. 2010;22(2):233.
Bornovalova MA, Huibregtse BM, Hicks BM, Keyes M, McGue M, Iacono W. Tests of a direct effect of childhood abuse on adult borderline personality disorder traits: a longitudinal discordant twin design. J Abnorm Psychol. 2013;122(1):180.
Bozzatello P, Bellino S, Bosia M, Rocca P. Early detection and outcome in borderline personality disorder. Front Psych. 2019;10:446813.
Bozzatello P, Garbarini C, Rocca P, Bellino S. Borderline personality disorder: risk factors and early detection. Diagnostics. 2021;11(11):2142.
Briscoe-Smith AM, Hinshaw SP. Linkages between child abuse and attention-deficit/hyperactivity disorder in girls: behavioral and social correlates. Child Abuse Negl. 2006;30(11):1239–55.
Calkins SD, Perry NB, Dollar JM. A biopsychosocial model of self-regulation in infancy. In: Child psychology. Psychology Press; 2016. p. 2–20.

Capaldi DM, Chamberlain P, Patterson GR. Ineffective discipline and conduct problems in males: association, late adolescent outcomes, and prevention. Aggress Violent Behav. 1997;2(4):343–53.

Cerutti R, Manca M, Presaghi F, Gratz KL. Prevalence and clinical correlates of deliberate self-harm among a community sample of Italian adolescents. J Adolesc. 2011;34(2):337–47.

Chapman AR, Bularga A, Mills NL. High-sensitivity cardiac troponin can be an ally in the fight against COVID-19. Circulation. 2020;141(22):1733–5.

Cicchetti D. How research on child maltreatment has informed the study of child development: perspectives from developmental psychopathology. In: Child maltreatment: theory and research on the causes and consequences of child abuse and neglect. Cambridge University Press; 1989. p. 377–431.

Cicchetti D. Socioemotional, personality, and biological development: illustrations from a multi-level developmental psychopathology perspective on child maltreatment. Annu Rev Psychol. 2016;67:187–211.

Cicchetti, D. (2006). Development and psychopathology. In D. Cicchetti & D. J. Cohen (Eds.), Developmental psychopathology: Theory and method. 2006 (2nd ed., pp. 1–23). John Wiley & Sons, Inc.

Courtney-Seidler EA, Klein D, Miller AL. Borderline personality disorder in adolescents. Clin Psychol Sci Pract. 2013;20(4):425.

Crick NR, Murray-Close DI, Woods K. Borderline personality features in childhood: a short-term longitudinal study. Dev Psychopathol. 2005;17(4):1051–70.

Crowell SE, Beauchaine TP, McCAULEY EL, Smith CJ, Stevens AL, Sylvers P. Psychological, autonomic, and serotonergic correlates of parasuicide among adolescent girls. Dev Psychopathol. 2005;17(4):1105–27.

Crowell SE, Beauchaine TP, Lenzenweger MF, Beauchaine T, Hinshaw S. The development of borderline personality disorder and self-injurious behavior. In: Child and adolescent psychopathology. Hoboken: John Wiley & Sons; 2008. p. 510–39.

Crowell SE, Beauchaine TP, Linehan MM. A biosocial developmental model of borderline personality: elaborating and extending Linehan's theory. Psychol Bull. 2009;135(3):495.

Crowell SE, Beauchaine TP, Hsiao RC, Vasilev CA, Yaptangco M, Linehan MM, McCauley E. Differentiating adolescent self-injury from adolescent depression: possible implications for borderline personality development. J Abnorm Child Psychol. 2012;40:45–57.

Crowell SE, Kaufman EA, Lenzenweger MF. The development of borderline personality and self-inflicted injury. In: Child and adolescent psychopathology; 2013. p. 577–609.

Crowell SE, Kaufman EA, Beauchaine TP. A biosocial model of BPD: theory and empirical evidence. In: Handbook of borderline personality disorder in children and adolescents. New York: Springer; 2014. p. 143–57.

Crowell SE, Kaufman EA. Development of self-inflicted injury: comorbidities and continuities with borderline and antisocial personality traits. Dev Psychopathol. 2016;28(4pt1):1071–88.

Crowell SE, Kaliush PR, Vlisides-Henry RD. Borderline personality disorder (BPD) Compass is a promising complementary intervention to dialectical behavior therapy: Comment on Sauer-Zavala; 2022.

De La Garza ÁG, Blanco C, Olfson M, Wall MM. Identification of suicide attempt risk factors in a national US survey using machine learning. JAMA Psychiatry. 2021;78(4):398–406.

Dick DM. Gene-environment interaction in psychological traits and disorders. Annu Rev Clin Psychol. 2011;7:383–409.

Dillahunt AK, Feldman DA, Thomas LR, Farstead BW, Frandsen SB, Lee S, Pazdera M, Galloway J, Bessette KL, Roberts H, Crowell SE. Self-injury in adolescence is associated with greater behavioral risk avoidance, not risk-taking. J Clin Med. 2022;11(5):1288.

Dixon-Gordon KL, Turner BJ, Rosenthal MZ, Chapman AL. Emotion regulation in borderline personality disorder: an experimental investigation of the effects of instructed acceptance and suppression. Behav Ther. 2016;48(6):750–64.

Dixon-Gordon KL, Turner BJ, Haliczer LA, Gratz KL, Tull MT, Chapman AL. Self-injury motives: a personcentered examination. Suicide Life Threat Behav. 2022;52(4):812–27.
Dixon-Gordon KL, Peters JR, Fertuck EA, Yen S. Emotional processes in borderline personality disorder: an update for clinical practice. J Psychother Integr. 2017;27(4):425.
Dixon-Gordon KL, Marsh NP, Balda KE, McQuade JD. Parent emotion socialization and child emotional vulnerability as predictors of borderline personality features. Res Child Adolesc Psychopathol. 2020;48:135–47.
Elzy MB. Emotional invalidation: an investigation into its definition, measurement, and effects, 2013.
Fisher WW, Saini V, Greer BD, Sullivan WE, Roane HS, Fuhrman AM, Craig AR, Kimball RT. Baseline reinforcement rate and resurgence of destructive behavior. J Exp Anal Behav. 2019;111(1):75–93.
Fonagy P, Target M, Bateman A. The mentalization based approach to psychotherapy for borderline personality disorder. In: The psychoanalytic therapy of severe disturbance. Routledge; 2018. p. 35–80.
Fruzzetti AE, Shenk C, Hoffman PD. Family interaction and the development of borderline personality disorder: a transactional model. Dev Psychopathol. 2005;17(4):1007–30.
Geselowitz B, Whalen DJ, Tillman R, Barch DM, Luby JL, Vogel A. Preschool age predictors of adolescent borderline personality symptoms. J Am Acad Child Adolesc Psychiatry. 2021;60(5):612–22.
Granic I, Patterson GR. Toward a comprehensive model of antisocial development: a dynamic systems approach. Psychol Rev. 2006;113(1):101.
Gratz KL, Tull MT, Reynolds EK, Bagge CL, Latzman RD, Daughters SB, Lejuez CW. Extending extant models of the pathogenesis of borderline personality disorder to childhood borderline personality symptoms: the roles of affective dysfunction, disinhibition, and self-and emotion-regulation deficits. Dev Psychopathol. 2009;21(4):1263–91.
Grove JL, Crowell SE. The Oxford handbook of dialectical behaviour therapy. New York: Oxford University Press; 2018.
Grove JL, Carlson SE, Parkhurst KA, O'Neill JC, Smith TW. Nonsuicidal self-injury, sleep quality, and shame response to a laboratory stress task. J Clin Psychol. 2023;79(3):871–85.
Gratz KL, Kiel EJ, Mann AJ, Tull MT. The prospective relation between borderline personality disorder symptoms and suicide risk: the mediating roles of emotion regulation difficulties and perceived burdensomeness. J Affect Disord. 2022;313:186–95.
Gratz KL, Richmond JR, Dixon-Gordon KL, Chapman AL, Tull MT. Multimodal assessment of emotional reactivity and regulation in response to social rejection among self-harming adults with and without borderline personality disorder. Personal Disord Theory Res Treat. 2019;10(5):395.
Gratz KL, Weiss NH, McDermott MJ, Dilillo D, Messman-Moore T, Tull MT. Emotion dysregulation mediates the relation between borderline personality disorder symptoms and later physical health symptoms. J Personal Disord. 2017;31(4):433–48.
Harned MS, Dimeff LA, Woodcock EA, Kelly T, Zavertnik J, Contreras I, Danner SM. Exposing clinicians to exposure: a randomized controlled dissemination trial of exposure therapy for anxiety disorders. Behav Ther. 2014a;45(6):731–44.
Harned MS, Korslund KE, Linehan MM. A pilot randomized controlled trial of dialectical behavior therapy with and without the dialectical behavior therapy prolonged exposure protocol for suicidal and self-injuring women with borderline personality disorder and PTSD. Behav Res Ther. 2014b;55:7–17.
Harned MS, Gallop RJ, Valenstein-Mah HR. What changes when? The course of improvement during a stage-based treatment for suicidal and self-injuring women with borderline personality disorder and PTSD. Psychother Res. 2018;28(5):761–75.
Harned MS, Gallop RJ, Schmidt SC, Korslund KE. The temporal relationships between therapist adherence and patient outcomes in dialectical behavior therapy. J Consult Clin Psychol. 2022;90(3):272.

Hooley JM. Expressed emotion and relapse of psychopathology. Annu Rev Clin Psychol. 2007;3:329–52.

Homan P, Reddan MC, Brosch T, Koenigsberg HW, Schiller D. Aberrant link between empathy and social attribution style in borderline personality disorder. J Psychiatr Res. 2017;94:163–71.

Hughes DJ, Kratsiotis IK, Niven K, Holman D. Personality traits and emotion regulation: a targeted review and recommendations. Emotion. 2020;20(1):63.

Hughes C, Devine RT. Parental influences on children's executive function: a differentiated approach. In: Executive function. Routledge; 2017. p. 160–71.

Hughes AE, Crowell SE, Uyeji L, Coan JA. A developmental neuroscience of borderline pathology: emotion dysregulation and social baseline theory. J Abnorm Child Psychol. 2012;40:21–33.

Jacob GA, Gutz L, Bader K, Lieb K, Tüscher O, Stahl C. Impulsivity in borderline personality disorder: impairment in self-report measures, but not behavioral inhibition. Psychopathology. 2010;43(3):180–8.

Jacob GA, Zvonik K, Kamphausen S, Sebastian A, Maier S, Philipsen A, Van Elst LT, Lieb K, Tüscher O. Emotional modulation of motor response inhibition in women with borderline personality disorder: an fMRI study. J Psychiatry Neurosci. 2013;38(3):164–72.

Jacobson CM, Muehlenkamp JJ, Miller AL, Turner JB. Psychiatric impairment among adolescents engaging in different types of deliberate self-harm. J Clin Child Adolesc Psychol. 2008;37(2):363–75.

Jaffee SR. Child maltreatment and risk for psychopathology in childhood and adulthood. Annu Rev Clin Psychol. 2017;13:525–51.

Kaufman EA, Puzia ME, Godfrey DA, Crowell SE. Physiological and behavioral effects of interpersonal validation: a multilevel approach to examining a core intervention strategy among self-injuring adolescents and their mothers. J Clin Psychol. 2020;76(3):559–80.

Kaufman EA, Victor SE, Hipwell AE, Stepp SD. Reciprocal influences of parent and adolescent borderline personality symptoms over 3 years. J Pers Disord. 2020;34(Supplement B): 130–45.

Kaufman SB, Yaden DB, Hyde E, Chirico A, Gaggioli A, Zhang JW, Keltner D. The development of the Awe Experience Scale (AWE-S): a multifactorial measure for a complex emotion. J Posit Psychol. 2019;14(4):474–88.

Kaufman EA, Crowell SE, Lenzenweger MF. The development of borderline personality and self-inflicted injury. In: Child and adolescent psychopathology. 3rd ed. Hoboken: Wiley; 2017a. p. 642–79.

Kaufman EA, Puzia ME, Mead HK, Crowell SE, McEachern A, Beauchaine TP. Children's emotion regulation difficulties mediate the association between maternal borderline and antisocial symptoms and youth behavior problems over 1 year. J Personal Disord. 2017b;31(2):170–92.

King-Casas B, Sharp C, Lomax-Bream L, Lohrenz T, Fonagy P, Montague PR. The rupture and repair of cooperation in borderline personality disorder. Science. 2008;321(5890):806–10.

Klonsky ED, Olino TM. Identifying clinically distinct subgroups of self-injurers among young adults: a latent class analysis. J Consult Clin Psychol. 2008;76(1):22.

Koppitz EM, De Moreau M. A comparison of emotional indicators on human figure drawings of children from Mexico and from the United States. Revista Interamericana de Psicología/ Interamerican. J Psychol. 1968;2(1)

Krause-Utz A, Cackowski S, Daffner S, Sobanski E, Plichta MM, Bohus M, Ende G, Schmahl C. Delay discounting and response disinhibition under acute experimental stress in women with borderline personality disorder and adult attention deficit hyperactivity disorder. Psychol Med. 2016;46(15):3137–49.

Krause-Utz A, Mertens LJ, Renn JB, Lucke P, Wöhlke AZ, van Schie CC, Mouthaan J. Childhood maltreatment, borderline personality features, and coping as predictors of intimate partner violence. J Interpers Violence. 2021;36(13–14):6693–721.

Kulacaoglu F, Solmaz M, Belli H, Ardic FC, Akin E, Kose S. The relationship between impulsivity and attention-deficit/hyperactivity symptoms in female patients with borderline personality disorder. Psychiatry Clin Psychopharmacol. 2017;27(3):249–55.

Lenzenweger MF, Clarkin JF, Levy KN, Yeomans FE, Kernberg OF. Predicting domains and rates of change in borderline personality disorder. Personal Disord Theory Res Treat. 2012;3(2):185.
Linehan MM. Dialectical behavior therapy in clinical practice. Guilford Publications; 2020.
Littlefield AK, Sher KJ, Wood PK. Do changes in drinking motives mediate the relation between personality change and "maturing out" of problem drinking? J Abnorm Psychol. 2010;119(1):93.
Linehan MM, Kehrer CA. Borderline personality disorder. In: Clinical handbook of psychological disorders, vol. 2; 1993.
Linehan MM. Skills training manual for treating borderline personality disorder. Guilford Press; 1993a.
Linehan MM. Behavior therapy: where we were, where we are and where we need to be going. Cogn Behav Pract. 2016;23(4):451–3.
Lobo FM, Lunkenheimer E. Understanding the parent-child coregulation patterns shaping child self-regulation. Dev Psychol. 2020;56(6):1121.
Luyten P, Fonagy P. The selfin depression. In: The self in understanding and treating psychological disorders. Cambridge University Press; 2016. p. 71.
Lynch TR, Rosenthal MZ, Kosson DS, Cheavens JS, Lejuez CW, Blair RJ. Heightened sensitivity to facial expressions of emotion in borderline personality disorder. Emotion. 2006;6(4):647.
Macfie J, Zvara BJ, Stuart GL, Kurdziel-Adams G, Kors SB, Fortner KB, Towers CV, Gorrondona AM, Noose SK. Pregnant women's history of childhood maltreatment and current opioid use: the mediating role of reflective functioning. Addict Behav. 2020;102:106134.
Mahan RM. Dyadic parent-adolescent role confusion dimensions: development and validation of an observational coding scale. University of Tennessee; 2020.
Martin S, Del-Monte J, Graziani P. Impulsivity issues in borderline personality disorder and it's links with insight: the role of urgency. Heliyon. 2019;5(10):e02564.
Meier MH, Slutske WS, Arndt S, Cadoret RJ. Impulsive and callous traits are more strongly associated with delinquent behavior in higher risk neighborhoods among boys and girls. J Abnorm Psychol. 2008;117(2):377.
Mendez I, Sintes A, Pascual JC, Puntí J, Lara A, Briones-Buixassa L, Nicolaou S, Schmidt C, Romero S, Fernández M, i Farrés CC. Borderline personality traits mediate the relationship between low perceived social support and nonsuicidal self-injury in a clinical sample of adolescents. J Affect Disord. 2022;302:204–13.
Miller MW, Resick PA. Internalizing and externalizing subtypes in female sexual assault survivors: implications for the understanding of complex PTSD. Behav Ther. 2007;38(1):58–71.
Miller CJ, Miller SR, Newcorn JH, Halperin JM. Personality characteristics associated with persistent ADHD in late adolescence. J Abnorm Child Psychol. 2008;36:165–73.
Muehlenkamp JJ, Ertelt TW, Miller AL, Claes L. Borderline personality symptoms differentiate non-suicidal and suicidal self-injury in ethnically diverse adolescent outpatients. J Child Psychol Psychiatry. 2011;52(2):148–55.
Neuhaus E, Beauchaine TP. Impulsivity and vulnerability to psychopathology. In: Child and adolescent psychopathology. 3rd ed; 2017. p. 178–212.
Oas P. Validity of a draw-A-person and Bender Gestalt tests as measures of impulsivity with adolescents. J Consult Clin Psychol. 1984;52(6):1011.
Oas P. The psychological assessment of impulsivity: a review. J Psychoeduc Assess. 1985;3(2):141–56.
Patterson GR, Capaldi DM. Antisocial parents: unskilled and vulnerable. In: Family transitions. Routledge; 2013. p. 195–218.
Paley B, Hajal NJ. Conceptualizing emotion regulation and coregulation as family-level phenomena. Clin Child Fam Psychol Rev. 2022;25(1):19–43.
Panlilio CC, Harden BJ, Harring J. School readiness of maltreated preschoolers and later school achievement: the role of emotion regulation, language, and context. Child Abuse Negl. 2018;75:82–91.

Paris J. The development of impulsivity and suicidality in borderline personality disorder. Dev Psychopathol. 2005;17(4):1091–104.

Petti TA, Vela RM. Borderline disorders of childhood: an overview. J Am Acad Child Adolesc Psychiatry. 1990;29(3):327–37.

Pohl S, Steuwe C, Mainz V, Driessen M, Beblo T. Borderline personality disorder and childhood trauma: exploring the buffering role of self-compassion and self-esteem. J Clin Psychol. 2021;77(3):837–45.

Porteus BD, Johnson RC. Children's responses to two measures of conscience development and their relation to sociometric nomination. Child Dev. 1965;36:703–11.

Ramos-Loyo J, González-Garrido AA, García-Aguilar G, Del Río-Portilla Y. The emotional content of faces interferes with inhibitory processing: an event related potential study. Int J Psychol Stud. 2012;5(2):52.

Rothbart MK, Ahadi SA, Evans DE. Temperament and personality: origins and outcomes. J Pers Soc Psychol. 2000;78(1):122.

Rufino KA, Ellis TE, Clapp J, Pearte C, Fowler JC. Variations of emotion dysregulation in borderline personality disorder: a latent profile analysis approach with adult psychiatric inpatients. Bord Personal Disord Emot Dysregul. 2017;4:1–9.

Sansone RA, Sellbom M, Songer DA. Borderline personality disorder and mental health care utilization: the role of self-harm. Personal Disord Theory Res Treat. 2018;9(2):188.

Sauer-Zavala S, Barlow DH. The case for borderline personality disorder as an emotional disorder: implications for treatment. Clin Psychol Sci Pract. 2014;21(2):118.

Schaich A, Braakmann D, Rogg M, Meine C, Ambrosch J, Assmann N, Borgwardt S, Schweiger U, Fassbinder E. How do patients with borderline personality disorder experience distress tolerance skills in the context of dialectical behavioral therapy?—a qualitative study. PLoS One. 2021a;16(6):e0252403.

Schaich A, Assmann N, Köhne S, Alvarez-Fischer D, Borgwardt S, Schweiger U, Klein JP, Faßbinder E. The mediating effect of difficulties in emotion regulation on the association between childhood maltreatment and borderline personality disorder. Eur J Psychotraumatol. 2021b;12(1):1934300.

Selby EA, Joiner TE Jr. Cascades of emotion: the emergence of borderline personality disorder from emotional and behavioral dysregulation. Rev Gen Psychol. 2009;13(3):219–29.

Selby EA, Joiner TE Jr. Emotional cascades as prospective predictors of dysregulated behaviors in borderline personality disorder. Personal Disord Theory Res Treat. 2013;4(2):168.

Shadara Z, Dehghani M, Heidari M, Mahmoud AM. Distress tolerance, impulsivity and aggression: the role of emotional dysregulation and reward sensitivity in individuals with borderline personality disorder features. Pract Clin Psychol. 2021;9(1):37–50.

Skodol AE, Gunderson JG, Pfohl B, Widiger TA, Livesley WJ, Siever LJ. The borderline diagnosis I: psychopathology, comorbidity, and personaltity structure. Biol Psychiatry. 2002;51(12):936–50.

Stead VE, Boylan K, Schmidt LA. Longitudinal associations between nonsuicidal self-injury and borderline personality disorder in adolescents: a literature review. Borderline Personal Disord Emot Dysregul. 2019;6:1–2.

Stepp SD, Scott LN, Morse JQ, Nolf KA, Hallquist MN, Pilkonis PA. Emotion dysregulation as a maintenance factor of borderline personality disorder features. Compr Psychiatry. 2014;55(3):657–66.

Stepp SD, Lazarus SA, Byrd AL. A systematic review of risk factors prospectively associated with borderline personality disorder: taking stock and moving forward. Personal Disord Theory Res Treat. 2016;7(4):316.

Stevens EM, Frank D, Codispoti M, Kypriotakis G, Cinciripini PM, Claiborne K, Deweese MM, Engelmann JM, Green CE, Karam-Hage M, Minnix JA. The late positive potentials evoked by cigarette-related and emotional images show no gender differences in smokers. Sci Rep. 2019;9(1):3240.

Trull TJ, Solhan MB, Tragesser SL, Jahng S, Wood PK, Piasecki TM, Watson D. Affective instability: measuring a core feature of borderline personality disorder with ecological momentary assessment. J Abnorm Psychol. 2008;117(3):647.
Vanwoerden S, Kalpakci A, Sharp C. The relations between inadequate parent-child boundaries and borderline personality disorder in adolescence. Psychiatry Res. 2017;257:462–71.
Vanwoerden S, Byrd AL, Vine V, Beeney JE, Scott LN, Stepp SD. Momentary borderline personality disorder symptoms in youth as a function of parental invalidation and youth-perceived support. J Child Psychol Psychiatry. 2022;63(2):178–86.
Vanwoerden S, McLaren V, Stepp SD, Sharp C. Are we thinking about the same disorder? A trifactor model approach to understand parents' and their adolescents' reports of borderline personality pathology. J Pers Assess. 2023;105(4):487–98.
Whalen DJ, Kiel EJ, Tull MT, Latzman RD, Gratz KL. Maternal borderline personality disorder symptoms and convergence between observed and reported infant negative emotional expressions. Personal Disord Theory Res Treat. 2015;6(3):229.
White CN, Gunderson JG, Zanarini MC, Hudson JI. Family studies of borderline personality disorder: a review. Harv Rev Psychiatry. 2003;11(1):8–19.
Wilson S, Durbin CE. Dyadic parent-child interaction during early childhood: contributions of parental and child personality traits. J Pers. 2012;80(5):1313–38.
Wilson ST, Stanley B, Brent DA, Oquendo MA, Huang YY, Haghighi F, Hodgkinson CA, Mann JJ. Interaction between tryptophan hydroxylase I polymorphisms and childhood abuse is associated with increased risk for borderline personality disorder in adulthood. Psychiatr Genet. 2012;22(1):15–24.
Zanarini MC, Frankenburg FR, Hennen J, Reich DB, Silk KR. Prediction of the 10-year course of borderline personality disorder. Am J Psychiatry. 2006;163(5):827–32.
Zanarini MC, Frankenburg FR, Hennen J, Silk KR. The longitudinal course of borderline psychopathology: 6-year prospective follow-up of the phenomenology of borderline personality disorder. Am J Psychiatry. 2003;160(2):274–83.

Chapter 8
The Emotional Cascade Model of Borderline Personality Disorder

Introduction

The emotional cascade model (ECM, Selby and Joiner Jr 2009; Selby et al. 2008, 2009, 2022) has been introduced to provide an explanation for the association between emotional and behavioral dysregulation, especially in cases of borderline personality disorder (BPD). The ECM, building on Linehan's biosocial model, aims to present a clarified understanding about the relationship between emotional reactivity and dysregulated behavioral experiences and how dynamic interactions between these emotional and behavioral patterns interact with an individual's environment, ultimately resulting in the emergence of a BPD diagnosis (Selby et al. 2014a, b).

As it has been mentioned, BPD is a severe disabling disorder manifested by highly problematic clinical features, that can disqualify all aspects of an individual's life (DAM-5-TR; APA 2022; Nolen-Hoeksema 2019; Martino et al. 2015). This disorder is characterized by dramatic emotional instability, disturbance in emotion, inappropriate and intense anger, marked reactivity of mood, experiencing out-of-control emotions, outbursts of anger, extremely persistent unstable patterns of interpersonal relationships, concern about abandonment, disturbed behaviors such as impulsivity, instability of self-concept, a deep feeling of emptiness, and self-destructive behaviors such as self-injury and recurrent suicidal behaviors and suicide attempts (DSM-5-TR; APA 2022). According to the *International Classification of Diseases* (ICD-10; World Health Organization (WHO) 2016), symptoms of BPD is defined as an emotionally unstable personality disorder (Chapman et al. 2020). Enormous social impairments (Zimmerman and Schunk 2012; Chapman et al. 2020; Nolen-Hoeksema 2020), interpersonal issues (e.g., Tomko et al. 2014), several comorbidity, and highly frequent self-destructive behaviors such as self-injuries (Dixon-Gordon et al. 2020; Bolton and Robinson 2010; Nolen-Hoeksema 2020; Chapman et al. 2020) have been demonstrated in BPD. As stated in previous

E. A. Selby, M. Salavati, *Theories of Borderline Personality Disorder*,
https://doi.org/10.1007/978-3-031-75503-3_8

chapters, emotion dysregulation is a core feature of BPD (e.g., Linehan 1993; Crowell et al. 2009; Dixon-Gordon et al. 2020; Trull et al. 2010).

Selby et al. (2009) proposed that individuals who suffer from BPD experience emotional instability, as well as, dysregulated behaviors, such as self-inflicted behaviors and binge eating (Selby et al. 2009). According to Selby (2007), a growing body of studies has been focused separately on emotion and cognitive regulation strategies, for instance, rumination (Nolen-Hoeksema and Morrow 1991; Nolen-Hoeksema et al. 2008) and thought suppression (Wegner et al. 1987), yet a few studies have been conducted to investigate these two forms of strategies together. In addition, several investigation have been done to demonstrate the role of emotion dysregulation in self-destructive behaviors (Selby 2007), such as nonsuicidal self-injury (e.g., Hasking et al. 2018; Mettler et al. 2023; Ahn and Lee 2024; Cuesta-Zamora et al. 2021; Wang et al. 2018, 2020, 2022), and eating issues (e.g., Kornacka et al. 2021; Rania et al. 2021; Verschueren et al. 2021), and other impulsive disorders (Kaufman et al. 2020; Stevens et al. 2018; Littlefield et al. 2010; Dillahunt et al. 2022). Pursuant to Selby (2007, 2011), Selby et al. (2008, 2009, 2012), Selby and Joiner Jr (2009), a crucial question has often remained unanswered: "*what is the specific nature of relationship between emotional and behavioral dysregulation?*"

Selby and Joiner Jr (2009) and Selby et al. (2008) conceptualized the ECM to elucidate the relationship between emotional and behavioral dysregulation via rumination, because severe rumination may initiate "emotional cascades" which can then contribute to behavioral dysregulation (Selby and Joiner Jr 2009; Selby et al. 2008). Selby et al. (2008) propounded a vicious cycle of rumination and affect (the emotional cascade) contribute to dysregulating behaviors that has a function to distract attention from intense negative emotions (Selby et al. 2008; Pelta 2021). In other words, Selby and Joiner Jr (2009) stated the ECM endeavors to propose a direct connection between emotion dysregulation and behavioral dysregulation in BPD based on a process called "emotional cascade model" (Selby and Joiner Jr 2009). The ECM elucidates the association between intense aversive emotions and dysregulated behaviors via a self-perpetuating cycle of rumination (described in more detail shortly), negative thoughts, and negative emotion (Jungmann et al. 2016; Pelta 2021). Selby et al. (2014a, b, c) elucidates that individual with BPD undergone to experience intense and recurrent negative emotions, which can contribute to subsequent behavioral dysregulation, as a result of emotional cascade (Selby et al. 2014a, b, c). Based on ECM, the reciprocal association between negative emotion and ruminative process can contribute to develop an" emotional cascade," which is generally commenced through an emotion-evoking event. The ruminative process is initiated because of exposure to an emotion-eliciting event and lead to amplifying the intensity of rumination, which contributes to exacerbate the intensity of emotion. In this state, individuals realized that turning attention from intense emotion and negative thoughts due to rumination is an extremely tough task. In turn, a vicious cycle will be shaped between rumination and negative affect, in which the result may be an increasingly and progressively intense, aversive emotional state, which can lead to escaping from experiencing of unpleasant and negative emotional state. In other words, BPD individuals attempt to distract attention from ruminative content and being involved in dysregulated behaviors to relief intense negative affect (see, Selby et al. 2009, 2014a, b, c; Selby and Joiner Jr 2009; Selby 2011; Hasking et al. 2018; Jungmann et al. 2016). Broadly speaking, there is a bidirectionality between emotional cascades and symptoms of BPD (Pelta 2021, p. 363).

To clarify and fully elucidate this model, it is crucial to explain some of the underlying core constructs of this model, including rumination, emotional cascade, dysregulated behavior, and invalidation. We will define these components in detail and in the following, ECM will be explained.

Core Constructs of Emotional Cascade Model

Rumination

A significant construct of ECM is a process named "rumination" (e.g., Martino et al. 2015), which is a form of repetitive thought focused on negative emotions and their reasons and consequences (Nolen-Hoeksema and Morrow 1991). Rumination refers to a continuous and repetitive thinking about signs and symptoms, reasons, and consequences of a negative emotional experience (Nolen-Hoeksema and Morrow 1991; Nolen-Hoeksema et al. 2008; Selby and Joiner Jr 2009). Most individuals utilize rumination to explore answers for personal life stressors and uncertainties, and they are often involved in ruminative thoughts about their distress. These people have a persistent tendency to maintain the belief that rumination will assist them in gaining insight into various aspects of their life (e.g., Rose et al. 2007; Papageorgiou and Wells 2002; Vine and Marroquín 2018; Wisco et al. 2018; Wisco and Harp 2021, 2023), yet some people have a strong tendency to ruminate habitually which may contribute to functional impairments and different manifestations of psychological disorders, such as depression and anxiety (Wisco et al. 2018; Wisco and Harp 2021, 2023; Watkins and Nolen-Hoeksema 2014). Repetitive thinking is recurrent thought about one's self, one's concerns, and one's experiences (see, Eisma et al. 2014a, b; Nolen-Hoeksema et al. 2008; Watkins 2009; Watkins and Roberts 2020). Rumination is a pattern of repetitive, self-focused thought in response to an emotional state (Pont et al. 2018; Thompson 2006), which has a crucial role in human life (Pont et al. 2018). "Rumination refers to repetitive thinking about an upsetting situation or an emotional experience, and about how the present situation relates to past problems or potential future problems" (Nolen-Hoeksema and Morrow 1991). Rumination is triggered in response to negative situations and can be considered as process amplifying negative emotions and can contribute to behavioral dysregulation (e.g., Martino et al. 2013, 2015; Caselli et al. 2013). Rumination comprises thinking repetitively about one's distress, its causes and consequences in a passive and repetitive form, without any attempts at solving a problem (Wisco et al. 2018; Wisco and Harp 2021, 2023; Nolen-Hoeksema et al. 2008).

In other words, rumination may lead an individual to take a passive and repetitive stance, and ignore an active approach to solve problems. This condition perpetuates experiencing of negative emotions, such as depression (Nolen-Hoeksema and Morrow 1991; Nolen-Hoeksema et al. 2008; Wisco and Harp 2021). The content of rumination consists of themes of self-worth and loss (Wisco et al. 2018; Wisco and Harp 2021, 2023), past-oriented subjects (Watkins et al. 2005), and is focused on past losses, which contribute to feeling of sadness and depressive symptoms (Nolen-Hoeksema et al. 2008; Wisco et al. 2018; Wisco and Harp 2021, 2023).

To fully appreciate the experience of rumination, it is essential to know two crucial components regarded as connected to rumination within cognitive behavioral approaches, including *reappraisal* and *problem-solving*, which are adaptive strategies to regulate emotions (e.g., Beck 1979; Cooper et al. 1992). Reappraisal includes producing without bias positive interpretation or perspectives about an event, especially a stressful situation, that contribute to reducing distress (Gross 1998, 2008, 2015). In line with this definition, there are maladaptive reappraisal in depression and anxiety, which may be the focus of psychotherapy in cognitive-behavioral therapies (see, Beck 1979; Beck and Clark 2010; Salkovskis et al. 1999; Beck and Clark 2010). In emotion regulation studies, adaptive reappraisal is a core strategy for those results in positive emotional responses in exposure to emotion-evoked situations (Gross 2015; Aldao et al. 2010, 2013). In contrast, suppression and avoidance are two significant maladaptive responses to stressful life events and are risk factors for psychological disorders especially depression and anxiety and self-destructive behaviors (Crowell et al. 2009; Aldao et al. 2010; Hill 2015; Nolen-Hoeksema and Aldao 2011). Several empirical and clinical investigations have been done to demonstrate the crucial role of suppression and avoidance in the development of psychopathology (Wenzlaff and Wegner 2000; Hill 2015; Franz et al. 2021). For instance, Franz et al. (2021) via utilizing the daily diary method through self-reports of stressful life events and suicidal thoughts suggested that expressive suppression can be an effective short-term emotion regulation strategy among individuals with suicidal behaviors. They found a higher levels of reappraisal, a lesser relationship between stress and suicidal thoughts, a higher level of expressive suppression, and a weaker association between stress and suicidal thoughts (Franz et al. 2021). Some individuals repetitively focus on their experience of emotion and its causes and consequences, or they become engaged in rumination, instead of avoiding or suppressing negative thoughts and mood (Aldao et al. 2010, 2013; Nolen-Hoeksema et al. 2008; Rusting and Nolen-Hoeksema 1998). According to core negative affect or thought arousing the repetitive thoughts, several investigations have identified different types of rumination, including depressive, grief, hostile, and angry ruminations (Zielinski et al. 2017; Papageorgiou and Wells 2004; Sukhodolsky et al. 2001; Eisma et al. 2014a, b). Across all of these types, rumination contributes to escalating negative emotions and thoughts, depression, anxiety, disturbed problem solving and making decision skills, and dysregulated and disinhibited behaviors (Zielinski et al. 2017; Nolen-Hoeksema et al. 2008).

As noted, rumination is the inclination to dwell on unpleasant thoughts and is exhibited on individual's negative affect and behaviors and the effects of one's depression (Nolen-Hoeksema 2001), and it is utilized as an emotion regulation strategy to exasperate depressive symptoms in adults and youth (Nolen-Hoeksema et al. 1994; Abela et al. 2002). Rumination most often begins in early adolescence because of the development of cognitive functions and escalated exposure to stressful life events (Buelens et al. 2019; Davey et al. 2008; Jose and Brown 2008). Vine and Marroquín (2018) indicated individuals rate themselves more insightful after experiencing rumination about a neutral subject, instead trying to distract themselves (Lyubomirsky and Nolen-Hoeksema 1993; Vine and Marroquín 2018). According to these finding, they suggested that experiencing of rumination may be similar to a process of achieving insight and a broader viewpoint to problems (Vine and Marroquín 2018). Several studies have illustrated that individuals tend to ruminate as a strategy to make sense of uncertainty about the future (e.g., Liao and Wei 2011; de Jong-Meyer et al. 2009), besides as a strategy for determining to resolve any inconsistency between current and ideal states while following their goals (Vine and Marroquín 2018; Watkins 2009; Watkins and Roberts 2020). Vine and Marroquín (2018) examined the utilization of rumination in association with the task of making sense of an uncertain state which is specifically related to the function of emotion regulation. They found that their study supports the point that sometimes rumination serves as a way of inspecting potential answers about emotional triggers. Furthermore, they debated implications for understanding the emotional issues perpetuating vicious cycles of rumination (Vine and Marroquín 2018).

Rumination has been investigated frequently in association with depression and sadness (e.g., Nolen-Hoeksema et al. 2008; Watkins 2009; Watkins and Roberts 2020; Wisco and Harp 2021). In other words, a wide range of studies about rumination is restricted to depressive rumination, anger rumination, stress reactive, and ruminative issues in interpersonal relationship (e.g., Peters et al. 2017; Ciesla et al. 2011a, b; Borders et al. 2010). Rumination is outstandingly correlated to negative cognitive style (Krahé et al. 2019), and this negative cognitive style modulate the association between rumination and symptoms of depression (Wisco and Harp 2021). Furthermore, investigations have shown rumination can be noticed as a mechanism through which interpretation biases and symptoms of depression are related to each other (Wisco and Harp 2021), as well as rumination mediates the association between these interpretation biases and depression symptoms (Everaert et al. 2017; Wisco et al. 2018, 2023; Wisco and Harp 2021). However, via a longitudinal investigation, Wisco and Harp (2021) examined rumination as a mechanism of the association between interpretation biases and depression symptoms, their results indicated antithetical findings that cognitive biases contribute to depression symptoms through rumination; therefore, based on these findings, more studies are needed to work on this complex interplay between cognitive biases, rumination, and depression (Wisco and Harp 2021).

Response style theory (Nolen-Hoeksema 2004) proposes an additional focus on what is termed *depressive rumination*, defining it as repetitive thinking about symptoms, causes, meanings, and consequences. Indeed, rumination in the context of experiencing stress seems to interfere with effective and functional problem-solving skills, as well as may forbid from making decision (Aldao et al. 2010; Ward et al.

2003; Wisco et al. 2018, 2023; Wisco and Harp 2021). Despite increasing negative thoughts during rumination, it should be considered that rumination is not defined just based on the content of thoughts, rather rumination should be regarded according to its repetitive and passive nature (Nolen-Hoeksema and Morrow 1991). *Self-focused rumination* is defined as an individual's attention and concentration on the negative emotion, and its causes and effects, besides self-evaluations associated with mood (Nolen-Hoeksema et al. 2008). On the contrary, *distraction* includes focusing attention away from the negative emotion via being involved in pleasant or neutral activities to thwart the mind from wondering the origin of negative emotion (Nolen-Hoeksema and Morrow 1991). This means distraction involves centering attention on nonemotional aspects of situation (Sheppes et al. 2011; Van Dillen and Koole 2007), or something completely different (Sauer et al. 2016). Sheppes et al. (2011, 2014) demonstrated that distraction was opposite to reappraisal in situations of high contrast low negative intensity. To clarify, stimuli with high and low intensity may be regulated before processing of emotional information. Yet, reappraisal can merely regulate the low-intensive information, whilst high-intensive information needs more cognitive resources (Sheppes et al. 2011, 2014; Sheppes and Meiran 2007, 2008). Moreover, through a systematic review and meta-analysis, Cano-López et al. (2021) proposed the development of rumination and its relations with depression is to some extent relies on metacognitive beliefs, based on metacognitive model of rumination and depression. Correspondent with the metacognitive model, based on the self-regulatory executive function (S-REF, Wells 2019; Wells and Matthews 1996), infers activation and retention of rumination, and its relation with depression, relies on metacognitive beliefs. Metacognitive beliefs attribute to this point that people have constant beliefs about their own cognitive system, which impress the control, monitoring, and appraisal of cognitions. Two metacognitive beliefs about rumination include positive beliefs (the utility of rumination) and negative beliefs (the uncontrollability and danger of rumination, and its negative interpersonal and social outcomes). Positive beliefs are triggered and being active in response to a negative mood or thought, contribute to utilizing rumination by an individual. It is assumed that rumination prevails the aversive negative situation and allows one to recognize and solve the problem. Yet, rumination is not always an adaptive strategy, instead it leads to intensified negative thoughts and exacerbates the negative emotion. Consequently, negative metacognitive beliefs relevant to the uncontrollability and danger of rumination and its aversive social and relational results appear, which contribute to appraising rumination as controllable and harmful thoughts, raising the accessibility of negative thoughts and emotions, and hence, boosting depressive signs and symptoms. In line with this perspective, metacognitive beliefs are causal factors in anticipating rumination and depression (Wells 2019; Michael et al. 2007; Papageorgiou and Wells 2003). In other words, Cano-López et al. (2021) concluded that metacognitive beliefs are associated factors in realizing the reasons for ruminating and getting depressed, consistent with the metacognitive model rumination and depression (Cano-López et al. 2021).

In building on this prior work on rumination, Selby et al. (2009) consider rumination as a potential construct that can afford a broader insight into understanding why individuals with BPD have a tendency to employ dysregulated behaviors in the case of exposure to unpleasant emotional state (Selby et al. 2009; Selby and Joiner Jr 2013). Rumination is defined as "the process of redirecting attention to causes and consequences of negative emotional response (Koster et al. 2013), which often has the effect of prolonging or maintaining the emotion (Young and Nolen-Hoeksema 2001)" (McRae and Zarolia 2020, p. 41; Beauchaine and Crowell 2020). Rumination is a form of repetitive thinking that redirect the person's attention to emotion-elicit stimuli (e.g., Nolen-Hoeksema and Morrow 1991; Jacobs et al. 2016), and can intensify negative emotions (Pelta 2021). Selby et al. (2009) suggest that rumination may be regarded as a process that leads to magnified sensitivity, heightened intensity, and prolonged duration of emotion in individual with BPD (Selby et al. 2009). Rumination is one of the most common forms of thinking process in individuals with BPD (Pelta 2021) and predicts several forms of behavioral dysregulation (Selby et al. 2009). Rumination is considered as a cognitive symptom associated to negative emotional states and is exhibited as a way of bypassing a difficulty and distressful situation and possible negative consequences, as opposed to deriving a solution (Nolan et al. 1998; Dell'Osso et al. 2019). Jungmann et al. (2016) considered intrusion as a mediator between rumination and dysregulated behavior and tested the ECM in 414 cases who suffer from OCD. Based on findings, it was concluded that intrusions strongly mediate the effect of rumination on behavioral dysregulation and compulsions. Furthermore, it was revealed that rumination may provoke intrusions, and in turn exacerbate dysregulated behaviors (Jungmann et al. 2016). According to the emotional cascade theory (Selby and Joiner Jr 2009), ruminative processes contribute to a vicious cycle resulting an intensive and severe aversive state of escalated negative emotion, which then requires potent and noticeable forms of distraction, such as dysregulated behaviors like binge eating, suicide, self-injury, and substance use (Selby and Joiner Jr 2009, 2013; Selby et al. 2009).

A wealth of data has shown that rumination is related to a host of negative consequences (Lyubomirsky et al. 2015; Pont et al. 2018), for instance, maladaptive coping styles, like negative attribution styles, hopelessness, pessimism, self-criticism, neediness, excessive investment in interpersonal relationship, neuroticism, and can predict depression (Lyubomirsky et al. 2015; Ciesla and Roberts 2002; Nolen-Hoeksema and Morrow 1993; Nolen-Hoeksema et al. 2008; Nolen-Hoeksema and Jackson 2001; Lyubomirsky and Nolen-Hoeksema 1995; Nolen-Hoeksema and Davis 1999; Spasojević and Alloy 2001). Furthermore, intensified rumination may contribute heightened anger and sadness (Thompson 2006), sleep issues (Thomsen et al. 2005; Selby et al. 2013), depressive disorder (Nolen-Hoeksema et al. 2007, 2008; Wisco and Harp 2021; Wisco et al. 2018, 2023), anxiety symptoms (Calmes and Roberts 2007), dysregulated behaviors and compulsions (Selby et al. 2008; Selby and Joiner Jr 2009, 2013; Jungmann et al. 2016), nonsuicidal self-injury (Hasking et al. 2018; Selby et al. 2010; Selby 2011, 2013a, b, c; Anestis and Selby 2015; Gardner et al. 2014; Hatzopoulos et al. 2022; Hilt et al. 2017; Tonta et al. 2022), internalizing and externalizing problems (Pont et al. 2018), suicidal ideation (Tucker et al. 2016; Joiner et al. 2007), eating behaviors (Selby et al. 2010; Kornacka et al. 2021; Arbuthnott et al. 2014), impulsive behaviors

(Selby et al. 2016), and BPD (Selby et al. 2008, 2010; Selby 2011, 2013a, b, c, 2016, 2020; Selby and Joiner Jr 2009, 2013).

A growing body of research is based on experimental investigation, which has been done through inducing rumination in participants to demonstrate its effects on depressed moods (see, Watkins 2009; Watkins and Roberts 2020; Nolen-Hoeksema and Morrow 1993, Nolen-Hoeksema et al. 2008; Wisco and Harp 2021). According to ongoing research, rumination can worsen negative emotions due to facilitating recall of negative events (e.g., Buelens et al. 2019). Rumination exacerbates negative mood-congruent thinking, interfere with problem solving, and instrumental behavior (Nolen-Hoeksema 2012). For instance, through inducing rumination, during thinking about past, present, and future, it has been demonstrated that dysphoric patients reported more focus on negative memories and more reports of experiencing negative events in their life in comparison with nondysphoric individuals (Lyubomirsky et al. 1998; McFarland and Buehler 1998). Moreover, there is typically greater focus on current issues, such as conflicts with others, and higher self-blaming and pessimistic about resolving these problems (Lyubomirsky and Nolen-Hoeksema 1995; Greenberg et al. 1995). In contrast, there is less focus on solutions for their interpersonal conflicts (Lyubomirsky and Nolen-Hoeksema 1995; Watkins and Moulds 2005), and less eager to participate in pleasant distracting activities (Lyubomirsky and Nolen-Hoeksema 1995). Additionally, dysphoric patients indicated higher levels of pessimism and lesser optimism with lower expectation to occur positive events for them in future (Lyubomirsky and Nolen-Hoeksema 1995). Rumination is proposed as a cognitive coping mechanism as well as regulates emotions in individuals with BPD (Gross 1998, 2015). Rumination with negative contents can intensify emotional distress (Sansone and Sansone 2012), and during rumination, negative emotion is amplified, as well as, the focus of attention may be directed to negative emotion, which results in emotional distress (Hill 2015), and rumination maintains and intensifies negative emotions such as depression (Brinker and Dozois 2009; Nolen-Hoeksema et al. 2008). Research has also considered rumination as a form of intrusions which may promote psychotherapeutic interventions for psychological matters via dysregulated behaviors and severe negative emotional states (Jungmann et al. 2016). According to Pelta (2021), there are different kinds of rumination, including pain rumination which is more frequent in BPD (Sansone et al. 2013), depressive rumination (Papageorgiou and Wells 2004; Baer and Sauer 2011), and anger rumination (Sauer-Zavala et al. 2013; Law et al. 2021). Through an empirical investigation examining the emotion regulation style and daily rumination, Zuzama et al. (2020) explored negative emotion regulation style and rumination as a mediator of the association between negative affect and depression, rather than merely utilizing rumination mediate the relationship between positive affect and depression. Furthermore, anxiety aggregation occurs due to negative affect, yet emotion regulation style does not significantly mediate this association. It can be concluded that both rumination use and negative emotion regulation style can mediate the relationship between negative affect and depression. In other words, rumination use has no effect on anxiety, while negative affect has a significant direct effect on anxiety (Zuzama et al. 2020).

Cognitive studies have revealed rumination may lead to intrusive thoughts (e.g., Santa Maria et al. 2012), consequently these unwanted negative thoughts may contribute to dysregulated behaviors, such as avoidance in posttraumatic stress disorder (PTSD) (Bryant et al. 2021; Michael et al. 2007), or being engaged in self-destructive behaviors (Selby and Joiner Jr 2013). Moreover, rumination may cause a general deficit in individual's competency for shifting from dysfunctional to functional strategies to accomplish a task, as well as is associated with biases in information processing, and a powerful propensity to be involved and remember negative information instead of attention to positive data (Nolen-Hoeksema et al. 2008). For instance, it has been revealed depressed ruminators display biases towards negative information in a task of basic attention and implicit memory, and more difficulties in inhibiting irrelevant negative information (Joormann and Tran 2009; Joormann et al. 2006; Siegle et al. 2002). Furthermore, studies have demonstrated ruminative response style are related to impulsive behaviors such as nonsuicidal self-injury (Hilt et al. 2017), binge eating and drinking (Nolen-Hoeksema et al. 2007, 2008; Nolen-Hoeksema and Harrell 2002). Trauma-related rumination have been proposed as a factor to perpetuate PTSD (e.g., Bryant et al. 2021). Ehring and Ehlers (2014) attempted to reveal that rumination mediate the relationship between emotion regulation ability among PTSD cases. In line with relationship between emotion regulation and PTSD, they concluded that low emotion regulation ability was significantly associated with PTSD symptom severity concurrently at 2 weeks post trauma, as well as 3- and 6-months posttrauma. Furthermore, consistent with the association between emotion regulation ability and rumination, they found considerable negative correlations between trauma-related rumination. Moreover, they showed that the relationship between low emotion regulation ability and PTSD was mediated by rumination (Ehring and Ehlers 2014). Several recent studies have demonstrated rumination is a strong predictor of persistent PTSD. Michael et al. (2007) revealed rumination both is utilized as a strategy to adapt with intrusive memories, and as a trigger for these memories. Rumination contributes to unproductive intrusive thoughts, is made up of "why" and "what if" questions, and higher levels of experiencing negative affects before and after rumination, were noticeably relevant to PTSD (Michael et al. 2007).

Rumination has also been found to be a risk factor for mood, anxiety, substance use, eating problems (e.g., Nolen-Hoeksema and Watkins 2011; Nolen-Hoeksema et al. 2007, 2008; Nolen-Hoeksema and Harrell 2002; Selby et al. 2008; Selby and Joiner Jr 2009, 2013). In a review about rumination done by Lyubomirsky et al. (2015) based on Nolen-Hoeksema's studies, they concluded rumination has a key role in maintaining, perpetuating, and exasperating depression (see, Nolen-Hoeksema and Morrow 1991; Nolen-Hoeksema et al. 2008), increasing the effects of depressed mood on negative thinking (see, Lyubomirsky and Nolen-Hoeksema 1993, 1995), interposing with efficient problem solving and instrumental behavior (see, Lyubomirsky and Nolen-Hoeksema 1993; Lyubomirsky et al. 1999, 2011, 2006a; Papageorgiou and Wells 2001, 2003), and declining social support (Nolen-Hoeksema and Davis 1999; Nolen-Hoeksema and Jackson 2001; McLaughlin and Nolen-Hoeksema 2012). Rumination amplifies both depression and the mechanisms that contribute to depression. Also, rumination intensifies a bidirectional circuit between negative mood and negative intrusive thoughts, lead to increasing emotional reactivity to unpleasant events. Moreover, rumination disrupts problem solving via leading an individual to contemplate more pessimistically and fatalistically. Since social support is dampened by rumination through providing adverse situations, rumination contributes to being rejected in any kind of potential helpmates. Finally, as mentioned, rumination interferes with instrumental behaviors which can lead a person to be unable in acting sufficiently, despite having potential capacity to behave effectively (Nolen-Hoeksema et al. 1999; Lyubomirsky et al. 2015). Furthermore, in anxious individuals, rumination can aggregate their anxiety, because rumination interposes with problem solving and instrumental behaviors which contributed to behavioral avoidance. In addition, rumination may lead to perceiving environmental stressors as threatening, such as prominent social threats contributing to social phobia, or in the case of an uncontrollable and unpredictable trauma, PTSD can be produced, as well as because of biological predisposition, such as dysfunctional fight-or-flight response, a heightened probability of rumination lead to panic attack may be occurred (Nolen-Hoeksema and Watkins 2011; Lyubomirsky et al. 2015; Michael et al. 2007).

In line with several studies, it has been documented that rumination is regarded as a maladaptive emotion regulation strategy, as well as, avoidance (Wenzlaff and Wegner 2000), concealing and suppression of expressions (e.g., Gross 1998, 2008, 2015; Nolen-Hoeksema et al. 2008), and worry (see, Nolen-Hoeksema and Aldao 2011; Lyubomirsky et al. 2015; Aldao and Nolen-Hoeksema 2012; Aldao et al. 2010; Hoyer et al. 2009). As mentioned by Aldao et al. (2010), there are three widely theorized adaptive emotion regulation strategies, including reappraisal, problem solving, and acceptance. Three strategies have been debated due their roles as risk factors for psychopathology consist with suppression (both expressive and thought suppression), avoidance (both experiential and behavioral avoidance), and rumination (Aldao et al. 2010). Miranda et al. (2013) found out that rumination and hopelessness mediate the association between emotion dysregulation and suicidal ideation. This means that perceived inability to utilize emotion regulation strategies may exacerbate vulnerability to suicidal thoughts via its consequences on rumination and hopelessness (Miranda et al. 2013). Gross's emotion regulation model (1998) includes antecedent-focused and response-focused emotion regulation strategies. In an antecedent-focused emotion regulation strategy, such as reappraisal, the focus is on moderating probability or experiencing a stressful event, to barricade or decline the amount of experienced distress. The main outcome in a response-focused emotion regulation strategy, like suppression, is to modulate an individual's emotional response to stressors once they have taken place (Gross 1998, 2015; Gross and Thompson 2007). In line with Nolen-Hoeksema et al. (2008), experimental investigations have revealed that rumination is related to a partially fragile problem-solving orientation, impaired problem solving, and more negative reappraisals of situations. Rumination has a significant positive correlation with suppression and avoidance of intensive distressful emotions and thoughts (e.g., Nolen-Hoeksema et al. 2008; Moulds et al. 2007). Individuals who ruminate attempt to search a way to get rid of aversive self-focused through suppressing negative emotions and thoughts cognitively or try to avoid self-awareness via engaging in different behaviors. Nolen-Hoeksema et al. (2008) demonstrated these endeavors to suppress or avoid ruminative thoughts intercede the association between rumination and binge eating, binge drinking, and self-inflicted behaviors (e.g., Nolen-Hoeksema et al. 2007, 2008; Selby et al. 2009, 2020; Miranda and Nolen-Hoeksema 2007). It has been indicated that inhibition and shifting data originated from neutral and computerized tasks, and questions data on emotion regulation and trait rumination in depressed and never-depressed women showed that depressed women whose executive function was intact were characterized via ruminative inclinations and more frequent utilize of expressive suppression. Moreover, trait rumination and expressive suppression were unrelated to executive functions in depressed women (Aker et al. 2014).

Based on Buelens et al. (2019, 2020), recent models have added cognitive constructs to dysregulated behaviors. In other words, rumination is associated with self-destructive and self-inflicted behaviors (Lyubomirsky et al. 2015; Selby et al. 2008, 2014a, b, c; Jungmann et al. 2016), such as NSSI (Hilt et al. 2017), reckless behaviors, like substance use and dangerous driving (Nolen-Hoeksema et al. 1999; Lyubomirsky et al. 2015). Selby et al. (2008) suggested that rumination is a cognitive element in developing behavioral dysregulation (Selby et al. 2008, 2014a, b, c, 2020; Buelens et al. 2019, 2020; Selby and Joiner Jr 2013).

Recent investigations have provided evidence to support some relationships between rumination, especially angry rumination, and borderline personality features (e.g., Smith et al. 2006; Selby et al. 2008, 2014a, b, c, 2020; Selby and Joiner Jr 2009, 2013; Hasking et al. 2017; Arbuthnott et al. 2014; Ramos-Cejudo et al. 2017). Angry rumination, as well as, depressive rumination may anticipate a wide range of borderline diagnostic features, such as aggression (Baer and Sauer 2011; Anestis et al. 2009; García-Sancho et al. 2016; White and Turner 2014), hostility (Anestis et al. 2009), anger experiences (Anestis et al. 2009), high levels of arousal (Pedersen et al. 2011), and decreasing the ability to manage anger and displace it with an aggressive behavior (García-Sancho et al. 2016; Ramos-Cejudo et al. 2017). Documented findings have revealed that anger rumination can significantly predict aggression proneness, and both BPD diagnosis and anger rumination are significant predictors of aggression susceptibility (Martino et al. 2015). Indeed, Selby et al. (2009) have shown angry rumination has a higher significant association with borderline features in comparison with depressive rumination. Gardner and Moore (2008) theorized that hostile rumination is associated with anger and is related to the emotion dysregulation characteristics of BPD (Gardner and Moore 2008; Zielinski et al. 2017). Selby et al. (2008) indicated that rumination is meaningfully related to binge eating, alcohol use, and social reassurance seeking in BPD and non-BPD groups. In addition, they posited rumination has an association with urgency (a desire to behave impulsively in the case of experiencing negative emotion) in both BPD and non-BPD cases. Selby et al. (2008) concluded these findings can show that ECM may be relevant to other types of behavioral dysregulations (Selby et al. 2008; Jungmann et al. 2016). DeShong et al. (2019) proposed dysregulated behaviors may be linked to rumination in BPD. Through an investigation about precursors of the ECM of BPD, they found neuroticism, childhood emotional vulnerability, and parental invalidation have significant roles in predicting rumination (DeShong et al. 2019). Among individuals with a biological predisposition, rumination can be led to substance and alcohol use to aggravate the negative moods caused by overthinking (Nolen-Hoeksema 2005), and in the case of environmental stressors, rumination is related to a great level of alcohol and substance use (Nolen-Hoeksema and Harrell 2002; Lyubomirsky et al. 2015). Furthermore, a ruminative response style is considered as a risk factor leading to eating problems, such as bulimic symptoms, comprising cycles of binge eating followed by a complex of efforts to purge the food consumed, like purging, via vomiting or taking laxatives. Selby et al. (2008) pointed out that an emotional cascade exists, whereby rumination amplifies negative affect, creating a strong urge in individual to binge eat (Selby et al. 2008). Various studies have demonstrated that rumination may be frequent in BPD, for instance, the association between rumination and neuroticism as a personality trait (e.g., Wupperman and Neumann 2006), negative emotional may be intensified by emotion contributed to behavioral dysregulation such as binge eating problems and self-inflicted injurious behaviors (Selby et al. 2008, 2009, 2013a, b, c, 2016, 2020; Selby and Joiner Jr 2009; Nolen-Hoeksema et al. 2007, 2008). Negative emotion is intensified through ruminative processes, which a BPD individual misinterprets this process as an insight into different problems. Hence, a great tendency toward utilizing rumination as a problem-solving strategy in BPD cases which may contribute to consider as a predictor of BPD (Baer and Sauer 2011). In terms of theoretical perspective, the ECM (Selby 2008) is consistent with this view. In other words, rumination can predict BPD traits, in which an individual with BPD has a high tendency to focus attention on interpersonal issues and negative emotions (Hill 2015; Baer et al. 2012).

Dysregulated Behavior

One of the core features of BPD is behavioral dysregulation, a broad range of behaviors that are difficult to control and detrimental for the individual (Selby et al. 2010). Selby et al. (2010) have indicated an association between BPD and alcohol misuse, substance use, hitting someone/breaking things, provoking fights/arguments, self-injury behaviors, overdosing, binge eating, impulsive spending, shoplifting/stealing, and risky sexual behaviors (Selby et al. 2010). Dysregulated behavior was presented by Selby and Joiner Jr (2009) in the ECM (Bresin 2020). Consistent with Selby et al. (2014a, b, c) "A dysregulated, or disinhibited behavior is engaged in by an individual that results in harmful consequences to that individual" (Selby et al. 2008, 2014a, b, c, p. 159). In line with Bresin (2020), dysregulated behaviors are defined as active behaviors with short-term advantages yet entail drastic recurrent long-term distress or impairment to the individual and/or those around them, including behaviors such as suicidal and nonsuicidal self-injury, aggression, impulsivity, and substance use (Bresin 2020). Dysregulated behaviors are overt behaviors that reciprocally interact with internal emotional experiences (Selby et al. 2014a, b, c). Behavioral dysregulation is assumed as a utilization of maladaptive behaviors recruited an individual to avoid, escape, or regulate distress, despite having potentially destructive consequences (Seah and Coifman 2022). Dysregulated behaviors are supposed to be a kind of behavioral avoidance. According to the point that dysregulated behaviors are overt actions, such as drinking alcohol and substance use, dysregulated behaviors can be differentiated from other forms of behavioral avoidance (Bresin 2020; Bresin and Mekawi 2022). Furthermore, Bresin (2020) provided four boundary conditions for dysregulated behaviors: (1) dysregulated behaviors and compulsive behaviors are different from each other, (2) dysregulated behaviors vary from sensation seeking behaviors, (3) dysregulated behaviors are a part of a larger group named behavioral avoidance, and (4) dysregulated behaviors are a subset of impulsive behaviors (Bresin and Mekawi 2022).

As mentioned, dysregulated behaviors comprise behaviors that are delicate to control and eventuate to functional disturbances in affected individuals (Selby and Joiner Jr 2009; Selby et al. 2010; Selby and Gardner 2015). Dysregulated behaviors, such as self-inflicted injuries, alcohol and substance use, binge eating and impulsivity, occur frequently and are composed of serious negative costs for individuals and society (Bresin and Mekawi 2022). Behavioral dysregulation refers to harmful and insufficient emotion regulation strategies, such as dysregulated behaviors and compulsions (Selby et al. 2008; Selby and Joiner Jr 2009, 2013; Jungmann et al. 2016), nonsuicidal self-injury (Hasking et al. 2018; Selby et al. 2010; Selby 2011, 2013a, b, c; Anestis and Selby 2015), internalizing and externalizing problems (Pont et al. 2018), suicidal behaviors (Tucker et al. 2016; Joiner et al. 2007), eating behaviors (Selby et al. 2010; Kornacka et al. 2021; Arbuthnott et al. 2014; Selby and Gardner 2015), impulsive behaviors (Selby et al. 2016), and extreme social reassurance seeking, self-inflicted behaviors (Jungmann et al. 2016; Selby and Gardner 2015).

Impulsivity, disinhibition, and hyperactivity are terms to define the impaired and insufficient control over behaviors (Neuhaus and Beauchaine 2017). *Nonsuicidal self-injury* (NSSI) refers to the deliberate and direct destruction or injury of body tissue with no intention for death, which are not socially sanctioned (Hasking et al. 2019; Glenn and Klonsky 2010; Whitlock et al. 2014; Selby and Gardner 2015). *Self-inflicted injury* (SII) is any behaviors of self-injury with the intention of causing bodily harm or death, such as NSSI, suicide attempt, and suicide (Crowell et al. 2014). *Self-injury behaviors* (SIB) or parasuicidal behaviors are described as deliberate and direct destruction of body tissues with or without intention for suicide (Gratz et al. 2017, 2019, 2022; Linehan 1993). Consistent with several studies, a positive association has been indicated between individual's dysregulated behaviors and impulsive traits (e.g., Bresin 2020; Bresin and Mekawi 2022; Berg et al. 2015), for instance, acting out with no delay in the face of negative emotion or negative urgency (Bresin and Mekawi 2022). Moreover, sensitivity to reward plays a substantial role in developing dysregulated behaviors (e.g., Carver and Harmon-Jones 2009), as well as a significant connection between some dysregulated behaviors and sensitivity to reward (e.g., Sadeh and Baskin-Sommers 2017). Furthermore, Selby and Joiner Jr (2009) proposed that individuals employ dysregulated behaviors to avoid, escape, or cope with turbulent intense emotions that are assumed to be out of control. It can be deduced that emotion dysregulation contributes to several forms of dysregulated behaviors, such as substance use (e.g., McHugh and Goodman 2019), broad types of psychopathologies (e.g., Cludius et al. 2020), self-injury and suicidal behaviors (Haywood et al. 2023; Selby et al. 2014a, b, c, 2016), and impulsive behaviors (e.g., Lynam et al. 2011; Selby and Joiner 2013).

Invalidation

Invalidating environments are another major factor that can influence emotional cascades. "Invalidation is the perception and actual experience of pervasive criticizing or trivializing of one's communication of internal experiences by others, as well as repeatedly being punished for appropriate emotional expression" (Linehan 1993; Selby et al. 2014a, b, c, p. 159). In invalidating environments, emotional experiences are often trivialized or disregard, any kind of displaying of negative affect will be punished, with a harsh control under any emotional expressiveness (Linehan 1993). Such scenarios frequently serve as fuel for ruminative experiences, many of which can become amplified into an emotional cascade.

Emotional Cascade Theory

Up to this point, emotional cascades have been described primarily in terms of momentary events that lead to intense negative emotional states which frequently are terminated or reduced by dysregulated behaviors. However, beyond this the ECM (Selby et al. 2008; Selby and Joiner Jr 2009) has provided an even more expansive model describing the reciprocation between intense negative emotions and dysregulated behaviors (Selby et al. 2020; Selby and Joiner Jr 2009), leading to various negative consequences and several psychopathology outcomes, including BPD (e.g., Gardner et al. 2014; Selby and Joiner Jr 2009, 2013; Selby et al. 2014a, b, c, 2016, 2020). The ECM proposes that the emotional turbulence and chaotic maladaptive behaviors in BPD may be related to rumination (DeShong et al. 2019). Individuals with BPD display a wide range of dysregulated behaviors, from interpersonal disputes in their relationships to life-threatening behaviors, such as NSSI and suicidal attempts (Selby et al. 2009). According to DSM-5-TR (2022), being engaged in different dysregulated behaviors is stressed as a major diagnostic criterion in individuals with BPD, such as involving in self-injury and suicidal behaviors, as well as, other emotion-elicited behaviors, like impulsivity and reckless, and other dysregulated behaviors (DSM-5-TR, APA 2022). Based on Selby and Joiner (2013), plenty of dysregulated behaviors have been manifested to have emotion regulating qualities, with different motivations for various behaviors, as well as, pursuant to individuals' reports, these behaviors are utilized to dampen or avoid the experience of negative emotions (Selby and Joiner 2013). Emotion dysregulation may lead to an inability to manage and control the emotion-dependent behaviors, or creating problems which contribute to engaging in goal-directed behaviors whilst experiencing distress (Dixon-Gordon et al. 2020). A growing body of investigation about emotion regulation strategies frequently have indicated that individual with BPD features show considerable difficulties in coping and response skillfully to distress situations, which lead to dysregulated behaviors in order to avoid or escape from experiencing intense negative emotions (e.g., Dixon-Gordon et al. 2011, 2018, 2020; Chapman et al. 2005, 2010, 2017; Gratz et al. 2014, 2017, 2019, 2022; Selby and Joiner Jr 2009, 2013; Selby et al. 2014a, b, c, 2016, 2020). For instance, it has been revealed that individuals with BPD engage in more impulsive behaviors after being induced fear in comparison to individuals with low BPD features (Chapman et al. 2010). Similarly, BPD is associated with dampening of willingness to endure emotional distress to follow goal-directed behaviors (Dixon-Gordon et al. 2020, 2024).

One of the most noticeable issues in the field of BPD research is attempting to understanding how dysregulated behaviors are developed and shaped over time. A growing body of studies have focused on elucidating various risk factors related to the development of dysregulated behaviors in BPD, such as biosocial theory (Linehan 1993), which explains BPD and dysregulated behaviors due to poor emotional recognition, and disturbed emotion regulation; developmental biosocial theory (Crowell et al. 2009; Crowell et al. 2014, 2022), which focuses on the role of emotion dysregulation and impulsivity in creating BPD symptoms; and emotion dysregulation (Gratz et al. 2014, 2017, 2019, 2022; Glenn and Klonsky 2005), which emphasizes on emotion dysregulation as a core risk factor to cause dysregulated behaviors. For instance, suicide is a dangerous, life-threatening behaviors, considered as a behavior opposed to life desire in people, yet paradoxically, a person who attempts suicide may do so specifically to escape from psychological pain (Selby et al. 2014a, b, c). Aiming at an overview of theories about suicide, Selby et al. (2014b) summarized theories of suicide composing of *biological theories, Sociological theory* (Day 1987), *Hopelessness theory* (Beck et al. 1989, 1993), *Psychache theory* (Shneidman 1998), *Escape theory* (Baumeister 1990), *Emotion Dysregulation theory* (Linehan 1993), and *interpersonal psychological theory* (Joiner 2005). The remarkably common point among many of these theories which is achieved through an overview is experiencing intensely aversive negative emotions before attempting suicide, and it seems suicidal attempts are a way to escape or avoid or be released from these intense emotions. In other words, Selby et al. (2014a, b, c) stated although each of these theories have their own unique viewpoints about factors contributed to recognize the motivations for and various forms of suicide, many of them have identical presupposes (Selby et al. 2014b). Based on Bresin and Mekawi (2022), studies have indicated notable shared variance across these dysregulated behaviors, as well as substantial overlap in different theories which provide explanations about the genesis of these behaviors (e.g., Sadeh and Baskin-Sommers 2017; Guo et al. 2017; Selby and Joiner Jr 2009).

Likewise, in their work on emotional cascades, Selby et al. (2014a, b, c) encapsulated functional models and theories of NSSI, including biological theories, social functions, psychodynamic theories (Carroll 1980), antisuicide model (Suyemoto 1998), affect regulation theories (Nock and Prinstein 2004; Nock et al. 2006), self-punishment hypothesis (Klonsky 2007), antidissociation theory (Gunderson 1984; Simpson 1994), feeling generation theory, experiential avoidance model (EAM, Chapman et al. 2005, 2006, 2017), and ECM (Selby et al. 2008; Selby and Joiner Jr 2009). In addition, elevated emotional and interpersonal distress (Klonsky et al. 2003; Klonsky and Muehlenkamp 2007; Klonsky and Olino 2008) elucidates why people tend to be involved in NSSI. Correspondingly, with a detailed and general overview, it can be found that the role of experiencing intense negative emotions which contribute to avoid or escape from these unpleasant emotions and as a reward engaging in NSSI. In other words, Selby et al. (2014a, b, c) posited that despite a wide array of theories of NSSI, which have their own terms and explanations, the question about why people engage in NSSI are unanswered and more investigations and experimental conceptualizations are needed (Selby et al. 2014a, b, c; Selby and Gardner 2015). Bresin and Mekawi (2022), through an investigation to distinguish core constructs of dysregulated behaviors, indicated no significant association between compulsive behaviors and dysregulated behaviors. Whereas strong and consistent evidence for impulsigenic manifestations across dysregulated behaviors was found, as well as, inconsistent evidence for correlation with reward sensitivity and emotion dysregulation. Furthermore, based on person-centered analysis, they demonstrated three groups that are specified by high dysregulated behavior, low dysregulated behavior, and aggressive self-harm behavior. They asserted being classified in these groups is different in line with impulsigenic traits and emotion dysregulation (Bresin and Mekawi 2022).

As mentioned, in line with Linehan's biosocial theory (1993), the core feature of BPD is emotion dysregulation, which caused through the transaction of invalidating environment and a biological-based emotional vulnerability. Emotion dysregulation can contribute to engaging in impulsive short-term emotion regulation strategies to cope with unpleasant negative emotions, such impulsive behaviors, self-inflicted injuries and binge eating (Linehan 1993). The most critical point in this process, which perpetuates dysregulated behaviors, is avoidance. Avoidance is used to reduce or escape from aversive negative emotions which leads to engaging in dysregulated behaviors (e.g., Selby et al. 2008, 2014a, b, c, 2016; Selby and Joiner Jr 2009, 2013; Chapman et al. 2005, 2017). Experiential avoidance and behaviors aimed to avoid or escape from negative emotions, thoughts and sensations, and have a crucial role in generating dysregulated behaviors (e.g., Hayes et al. 1996; Linehan 1993; Crowell et al. 2009, 2017). A wealth body of studies have documented that individuals with BPD diagnosis and BPD traits have a great tendency to avoid any experiences of unwanted, aversive, and negative emotions, constituting emotional avoidance and engaging in dysregulated behaviors, rather utilizing more effective alternatives regulating strategies (e.g., Chapman et al. 2005, 2017; Rosenthal et al. 2005; Aldao and Dixon-Gordon 2014; Crowell et al. 2014; Selby et al. 2008, 2014a, b, c, 2016, 2020; Selby and Joiner Jr 2009, 2013; Sheppes and Levin 2013; Stevens et al. 2020;

Sheppes et al. 2011). This inclination toward emotional avoidance is supposed to be maladaptive which lead to the development of a wide range of various psychopathology (Aldao et al. 2010; Chapman et al. 2017, 2019). According to empirically experimental investigations, individuals with BPD have a lower tendency to accept emotional state and utilizing acceptance-based emotion regulation strategies (Sachse et al. 2011), and these deficiencies among effective strategies modulate the association between BPD symptoms and dysregulated behaviors (Wupperman et al. 2013; Chapman et al. 2017, 2019). In the same way, through assessing the effects of avoidance-versus acceptance-oriented emotion regulation instructions in individuals with BPD, MDD, and nonpsychiatric control, it has been demonstrated avoidance from negative emotions can have short-term benefits for individuals with BPD. However, BPD patients may utilize insufficient skills and maladaptive behaviors to avoid or distract from negative emotions (Chapman et al. 2017, 2019). In other words, according to the EAM (Chapman et al. 2006), nonsuicidal self-injury may be engaged in as a distraction from unwanted, negative thoughts, emotions and somatic sensations, or other distressing or unpleasant internal experiences, which may be reinforced negatively (Selby et al. 2009), and provide strong reinforcement for NSSI, in spite of negative results in long-term (Turner et al. 2013).

As mentioned, the ECM proposed by Selby et al. (2008) and Selby and Joiner Jr (2009) to provide a broad model for understanding the association between aversive negative emotional states and a wide array of dysregulated behaviors (Selby and Coniglio 2020). In other words, ECM (Selby and Joiner Jr 2009) endeavors to propose a direct link between emotion dysregulation and behavioral dysregulation in BPD via explaining a process named an "emotional cascade" (Selby 2011). It can be claimed that ECM is a unique one to explain the interplay between emotion dysregulation and behavioral dysregulation for several reasons. The emotional cascade suggests the association between unpleasantly aversive emotions and behavioral dysregulation is elucidated by a vicious self-perpetuating cycle of rumination, negative thoughts, and negative emotion (Jungmann et al. 2016; Selby et al. 2008, 2009, 2013a, b, c, 2014a, b, c, 2020; Selby and Joiner Jr 2009, 2013; Tuna and Bozo 2014; Hasking et al. 2017). Significantly, ECM focuses on the key role of rumination to response to negative emotions (Selby et al. 2008, 2014a, b, c, 2020; Selby and Joiner Jr 2009, 2013). In order to understand ECM, it is preferable to follow Selby's line of thinking. Through this process, it can be found that the most challenging question for him was "*what is the connection between emotional and behavioral dysregulation; why does emotion dysregulation appear to result in behavioral dysregulation?*" (Selby 2007). In other words, he attempts to answer why only some people experiencing negative life events or escalated levels of distress developed clinically associated behavioral dysregulation (Selby et al. 2009; Selby 2011). Selby (2007) posits that there are some specific cognitive emotion regulations which may underlie this connection contributed to exacerbating the intensity of negative emotions, and cause an individual being engaged in dysregulated behaviors, maladaptive behavioral emotion regulation strategies, in order to dampen this intense of unwanted emotion. Selby (2007) proposes that self-inflicted injuries (e.g., Nock and Prinstein 2004), binge eating issues (e.g., Agras and Telch 1998), and reassurance seeking in social situation (Joiner Jr and Schmidt 1998) are instances of dysregulated behaviors which lead to reducing the intensity of negative emotions. Behavioral dysregulation in BPD is considered as a sequence of methods of "distraction" that split-up the emotional cascade process (Selby 2011). Furthermore, He states that despite impulsive behaviors can be hypothesized to have similar underlying problems with other forms of dysregulated behaviors, some specific impulsive behaviors can be generated by different predisposition factors. Selby (2007) proposes four reasons for engaging in impulsive behaviors based on Whiteside and Lynam (2001), comprising sensation seeking, lack of premeditation, lack of perseverance, and urgency (feeling the necessity to act in the case of exposure to emotional distress). One of the most noticeable factors which has been found as a factor in engaging in dysregulated behaviors is urgency, for example, bulimia (Claes et al. 2005, 2018), alcohol use (Tsey et al. 2003), and BPD (Whiteside et al. 2005). Based on Selby (2007), individuals who exhibits high levels of urgency may be more likely to be involved in dysfunctional behaviors, such as impulsive shopping and substance use because of emotion dysregulation. In addition, Selby (2007) emphasizes the role of *rumination* as a cognitive emotion regulation strategy, which based on a body of investigations, can intensify and perpetuate negative emotion (e.g., Rusting and Nolen-Hoeksema 1998). *Thought suppression* is another emotion regulation strategy proposed by Selby (2007). Thought suppression refers to intentional attempts to decline the frequency and intensity of unwanted cognitions, which contribute to negative psychological consequences, such as a paradoxical "rebound" effect in which the frequency of unpleasant thoughts raises following efforts to suppress (e.g., Abramowitz et al. 2001; Rosenthal et al. 2005). Moreover, catastrophizing is supposed by Selby (2007) as another cognitive emotion regulation strategy: *a tendency to think precedingly about how disastrous a situation can be and about the worst consequences of current situation in the future.* Correspondingly, catastrophizing can exacerbate the frequency and intensity of emotional distress (Sullivan et al. 1995), and is a specific form of rumination alike to worry. All of these mentioned cognitive emotion regulation strategies seem to have a shared theme: "*focusing attention usually on stimuli which are emotionally negative and unpleasant.*" These shifts in attention to negative emotions can be contributed by ruminative processes which lead to amplify the effect of negative affect. In other words, according to Selby (2007), this inclination toward rumination on negative emotional thoughts exacerbates levels of negative affect, and in turn, an escalation in negative affect raises levels of rumination. As stated, rumination has been experimentally investigated associated with BPD (e.g., Abela et al. 2003; Selby et al. 2013a, b, c; Martino et al. 2015; DeShong et al. 2019), as well as, the role of rumination in suicidal behaviors (e.g., Selby and Gardner 2015), and NSSI (e.g., Selby et al. 2010; Selby 2011; Selby and Gardner 2015; Arbuthnott et al. 2014; Tonta et al. 2022). Based on Selby and Joiner Jr (2009), rumination is a key feature of the ECM. This theoretical model posits that intense emotion contribute to an "emotional cascade," which lead to focusing more attention on negative emotion, and steadily contributing to more intense rumination (see, Gardner et al. 2014). In other words, whilst rumination escalates negative emotion, there is some evidence that negative emotion exacerbates rumination (Selby et al. 2016). According to ECM, individuals ruminate intensely about an event that inaugurates feeling of negative emotion (Selby et al. 2008; Selby and Joiner 2013). In other words, the reciprocal association between negative emotion and ruminative processes generate an "emotional cascade," which is commenced by an emotion eliciting event (Selby et al. 2008, 2015a, b; Selby and Joiner Jr 2009, 2013). In keeping with overview of relevant studies, he proposes that intense levels of rumination may contribute to extremely high level of negative affect, where slightest negative emotional stimuli are followed by a flood of racing negative emotional thoughts. This racing flow of thoughts exacerbates levels of negative emotion in a vicious repetitive cycle: *an emotional cascade*. This positive feedback cycle increased levels of negative emotions; therefore, in order to disconnect this vicious loop, an individual may engage in behaviors which assist to distract from emotional thoughts, but are relatively effective in short-term and then maladaptive toward overall mental and physical health over time (Selby 2007; Selby et al. 2008; Selby and Joiner Jr 2009, 2013).

Selby and colleagues (2011) describe the ECM (Selby and Joiner Jr 2009) as a turbulent disturbed emotional experience in individual with BPD is a result of emotional cascade, a damaged cycle of escalating rumination and negative emotion. Therefore, dysregulated behaviors may provide powerful means of distraction from rumination because of the noticeable physical sensations resulted of these types of behaviors, such as pain from self-injury. It means, this distraction "short-circuits" the emotional cascade, stopping the escalation and intensity of negative emotions and permitting these negative emotions to descend because attention is no longer on negative emotions. As a result, it can be concluded that a dysregulated behavior interferes with the ruminative process by providing negative feedback to emotional cascade. An emotional cascade initiates when an individual experiences an upsetting event, which lead him/her to ruminate about that unpleasant situation. Then, as mentioned, during an individual is ruminating, an escalation in negative emotion occurs, which in turn contributes to an increasing in rumination level, thus reciprocally rumination and negative emotion intensify each other (Selby et al. 2014a, b, c). This process leads to a self-amplifying positive feedback loop of intense rumination and negative emotion that led to a steadily more intense, unwanted, and aversive emotional state named "emotional cascade" (Selby et al. 2008, 2009, 2014a, b, c, 2016, 2020; Selby and Joiner Jr 2009, 2013; Gardner et al. 2014). Therefore, final consequence of an emotional cascade is an extremely aversive state of negative affect (Selby et al. 2009, 2014a, b, c, 2016, 2020; Selby 2011; Selby and Joiner Jr 2009, 2013). Overall, there may be a pernicious bidirectional-compounding effects of rumination and negative emotion which contribute to dysregulated behaviors such as impulsivity (Selby et al. 2009, 2016). Selby et al. (2016) propose that there is a linear relationship between rumination and negative emotion. They point out that the ECM presents two significant modifications of this relationship among impulsive people: (1) the experience of both rumination and negative emotion has a synergistic effect on subsequent negative emotion and rumination, which leads to a sharp elevating aversive experience relevant to when only one of these two factors is escalated and (2) due to this synergistic effect, the temporal relationship between rumination and negative emotion can be better described as exponential rather than linear (Selby et al. 2016). As stated, the ECM (Selby et al. 2009; Selby and Joiner Jr 2009) posits that individuals with BPD experience frequent and severe peak in negative emotion, which may contribute to pursuant dysregulated behaviors, as a result of emotional cascade (Selby et al. 2014a, b, c, 2016). This emotional cascade results in excessive, aversive emotions and debilitates the ability to shift an individual's attention away from it (see, Jungmann et al. 2016; Meaney et al. 2016; Arbuthnott et al. 2014; Selby and Joiner Jr 2009, 2013). Subsequently, these emotions can be enormous and overwhelming, which can be a hard task to manage them via safe and harmless methods, such as reappraisal and distraction (Jungmann et al. 2016). At the peak of this emotional cascade, dysregulated behaviors are more likely to take place (Selby et al. 2014a, b, c). In other words, at the height peak of this emotional cascade, dysregulated behaviors play the most prominent role (Selby et al. 2016, 2020; Selby and Joiner Jr 2009), and as a substitute, people may tend to utilize the maladaptive types of behavioral emotion regulation to distract from rumination, which are adverse means (e.g., Jungmann et al. 2016; Selby and Joiner Jr 2009, 2013; Selby et al. 2009, 2014a, b, c, 2016, 2020), such as binge eating (e.g., Selby and Coniglio 2020; Arbuthnott et al. 2014), NSSI (e.g., Arbuthnott et al. 2014; Hatzopoulos et al. 2022), and impulsivity (Selby et al. 2016).

The ECM attempts to elucidate why minor negative emotional stimuli may be followed by emotional experiences that become out of control (Selby 2011; Selby and Joiner Jr 2009, 2013). The ECM proposes that aversive emotional conditions and experiences produce rumination, which in turn, leads to the escalation the intensity and severity of emotional distress. Meaney et al. (2016) cited that in consistence with ECM, rumination has an interaction with emotional instability to forecast self-injury (Selby et al. 2013a, b, c), has a moderator role in the association between psychological distress and self-injury (Voon et al. 2013), and an interaction with BPD symptoms to predict dysregulated behaviors (Selby and Joiner Jr 2013), and is associated with BPD symptom severity (Selby and Joiner Jr 2009; Selby et al. 2009; Steenkamp et al. 2022). Selby (2011) indicated that high levels of rumination have an exponential effect on predicting future engagement in dysregulated behaviors, especially in individuals with BPD (Selby 2011). Consequently, this heightened emotional distress contributes to employing dysregulated behaviors as a mechanism of downregulating or lessening emotional disturbances. In line with this theoretical model, the presence of BPD symptoms is produced because of problematic regulatory cognitive strategies such as rumination, which may intensify aversive negative emotional state; therefore, a BPD individual employs ineffective emotion regulation strategies to damp and moderate disturbed affective state (Selby et al. 2008; Selby and Joiner Jr 2009, 2013; Meaney et al. 2016). These behaviors are utilized to provide distraction from the rumination elements of an emotional cascade, by causing intense physical sensations to focus on instead of ruminating on the problem (Selby et al. 2014a, b, c), such as feeling of pain (Selby et al. 2019a, b), the sight of blood in NSSI (Selby et al. 2019a, b; Nock et al. 2006, 2018), physical sensations induced by substance use (Selby et al. 2014a, b, c). Selby et al. (2014a, b, c) posit because of this powerful physical sensations, dysregulated behaviors may short-circuit the emotional cascade. This may occur because of reducing rumination, which contribute to a pursuant decline in negative emotion and a subsequent escalation in feelings of alleviation (Selby et al. 2014a, b, c). Since these dysregulated behaviors are significantly major forms of distraction, may hamper the emotional cascade, because of their sensory effects of these behaviors process, such as taste/fullness in binge eating. Moreover, these dysregulated behaviors have emotion regulatory effects because the individuals believe these behaviors have (Selby et al. 2009). Once an emotional cascade is in a full-generating cycle, stopping this cascade is a tough task for the individual, and further, simple distractions may be less potent and cognitive efforts at pulling attention away from problem works insufficiently, and as a consequence, it may be difficult for some activities or skills to stop the cascading cycle (Selby et al. 2014a, b, c). In other words, behaviors which assist distract someone from with low levels of rumination, such as taking a cold shower, are not able to damp and pull attention from intense rumination; alternatively, instead the individuals engage in dysregulated behaviors that result in intense physical sensations, like pain or the sight of blood during NSSI (Selby et al. 2009) to interfere with the cascade process. This may elucidate why a range of more adaptive behaviors are not utilized to distract from negative thoughts and emotions by the individual (Selby et al. 2014a, b, c). Substance use, NSSI, suicidal behaviors, binge eating, and problematic interpersonal behaviors are more frequent dysregulated behaviors that individuals with BPD engage them (e.g., Selby et al. 2009, 2010; Arbuthnott et al. 2014; Hatzopoulos et al. 2022). It should be noted that behavioral dysregulation have provisional effects, and even some dysregulated behaviors can arouse another cascade of emotions, due to specific unwanted emotions, such as embarrassment (Selby et al. 2009). For instance, the mechanism of distraction from negative emotions in NSSI has been clarified by the ECM, in which NSSI is considered a difficult to control behavior resulting from emotional cascades (Selby et al. 2013a, b, c). Then, this interference turns to the system of dysregulation in emotion into a more stable condition of lower negative emotion. Selby (2011) emphasizes that this similar pattern of behavioral distraction may expand to different forms of dysregulated behaviors in BPD, including aggressive and problematic interpersonal behaviors (Selby 2011). Emotion dysregulation and dysregulated behaviors are two significant elements of BPD psychopathology (Selby and Joiner Jr 2009).

To reach to a deep understanding of the ECM, it should be mentioned that the model helps address a particularly challenging question for those with behavioral dysregulation and/or BPD: *If distraction is helpful and useful to reduce unwanted emotional state and regulate negative emotion, then why is that the other types of distraction, especially adaptive behaviors such as taking a cold shower are not as effective as extreme forms dysregulated behaviors such as NSSI and substance use?* (Selby 2011). To answer this critical question, ECM emphasizes the core role of rumination to response to negative emotions, and essentially, rumination may lead to and become a part of a subsequent emotional cascade (Selby et al. 2008, 2014a, b, c, 2020; Selby and Joiner Jr 2009, 2013; Selby 2011), but it should be noticed that this model endeavors to establish a novel perspective on and expand the traditional construct of rumination (Nolen-Hoeksema and Morrow 1991; Nolen-Hoeksema et al. 2008), rather that redefine it (Selby et al. 2009, 2016), through highlighting a dynamic process that unravels this concept that although rumination is necessary, it is finally insufficient and dysfunctional component (Selby et al. 2016). A growing body of studies have demonstrated rumination contributes to aggravating negative emotions; nevertheless, it has not been clarified whether synergistic increases in rumination and negative emotion besides increase rumination, if this process pursues in a steadily manner during the time to finally contribute to exceeding emotional experiences (Selby et al. 2016). Moreover, several studies have mentioned that dysregulated behaviors are recruited to avoid or escape from ruminative thoughts (Nolen-Hoeksema et al. 2007, 2008); meanwhile, the ECM proposes that rumination is a major driving force in generating dysregulated behaviors (Selby et al. 2009), yet it should be pointed out that rumination has been associated with many psychological disorders and mental difficulties, such as depression, anxiety disorders, and personality disorders (Aldao et al. 2010), as well as, dysregulated behaviors, such as drinking alcohol (e.g., Selby et al. 2008, 2009) and NSSI (e.g., Selby and Gardner 2015), but not all individuals who ruminate engage in behavioral dysregulation. This may be due to severity and intensity of experiencing rumination. It means experiencing less intense rumination may contribute to disorders such as depression and experiencing more intense rumination may lead to BPD features, especially dysregulated behaviors (Selby 2011). Furthermore, a growing body of models attempt to describe rumination as a static phenomenon, in which negative emotions are increased and maintained in a stable level by rumination (Raikes and Thompson 2006; Fredrickson and Branigan 2005), rather, the ECM regards a reciprocal interaction between rumination and negative affect, which causes to perpetuate and exacerbate the vicious cycle that lead an individual to distract attention from rumination in order to reduce the intense emotional experiences (Selby et al. 2008, 2009, 2013a, b, c, 2016, 2020; Selby 2011).

In line with Selby et al. (2016), several investigations have manifested both the reciprocal relationship between rumination and levels of negative emotion (e.g., Carver et al. 1979), as well as predicting rumination and negative emotions based on momentary assessment (Moberly and Watkins 2008, Pechtel et al. 2022; Selby et al. 2008). Bresin and Verona (2016) indicated whether pain disintegrates the link between rumination and negative affect, as suggested by ECM, via utilizing a novel task which measured astonishing magnitude and self-report unpleasantness whilst rumination and distraction, besides, before, and after experiencing a painful and non-painful stimulus. They reached the conclusion that pain associated with non-painful stimuli would decline negative affect during rumination, and pain-related reduction in negative affect may be higher in rumination in comparison with distraction in both measures (Bresin and Verona 2016). Along these lines, Salovey (1992) identified that elevations in happiness or sadness increased self-focused attention, which can contribute to rumination (Watkins 2009; Watkins and Roberts 2020).

The Emergence of Borderline Personality Disorder

Selby and Joiner Jr (2009) postulated that since BPD is characterized by a broad range of frequent emotional instability and dysregulated behaviors, BPD can be assumed as the extreme continuum of emotional cascades (Selby and Joiner Jr 2009, 2013). The ECM proposes a significant perspective about the development of BPD (Selby et al. 2009, 2016, 2020; Selby and Joiner Jr 2009, 2013), suggesting that experiencing multiple emotional cascades lead to the emergence and progression of BPD during time (Selby et al. 2014a, b, c). Selby and Joiner Jr (2009) integrated two crucial factors, consisting of time and development, into their model, to note several factors, may contribute to the eventual development of emotional cascades (Selby and Joiner Jr 2009; Selby et al. 2014a, b, c). In other words, emotional cascades have been introduced according to a real-time phenomenon, in which there is an event, an emotional cascade, and dysregulated behaviors. The most significant question for Selby and Joiner Jr (2009) was: "*based on considering emotional cascades as merely real-time phenomenon, so how do real-time emotional cascades result in such a complex disorder?*". To answer, they proposed a framework that integrates several elements that are involved in the development of BPD. They accentuate all of these factors are tied together through emotional cascades and behavioral dysregulation: two core components in ECM (Selby and Joiner Jr 2009). In keeping with this model, BPD is emerged through a complex interaction between core multiple factors: time, emotional cascade, and dysregulated behaviors. According to ECM, the core psychopathology in BPD is eventuated from emotional cascades (Selby et al. 2016). These emotional cascades occur more frequently and intensely in BPD individuals in comparison with other externalizing disorders, such as eating disorder (Selby and Joiner Jr 2009). Based on ECM, there are a reciprocal association between negative emotion and ruminative processes which leads to a "cascade of emotion," which is commenced via an emotion-elicited event. This event entails an individual to ruminate intensely, which contribute to exacerbating the intensity of emotion. While the intensity of emotion rises, it becomes a hard task for an individual with BPD to elude from emotional experience through distracting attention, and in turn, individuals' attention may be focused on emotional stimuli (Salovey 1992). Therefore, a positive feedback loop between rumination and negative affect will be generated (Selby and Joiner Jr 2009, 2013; Selby et al. 2008, 2014a, b, c, 2020; Pelta 2021). This emotional cascade contributes to emerging compound disorders, such as BPD (Pelta 2021; Selby and Joiner Jr 2009, 2013) (Fig. 8.1).

As it has been displayed in Fig. 8.1, several significant constructs and risk factors are involved in the development and shaping BPD, through generating emotional cascades, which is the heart of this interacting network (Selby et al. 2014a, b, c; Selby and Joiner Jr 2009). Lewin (1992) referred to emergence as a phenomenon of intricate system rising from the collaborative interactions of a network components. Consistent with this definition, Selby and Joiner Jr (2009) propose that BPD may emerge from the interacting network of components, by focusing on emotional cascades as core aspect of the network (Selby and Joiner Jr 2009). As it has been

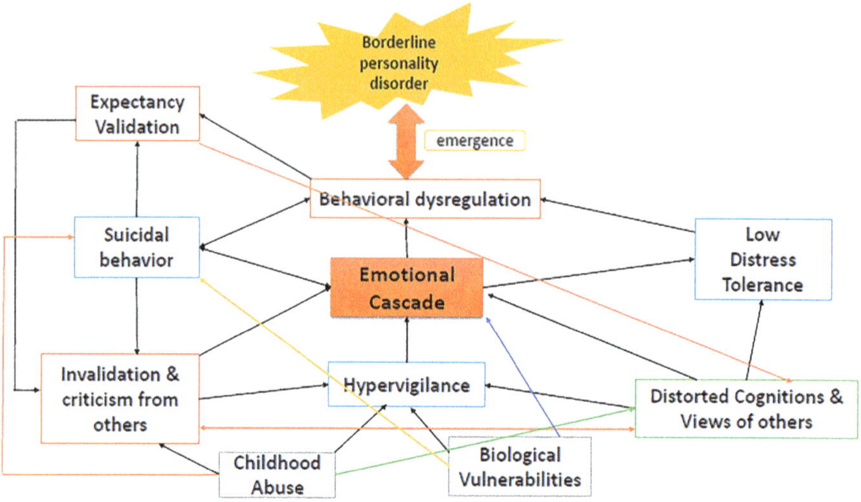

Fig. 8.1 Emotional cascade model and the emergence of BPD. (Source: Adapted from Selby et al. (2014a, b, c, p. 161))

illustrated in Fig. 8.1, many factors such as cognitive distortions and perceived invalidation lead to the development of emotional cascades (Selby et al. 2014a, b, c). It means that the synthesis of these various interactions between constructs and a pattern of emotional cascades and behavioral dysregulation may be what results in the development of BPD over time. Supposing BPD as an emergent phenomenon permits us to conceptualize for making an integrative formulation of *biological vulnerabilities and environmental* issues (child abuse and invalidation and criticism from others), with *cognitive* factors (distorted cognitions and views of others), and *behavioral* elements (dysregulated behaviors), which perpetuate this complicated disorder: bottom-up and top-down effects on the maintenance of BPD (Selby and Joiner Jr 2009). As mentioned by Selby et al. (2014a, b, c), BPD may be compromised of various biological, cognitive, social, and environmental factors, that interact with each other through emotional cascades (Selby et al. 2014a, b, c). It should be noticed that there is a bidirectional causation of these factors which permits the model to be able to foresee the proximal components, such as cognitive distortions. Distorted cognitions not only have an impact on emotional cascades, but also the resultant behavioral dysregulation can modify distorted cognitions. For instance, child abuse may have an impact on subsequent distorted cognitions and hypervigilance toward others, that can be contribute to emotional cascades (Selby and Joiner Jr 2009). In fact, by Selby et al. (2014a, b, c) mention that repeated experiences with emotional cascades and dysregulated behaviors may subsequently escalate these core factors, such that new type of cognitive distortions shaping and being exposed to highly invalidating situations from other people in their interpersonal communications (Selby et al. 2014a, b, c). Selby and Joiner Jr (2009) highlight that as individuals with BPD being engaged in dysregulated behaviors, individuals around them may begin to reply in a negative and inappropriate way, such as criticizing them, which lead to intensifying the emotional cascades. They assert this top-down interaction can be named "expectancy validation": *a process that may magnify distorted cognitions about others and create new cognitive distortions* (Selby and Joiner Jr 2009). Subsequently, during the time, several issues may rise in response to emotional cascades, including exacerbation in invalidation, lower levels of distress tolerance, and self-destructive behaviors, especially suicidal behaviors (Selby et al. 2014a, b, c). In other words, due to these problematic matters, such as decreasing distress tolerance levels with the experience of more emotional cascades, individuals with BPD may experience a decreased threshold for dysregulated behaviors (Selby and Joiner Jr 2009): *a synthesis of these diverse interactions between constructs which leads to the emergence of BPD* (Selby et al. 2014a, b, c).

Investigation Supporting the Emotional Cascade Model

A growing body of studies have been done to support the validity of the ECM. Some evidence has been acquired for the role of rumination in generating emotional cascade, as well as, emotional cascades in dysregulated behaviors, such as alcohol use, being eating and purging, NSSI, suicidal attempts, and seeking reassurance excessively (e.g., Selby and Joiner Jr 2009, 2013; Selby et al. 2008, 2009, 2010, 2013a, b, c, 2014a, b, c, 2016, 2020; Arbuthnott et al. 2014; Meaney et al. 2016; Hatzopoulos et al. 2022; DeShong et al. 2019; Hasking et al. 2018; Tunta and Bozo 2014; Martino et al. 2015). Hasking et al. (2018) indicated that both self-report (Selby et al. 2013a, b, c; Slabbert et al. 2018) and empirical studies (Arbuthnott et al. 2014) support ECM, with rumination differentiating between individuals who engage in NSSI and who do not, and escalating the association between negative emotion and NSSI (e.g., Arbuthnott et al. 2015; Selby et al. 2013a, b, c; Nicolai et al. 2016; Victor and Klonsky 2014). Selby et al. (2013a, b, c) demonstrated the emotional cascades can be featured by instability of rumination and negative emotion, where there are sharp fluctuations in the levels of rumination and negative emotions throughout a day, opposite to average levels of rumination and negative emotion (Selby et al. 2013a, b, c). Jungmann et al. (2016) demonstrated that unwanted negative thoughts may act as a mediator between rumination and commence of dysregulated behavioral responses which suggested by ECM (Jungmann et al. 2016). In addition, a body of investigations have displayed associations between greater levels of negative emotional intensity and psychological distress (Bornovalova et al. 2011), anxiety (Brumariu and Kerns 2013), and anxiety reactivity and perseveration (Rudaizky and MavLeod 2014; Jungmann et al. 2016). Selby et al. (2013a, b, c) examined the role of trait rumination, and momentary instability of rumination. The findings indicated an interaction between rumination instability and negative emotion instability notably predicted NSSI, besides the powerful effects occurring for sadness and rumination about past, consistent with ECM (Selby et al. 2013a, b, c). In one study about bidirectional-compounding effects of rumination and negative emotion in predicting impulsive behavior and testing emotional cascades, it has been revealed rumination can predict subsequent aggregating in rumination that lasted over remained over prolonged periods of time. Moreover, research results demonstrated that rumination and negative emotion had an important role in the prediction of escalated levels of each other, and, a synergistic effect between rumination and negative emotion has been found, which may foresee broader elevations in further rumination and negative emotion than when one variable alone was elevated. Ultimately, synergistic effects of rumination and negative emotion were obtained in predicting number of impulsive behaviors (Selby et al. 2014a, b, c). DeShong et al. (2019) examined whether the constructs of the ECM associate with other constructs within the BPD nomological network. Specially, neuroticism, childhood emotional vulnerability, and parental invalidation were assessed in order to find out the association between these factors and the ruminative process and engagement in maladaptive behaviors as described in ECM, among students. Based on the results, it was demonstrated that neuroticism predicted rumination 1 months later in both samples, and also, childhood emotional vulnerability and parental invalidation predicted rumination 2 months later in one sample (DeShong et al. 2019). Hatzopoulos et al. (2022) studied the moderating role of rumination in the association between reactivity, intensity, and perseveration of emotion and NSSI. They found rumination was associated with NSSI yet did not moderate relationships between dimensions of negative emotion and NSSI; however, rumination played as a moderator in the association between perseveration of positive emotion and history of NSSI (Hatzopoulos et al. 2022).

A body of research has demonstrated that rumination leads to intrusive thoughts (e.g., Santa Maria et al. 2012), dysfunctional behaviors, such as avoidance in PTSD (Horowitz et al. 1982), and can be considered as a risk factor for self-destructive behaviors (Batey et al. 2010). In spite of being considered this point that ECM has a great emphasis on the intensity (the strength of emotional responses) of emotion, which is supposed the core factor in NSSI, there are several studies which demonstrated that other dimensions of emotion are influenced. These dimensions constitute salient characteristics of emotional responses, comprising reactivity (the possibility of experiencing an emotional response), and perseveration (the duration of emotional responses one evoked). A growing body of studies have indicated that these dimensions have key roles in psychopathology (Hatzopoulos et al. 2022). Selby et al. (2010) highlighted individuals with BPD displayed greater reactivity and intensity of negative emotion following the rumination induction than control group (Selby et al. 2009). Hasking et al. (2018) investigated whether rumination and multisensory imagery-based cognitions moderated the associations between emotion and NSSI, and frequency of the behavior. Their findings suggested that although elements of ECM may usefully propose an explanation for NSSI, various factors are associated with the odds of engaging in NSSI, and the frequency of the behavior among individuals be involved in self-injurious behaviors. Moreover, they demonstrated none of the potential moderators, comprising rumination and imagery, were directly associated with NSSI. Rather the frequency of engaging in self-injury behaviors and the odds of engaging in NSSI, can be best conceptualized as a complicated interaction between emotion and cognitions (Hasking et al. 2018). Selby et al. (2010) hypothesized both high rumination and habituation to the fear of pain may have a strong influence on NSSI because among individuals who lack a fear of pain and ruminate intensely will not be afraid to inflict physical pain as a way to distract from negative affect. Based on their results, the interaction effect of rumination and painful/provocative experiences on the frequency of NSSI have been revealed. In addition, they pointed out despite the point that this interaction remarkably predicted NSSI, it could not foresee dysregulated behaviors and drinking as a coping mechanism (Selby et al. 2010).

More recently, Selby et al. (2020) conducted *Temporal Bayesian Network* (TBN) modeling, in which the associations between multiple subcomponents of a model can be specified and examined over a dynamic time frame, to evaluate the ECM in BPD adolescents and young adults with nonsuicidal self-injury. According to their findings the ECM has considerably a predictive utility, indicating remarkable accuracy (90%) in forecasting BPD diagnosis, and momentary prediction of rumination, negative emotion, and dysregulated behaviors. They asserted that these findings support and validate the point that BPD may appear from a dynamic interaction between emotional cascades and dysregulated behaviors (Selby et al. 2020). Furthermore, based on structural equation modeling, Selby et al. (2009) indicated that emotional cascades completely mediated the association BPD symptoms and a behavioral dysregulation latent variable (excessive reassurance seeking, bulimic behaviors, drinking to cope, NSSI, and suicidal symptoms) (Selby et al. 2009). Selby and Joiner Jr (2013) examined the potential for emotional cascades to prospectively predict the occurrence of dysregulated behaviors in daily life. Their findings demonstrated a significant three-way interaction, displayed via high levels of negative emotion and rumination in individuals with BPD, had an escalated possibility of engaging in a dysregulated behavior beyond those with low levels of BPD symptoms. They highlighted these findings propose a major part of ECM (Selby and Joiner Jr 2013). Gardner et al. (2014) examined the ECM in adult male offenders with borderline personality traits. Findings suggest that emotional cascade, measured as rumination, may have a significant role in NSSI and suicidal behaviors in adult male offenders. In addition, this investigation accentuates the benefits of targeting rumination to manage the risk of NSSI and suicidal behaviors in custodial settings (Gardner et al. 2014). Selby et al. (2013b) supposed nightmares as the experience of emotional cascades that occur during sleep. They assert these cascades may transfer from a stressful day and contribute to increased cognitive activity during sleep, as well as nightmare-like phenomena. To investigate, negative emotion, rumination, and number of nightmares were assessed daily during 2 weeks in individuals with BPD. Findings revealed that BPD group experienced more frequent nightmares. In addition, they found an interaction between BPD diagnosis and baseline trait rumination to prospectively predict number of nightmares, and daily experience of emotional cascade predicted further number of nightly nightmares (Selby et al. 2013b).

References

Abela JR, Brozina K, Haigh EP. An examination of the response styles theory of depression in third-and seventh-grade children: a short-term longitudinal study. J Abnorm Child Psychol. 2002;30:515–27.

Abela JR, Payne AV, Moussaly N. Cognitive vulnerability to depression in individuals with borderline personality disorder. J Personal Disord. 2003;17(4):319–29.

Abramowitz JS, Tolin DF, Street GP. Paradoxical effects of thought suppression: a meta-analysis of controlled studies. Clin Psychol Rev. 2001;21(5):683–703.

Agras WS, Telch CF. The effects of caloric deprivation and negative affect on binge eating in obese binge-eating disordered women. Behav Ther. 1998;29(3):491–503.

Ahn CY, Lee JS. Digital phenotyping for real-time monitoring of nonsuicidal self-injury: protocol for a prospective observational study. JMIR Res Protoc. 2024;13(1):e53597.

Aldao A, Dixon-Gordon KL. Broadening the scope of research on emotion regulation strategies and psychopathology. Cogn Behav Ther. 2014;43(1):22–33.

Aldao A, Nolen-Hoeksema S, Schweizer S. Emotion-regulation strategies across psychopathology: a meta-analytic review. Clin Psychol Rev. 2010;30(2):217–37.

Aldao A, Nolen-Hoeksema S. When are adaptive strategies most predictive of psychopathology? J Abnorm Psychol. 2012;121(1):276.

Aldao A, Mennin DS, McLaughlin KA. Differentiating worry and rumination: evidence from heart rate variability during spontaneous regulation. Cogn Ther Res. 2013;37:613–9.

Aker M, Harmer C, Landrø NI. More rumination and less effective emotion regulation in previously depressed women with preserved executive functions. BMC Psychiatry. 2014;14:1.

American Psychiatric Association. Diagnostic and statistical manual of mental disorders. 5th ed. Text Revised (DSM-5-TR). American Psychiatric Association; 2022.

Anestis MD, Selby EA. Grit and perseverance in suicidal behavior and nonsuicidal self-injury. Death Stud. 2015;39(4):211–8.

Anestis MD, Anestis JC, Selby EA, Joiner TE. Anger rumination across forms of aggression. Personal Individ Differ. 2009;46(2):192–6.

Arbuthnott AE, Lewis SP, Bailey HN. Rumination and emotions in nonsuicidal self-injury and eating disorder behaviors: a preliminary test of the emotional cascade model. J Clin Psychol. 2015;71(1):62–71.

Arbuthnott KD, Arbuthnott DW, Thompson VA. The mind in therapy: cognitive science for practice. Routledge; 2014.

Baer RA, Sauer SE. Relationships between depressive rumination, anger rumination, and borderline personality features. Personal Disord Theory Res Treat. 2011;2(2):142.

Baer RA, Peters JR, Eisenlohr-Moul TA, Geiger PJ, Sauer SE. Emotion-related cognitive processes in borderline personality disorder: a review of the empirical literature. Clin Psychol Rev. 2012;32(5):359–69.

Batey M, Chamorro-Premuzic T, Furnham A. Individual differences in ideational behavior: can the big five and psychometric intelligence predict creativity scores? Creat Res J. 2010;22(1):90–7.

Baumeister RF. Suicide as escape from self. Psychol Rev. 1990;97(1):90.

Beauchaine TP, Crowell SE, editors. The Oxford handbook of emotion dysregulation. Oxford University Press; 2020.

Beck AT, editor. Cognitive therapy of depression. Guilford Press; 1979.

Beck AT, Brown G, Steer RA. Prediction of eventual suicide in psychiatric inpatients by clinical ratings of hopelessness. J Consult Clin Psychol. 1989;57(2):309.

Beck AT, Steer RA, Beck JS, Newman CF. Hopelessness, depression, suicidal ideation, and clinical diagnosis of depression. Suicide Life Threat Behav. 1993;23(2):139–45.

Beck AT, Clark DA. Cognitive theory and therapy of anxiety and depression: convergence with neurobiological findings. Trends Cogn Sci. 2010;14(9):418–24.

Berg JM, Latzman RD, Bliwise NG, Lilienfeld SO. Parsing the heterogeneity of impulsivity: a meta-analytic review of the behavioral implications of the UPPS for psychopathology. Psychol Assess. 2015;27(4):1129.

Bolton JM, Robinson J. Population-attributable fractions of Axis I and Axis II mental disorders for suicide attempts: findings from a representative sample of the adult, noninstitutionalized US population. Am J Public Health. 2010;100(12):2473–80.

Bornovalova MA, Tull MT, Gratz KL, Levy R, Lejuez CW. Extending models of deliberate self-harm and suicide attempts to substance users: exploring the roles of childhood abuse, posttraumatic stress, and difficulties controlling impulsive behavior when distressed. Psychol Trauma Theory Res Pract Policy. 2011;3(4):349.

Borders A, Earleywine M, Jajodia A. Could mindfulness decrease anger, hostility, and aggression by decreasing rumination? Aggress Behav. 2010;36(1):28–44.

Bresin K, Verona E. Pain, affect, and rumination: an experimental test of the emotional cascade theory in two undergraduate samples. J Exp Psychopathol. 2016;7(2):205–24.

Bresin K. Toward a unifying theory of dysregulated behaviors. Clin Psychol Rev. 2020;80:101885.

Bresin K, Mekawi Y. Unpacking the construct of dysregulated behaviors using variable-centered and person-centered analytic approaches. Subst Use Misuse. 2022;57(4):603–12.

Brinker JK, Dozois DJ. Ruminative thought style and depressed mood. J Clin Psychol. 2009;65(1):1–9.

Brumariu LE, Kerns KA. Pathways to anxiety: contributions of attachment history, temperament, peer competence, and ability to manage intense emotions. Child Psychiatry Hum Dev. 2013;44:504–15.

Bryant RA, Williamson T, Erlinger M, Felmingham KL, Malhi G, Hinton M, Williams L, Korgaonkar MS. Neural activity during response inhibition associated with improvement of dysphoric symptoms of PTSD after trauma-focused psychotherapy—an EEG-fMRI study. Transl Psychiatry. 2021;11(1):218.

Buelens T, Luyckx K, Gandhi A, Kiekens G, Claes L. Nonsuicidal self-injury in adolescence: longitudinal associations with psychological distress and rumination. J Abnorm Child Psychol. 2019;47:1569–81.

Buelens T, Luyckx K, Kiekens G, Gandhi A, Muehlenkamp JJ, Claes L. Investigating the DSM-5 criteria for nonsuicidal self-injury disorder in a community sample of adolescents. J Affect Disord. 2020;260:314–22.

Calmes CA, Roberts JE. Repetitive thought and emotional distress: rumination and worry as prospective predictors of depressive and anxious symptomatology. Cogn Ther Res. 2007;31:343–56.

Cano-López JB, Salguero JM, García-Sancho E, Ramos-Cejudo J. Testing the metacognitive model of rumination and depression in non-clinical population: new data about PBRS and NBRS scales. J Psychopathol Behav Assess. 2021;43(2):240–50.

Carroll JB. Individual difference relations in psychometric and experimental cognitive tasks. Chapel Hill: LL Thurstone Psychometric Laboratory, University of North Carolina; 1980.

Carver CS, Blaney PH, Scheier MF. Focus of attention, chronic expectancy, and responses to a feared stimulus. J Pers Soc Psychol. 1979;37(7):1186.

Carver CS, Harmon-Jones E. Anger is an approach-related affect: evidence and implications. Psychol Bull. 2009;135(2):183.

Caselli G, Gemelli A, Querci S, Lugli AM, Canfora F, Annovi C, Rebecchi D, Ruggiero GM, Sassaroli S, Spada MM, Watkins ER. The effect of rumination on craving across the continuum of drinking behaviour. Addict Behav. 2013;38(12):2879–83.

Chapman AL, Specht MW, Cellucci T. Borderline personality disorder and deliberate self-harm: does experiential avoidance play a role? Suicide Life Threat Behav. 2005;35(4):388–99.

Chapman AL, Gratz KL, Brown MZ. Solving the puzzle of deliberate self-harm: the experiential avoidance model. Behav Res Ther. 2006;44(3):371–94.

Chapman AL, Dixon-Gordon KL, Layden BK, Walters KN. Borderline personality features moderate the effect of a fear induction on impulsivity. Personal Disord Theory Res Treat. 2010;1(3):139.
Chapman AL, Rosenthal MZ, Dixon-Gordon KL, Turner BJ, Kuppens P. Borderline personality disorder and the effects of instructed emotional avoidance or acceptance in daily life. J Personal Disord. 2017;31(4):483–502.
Chapman AL. Borderline personality disorder and emotion dysregulation. Dev Psychopathol. 2019;31(3):1143–56.
Chapman AL, Hope NH. Dialectical behavior therapy and treatment of emotion dysregulation. In: The Oxford handbook of emotion dysregulation; 2020. p. 463.
Ciesla JA, Roberts JE. Self-directed thought and response to treatment for depression: a preliminary investigation. J Cogn Psychother. 2002;16(4):435–53.
Ciesla JA, Dickson KS, Anderson NL, Neal DJ. Negative repetitive thought and college drinking: angry rumination, depressive rumination, co-rumination, and worry. Cogn Ther Res. 2011a;35:142–50.
Ciesla JA, Felton JW, Roberts JE. Testing the cognitive catalyst model of depression: does rumination amplify the impact of cognitive diatheses in response to stress? Cognit Emot. 2011b;25(8):1349–57.
Claes R, Beheydt C, Lemmens B. Unidimensionality of abbreviated proactive personality scales across cultures. Appl Psychol. 2005;54(4):476–89.
Claes L, Bouman WP, Witcomb GL, Arcelus J. Non-suicidal self-injury and suicidality in trans people: a systematic review of the literature. In: Gender dysphoria and gender incongruence; 2018. p. 70–81.
Cludius B, Mennin D, Ehring T. Emotion regulation as a transdiagnostic process. Emotion. 2020;20(1):37.
Cooper ML, Russell M, Skinner JB, Frone MR, Mudar P. Stress and alcohol use: moderating effects of gender, coping, and alcohol expectancies. J Abnorm Psychol. 1992;101(1):139.
Crowell SE, Beauchaine TP, Linehan MM. A biosocial developmental model of borderline personality: elaborating and extending Linehan's theory. Psychol Bull. 2009;135(3):495.
Crowell D, Madigan DJ. Perfectionistic concerns cognitions predict burnout in college athletes: a three-month longitudinal study. Int J Sport Exerc Psychol. 2022;20(2):532–50.
Crowell SE, Price CJ, Puzia ME, Yaptangco M, Cheng SC. Emotion dysregulation and autonomic responses to film, rumination, and body awareness: extending psychophysiological research to a naturalistic clinical setting and a chemically dependent female sample. Psychophysiology. 2017;54(5):713–23.
Crowell SE, Baucom BR, Yaptangco M, Bride D, Hsiao R, McCauley E, Beauchaine TP. Emotion dysregulation and dyadic conflict in depressed and typical adolescents: evaluating concordance across psychophysiological and observational measures. Biol Psychol. 2014;98:50–8.
Cuesta-Zamora C, González-Martí I, García-López LM, Ros L, Plateau CR, Ricarte JJ. Emotion dysregulation as a mediator of the relationship between anxiety, compulsive exercise and eating disorder symptoms in adolescents. Children. 2021;8(12):1088.
Day LH. Durkheim on religion and suicide-a demographic critique. Sociology. 1987;21(3):449–61.
Davey CG, Yücel M, Allen NB. The emergence of depression in adolescence: development of the prefrontal cortex and the representation of reward. Neurosci Biobehav Rev. 2008;32(1):1–9.
de Jong-Meyer R, Beck B, Riede K. Relationships between rumination, worry, intolerance of uncertainty and metacognitive beliefs. Personal Individ Differ. 2009;46(4):547–51.
Dell'Osso L, Cremone IM, Carpita B, Dell'Oste V, Muti D, Massimetti G, Barlati S, Vita A, Fagiolini A, Carmassi C, Gesi C. Rumination, posttraumatic stress disorder, and mood symptoms in borderline personality disorder. Neuropsychiatr Dis Treat. 2019:1231–8.
DeShong HL, Grant DM, Mullins-Sweatt SN. Precursors of the emotional cascade model of borderline personality disorder: the role of neuroticism, childhood emotional vulnerability, and parental invalidation. Personal Disord Theory Res Treat. 2019;10(4):317.

Dillahunt AK, Feldman DA, Thomas LR, Farstead BW, Frandsen SB, Lee S, Pazdera M, Galloway J, Bessette KL, Roberts H, Crowell SE. Self-injury in adolescence is associated with greater behavioral risk avoidance, not risk-taking. J Clin Med. 2022;11(5):1288.

Dixon-Gordon KL, Gratz KL, McDermott MJ, Tull MT. The role of executive attention in deliberate self-harm. Psychiatry Res. 2014;218(1–2):113–7.

Dixon-Gordon KL, Weiss NH, Brick LA, Goldstein SC, Schick MR, Laws H, Kiefer R, Contractor AA, Sullivan TP. Measuring emotion dysregulation in daily life: an experience sampling study. Anxiety Stress Coping. 2024:1–9.

Dixon-Gordon KL, Haliczer LA, Conkey LC, Whalen DJ. Difficulties in interpersonal emotion regulation: initial development and validation of a self-report measure. J Psychopathol Behav Assess. 2018;40:528–49.

Dixon-Gordon KL, Marsh NP, Balda KE, McQuade JD. Parent emotion socialization and child emotional vulnerability as predictors of borderline personality features. Res Child Adolesc Psychopathol. 2020;48:135–47.

Ehring T, Ehlers A. Does rumination mediate the relationship between emotion regulation ability and posttraumatic stress disorder? Eur J Psychotraumatol. 2014;5(1):23547.

Eisma MC, Stroebe MS, Schut HA, Van Den Bout J, Boelen PA, Stroebe W. Development and psychometric evaluation of the Utrecht Grief Rumination Scale. J Psychopathol Behav Assess. 2014a;36:165–76.

Eisma MC, Schut HA, Stroebe MS, van den Bout J, Stroebe W, Boelen PA. Is rumination after bereavement linked with loss avoidance? Evidence from eye-tracking. PLoS One. 2014b;9(8):e104980.

Everaert J, Grahek I, Duyck W, Buelens J, Van den Bergh N, Koster EH. Mapping the interplay among cognitive biases, emotion regulation, and depressive symptoms. Cognit Emot. 2017;31(4):726–35.

Franz MR, Brock RL, DiLillo D. Trauma symptoms contribute to daily experiential avoidance: does partner support mitigate risk? J Soc Pers Relat. 2021;38(1):322–41.

Fredrickson BL, Branigan C. Positive emotions broaden the scope of attention and thought-action repertoires. Cognit Emot. 2005;19(3):313–32.

García-Sancho E, Salguero JM, Fernández-Berrocal P. Angry rumination as a mediator of the relationship between ability emotional intelligence and various types of aggression. Personal Individ Differ. 2016;89:143–7.

Gardner FL, Moore ZE. Understanding clinical anger and violence: the anger avoidance model. Behav Modif. 2008;32(6):897–912.

Gardner KJ, Dodsworth J, Selby EA. Borderline personality traits, rumination, and self-injurious behavior: an empirical test of the emotional cascades model in adult male offenders. J Forensic Psychol Pract. 2014;14(5):398–417.

Glenn CR, Klonsky ED. A multimethod analysis of impulsivity in nonsuicidal self-injury. Personal Disord Theory Res Treat. 2010;1(1):67.

Gratz KL, Kiel EJ, Latzman RD, Elkin TD, Moore SA, Tull MT. Emotion: empirical contribution: maternal borderline personality pathology and infant emotion regulation: examining the influence of maternal emotion-related difficulties and infant attachment. J Personal Disord. 2014;28(1):52–69.

Gratz KL, Weiss NH, McDermott MJ, Dilillo D, Messman-Moore T, Tull MT. Emotion dysregulation mediates the relation between borderline personality disorder symptoms and later physical health symptoms. J Personal Disord. 2017;31(4):433–48.

Gratz KL, Richmond JR, Dixon-Gordon KL, Chapman AL, Tull MT. Multimodal assessment of emotional reactivity and regulation in response to social rejection among self-harming adults with and without borderline personality disorder. Personal Disord Theory Res Treat. 2019;10(5):395.

Gratz KL, Kiel EJ, Mann AJ, Tull MT. The prospective relation between borderline personality disorder symptoms and suicide risk: the mediating roles of emotion regulation difficulties and perceived burdensomeness. J Affect Disord. 2022;313:186–95.

Greenberg MT, Kusche CA, Cook ET, Quamma JP. Promoting emotional competence in school-aged children: the effects of the PATHS curriculum. Dev Psychopathol. 1995;7(1):117–36.
Gross JJ. The emerging field of emotion regulation: an integrative review. Rev Gen Psychol. 1998;2(3):271–99.
Gross JJ. Emotion and emotion regulation: personality processes and individual differences; 2008.
Gross JJ. Emotion regulation: current status and future prospects. Psychol Inq. 2015;26(1):1–26.
Gross, J. J., & Thompson, R. A. (2007). Emotion Regulation: Conceptual Foundations. In J. J. Gross (Ed.), Handbook of emotion regulation (pp. 3–24). The Guilford Press.
Gunderson K. Leibnizian privacy and Skinnerian privacy. Behav Brain Sci. 1984;7(4):628–9.
Guo M, Li C, Lei Y, Xu S, Zhao D, Lu XY. Role of the adipose PPARγ-adiponectin axis in susceptibility to stress and depression/anxiety-related behaviors. Mol Psychiatry. 2017;22(7):1056–68.
Hasking P, Whitlock J, Voon D, Rose A. A cognitive-emotional model of NSSI: using emotion regulation and cognitive processes to explain why people self-injure. Cognit Emot. 2017;31(8):1543–56.
Hasking PA, Di Simplicio M, McEvoy PM, Rees CS. Emotional cascade theory and nonsuicidal self-injury: the importance of imagery and positive affect. Cognit Emot. 2018;32(5):941–52.
Hasking P, Boyes ME, Finlay-Jones A, McEvoy PM, Rees CS. Common pathways to NSSI and suicide ideation: the roles of rumination and self-compassion. Arch Suicide Res. 2019;23(2):247–60.
Hatzopoulos K, Boyes M, Hasking P. Relationships between dimensions of emotional experience, rumination, and nonsuicidal self-injury: an application of the emotional cascade model. J Clin Psychol. 2022;78(4):692–709.
Hayes SC, Wilson KG, Gifford EV, Follette VM, Strosahl K. Experiential avoidance and behavioral disorders: a functional dimensional approach to diagnosis and treatment. J Consult Clin Psychol. 1996;64(6):1152.
Haywood SB, Hasking P, Boyes ME. Associations between nonsuicidal self-injury and experiential avoidance: a systematic review and Robust Bayesian Meta-analysis. J Affect Disord. 2023;325:470–9.
Hill R. Rumination as a mediator between Borderline Personality Disorder (BPD) traits and the cognitive and behaviour dysregulation symptoms in bulimia; 2015.
Hilt LM, Sladek MR, Doane LD, Stroud CB. Daily and trait rumination: diurnal cortisol patterns in adolescent girls. Cognit Emot. 2017;31(8):1757–67.
Horowitz LM, French RD, Anderson CA. The prototype of a lonely person. Loneliness: a sourcebook of current theory, research, and therapy; 1982. p. 183–205.
Hoyer J, Beesdo K, Gloster AT, Runge J, Höfler M, Becker ES. Worry exposure versus applied relaxation in the treatment of generalized anxiety disorder. Psychother Psychosom. 2009;78(2):106–15.
Jacobs RH, Watkins ER, Peters AT, Feldhaus CG, Barba A, Carbray J, Langenecker SA. Targeting ruminative thinking in adolescents at risk for depressive relapse: rumination-focused cognitive behavior therapy in a pilot randomized controlled trial with resting state fMRI. PLoS One. 2016;11(11):e0163952.
Joiner TE Jr, Sachs-Ericsson NJ, Wingate LR, Brown JS, Anestis MD, Selby EA. Childhood physical and sexual abuse and lifetime number of suicide attempts: a persistent and theoretically important relationship. Behav Res Ther. 2007;45(3):539–47.
Joiner TE Jr, Schmidt NB. Excessive reassurance-seeking predicts depressive but not anxious reactions to acute stress. J Abnorm Psychol. 1998;107(3):533.
Joiner TE Jr, Brown JS, Wingate LR. The psychology and neurobiology of suicidal behavior. Annu Rev Psychol. 2005;56:287–314.
Joormann J, Tran TB. Rumination and intentional forgetting of emotional material. Cognit Emot. 2009;23(6):1233–46.
Joormann J, Dkane M, Gotlib IH. Adaptive and maladaptive components of rumination? Diagnostic specificity and relation to depressive biases. Behav Ther. 2006;37(3):269–80.

Jose PE, Brown I. When does the gender difference in rumination begin? Gender and age differences in the use of rumination by adolescents. J Youth Adolesc. 2008;37:180–92.

Jungmann SM, Vollmer N, Selby EA, Witthöft M. Understanding dysregulated behaviors and compulsions: an extension of the emotional cascade model and the mediating role of intrusive thoughts. Front Psychol. 2016;7:149408.

Kaufman EA, Perez J, Lazarus S, Stepp SD, Pedersen SL. Understanding the association between borderline personality disorder and alcohol-related problems: an examination of drinking motives, impulsivity, and affective instability. Personal Disord Theory Res Treat. 2020;11(3):213.

Klonsky ED, Oltmanns TF, Turkheimer E. Deliberate self-harm in a nonclinical population: prevalence and psychological correlates. Am J Psychiatry. 2003;160(8):1501–8.

Klonsky ED. The functions of deliberate self-injury: a review of the evidence. Clin Psychol Rev. 2007;27(2):226–39.

Klonsky ED, Muehlenkamp JJ. Self-injury: a research review for the practitioner. J Clin Psychol. 2007;63(11):1045–56.

Klonsky ED, Olino TM. Identifying clinically distinct subgroups of self-injurers among young adults: a latent class analysis. J Consult Clin Psychol. 2008;76(1):22.

Knowles R, Tai S, Christensen I, Bentall R. Coping with depression and vulnerability to mania: a factor analytic study of the Nolen-Hoeksema (1991) response styles questionnaire. Br J Clin Psychol. 2005;44(1):99–112.

Kornacka M, Czepczor-Bernat K, Napieralski P, Brytek-Matera A. Rumination, mood, and maladaptive eating behaviors in overweight and healthy populations. Eat Weight Disord Stud Anorexia Bulimia Obes. 2021;26:273–85.

Koster EH, De Lissnyder E, De Raedt R. Rumination is characterized by valence-specific impairments in switching of attention. Acta Psychol. 2013;144(3):563–70.

Krahé C, Whyte J, Bridge L, Loizou S, Hirsch CR. Are different forms of repetitive negative thinking associated with interpretation bias in generalized anxiety disorder and depression? Clin Psychol Sci. 2019;7(5):969–81.

Law KC, Rogers ML, Tucker RP, Bauer BW, Capron DW, Anestis MD, Joiner TE. Rumination in the context of anger and sadness: differential effects on state agitation. J Affect Disord. 2021;280:89–96.

Lewin M. The impact of Kurt Lewin's life on the place of social issues in his work. J Soc Issues. 1992;48(2):15–29.

Liao KY, Wei M. Intolerance of uncertainty, depression, and anxiety: the moderating and mediating roles of rumination. J Clin Psychol. 2011;67(12):1220–39.

Linehan MM. Cognitive-behavioral treatment of borderline personality disorder. Enskede: TPB; 1993.

Littlefield AK, Sher KJ, Steinley D. Developmental trajectories of impulsivity and their association with alcohol use and related outcomes during emerging and young adulthood I. Alcohol Clin Exp Res. 2010;34(8):1409–16.

Lynam DR, Miller JD, Miller DJ, Bornovalova MA, Lejuez CW. Testing the relations between impulsivity-related traits, suicidality, and nonsuicidal self-injury: a test of the incremental validity of the UPPS model. Personal Disord Theory Res Treat. 2011;2(2):151.

Lyubomirsky S, Lepper HS. A measure of subjective happiness: preliminary reliability and construct validation. Soc Indic Res. 1999;46:137–55.

Lyubomirsky S, Dickerhoof R, Boehm JK, Sheldon KM. Becoming happier takes both a will and a proper way: an experimental longitudinal intervention to boost well-being. Emotion. 2011;11(2):391.

Lyubomirsky S, Tkach C, DiMatteo MR. What are the differences between happiness and self-esteem. Soc Indic Res. 2006;78:363–404.

Lyubomirsky S, Nolen-Hoeksema S. Self-perpetuating properties of dysphoric rumination. J Pers Soc Psychol. 1993;65(2):339.

Lyubomirsky S, Nolen-Hoeksema S. Effects of self-focused rumination on negative thinking and interpersonal problem solving. J Pers Soc Psychol. 1995;69(1):176.
Lyubomirsky S, Caldwell ND, Nolen-Hoeksema S. Effects of ruminative and distracting responses to depressed mood on retrieval of autobiographical memories. J Pers Soc Psychol. 1998;75(1):166.
Lyubomirsky S, Layous K, Chancellor J, Nelson SK. Thinking about rumination: the scholarly contributions and intellectual legacy of Susan Nolen-Hoeksema. Annu Rev Clin Psychol. 2015;11:1–22.
Martino F, Caselli G, Berardi D, Fiore F, Marino E, Menchetti M, Prunetti E, Ruggiero GM, Sasdelli A, Selby E, Sassaroli S. Anger rumination and aggressive behaviour in borderline personality disorder. Personal Ment Health. 2015;9(4):277–87.
McFarland C, Buehler R. The impact of negative affect on autobiographical memory: the role of self-focused attention to moods. J Pers Soc Psychol. 1998;75(6):1424.
Martino ML, Freda MF, Camera F. Effects of Guided Written Disclosure Protocol on mood states and psychological symptoms among parents of off-therapy acute lymphoblastic leukemia children. Journal of Health Psychology. 2013 Jun;18(6):727–36.
McHugh RK, Goodman FR. Are substance use disorders emotional disorders? Why heterogeneity matters for treatment. 2019.
McLaughlin KA, Nolen-Hoeksema S. Interpersonal stress generation as a mechanism linking rumination to internalizing symptoms in early adolescents. J Clin Child Adolesc Psychol. 2012;41(5):584–97.
McRae K, Zarolia P. Cognition and emotion in emotion dysregulation. In: The Oxford handbook of emotion dysregulation. Oxford University Press; 2020. p. 39–52.
Meaney R, Hasking P, Reupert A. Prevalence of borderline personality disorder in university samples: systematic review, meta-analysis and meta-regression. PLoS One. 2016;11(5):e0155439.
Mettler J, Cho S, Stern M, Heath NL. Negative and positive emotional reactivity in women with and without a history of self-injury. Psychol Rep. 2023:00332941231180118.
Michael T, Halligan SL, Clark DM, Ehlers A. Rumination in posttraumatic stress disorder. Depress Anxiety. 2007;24(5):307–17.
Miranda R, Nolen-Hoeksema S. Brooding and reflection: rumination predicts suicidal ideation at 1-year follow-up in a community sample. Behav Res Ther. 2007;45(12):3088–95.
Miranda R, Polanco-Roman L, Tsypes A, Valderrama J. Perceived discrimination, ruminative subtypes, and risk for depressive symptoms in emerging adulthood. Cult Divers Ethn Minor Psychol. 2013;19(4):395.
Moberly NJ, Watkins ER. Ruminative self-focus, negative life events, and negative affect. Behav Res Ther. 2008;46(9):1034–9.
Moulds ML, Kandris E, Starr S, Wong AC. The relationship between rumination, avoidance and depression in a non-clinical sample. Behav Res Ther. 2007;45(2):251–61.
Neuhaus E, Beauchaine TP. Impulsivity and vulnerability to psychopathology. In: Child and adolescent psychopathology. 3rd ed. Hoboken: Wiley; 2017. p. 178–212.
Nicolai KA, Wielgus MD, Mezulis A. Identifying risk for self-harm: rumination and negative affectivity in the prospective prediction of nonsuicidal self-injury. Suicide Life Threat Behav. 2016;46(2):223–33.
Nock MK, Prinstein MJ. A functional approach to the assessment of self-mutilative behavior. J Consult Clin Psychol. 2004;72(5):885.
Nock MK, Joiner TE Jr, Gordon KH, Lloyd-Richardson E, Prinstein MJ. Nonsuicidal self-injury among adolescents: diagnostic correlates and relation to suicide attempts. Psychiatry Res. 2006;144(1):65–72.
Nock MK, Millner AJ, Joiner TE, Gutierrez PM, Han G, Hwang I, King A, Naifeh JA, Sampson NA, Zaslavsky AM, Stein MB. Risk factors for the transition from suicide ideation to suicide attempt: results from the Army study to assess risk and resilience in Servicemembers (Army STARRS). J Abnorm Psychol. 2018;127(2):139.
Nolen-Hoeksema, S. Abnormal Psychology. Paperback. 2019.

Nolan SA, Roberts JE, Gotlib IH. Neuroticism and ruminative response style as predictors of change in depressive symptomatology. Cogn Ther Res. 1998;22(5):445–55.
Nolen-Hoeksema S, Harrell ZA. Rumination, depression, and alcohol use: tests of gender differences. J Cogn Psychother. 2001;16(4):391–403.
Nolen-Hoeksema S. Emotion regulation and psychopathology: the role of gender. Annu Rev Clin Psychol. 2012;8(1):161–87.
Nolen-Hoeksema S. The response styles theory. In: Depressive rumination: nature, theory and treatment, vol. 1; 2004. p. 105–23.
Nolen-Hoeksema S, Aldao A. Gender and age differences in emotion regulation strategies and their relationship to depressive symptoms. Personal Individ Differ. 2011;51(6):704–8.
Nolen-Hoeksema S, Harrell ZA. Rumination, depression, and alcohol use: tests of gender differences. J Cogn Psychother. 2002;16(4):391–403.
Nolen-Hoeksema S, Jackson B. Mediators of the gender difference in rumination. Psychol Women Q. 2001;25(1):37–47.
Nolen-Hoeksema S, Morrow J. A prospective study of depression and posttraumatic stress symptoms after a natural disaster: the 1989 Loma Prieta Earthquake. J Pers Soc Psychol. 1991;61(1):115.
Nolen-Hoeksema S, Morrow J. Effects of rumination and distraction on naturally occurring depressed mood. Cognit Emot. 1993;7(6):561–70.
Nolen-Hoeksema S, Parker LE, Larson J. Ruminative coping with depressed mood following loss. J Pers Soc Psychol. 1994;67(1):92.
Nolen-Hoeksema S, Larson J, Grayson C. Explaining the gender difference in depressive symptoms. J Pers Soc Psychol. 1999;77(5):1061.
Nolen-Hoeksema S, Stice E, Wade E, Bohon C. Reciprocal relations between rumination and bulimic, substance abuse, and depressive symptoms in female adolescents. J Abnorm Psychol. 2007;116(1):198.
Nolen-Hoeksema S, Wisco BE, Lyubomirsky S. Rethinking rumination. Perspect Psychol Sci. 2008;3(5):400–24.
Nolen-Hoeksema S, Watkins ER. A heuristic for developing transdiagnostic models of psychopathology: explaining multifinality and divergent trajectories. Perspect Psychol Sci. 2011;6(6):589–609.
Papageorgiou C, Wells A. Positive beliefs about depressive rumination: development and preliminary validation of a self-report scale. Behav Ther. 2001;32(1):13–26.
Papageorgiou C, Wells A. An empirical test of a clinical metacognitive model of rumination and depression. Cogn Ther Res. 2002;27:261–73.
Papageorgiou C, Wells A. An empirical test of a clinical metacognitive model of rumination and depression. Cogn Ther Res. 2003;27:261–73.
Papageorgiou C, Wells A, editors. Depressive rumination: nature, theory and treatment. Wiley; 2004.
Pechtel P, Harris J, Karl A, Clunies-Ross C, Bower S, Moberly NJ, Pizzagalli DA, Watkins ER. Emerging ecophenotype: reward anticipation is linked to high-risk behaviours after sexual abuse. Soc Cogn Affect Neurosci. 2022;17(11):1035–43.
Pedersen WC, Denson TF, Goss RJ, Vasquez EA, Kelley NJ, Miller N. The impact of rumination on aggressive thoughts, feelings, arousal, and behaviour. Br J Soc Psychol. 2011;50(2):281–301.
Pelta C. Emotional cascade model and deep learning. Int J Adv Comput Sci Appl. 2021;12(8):363.
Peters JR, Eisenlohr-Moul TA, Upton BT, Talavera NA, Folsom JJ, Baer RA. Characteristics of repetitive thought associated with borderline personality features: a multimodal investigation of ruminative content and style. J Psychopathol Behav Assess. 2017;39(3):456–66.
Pont A, Rhee SH, Corley RP, Hewitt JK, Friedman NP. Rumination and psychopathology: are anger and depressive rumination differentially associated with internalizing and externalizing psychopathology? Clin Psychol Sci. 2018;6(1):18–31.
Ramos-Cejudo J, Salguero JM, Kannis-Dymand L, García-Sancho E, Love S. Anger rumination in Australia and Spain: validation of the Anger Rumination Scale. Aust J Psychol. 2017;69(4):293–302.

Rania M, Monell E, Sjölander A, Bulik CM. Emotion dysregulation and suicidality in eating disorders. Int J Eat Disord. 2021;54(3):313–25.
Raikes HA, Thompson RA. Family emotional climate, attachment security and young children's emotion knowledge in a high risk sample. Br J Dev Psychol. 2006;24(1):89–104.
Rose AJ, Carlson W, Waller EM. Prospective associations of co-rumination with friendship and emotional adjustment: considering the socioemotional trade-offs of co-rumination. Dev Psychol. 2007;43(4):1019.
Rosenthal MZ, Cheavens JS, Lejuez CW, Lynch TR. Thought suppression mediates the relationship between negative affect and borderline personality disorder symptoms. Behav Res Ther. 2005;43(9):1173–85.
Rudaizky D, MacLeod C. Anxiety reactivity and anxiety perseveration represent independent dimensions of anxiety vulnerability: an in vivo study. Anxiety Stress Coping. 2014;27(4):361–75.
Rusting CL, Nolen-Hoeksema S. Regulating responses to anger: effects of rumination and distraction on angry mood. J Pers Soc Psychol. 1998;74(3):790.
Sachse S, Keville S, Feigenbaum J. A feasibility study of mindfulness-based cognitive therapy for individuals with borderline personality disorder. Psychol Psychother Theory Res Pract. 2011;84(2):184–200.
Sadeh N, Baskin-Sommers A. Risky, impulsive, and self-destructive behavior questionnaire (RISQ): a validation study. Assessment. 2017;24(8):1080–94.
Salkovskis P, Shafran R, Rachman S, Freeston MH. Multiple pathways to inflated responsibility beliefs in obsessional problems: possible origins and implications for therapy and research. Behav Res Ther. 1999;37(11):1055–72.
Salovey P. Mood-induced self-focused attention. J Pers Soc Psychol. 1992;62(4):699.
Sansone RA, Sansone LA. Rumination: relationships with physical health. Innov Clin Neurosci. 2012;9(2):29.
Sansone RA, Watts DA, Wiederman MW. Pain and pain catastrophizing among internal medicine outpatients with borderline personality symptomatology: a cross-sectional self-report survey. Prim Care Companion CNS Disord. 2013;15(5):27071.
Santa Maria A, Reichert F, Hummel SB, Ehring T. Effects of rumination on intrusive memories: does processing mode matter? J Behav Ther Exp Psychiatry. 2012;43(3):901–9.
Sauer C, Sheppes G, Lackner HK, Arens EA, Tarrasch R, Barnow S. Emotion regulation choice in female patients with borderline personality disorder: findings from self-reports and experimental measures. Psychiatry Res. 2016;242:375–84.
Sauer-Zavala SE, Geiger PJ, Baer RA. The effect of anger rumination in the relationship between borderline personality disorder symptoms and precursors. J Personal Disord. 2013;27(4):465–72.
Seah TH, Coifman KG. Emotion differentiation and behavioral dysregulation in clinical and nonclinical samples: a meta-analysis. Emotion. 2022;22(7):1686.
Selby EA. Understanding the relationship between emotional and behavioral dysregulation: a cascade of emotions; 2007.
Selby EA. A real-time evaluation of emotional cascades in borderline personality disorder. Doctoral dissertation, The Florida State University; 2011.
Selby EA, Gardner K. A latent profile analysis of suicidal and self-injurious behavior, other dysregulated behaviors, and borderline personality disorder symptoms. J Exp Psychopathol. 2015;6(4):356–68.
Selby EA, Joiner TE Jr. Cascades of emotion: the emergence of borderline personality disorder from emotional and behavioral dysregulation. Rev Gen Psychol. 2009;13(3):219–29.
Selby EA, Joiner TE Jr. Emotional cascades as prospective predictors of dysregulated behaviors in borderline personality disorder. Personal Disord Theory Res Treat. 2013;4(2):168.
Selby EA, Anestis MD, Joiner TE. Understanding the relationship between emotional and behavioral dysregulation: emotional cascades. Behav Res Ther. 2008;46(5):593–611.
Selby EA, Anestis MD, Bender TW, Joiner TE Jr. An exploration of the emotional cascade model in borderline personality disorder. J Abnorm Psychol. 2009;118(2):375.

Selby EA, Smith AR, Bulik CM, Olmsted MP, Thornton L, McFarlane TL, Berrettini WH, Brandt HA, Crawford S, Fichter MM, Halmi KA. Habitual starvation and provocative behaviors: two potential routes to extreme suicidal behavior in anorexia nervosa. Behav Res Ther. 2010;48(7):634–45.

Selby EA, Connell LD, Joiner TE. The pernicious blend of rumination and fearlessness in nonsuicidal self-injury. Cogn Ther Res. 2010;34:421–8.

Selby EA, Bender TW, Gordon KH, Nock MK, Joiner TE Jr. Non-suicidal self-injury (NSSI) disorder: a preliminary study. Pers Disord Theory Res Treat. 2012a;3:167–75.

Selby EA, Doyle P, Crosby RD, Wonderlich SA, Engel SG, Mitchell JD, Le Grange D. Momentary emotion surrounding bulimic behaviors in women with bulimia nervosa and borderline personality disorder. J Psychiatr Res. 2012b;46(11):1492–500.

Selby EA, Franklin J, Carson-Wong A, Rizvi SL. Emotional cascades and self-injury: investigating instability of rumination and negative emotion. J Clin Psychol. 2013a;69(12):1213–27.

Selby EA, Ribeiro JD, Joiner TE Jr. What dreams may come: emotional cascades and nightmares in borderline personality disorder. Dreaming. 2013b;23(2):126.

Selby EA, Yen S, Spirito A. Time varying prediction of thoughts of death and suicidal ideation in adolescents: weekly ratings over 6-month follow-up. J Clin Child Adolesc Psychol. 2013c;42(4):481–95.

Selby EA, Kranzler A, Panza E. Development of emotional cascades in borderline personality disorder. In: Handbook of borderline personality disorder in children and adolescents. New York: Springer New York; 2014a. p. 159–76.

Selby EA, Joiner TE Jr, Ribeiro JD. Comprehensive theories of suicidal. In: The Oxford handbook of suicide and self-injury. Oxford University Press; 2014b. p. 286.

Selby EA, Nock MK, Kranzler A. How does self-injury feel? Examining automatic positive reinforcement in adolescent self-injurers with experience sampling. Psychiatry Res. 2014c;215(2):417–23.

Selby EA, Cornelius T, Fehling KB, Kranzler A, Panza EA, Lavender JM, Wonderlich SA, Crosby RD, Engel SG, Mitchell JE, Crow SJ. A perfect storm: examining the synergistic effects of negative and positive emotional instability on promoting weight loss activities in anorexia nervosa. Front Psychol. 2015a;6:1260.

Selby EA, Kranzler A, Fehling KB, Panza E. Nonsuicidal self-injury disorder: the path to diagnostic validity and final obstacles. Clin Psychol Rev. 2015b;38:79–91.

Selby EA, Fehling KB, Panza EA, Kranzler A. Rumination, mindfulness, and borderline personality disorder symptoms. Mindfulness. 2016;7:228–35.

Selby EA, Kranzler A, Lindqvist J, Fehling KB, Brillante J, Yuan F, Gao X, Miller AL. The dynamics of pain during nonsuicidal self-injury. Clin Psychol Sci. 2019a;7(2):302–20.

Selby EA, Panza E, Plasencia M. Positive emotion dysregulation in eating disorders and obesity. In: The Oxford handbook of positive emotion and psychopathology. Oxford University Press; 2019b. p. 424–43.

Selby EA, Coniglio KA. Positive emotion and motivational dynamics in anorexia nervosa: a positive emotion amplification model (PE-AMP). Psychol Rev. 2020;127(5):853.

Selby EA, Harnedy LE, Hiner M, Kim J. Developmental and momentary dynamics in the onset and maintenance of nonsuicidal self-injurious behavior and borderline personality disorder. Curr Psychiatry Rep. 2022;24(12):897–909.

Sheppes G, Meiran N. Better late than never? On the dynamics of online regulation of sadness using distraction and cognitive reappraisal. Personal Soc Psychol Bull. 2007;33(11):1518–32.

Sheppes G, Meiran N. Divergent cognitive costs for online forms of reappraisal and distraction. Emotion. 2008;8(6):870.

Sheppes G, Levin Z. Emotion regulation choice: selecting between cognitive regulation strategies to control emotion. Front Hum Neurosci. 2013;7:179.

Sheppes G, Scheibe S, Suri G, Gross JJ. Emotion-regulation choice. Psychol Sci. 2011;22(11):1391–6.

Sheppes G, Brady WJ, Samson AC. In (visual) search for a new distraction: the efficiency of a novel attentional deployment versus semantic meaning regulation strategies. Front Psychol. 2014;5:77367.

Shneidman ES. The suicidal mind. USA: Oxford University Press; 1998.

Siegle GJ, Steinhauer SR, Thase ME, Stenger VA, Carter CS. Can't shake that feeling: event-related fMRI assessment of sustained amygdala activity in response to emotional information in depressed individuals. Biol Psychiatry. 2002;51(9):693–707.

Simpson WB. Borderline personality disorder: dimension or category? A maximum covariance analysis. Boston University; 1994.

Slabbert A, Hasking P, Boyes M. Riding the emotional roller coaster: the role of distress tolerance in nonsuicidal self-injury. Psychiatry Res. 2018;269:309–15.

Smith SD, Most SB, Newsome LA, Zald DH. An emotion-induced attentional blink elicited by aversively conditioned stimuli. Emotion. 2006;6(3):523.

Spasojević J, Alloy LB. Rumination as a common mechanism relating depressive risk factors to depression. Emotion. 2001;1(1):25.

Steenkamp L, Weijers J, Gerrmann J, Eurelings-Bontekoe E, Selten JP. The relationship between childhood abuse and severity of psychosis is mediated by loneliness: an experience sampling study. Schizophr Res. 2022;241:306–11.

Stevens R, Dykstra J, Everette WK, Chapman J, Bladow G, Farmer A, Halliday K, Mazurek ML. Compliance cautions: investigating security issues associated with US Digital-Security Standards. In: NDSS; 2020.

Stevens AK, Blanchard BE, Littlefield AK. Impulsive dispositions and alcohol: what we know, how we know it, and where to go from here. Borderline Pers Disord Emot Dysregul. 2018;5:1–10.

Sukhodolsky DG, Golub A, Cromwell EN. Development and validation of the anger rumination scale. Personal Individ Differ. 2001;31(5):689–700.

Sullivan MJ, Bishop SR, Pivik J. The pain catastrophizing scale: development and validation. Psychol Assess. 1995;7(4):524.

Suyemoto KL. The functions of self-mutilation. Clin Psychol Rev. 1998;18(5):531–54.

Thompson B. Foundations of behavioral statistics: an insight-based approach. Guilford Press; 2006.

Thomsen DK, Mehlsen MY, Viidik A, Sommerlund B, Zachariae R. Age and gender differences in negative affect—is there a role for emotion regulation? Personal Individ Differ. 2005;38(8):1935–46.

Tomko RL, Trull TJ, Wood PK, Sher KJ. Characteristics of borderline personality disorder in a community sample: comorbidity, treatment utilization, and general functioning. J Personal Disord. 2014;28(5):734–50.

Tonta KE, Boyes M, Howell J, McEvoy P, Johnson A, Hasking P. Modeling pathways to nonsuicidal self-injury: the roles of perfectionism, negative affect, rumination, and attention control. J Clin Psychol. 2022;78(7):1463–77.

Trull TJ, Tomko RL, Brown WC, Scheiderer EM. Borderline personality disorder in 3-D: dimensions, symptoms, and measurement challenges. Soc Personal Psychol Compass. 2010;4(11):1057–69.

Tsey K, Whiteside M, Deemal A, Gibson T. Social determinants of health, the 'control factor'and the Family Wellbeing Empowerment Program. Australas Psychiatry. 2003;11(supl):S34–9.

Tucker RP, Lengel GJ, Smith CE, Capron DW, Mullins-Sweatt SN, Wingate LR. Maladaptive five factor model personality traits associated with borderline personality disorder indirectly affect susceptibility to suicide ideation through increased anxiety sensitivity cognitive concerns. Psychiatry Res. 2016;246:432–7.

Tuna E, Bozo Ö. Exploring the link between emotional and behavioral dysregulation: a test of the emotional cascade model. J Gen Psychol. 2014;141(1):1–7.

Turner BJ, Layden BK, Butler SM, Chapman AL. How often, or how many ways: clarifying the relationship between nonsuicidal self-injury and suicidality. Arch Suicide Res. 2013;17(4):397–415.

Van Dillen LF, Koole SL. Clearing the mind: a working memory model of distraction from negative mood. Emotion. 2007;7(4):715.

Verschueren M, Claes L, Palmeroni N, Raemen L, Buelens T, Moons P, Luyckx K. Identity functioning and eating disorder symptomatology: the role of cognitive emotion regulation strategies. Front Psychol. 2021;12:667235.

Victor SE, Klonsky ED. Correlates of suicide attempts among self-injurers: a meta-analysis. Clin Psychol Rev. 2014;34(4):282–97.

Vine V, Marroquín B. Affect intensity moderates the association of emotional clarity with emotion regulation and depressive symptoms in unselected and treatment-seeking samples. Cogn Ther Res. 2018;42:1–5.

Voon V, Ekanayake V, Wiggs E, Kranick S, Ameli R, Harrison NA, Hallett M. Response inhibition in motor conversion disorder. Mov Disord. 2013;28(5):612–8.

Wang S, Leviston Z, Hurlstone M, Lawrence C, Walker I. Emotions predict policy support: why it matters how people feel about climate change. Glob Environ Chang. 2018;50:25–40.

Wang Z, Ho SB, Cambria E. A review of emotion sensing: categorization models and algorithms. Multimed Tools Appl. 2020;79:35553–82.

Wang YJ, Li X, Ng CH, Xu DW, Hu S, Yuan TF. Risk factors for nonsuicidal self-injury (NSSI) in adolescents: a meta-analysis. EClinicalMedicine. 2022;46:101350.

Ward A, Lyubomirsky S, Sousa L, Nolen-Hoeksema S. Can't quite commit: rumination and uncertainty. Personal Soc Psychol Bull. 2003;29(1):96–107.

Watkins ER. Depressive rumination: investigating mechanisms to improve cognitive behavioural treatments. Cogn Behav Ther. 2009;38(S1):8–14.

Watkins ER, Roberts H. Reflecting on rumination: consequences, causes, mechanisms and treatment of rumination. Behav Res Ther. 2020;127:103573.

Watkins ED, Moulds M, Mackintosh B. Comparisons between rumination and worry in a nonclinical population. Behav Res Ther. 2005;43(12):1577–85.

Watkins ED, Moulds M. Distinct modes of ruminative self-focus: impact of abstract versus concrete rumination on problem solving in depression. Emotion. 2005;5(3):319.

Watkins ER, Nolen-Hoeksema S. A habit-goal framework of depressive rumination. J Abnorm Psychol. 2014;123(1):24.

Wegner DM, Schneider DJ, Carter SR, White TL. Paradoxical effects of thought suppression. J Pers Soc Psychol. 1987;53(1):5.

Wells A, Matthews G. Modelling cognition in emotional disorder: the S-REF model. Behav Res Ther. 1996;34(11–12):881–8.

Wells A. Breaking the cybernetic code: understanding and treating the human metacognitive control system to enhance mental health. Front Psychol. 2019;10:480104.

Wenzlaff RM, Wegner DM. Thought suppression. Annu Rev Psychol. 2000;51(1):59–91.

White BA, Turner KA. Anger rumination and effortful control: mediation effects on reactive but not proactive aggression. Personal Individ Differ. 2014;56:186–9.

Whiteside SP, Lynam DR. The five factor model and impulsivity: using a structural model of personality to understand impulsivity. Personal Individ Differ. 2001;30(4):669–89.

Whiteside U, Richards J, Martina Fruhbauerova MS, Ghazaleh Shokouhaghaei MA. "I didn't wake up in the morning and think that I was going to kill myself": conceptual model of and intervention development for unplanned suicide attempts. 2005.

Whitlock J, Exner-Cortens D, Purington A. Assessment of nonsuicidal self-injury: development and initial validation of the Nonsuicidal Self-Injury–Assessment Tool (NSSI-AT). Psychol Assess. 2014;26(3):935.

Wisco BE, Harp DR. Rumination as a mechanism of the association between interpretation bias and depression symptoms: a longitudinal investigation. J Exp Psychopathol. 2021;12(2):20438087211015233.

Wisco BE, Plate AJ, May CL, Aldao A. A latent profile analysis of repetitive negative thinking: distinguishing ruminators from worriers. J Exp Psychopathol. 2018;9(4):2043808718811428.

Wisco BE, Vrshek-Schallhorn S, May CL, Campbell AA, Nomamiukor FO, Pugach CP. Effects of trauma-focused rumination among trauma-exposed individuals with and without posttraumatic stress disorder: an experiment. J Trauma Stress. 2023;36(2):285–98.

Wupperman P, Neumann CS. Depressive symptoms as a function of sex-role, rumination, and neuroticism. Personal Individ Differ. 2006;40(2):189–201.

Wupperman P, Fickling M, Klemanski DH, Berking M, Whitman JB. Borderline personality features and harmful dysregulated behavior: the mediational effect of mindfulness. J Clin Psychol. 2013;69(9):903–11.

Young EA, Nolen-Hoeksema S. Effect of ruminations on the saliva cortisol response to a social stressor. Psychoneuroendocrinology. 2001;26(3):319–29.

Zielinski MJ, Veilleux JC, Winer ES, Nadorff MR. A short-term longitudinal examination of the relations between depression, anhedonia, and self-injurious thoughts and behaviors in adults with a history of self-injury. Compr Psychiatry. 2017;73:187–95.

Zimmerman BJ, Schunk DH. Motivation: an essential dimension of self-regulated learning. In: Motivation and selfregulated learning. Routledge; 2012. p. 1–30.

Zuzama N, Fiol-Veny A, Roman-Juan J, Balle M. Emotion regulation style and daily rumination: potential mediators between affect and both depression and anxiety during adolescence. Int J Environ Res Public Health. 2020;17(18):6614.

Chapter 9
The Schema Model of Borderline Personality Disorder

Introduction

Schema therapy, developed originally as an individual psychotherapy by Jeffry Young et al. (1996, 2003, 2006, 2008), is an integrative psychotherapy approach indicated to be effective in overcoming the clinical challenges with moderate to severe personality issues and chronic complicated psychiatric disorders (Jacob and Arntz 2013; Edwards 2022; Young et al. 2003, 2006; Farrell et al. 2009, 2012, 2014; Dadomo et al. 2016, 2022; Arntz et al. 2021, 2022, 2023; Rafaeli et al. 2010), which was first applied for patients diagnosed borderline personality disorder over 20 years ago (Taylor et al. 2017). The concept of schema model and schema therapy has been extending at an increasingly fast pace over the past 30 years (Arntz et al. 2021, 2022, 2023; Chan and Tan 2019; Jacob and Arntz 2012). Schema therapy has been designed for treating the chronic characterological facets of disorders and personality disorders, not acute full-blown psychiatric disorders (Young et al. 2006; Farrell and Shaw 2017; Arntz et al. 2021, 2022, 2023), and is an innovative psychotherapy that has not only been shown to have significant efficacy in the treatment of personality disorders but exhibits effectiveness for other complex psychiatric issues (Skewes et al. 2015). This approach is focused on patients who are not being helped by traditional cognitive behavior considered as the "treatment failures," and has been developed as a systematic therapeutic approach via integrating techniques drawn from several various schools of therapy, including cognitive-behavioral, attachment, Gestalt, object relations, constructivist, and psychoanalytic schools (Young et al. 2006; Lobbestael et al. 2008; Flanagan 2014; Flanagan et al. 2020; Bach and Farrell 2018), and is a theoretically comprehensive model (Farrell and Shaw 2017). Substantially growing body of studies have demonstrated the association between the core constructs of schema model and mental issues, as well as the efficacy of schema therapy in various psychiatric disorders (e.g., Skewes et al. 2015; Van Dijk et al. 2019, 2023; Josek et al. 2023; Arntz et al. 2022; Khasho et al. 2023;

E. A. Selby, M. Salavati, *Theories of Borderline Personality Disorder*,
https://doi.org/10.1007/978-3-031-75503-3_9

Van Donzel et al. 2021), encompassing *borderline personality disorder* (Frías et al. 2018; Bach et al. 2018; Wibbelink et al. 2022; Dickhaut and Arntz 2014; Fassbinder et al. 2016a, b; Wetzelaer et al. 2014; Koppeschaar et al. 2023; May Tan et al. 2018; Josek et al. 2023; Arntz et al. 2022; Khasho et al. 2023; Schaich et al. 2020; de Klerk et al. 2017; Hilden et al. 2021; Jacob et al. 2018; van der Linde et al. 2023a, b; Esmaeilian et al. 2022; Khasho et al. 2023), *bipolar disorders* (Khosravani et al. 2021; Rezaei et al. 2017, 2021; Hawke and Provencher 2012; Nilsson et al. 2012; Videler et al. 2014; Ociskova et al. 2022; Özdin et al. 2018), *depressive disorder* (Mavroeides et al. 2024; Dinger et al. 2015; Videler et al. 2014; Malogiannis et al. 2014; Lim et al. 2018; Özdin et al. 2018; Flink et al. 2018; Davoodi et al. 2018), *anxiety disorders* (Tariq et al. 2021; Taylor et al. 2017; Gewelt 2017; Penney and Norton 2022; Varmazyar et al. 2021), *eating disorders* (Maher et al. 2022; Unoka et al. 2010; George and Franko 2010; Simpson et al. 2010; Huckstepp et al. 2023; Spirou et al. 2022a, b), *personality disorders* (Jacobs et al. 2019; Yakın and Arntz 2023; Renner et al. 2013; Skewes et al. 2015; Bamelis et al. 2014; Salgó et al. 2021; Van Dijk et al. 2019, 2023; Van Donzel et al. 2021; Haeyen 2019; Videler et al. 2017, 2019; Koppers et al. 2020; Marissink 2021), *antisocial personality disorder and violent PD offenders* (Doroszczyk and Talarowska 2023; Bernstein et al. 2023; Schilder et al. 2019), *obsessive compulsive disorder* (Semeniuc et al. 2023; Khosravani et al. 2017a, b; Kwak and Lee 2015; Peeters et al. 2022; Sunde et al. 2019), *narcissistic personality disorder* (Mącik 2024), *internalizing and externalizing behaviors* (Van Wijk-Herbrink et al. 2017, 2018; Van Vilerberghe et al. 2017, 2023; Nijhof et al. 2011; Roelofs et al. 2016), *suicidal behaviors and nonsuicidal self-injury* (Grażka and Strzelecki 2023; Pilkington et al. 2021; Nilsson 2016; Flink et al. 2017; Ha and Park 2022; Grażka and Strzelecki 2023), *trauma-related disorders* (Dutra et al. 2008; Brand and Webermann 2015; Cockram et al. 2010; Peeters et al. 2022; van den End et al. 2023; Lian et al. 2024), *attachment issues* (Langhinrichsen-Rohling et al. 2017), *schizophrenia* (Azadi et al. 2019; Bortolon et al. 2013), *substance use disorders* (Khosravani et al. 2017a, b; Khosravani et al. 2021; Shorey et al. 2015; Boog et al. 2018; Boog and Tibboel 2023; Gerges et al. 2024), *emotion regulation issues* (Dadomo et al. 2016, 2022; Fassbinder et al. 2016a, b; Yakın et al. 2020; Salgó et al. 2021; Csukly et al. 2023), *dissociative identity disorder* (Bachrach et al. 2023; van der Linde et al. 2023a, b), *autism spectrum disorder* (Oshima et al. 2015), *hyperactive attention-deficit disorder* (Philipsen et al. 2017; Kiraz and Sertçelik 2021), and *childhood maltreatment and abuse* (Mertens et al. 2020; Lobbestael et al. 2005; Khosravi 2020).

The term "Schema" has been used in several fields of investigation. Generally, schema refers to a structure, framework, or outline. At a cognitive level, the word "schema" has been utilized in psychology chiefly in the field of cognitive development, especially associated with Piaget's work on schemata (Young et al. 2006). The term "schema" has been derived from information processing theory, a theory describing the storage of cognitive and perceptual information in human memory by theme (Williams 2019; Vonk 1999; Van Genderen et al. 2012). Schemas are the cognitive structures in which various data from early childhood experiences are maintained in autobiographical memory (Louis et al. 2021; Louis 2024; Conway and Pleydell-Pearce 2000). In line with the information processing theory, the experiences are retained in human autobiographical memory by means of diagrams from the early stages of life (Conway and Pleydell-Pearce 2000), and schemas act as filters guiding individuals to order, interpret, and predict the world (Carr and Francis 2010; Van Genderen et al. 2012). In psychology parlance, schema is defined as a pattern established on reality or experience to assist individuals elucidate and mediate their perception and formulate their responses. Schema appertains to an abstract representation of the specified features of an event, a type of blueprint of its prominent components (Young et al. 2006). A schema is an organized structure of knowledge developing in early life and presents in emotions, thoughts, and behaviors (Arntz 2018; Renner et al. 2018; Arntz and Van Genderen 2020), and are relevant to an individual's core conceptions of self, others, and the world (Van Dijk et al. 2019, 2023).

In the early stages of schema therapy establishment, Young et al. (2003) emphasized on the role of early maladaptive schemas (EMSs) as a central pathological structure in the development of personality pathology (Arntz et al. 2021, 2022, 2023; Jacobs et al. 2019). Early maladaptive schemas are presented as the unconditional and dysfunctional underlying beliefs including beliefs about self and interpersonal relationships with each other developing during early stage of life and provide a selective filter for incoming experiences (Young et al. 2003; Lobbestael et al. 2008), are developed at an early stages of child's life resulted by the interaction among the child's temperament, the parenting style of parents, and different traumatic experiences (Young and Brown 2005; Van Genderen et al. 2012; Louis et al. 2021, Louis 2024; Farrell and Shaw 2017. EMSs are defined as "a broad, pervasive theme or pattern, compromised of memories, emotions, cognitions, bodily sensations, regarding oneself and one's relationships with others, developed during childhood or adolescence, elaborated throughout one's lifetime and dysfunctional to a significant degree" (Young et al. 2003, p. 7). Early maladaptive schemas are adaptive and healthy in childhood; as the child grows older, schemas can become maladaptive due to development of EMSs (Young et al. 2003, 2006). In accordance with Young et al. (2006), maladaptive schemas are self-destructive emotional and cognitive patterns which begin in the early stages of human development and repeat during later life. Although experiencing childhood or mistreatment trauma is not necessary for the development of early maladaptive schemas, all of them are destructive in nature, and most of them are made by harmful experiences that are repeated regularly throughout childhood and adolescence. Due to the cumulative quality of these toxic experiences during early phases of life, a full-blown schema emerges (Young et al. 2006). Through a systematic review, found prominent relevance of early maladaptive schema modes for clinical psychiatric disorders beyond personality disorders was found, and EMSs have a central role in vulnerability toward various mental issues (Bär et al. 2023).

Young et al. (2006) asserted that early maladaptive schemas are caused by unmet core emotional needs in childhood. At first core, emotional needs was defined by Young et al. (2003) and Lockwood et al. (Lockwood and Perris 2012; Lockwood and Samson 2020), and recently these needs have been studied and conceptualized by Bach et al. (2018) and Louis et al. (2020). In line with Young et al. (2006), core emotional needs for people encompasses five domains, including (1) Secure Attachment to others comprising Safety, Stability, Nurturance, and Acceptance; (2) Autonomy, Competence, and Sense of Identity; (3) Freedom to Express Valid Needs and Validation of Emotions and Needs; (4) Spontaneity and Play; and (5) Realistic Limits to Foster Self-Control (Young et al. 2006; Farrell and Shaw 2017; Brockman et al. 2023; Arntz et al. 2021, 2022, 2023). Arntz et al. (2018) proposed that the basic needs of children consist of safety, autonomy, self-appreciation, self-expression, and realistic limits (Arntz and Van Genderen 2020). Empirically supported investigations have revealed four categories of EMSs that originated from the frustration of core emotional needs related with maladaptive parental styles (Bach et al. 2018; Louis et al. 2020). Additionally, two emotional needs were added to the original five core needs that lead to the development of early maladaptive schemas (EMSs), including the need for Self-Coherence, and the need for Fairness, contributing to three new EMSs, and Lack of a Coherent Identity, Lack of a Meaningful World, and Unfairness (Arntz et al. 2021, 2022, 2023). Consistent with the schema model and schema therapy, individuals may not only experience adverse childhood experiences, but they also may be completely sheltered and overprotected throughout childhood in ways that contribute to the development of early maladaptive schemas (Young et al. 2006). According to schema model, characterological issues is caused by not adequately fulfillment of core emotional needs during early stages of life, especially in childhood (Arntz et al. 2021, 2022, 2023). Whenever the emotional core needs are partially or not met, whether due to traumatic experiences in the child's environment, or related to parental influence such as childhood maltreatment, in interaction with the child's temperament, may contribute to the failure to fulfill emotional core needs. This maladaptive process results to the development of early maladaptive schemas and dysfunctional coping styles (Arntz and Van Genderen 2020; Farrell and Shaw 2017). Based on meta-analytic findings, substantial associations were revealed between childhood experiences of unmet needs with the development of EMSs in adolescence and adulthood. Additionally, recollections of maternal overprotective parenting styles demonstrated relations with schemas pertained to disconnection and rejection, and impaired autonomy and performance (Bruysters and Pilkington 2023).

Young et al. (2006) introduced 18 early maladaptive schemas with five domains and three coping styles. These EMSs and associated schema domain include*:*

1. **Disconnection and Rejection**, *including Abandonment/Instability, Mistrust/Abuse, Emotional Deprivation consisting of Deprivation of Nurturance, Deprivation of Empathy, Deprivation of Protection), Defectiveness/Shame, and Social Isolation/Alienation;*
2. **Impaired Autonomy and Performance**, *consisting of Dependence/Incompetence, Vulnerability or Harm or Illness, Enmeshment/Undeveloped Self, and Failure;*
3. **Impaired Limits** *encompassing Entitlement/Grandiosity, and Insufficient Self-Control/Self-Discipline;*

4. **Other-Directedness**, *consisting of Subjugation (Subjugation of needs, Subjugation of emotions), Self-Sacrifice, and Approval-Seeking/Recognition-Seeking; and.*
5. **Over-vigilance and Inhibition**, *including Negative/Pessimism, Emotional Inhibition, Unrelenting Standards/Hypercriticism, and Punitiveness.*

Furthermore, Young et al. (2003, 2006) identified three maladaptive coping styles and responses that apply to perpetuate the EMSs, comprising *schema overcompensation* (they fight schema via thoughts, emotions, actions as if the opposite of schema is true), *schema avoidance* (they avoid the schema to be triggered and try never schema be activated without awareness), *schema surrender* (they do not avoid schema as if schema is true) (Young et al. 2003, Young et al. 2006; Lobbestael et al. 2008; Brockman et al. 2023; Farrell and Shaw 2017). According to the schema model, maladaptive schemas are activated in situations associated with the content of the schema, contributing to the emergence of strong emotional parts of schemas. During this condition, an individual experiences the situation emotionally like a child, not cognitively, and also coping style is the same as has been thought during childhood (Ke and Barlas 2020; Mącik 2024; Roediger et al. 2021). Young et al. (2003) proposed that diagnostic symptoms for personality disorders can be identified as a list of coping strategies (Young et al. 2003).

Over time, a second core construct of the schema model was proposed by Young et al. (2003), named *schema mode* to provide knowledge about the development of maladaptive emotional states triggered by the activation of trauma memory (Lian et al. 2024; Brockman et al. 2023; Jacobs et al. 2019), and are an important part of schema therapy (Lobbestael et al. 2008; Farrell and Shaw 2017; Roediger et al. 2021). Because of the presence of several schemas and coping styles in individuals met BPD criteria leading to the complicated clinical manifestations, especially rapid shifts in their behaviors and emotions, applying the schema model would be an overwhelming for both the patient and the therapist to overcome all at one time (Young et al. 2006; Arntz and Van Genderen 2020). Therefore, substantial emotional fluctuations in individuals with BPD contribute to highly undistinguishable problems which made their psychological states more complicated. The construct of "schema mode" was presented by Young et al. (2003) (Lobbestael et al. 2008), which is associated with one or several early maladaptive schemas (Spirou et al. 2022a, b). In line with Young et al. (2006), the term schema mode is the most complicated concept of schema theory due to encompassing several components. Schema modes are presented as moment-to-moment emotional states and adaptive or maladaptive coping responses experienced by people (Young et al. 2006), in which working with BPD would be challenging by the basic schema model (Brockman et al. 2023). Schema mode is defined as "the dominant emotional states, coping patterns and reactions which are activated at a specific time" (Rafaeli et al. 2010; Lobbestael et al. 2008). Schema modes are the current states of emotional, cognitive, behavioral, and neurological conditions experienced by an individual, and are the reflection of partially disintegrated states of self (Farrell and Shaw 2017). Schema modes are presented as the emotional states and behavioral coping responses activated when a traumatic memory is triggered (Jhonston and Vanderstoep 2009), and are a set of schemas and processes which influence an individual's thoughts, emotions, and behaviors in a certain situation (Arntz and Van Genderen 2020). However, there is no fundamental difference between schema theory and schema mode model (Arntz and Van Genderen 2020), early maladaptive schemas are considered as states while schema modes have been assumed as the properties of states, it means that schema modes describe the momentary emotional-cognitive-behavioral *state* of an individual while early maladaptive schemas are more *trait* like (Arntz et al. 2021, 2022, 2023; Spirou et al. 2022a, b), and updated schema mode model has supported the conceptualization of state-based modes rather than trait-based EMSs (Jacob and Arntz 2013). Whenever early maladaptive schemas or coping responses are activated by situations, thoughts, feelings, and memories, schema modes are triggered which may contribute to the development of intense emotional states, avoidance responses, or self-destructive behaviors which control an individual's functioning (Young et al. 2003; Young et al. 2006; Farrell and Shaw 2017). Schema modes have been presented to formulate the complicated combination of individual's severely prevalent emotional states, schemas, and coping responses (Yakın and Arntz 2023; Keulen-de Vos et al. 2017; Roediger et al. 2021).

Schema modes were categorized to three dysfunctional modes and two functional modes by Young et al. (2003), consisting of **Child Modes** (*in which an individual thinks, feels, and acts as a child*), **internalized Parent Modes** (*states in which an individual experiences excessively severe self-punishment and highly extreme demand for achievement and idea standard due to dysfunctional moral criteria and demanding behaviors of parents/caregivers*), **Dysfunctional Coping Modes** (*states in which a person attempts to avoid, escape, or compensate EMSs*), and **Functional Modes** (*Healthy Adult Mode and Child Mode*) (Young et al. 2003; Young et al. 2006; Farrell and Shaw 2017; Arntz et al. 2021, 2022, 2023; Stavropoulos et al. 2020; Jacobs et al. 2019). Schema modes encompass three paths of experiencing the self: emotional memories of oneself as a child (child modes), memories of internalized significant others (prenatal modes), and an inclination to protect oneself (coping modes) (Mącik 2024). Additionally, Young et al. (2003) proposed three dysfunctional coping modes including the Compliant Surrenderer, the Detached Protector, and the Over-compensator (Young and Lindemann 2002; Young et al. 2006; Arntz and Van Genderen 2020; Brockman et al. 2023; Lobbestael et al. 2008; Roediger et al. 2021). It should be noticed that schema modes, similar to schemas, are not only identified among people who met personality disorder criteria, but play a role in everybody. Significantly, the degree to which a mode works independently from other modes and also the strength of a mode distinguishes a pathological mode. In a mentally healthier individual, schema modes are more independent and less maladaptive modes are dominant (Van Genderen et al. 2012). It should be stressed that schemas are appraised according to their intensity, whereas schema modes are assessed based on their frequency (Bach and Farrell 2018). A healthier person can experience a range of negative emotions, such as grief and sadness in an unpleasant circumstance, and can control and regulate intense negative emotions and behaviors. Whereas an individual with abnormal personality traits is faced with various difficult issues across different situations (Van Genderen et al. 2012). In the condition of detrimental circumstances such as adverse childhood experiences (Koppeschaar et al. 2023), early maladaptive schemas and schema modes are developed that are pertinent to coping styles to survive emotionally, contributing to the development of interpersonal dysfunctional coping and instability in emotional states (Van Dijk et al. 2019, 2023). Schema modes are triggered via activation of early maladaptive schemas which resulted in adversely intense emotions, and three dysfunctional coping styles will be developed to deal with these severely painful emotions (Young et al. 2003; Arntz and Van Genderen 2020).

According to modern theoretical investigations, schema modes are comprised of: **(1) Child Modes**: *Vulnerable Child, Angry Child, Enraged Child, Impulsive Child, Undisciplined Child, Happy Child*; **(2) Coping Modes**: *Surrender/Resignation Coping Modes* (Compliant Surrenderer, Helpless Surrenderer, Self-Pity Victim), *Avoidance Coping Modes* (Detached Protector, Detached Self-Soother, Avoidant Protector, Angry Protector), *Overcompensation/Inversion Modes* (Approval/Recognition Seeker, Self-Aggrandizer, Over-controller Modes: *perfectionistic, suspicious, overanalyzing, Scolding and Flagellating over-controller*, Bully and Attack, Conning and Manipulative, and Predator), **(3) Maladaptive Inner Critic/Parent Modes** (Punitive Critic, Demanding Critic, Guilt-Inducing Critic), and **(4) Healthy Adult Mode** (Brockman et al. 2023; Arntz et al. 2021, 2022, 2023; Talbot et al. 2015; Stavropoulos et al. 2020; Jacobs et al. 2019; Roediger et al. 2021).

Maladaptive Child Modes are featured by regression to emotional-behavioral state which have appeared in response to unmet needs (Flanagan et al. 2020; Brockman et al. 2023; Arntz et al. 2021, 2022, 2023). Whenever a person experiences intensely adverse emotions, such as sadness, shame, hopelessness, because of various frustrations in the fulfillment of emotional core needs, dysfunctional child modes encompassing vulnerable child mode, and angry/impulsive child mode, will be activated (Fassbinder et al. 2016a, b; Flanagan et al. 2020; Aalders and van Dijk 2012; Salgó et al. 2021).

Maladaptive Parent Modes present introjected harmful behaviors of significant others toward the patient as a child, as well as introjection of parental norms, expectations, and standards (Jacobs et al. 2019; Arntz et al. 2021, 2022, 2023; Edwards 2022; Van Wijk-Herbrink et al. 2017). Dysfunctional punitive/demanding parent child mode are pertinent wit self-blame, self-devaluation, self-hate, guilt feeling, shame, and extremely high standards. This mode regards to internalized negative beliefs about self and sever standards which have been acquired in childhood relevant to self-destructive messages from significant others, especially parents (Fassbinder et al. 2016a, b; Salgó et al. 2021).

Maladaptive Coping Modes include dysfunctional coping responses to early maladaptive schemas (Jacobs et al. 2019; Arntz et al. 2021, 2022, 2023). These maladaptive regulatory strategies decline the impact of the emotional responses to core emotional unmet needs, but since these coping mechanisms do not contribute to the satisfaction of core needs, can lead to the development of dysfunctional emotion regulation strategies (Salgó et al. 2021). Rafaeli et al. (2016, p. 268) stated "where child modes and particularly the Vulnerable Child capture the helpless and muted emotional reactions of the child, coping modes develop out of a child's basic survival operations: they are primarily automatic adaptation-promoting measures taken in order to survive in an emotionally negligent or otherwise noxious environment."

In *Healthy Modes*, an individual feels loved, acceptance, protection, and understanding, behaves playfully, manifest functional cognitions and emotions, promoted well-being, self-regulation, sense of identity, sufficient activities, and healthy interpersonal relationships (Jacobs et al. 2019; Arntz et al. 2021, 2022, 2023; Edwards 2022; Van Wijk-Herbrink et al. 2017; Aalbers et al. 2021; Roediger et al. 2021). Healthy Modes, comprising the Healthy Adult Mode and the Happy Child Mode. The Healthy Adult Modes consist of integrated adaptive thoughts, cognitions, and behaviors contributing to well-stabilized emotion regulation strategies (Salgó et al. 2021), solving problems and developing health interpersonal relationship (Fassbinder et al. 2016a, b). Whereas the Happy Child Mode encompasses a mode where the core emotional needs are met contributing the feeling of love, joy, play, acceptance, spontaneity (Salgó et al. 2021; Fassbinder et al. 2016a, b).

Schema Model Conceptualization of Borderline Personality Disorder

Borderline personality disorder (BPD) is a severe and serious mental health issue characterized by pervasive patterns of emotional instability, difficulties in emotion regulation, disturbed self-image and identity formulation, difficulties in interpersonal relationships, impulse control issues, problems in identity, and self-destructive behaviors (Streit et al. 2024; Selby et al. 2022; APA, DSM-5-TR, 2022). As stated, Young et al. (2003) introduced EMSs, in five domains, which represent a one-dimensional theme, whereas a schema mode reflected a constellation of schemas and coping styles that are active at a moment of time (Young et al. 2006; Lobbestael et al. 2007). Young et al. (2003) provided this idea that BPD may be characterized by almost 18 schemas (Young et al. 2003, 2006), while recent findings have revealed the primary significance of Abandonment/Instability, Mistrust/Abuse, Defectiveness/Shame, Insufficient Self-Control, Emotional Deprivation, Subjugation, and Punitiveness (Jacob and Arntz 2012; Bach and Farrell 2018). An increasing amount of empirical and clinical studies have documented the key role of early maladaptive schemas and schema modes in personality pathology, especially in BPD (e.g., Carr and Francis 2010; Cohen et al. 2016; Arthurs and Tan 2017; Aloi et al. 2020; Ashiq et al. 2018). Young et al. (2003) emphasized that schemas are stable underlying themes in BPD that are not active at moment, in comparison with schema modes that are active at any given moment and caused moment-to-moment fluctuation (Bach and Farrell 2018). In addition, some studies have identified the association between schemas and the pathologic traits of personality based on the alternative model in DSM-5 (Bach and Lobbestael 2019; Aloi et al. 2020; Bach and Bernstein

2019). In spite the growing body of studies regarding to the relationships between the constructs of schema model and personality disorders, there is no confirmed agreement about the number of schemas recognizing as the prototypical personality type (Mącik 2024). As explained above, there are numerous EMS in patients with BPD presented at the same time leading to a confusing situation both for patient and therapist. These schema shifts in emotional states and behaviors occur very quickly, so that makes the situation incomprehensible for patients and individuals around them. As mentioned, schema therapy was originally developed by Young et al. (2003) to overcome several challenges in psychotherapy with characterological disorders, especially BPD based on concepts of EMSs and schema modes (Young et al. 2006; Arntz and Van Genderen 2020). The combination of 18 early maladaptive schemas and three coping styles contribute to 54 possible conditions which lead to the complicated task of recognizing and formulating the patient's problems based on the schema model (Arntz and Van Genderen 2020). In previous sections, this complex problem was part of what led to the development of "schema mode," also known as a "schema state" by McGinn and Young et al. (1996). Referent to schema modes, Young et al. (2003) concentrated on BPD by focusing on their flipping of schemas, reactions, defense mechanisms, and coping styles. Young et al. (2006) proposed that BPD personality is influenced by five schema modes, the aspects of self, encompassing (1) abandoned and abused child; (2) angry and impulsive child mode; (3) detached protector mode; (4) punitive parent mode; and (5) healthy adult mode. Young et al. (2003) assumed these constructs have contributing roles in the development of BPD (Van Genderen et al. 2012; Flanagan et al. 2020). Alternatively, Farrell et al. (2012) proposed that all 14 schema modes are involved in the development of BPD (Farrell et al. 2009, 2012, 2014). Recent studies have demonstrated that the schema modes presented in BPD encompassing the Abandoned/Abused Child Mode related to intense emotion including sadness, loneliness, and fears of abandonment; the Angry, Impulsive Child Mode manifested in the outburst of anger, hostility, or impulsive behaviors; the Punitive Parent Mode presented by attempt to be detached from emotional pain through keeping distance people and avoiding or distracting from intensely negative emotions, for instance self-inflicted self-injury, dissociation, eating issues; and the Health Adult Mode associated with healthy functions and healthy interpersonal relationships (Josek et al. 2023; Van Genderen et al. 2012). Recently, extra significant modes have been introduced that are weak in BPD, including the Happy Child Mode, Undisciplined/Impulsive Child Mode, and Angry Child Mode (Arntz and Van Genderen 2020). Additionally, van der Wijngaart and Hayes (2018) presented six prominent modes in BPD, encompassing the Angry-Impulsive Child Mode; the Abandoned/Abused Child Mode; the Punitive Parent Mode; the Healthy Adult Mode (weak); and the Healthy Child Mode (weak). According to Farrell and Shaw (2017), modes profile in BPD encompasses the Abandoned Child Mode, the Angry Child Mode, the Detached Protector, Bully and Attack coping, Punitive Parent modes, and weak Health Adult Mode.

Recent Empirical and Clinical Research

To date, mixed results have been obtained from experimental research about schema and schema modes pertinent to BPD (e.g., Bach et al. 2018; Cohen et al. 2016; Bach and Farrell 2018; Lobbestael et al. 2008). Arntz et al. (2005) claimed that BPD cases tend to switch between four modes encompassing Angry or Enraged Child Mode, Impulsive Child Mode, and Punitive Parent Mode (Bach and Lobbestael 2019), while Young et al. (2003) introduced six modes including Angry or Enraged Child Mode, Impulsive Child Mode, Punitive Parent Mode, Detached Protector, and Abandoned Child Mode (Bach and Farrell 2018). Barazandeh et al. (2018) emphasized on the significance of Demanding Parent Mode, Vulnerable Child Mode, and Detached Protector Mode. Barazandeh et al. (2018) identified which modes were regarded to dissociative experiences among individuals met BPD criteria. According to their findings, a significant correlation was revealed between dissociative experiences and the modes Angry Child, Impulsive Child, and Detached Protector among adolescent BPD. Specifically, 58% of the variance in dissociative experiences in BPD were explained by the modes Detached Protector and Impulsive Child Mode (Barazandeh et al. 2018). Lee et al. (2015) examined early maladaptive schemas scores among individuals with and without personality disorders, and concluded that patients with personality disorders reported significantly higher scores of EMSs in comparison with patients without personality disorders (Lee et al. 2015).

Mącik (2024) investigated whether the schema modes are applicable and appropriate for elucidating borderline and narcissistic behaviors, in which they assessed the mutual association between the schema modes to recognize clearly borderline and narcissistic behavioral issues among 467 healthy adults. The findings supported the importance of this theoretically important assumption and indicated that the most significant modes for both borderline and narcissistic behaviors were the Punitive Parent Mode, the Angry Child Mode, and the Enraged Child Modes. The most considerable coping style for borderline behaviors was the Detached Protector Coping Mode which associated with a sense of emptiness and furthermore, narcissistic behaviors was relevant to Bully and Attack, and Self-Aggrandizer Modes which were regarded to aggressive and dominant behavior. The results elucidated 47% of the variance in borderline and 44% in narcissistic behaviors (Mącik 2024).

Since no investigation to date has simultaneously assessed whether EMSs and schema modes can distinguish patients who met criteria for a BPD diagnosis, Bach and Farrell (2018) examined the utility of schema therapy constructs to differentiate BPD patients from other personality disorders and healthy controls. Additionally, they identified whether some combinations of schemas and schema modes are unique to patients with BPD. Findings demonstrated that schemas of Mistrust/Abuse, and Defectiveness/Shame along with modes of Angry Child, Impulsive Child, and low Happy Child uniquely differentiated BPD from other personality disorder group. Furthermore, schemas of Mistrust/Abuse, Defectiveness/Shame, and Insufficient Self-Control along with modes of Vulnerable Child, Enraged Child, and low Happy Child uniquely differentiated BPD from a healthy control group (Bach and Farrell 2018).

Extreme shifts in emotions, cognitions, and behaviors occur in dissociative identity disorder which emerge in other severe mental issues, especially BPD due to adverse childhood experiences, which schema model have conceptualized and elucidated (Lobbestael et al. 2005; Bachrach et al. 2023). Khosravi (2020) investigated the mediating role of EMSs in the association between experiencing of childhood maltreatment and dissociation among 152 patients with BP pathology. The results indicated the key role of schema therapy in declining dissociative symptoms to emotional stimuli related to emotional neglect, vulnerability to harm, and defectiveness/shame (Khosravi 2020). In line with cross-sectional research, Van Wijk-Herbrink et al. (2017) studied the association between adolescent internalizing and externalizing behaviors and EMSs, coping responses, and schema modes among 699 adolescents. They concentrated on EMSs pertained to experiences of disconnection and rejection encompassing vulnerable emotions including shame, mistrust, deprivation, abandonment, and isolation/alienation. The findings showed association between experiencing of abandonment and rejection with both externalizing and internalizing behavioral problems, and also coping styles and schema modes indicated a mediating role in these associations (Van Wijk-Herbrink et al. 2017).

in one final note, a systematic review across mental health disorders conducted by Taylor et al. (2017), it was found that schema therapy can be considered as an effective and efficient psychotherapy to mitigate EMSs and symptoms of a wide range of psychiatric disorders and personality disorders, especially BPD. Based on these meta-analytic results, schema therapy exerts a considerable reduction in EMSs and is effective in ameliorating symptoms of personality disorders (Taylor et al. 2017). Furthermore, Koppers et al. (2020) showed EMS and schema modes together anticipated enhancements in global distress after psychotherapy (Koppers et al. 2020). Therefore, work on the underlying role of maladaptive schemas in the development of BPD should continue, as well as further investigation on the utility and treatment mechanisms of schema therapy in helping those with BPD.

To sum up, early maladaptive schemas (EMSs) have been presented as a core psychopathological structure in the development of personality pathology, especially BPD. As stated earlier, early maladaptive schemas encompass five domains including 18 EMS which have shown substantially key roles in the development and maintenance of self-destructive emotional and cognitive patterns among individuals with BPD. In addition, it was shown that early maladaptive schema modes have key roles in the etiology of other psychiatric disorders, and personality disorders, as well. It has been found that different complicated manifestations of BPD can be elucidated through schema and schema mode models, including rapid mood turbulences, shifts in their behavior's patterns, and remarkable fluctuations in emotional and psychological states of BPD patients. Moreover, based on several empirical and clinical investigations, schema therapy and schema mode therapy have indicated significant effectiveness in decreasing the severity and frequency of BPD clinical features, such as fear of abandonment, impulsivity, and self-destructive behaviors.

References

Aalbers G, Engels T, Haslbeck JM, Borsboom D, Arntz A. The network structure of schema modes. Clin Psychol Psychother. 2021;28(5):1065–78.
Aalders H, van Dijk J. Schema therapy in a psychodynamic group. In: The Wiley-Blackwell handbook of schema therapy: theory, research, and practice; 2012. p. 383–90.
Aloi M, Verrastro V, Rania M, Sacco R, Fernández-Aranda F, Jiménez-Murcia S, De Fazio P, Segura-Garcia C. The potential role of the early maladaptive schema in behavioral addictions among late adolescents and young adults. Front Psychol. 2020;10:3022.
American Psychiatric Association. Diagnostic and statistical manual of mental disorders. 5th ed. Text Revised (DSM-5-TR); 2022.
Arntz A, Klokman J, Sieswerda S. An experimental test of the schema mode model of borderline personality disorder. J Behav Ther Exp Psychiatry. 2005;36(3):226–39.
Arntz A. Schema therapy. In: Science and practice in cognitive therapy: foundations, mechanisms, and applications. Guilford Publications; 2018. p. 65–86.
Arntz A, Van Genderen H. Schema therapy for borderline personality disorder. John Wiley & Sons; 2020.
Arntz A, Lobbestael J, Livesley JW, Larstone R. Cognitive structures and processes in personality disorders. In: Handbook of personality disorders: theory, research, and treatment. Guilford Publications; 2018. p. 141–54.
Arntz A, Rijkeboer M, Chan E, Fassbinder E, Karaosmanoglu A, Lee CW, Panzeri M. Towards a reformulated theory underlying schema therapy: position paper of an international workgroup. Cogn Ther Res. 2021;1:1–4.
Arntz A, Jacob GA, Lee CW, Brand-de Wilde OM, Fassbinder E, Harper RP, Lavender A, Lockwood G, Malogiannis IA, Ruths FA, Schweiger U. Effectiveness of predominantly group schema therapy and combined individual and group schema therapy for borderline personality disorder: a randomized clinical trial. JAMA Psychiatry. 2022;79(4):287–99.
Arntz A, Mensink K, Cox WR, Verhoef RE, van Emmerik AA, Rameckers SA, Badenbach T, Grasman RP. Dropout from psychological treatment for borderline personality disorder: a multilevel survival meta-analysis. Psychol Med. 2023;53(3):668–86.
Arthurs SD, Tan JC. Personality traits, early maladaptive schemas, and severity of nonsuicidal self-injury. Psi Chi J Psychol Res. 2017;22(3):181–92.
Ashiq A, Riaz MN, Riaz MA. Direct and indirect effect of childhood traumatic experiences on cluster-B personality disorders in adults. Pak J Med Res. 2018;57(4):160.
Azadi S, Khosravani V, Naragon-Gainey K, Bastan FS, Mohammadzadeh A, Ghorbani F. Early maladaptive schemas are associated with increased suicidal risk among individuals with schizophrenia. Int J Cogn Ther. 2019;12(4):274–91.
Bach B, Farrell JM. Schemas and modes in borderline personality disorder: the mistrustful, shameful, angry, impulsive, and unhappy child. Psychiatry Res. 2018;259:323–9.
Bach B, Bernstein DP. Schema therapy conceptualization of personality functioning and traits in ICD-11 and DSM-5. Curr Opin Psychiatry. 2019;32(1):38–49.
Bach B, Lobbestael J. Elucidating DSM-5 and ICD-11 diagnostic features of borderline personality disorder using schemas and modes. Psychopathology. 2019;51(6):400–7.
Bach B, Lockwood G, Young JE. A new look at the schema therapy model: organization and role of early maladaptive schemas. Cogn Behav Ther. 2018;47(4):328–49.
Bachrach N, Rijkeboer MM, Arntz A, Huntjens RJ. Schema therapy for dissociative identity disorder: a case report. Front Psych. 2023;14:1151872.
Bamelis LL, Evers SM, Spinhoven P, Arntz A. Results of a multicenter randomized controlled trial of the clinical effectiveness of schema therapy for personality disorders. Am J Psychiatry. 2014;171(3):305–22.
Bär A, Bär HE, Rijkeboer MM, Lobbestael J. Early maladaptive schemas and schema modes in clinical disorders: a systematic review. Psychol Psychother Theory Res Pract. 2023;96(3): 716–47.

Barazandeh H, Kissane DW, Saeedi N, Gordon M. Schema modes and dissociation in borderline personality disorder/traits in adolescents or young adults. Psychiatry Res. 2018;261:1–6.

Bernstein DP, Keulen-de Vos M, Clercx M, De Vogel V, Kersten GC, Lancel M, Jonkers PP, Bogaerts S, Slaats M, Broers NJ, Deenen TA. Schema therapy for violent PD offenders: a randomized clinical trial. Psychol Med. 2023;53(1):88–102.

Boog M, Tibboel H. Automaticity: schema modes in addiction. Front Psych. 2023;14:1158067.

Boog M, Van Hest KM, Drescher T, Verschuur MJ, Franken IH. Schema modes and personality disorder symptoms in alcohol-dependent and cocaine-dependent patients. Eur Addict Res. 2018;24(5):226–33.

Bortolon C, Capdevielle D, Boulenger JP, Gely-Nargeot MC, Raffard S. Early maladaptive schemas predict positive symptomatology in schizophrenia: a cross-sectional study. Psychiatry Res. 2013;209(3):361–6.

Brand BL, Webermann AR. An update on treatment research for severe dissociative disorders. In: Becoming more disability friendly: trauma psychology and people with disabilities; 2015. p. 9.

Brockman RN, Simpson S, Hayes C, van der Wijngaart R, Smout M. Cambridge guide to schema therapy. Cambridge University Press; 2023.

Bruysters NY, Pilkington PD. Overprotective parenting experiences and early maladaptive schemas in adolescence and adulthood: a systematic review and meta-analysis. Clin Psychol Psychother. 2023;30(1):10–23.

Carr SN, Francis AJ. Early maladaptive schemas and personality disorder symptoms: an examination in a non-clinical sample. Psychol Psychother Theory Res Pract. 2010;83(4):333–49.

Chan EW, Tan HJ. Positive psychology couple schema therapy: a new model of couple therapy focusing on reigniting couple attraction via schema therapy and positive psychology. J ReAtt Ther Dev Divers. 2019;2(2):61–9.

Cockram DM, Drummond PD, Lee CW. Role and treatment of early maladaptive schemas in Vietnam veterans with PTSD. Clin Psychol Psychother. 2010;17(3):165–82.

Cohen LJ, Tanis T, Ardalan F, Yaseen Z, Galynker I. Maladaptive interpersonal schemas as sensitive and specific markers of borderline personality disorder among psychiatric inpatients. Psychiatry Res. 2016;242:395–403.

Conway MA, Pleydell-Pearce CW. The construction of autobiographical memories in the self-memory system. Psychol Rev. 2000;107(2):261.

Csukly G, Farkas K, Fodor T, Unoka Z, Polner B. Stronger coupling of emotional instability with reward processing in borderline personality disorder is predicted by schema modes. Psychol Med. 2023;53(14):6714–23.

Dadomo H, Grecucci A, Giardini I, Ugolini E, Carmelita A, Panzeri M. Schema therapy for emotional dysregulation: theoretical implication and clinical applications. Front Psychol. 2016;7:209621.

Dadomo H, Salvato G, Lapomarda G, Ciftci Z, Messina I, Grecucci A. Structural features predict sexual trauma and interpersonal problems in borderline personality disorder but not in controls: a multi-voxel pattern analysis. Front Hum Neurosci. 2022;16:773593.

Davoodi E, Wen A, Dobson KS, Noorbala AA, Mohammadi A, Farahmand Z. Early maladaptive schemas in depression and somatization disorder. J Affect Disord. 2018;235:82–9.

de Klerk N, Abma TA, Bamelis LL, Arntz A. Schema therapy for personality disorders: a qualitative study of patients' and therapists' perspectives. Behav Cogn Psychother. 2017;45(1):31–45.

Dickhaut V, Arntz A. Combined group and individual schema therapy for borderline personality disorder: a pilot study. J Behav Ther Exp Psychiatry. 2014;45(2):242–51.

Dinger U, Barrett MS, Zimmermann J, Schauenburg H, Wright AG, Renner F, Zilcha-Mano S, Barber JP. Interpersonal problems, dependency, and self-criticism in major depressive disorder. J Clin Psychol. 2015;71(1):93–104.

Doroszczyk M, Talarowska M. Young's early maladaptive schemas versus psychopathic traits in a non-clinical population. Adv Psychiatry Neurol/Postepy Psychiatr Neurol. 2023;32(2):83–91.

Dutra L, Callahan K, Forman E, Mendelsohn M, Herman J. Core schemas and suicidality in a chronically traumatized population. J Nerv Ment Dis. 2008;196(1):71–4.

Edwards C. Personality disorders. In: Mental health care for elite athletes, vol. 6. Cham: Springer International Publishing; 2022. p. 97–103.
Esmaeilian N, Hoorelbeke K, Naderzadeh S, Koster EH. Associations between borderline personality disorder features, early maladaptive schemas, and schema modes: a network analysis in a nonclinical sample. Personal Individ Differ. 2022;195:111674.
Farrell JM, Shaw IA, Webber MA. A schema-focused approach to group psychotherapy for outpatients with borderline personality disorder: a randomized controlled trial. J Behav Ther Exp Psychiatry. 2009;40(2):317–28.
Farrell JM, Shaw IA, Shaw I. Group schema therapy for borderline personality disorder: a step-by-step treatment manual with patient workbook. Wiley; 2012.
Farrell JM, Reiss N, Shaw IA. The schema therapy clinician's guide: a complete resource for building and delivering individual, group and integrated schema mode treatment programs. Wiley; 2014.
Farrell JM, Shaw IA. Experiencing schema therapy from the inside out: a self-practice/self-reflection workbook for therapists. Guilford Publications; 2017. p. 12.
Fassbinder E, Schuetze M, Kranich A, Sipos V, Hohagen F, Shaw I, Farrell J, Arntz A, Schweiger U. Feasibility of group schema therapy for outpatients with severe borderline personality disorder in Germany: a pilot study with three year follow-up. Front Psychol. 2016a;7:1851.
Fassbinder E, Schweiger U, Martius D, Brand-de Wilde O, Arntz A. Emotion regulation in schema therapy and dialectical behavior therapy. Front Psychol. 2016b;7:1373.
Flanagan CM. Unmet needs and maladaptive modes: a new way to approach longer-term problems. J Psychother Integr. 2014;24(3):208.
Flanagan C, Atkinson T, Young J. An introduction to schema therapy: origins, overview, research status and future directions. In: Creative methods in schema therapy. Routledge; 2020. p. 1–6.
Flink N, Lehto SM, Koivumaa-Honkanen H, Viinamäki H, Ruusunen A, Valkonen-Korhonen M, Honkalampi K. Early maladaptive schemas and suicidal ideation in depressed patients. Eur J Psychiatry. 2017;31(3):87–92.
Flink N, Honkalampi K, Lehto SM, Leppänen V, Viinamäki H, Lindeman S. Comparison of early maladaptive schemas between borderline personality disorder and chronic depression. Clin Psychol Psychother. 2018;25(4):532–9.
Frías Á, Navarro S, Palma C, Farriols N, Aliaga F, Salvador A, Aluco E, Martínez B, Solves L. Early maladaptive schemas associated with dimensional and categorical psychopathology in patients with borderline personality disorder. Clin Psychol Psychother. 2018;25(1):e30–41.
George JB, Franko DL. Cultural issues in eating pathology and body image among children and adolescents. J Pediatr Psychol. 2010;35(3):231–42.
Gerges S, Hallit S, Malaeb D, Laghi F, Obeid S. Drunkorexia among a sample of Lebanese adults: the role of early maladaptive schemas. Psychol Rep. 2024;127(3):1175–200.
Gewelt SE. Early maladaptive schemas in anxiety disorders-an investigation of schemas' relation to symptoms in a complex sample (Master's thesis), 2017.
Grażka A, Strzelecki D. Early maladaptive schemas and schema modes among people with histories of suicidality and the possibility of a universal pattern: a systematic review. Brain Sci. 2023;13(8):1216.
Ha J, Park D. Suicidal ideation and suicide attempts among university students in South Korea during the COVID-19 pandemic: the application of interpersonal-psychological theory and early maladaptive schema. PeerJ. 2022;10:e13830.
Haeyen S. Strengthening the healthy adult self in art therapy: using schema therapy as a positive psychological intervention for people diagnosed with personality disorders. Front Psychol. 2019;10:445514.
Hawke LD, Provencher MD. Early maladaptive schemas among patients diagnosed with bipolar disorder. J Affect Disord. 2012;136(3):803–11.
Hilden HM, Rosenström T, Karila I, Elokorpi A, Torpo M, Arajärvi R, Isometsä E. Effectiveness of brief schema group therapy for borderline personality disorder symptoms: a randomized pilot study. Nord J Psychiatry. 2021;75(3):176–85.

Huckstepp TJ, Allen A, Maher AL, Houlihan C, Mason J. Factor structure of the Young Positive Schema Questionnaire in an eating disorder sample. Eat Weight Disord Stud Anorexia Bulimia Obes. 2023;28(1):13.

Jacob GA, Arntz A. Emotion-focused techniques in schema therapy and the role of exposure techniques. In: Exposure therapy: rethinking the model-refining the method. New York: Springer New York; 2012. p. 167–81.

Jacob GA, Arntz A. Schema therapy for personality disorders—a review. Int J Cogn Ther. 2013;6(2):171–85.

Jacob GA, Hauer A, Köhne S, Assmann N, Schaich A, Schweiger U, Fassbinder E. A schema therapy–based eHealth program for patients with borderline personality disorder (priovi): naturalistic single-arm observational study. JMIR Ment Health. 2018;5(4):e10983.

Jacobs I, Lenz L, Dörner S, Wegener B. How do schema modes and mode factors align with defense styles and personality disorder symptoms? Personal Disord Theory Res Treat. 2019;10(5):427.

Jhonston DD, Vanderstoep SW. Research methods for everyday life. San Francisco: Jossey-Bass; 2009.

Josek AK, Schaich A, Braakmann D, Assmann N, Jauch-Chara K, Arntz A, Schweiger U, Fassbinder E. Chairwork in schema therapy for patients with borderline personality disorder—a qualitative study of patients' perceptions. Front Psych. 2023;14:1180839.

Ke T, Barlas J. Thinking about feeling: using trait emotional intelligence in understanding the associations between early maladaptive schemas and coping styles. Psychol Psychother Theory Res Pract. 2020;93(1):1–20.

Keulen-de Vos M, Bernstein DP, Clark LA, de Vogel V, Bogaerts S, Slaats M, Arntz A. Validation of the schema mode concept in personality disordered offenders. Leg Criminol Psychol. 2017;22(2):420–41.

Khasho DA, van Alphen SP, Ouwens MA, Arntz A, Heijnen-Kohl SM, Videler AC. The effectiveness of individual schema therapy in older adults with borderline personality disorder: a multiple-baseline case series design. Clin Psychol Psychother. 2023;30(6):1313–23.

Khosravani V, Ardestani MS, Bastan FS, Kamali Z. The relationship between alexithymia and symptom dimensions in patients with obsessive-compulsive disorder. J Obsessive Compuls Relat Disord. 2017a;14:127–33.

Khosravani V, Alvani A, Seidisarouei M, Amirinezhad A, Shojaee D. Early maladaptive schemas, behavioral inhibition/approach systems, and defense styles in the users of natural and synthetic substances and healthy subjects. J Subst Abus. 2017b;22(2):168–75.

Khosravani V, Samimi Ardestani SM, Mohammadzadeh A, Sharifi Bastan F, Amirinezhad A. The emotional schemas and obsessive-compulsive symptom dimensions in people with obsessive-compulsive disorder. Int J Cogn Ther. 2020;13:341–57.

Khosravi M. Child maltreatment-related dissociation and its core mediation schemas in patients with borderline personality disorder. BMC Psychiatry. 2020;20:1–9.

Khosravi M. Lewy body dementia in an elderly patient with bipolar disorder: challenges and treatment options. Bipolar Disord. 2021;23:736.

Kiraz S, Sertçelik S. Adult attention deficit hyperactivity disorder and early maladaptive schemas. Clin Psychol Psychother. 2021;28(5):1055–64.

Koppers D, Van H, Peen J, Alberts J, Dekker J. The influence of depressive symptoms on the effectiveness of a short-term group form of schema cognitive behavioural therapy for personality disorders: a naturalistic study. BMC Psychiatry. 2020;20:1.

Koppeschaar A, Bachrach N, Arntz A. Timing of imagery rescripting during schema therapy for borderline personality disorder: the LUCY trial. Front Psych. 2023;14:1204439.

Kwak KH, Lee SJ. A comparative study of early maladaptive schemas in obsessive–compulsive disorder and panic disorder. Psychiatry Res. 2015;230(3):757–62.

Langhinrichsen-Rohling J, Thompson K, Selwyn C, Finnegan H, Misra T. Maladaptive schemas mediate poor parental attachment and suicidality in college students. Death Stud. 2017;41(6):337–44.

Lee SJ, Choi YH, Rim HD, Won SH, Lee DW. Reliability and validity of the Korean Young Schema Questionnaire-Short Form-3 in medical students. Psychiatry Investig. 2015;12(3):295.
Lim CR, Barlas J, Ho RC. The effects of temperament on depression according to the schema model: a scoping review. Int J Environ Res Public Health. 2018;15(6):1231.
Lian AE, Chooi WT, Bono SA. The development and the effectiveness of schema therapy on Malaysian female young adults who experienced continuous trauma and post-traumatic stress disorder. Eur J Trauma Dissoc. 2024;12:100427.
Lobbestael J, van Vreeswijk M, Arntz A. Netherlands Journal of Psychology, 2007, number 3 Shedding light on schema modes: a clarification of the mode concept and its current research status. Neth J Psychol. 2007;63:69–78.
Lobbestael J, Arntz A, Sieswerda S. Schema modes and childhood abuse in borderline and antisocial personality disorders. J Behav Ther Exp Psychiatry. 2005;36(3):240–53.
Lobbestael J, Van Vreeswijk MF, Arntz A. An empirical test of schema mode conceptualizations in personality disorders. Behav Res Ther. 2008;46(7):854–60.
Lockwood G, Perris P. A new look at core emotional needs. In: The Wiley-Blackwell handbook of schema therapy: theory, research, and practice. John Wiley & Sons; 2012. p. 41–66.
Lockwood G, Samson R. Understanding and meeting core emotional needs. In: Creative methods in schema therapy. Routledge; 2020. p. 76–90.
Louis JP, Wood AM, Lockwood G. Development and validation of the Positive Parenting Schema Inventory (PPSI) to complement the Young Parenting Inventory (YPI) for schema therapy (ST). Assessment. 2020;27(4):766–86.
Louis CC. Worry and working memory function: investigating interactive effects of worry, basal dopamine, and estradiol on theta-gamma coupling in a female sample (Doctoral dissertation, Michigan State University), 2024.
Louis CC, D'Esposito M, Moser JS. Investigating interactive effects of worry and the catechol-o-methyltransferase gene (COMT) on working memory performance. Cogn Affect Behav Neurosci. 2021;21(6):1153–63.
Mącik D. Are the schema modes suitable for explaining borderline and narcissistic behaviours? Curr Psychol. 2024;43(4):3070–9.
Maher A, Cason L, Huckstepp T, Stallman H, Kannis-Dymand L, Millear P, Mason J, Wood A, Allen A. Early maladaptive schemas in eating disorders: a systematic review. Eur Eat Disord Rev. 2022;30(1):3–22.
Malogiannis IA, Arntz A, Spyropoulou A, Tsartsara E, Aggeli A, Karveli S, Vlavianou M, Pehlivanidis A, Papadimitriou GN, Zervas I. Schema therapy for patients with chronic depression: a single case series study. J Behav Ther Exp Psychiatry. 2014;45(3):319–29.
Marissink S. Schema modes and patient characteristics as predictors of treatment outcome in a schema therapy-based treatment for inpatients with personality disorders (Master's thesis, University of Twente), 2021.
Mavroeides G, Basta M, Vgontzas A, Karademas E, Simos P, Koutra K. Early maladaptive schema domains and suicide risk in major depressive disorder: the mediating role of patients' illness-related self-regulation processes and symptom severity. Curr Psychol. 2024;43(5):4751–65.
Mertens Y, Yılmaz M, Lobbestael J. Schema modes mediate the effect of emotional abuse in childhood on the differential expression of personality disorders. Child Abuse Negl. 2020;104:104445.
Nijhof KS, Vermulst A, Scholte RH, van Dam C, Veerman JW, Engels RC. Psychopathic traits of Dutch adolescents in residential care: identifying subgroups. J Abnorm Child Psychol. 2011;39:59–70.
Nilsson KK. Early maladaptive schemas in bipolar disorder patients with and without suicide attempts. J Nerv Ment Dis. 2016;204(3):236–9.
Nilsson KK, Straarup KN, Jørgensen CR, Licht RW. Affective temperaments' relation to functional impairment and affective recurrences in bipolar disorder patients. J Affect Disord. 2012;138(3):332–6.

Ociskova M, Prasko J, Kantor K, Hodny F, Kasyanik P, Holubova M, Vanek J, Slepecky M, Nesnidal V, Belohradova KM. Schema therapy for patients with bipolar disorder: theoretical framework and application. Neuropsychiatr Dis Treat. 2022;18:29.

Oshima F, Iwasa K, Nishinaka H, Shimizu E. Early maladaptive schemas and autism spectrum disorder in adults. J Evid-Based Psychot. 2015;15(2):191–205.

Özdin S, Sarisoy G, Şahin AR, Arik AC, Özyıldız Güz H, Böke Ö, Karabekiroğlu A. Early maladaptive schemas in patients with bipolar and unipolar disorder. Int J Psychiatry Clin Pract. 2018;22(2):151–6.

Peeters N, van Passel B, Krans J. The effectiveness of schema therapy for patients with anxiety disorders, OCD, or PTSD: a systematic review and research agenda. Br J Clin Psychol. 2022;61(3):579–97.

Penney ES, Norton AR. A novel application of the schema therapy mode model for social anxiety disorder: a naturalistic case study. Clin Case Stud. 2022;21(1):34–47.

Philipsen A, Lam AP, Breit S, Lücke C, Müller HH, Matthies S. Early maladaptive schemas in adult patients with attention deficit hyperactivity disorder. Atten Defic Hyperact Disord. 2017;9:101–11.

Pilkington P, Younan R, Bishop A. Early maladaptive schemas, suicidal ideation, and self-harm: a meta-analytic review. J Affect Disord Rep. 2021;3:100051.

Rafaeli E, Bernstein DP, Young J. Schema therapy: distinctive features. Routledge; 2010.

Rafaeli E, Maurer O, Lazarus G, Thoma NC. The self inschematherapy. The self in understanding and treating psychological disorders. 2016;59.

Renner F, Arntz A, Leeuw I, Huibers M. Treatment for chronic depression using schema therapy. Clin Psychol Sci Pract. 2013;20(2):166.

Renner F, DeRubeis R, Arntz A, Peeters F, Lobbestael J, Huibers MJ. Exploring mechanisms of change in schema therapy for chronic depression. J Behav Ther Exp Psychiatry. 2018;58:97–105.

Rezaei M, Rahmani S, Hashemi SR, Farnia V. Bipolar mood disorder cases hospitalized in Farabi hospital of Kermanshah city (western part of Iran): 15-years survey (2001–15). J Fundam Ment Health. 2017;19(5):575–80.

Rezaei M, Hashemi SR, Farnia V, Rahmani S. Recurrent events model application in determining the risk factors of bipolar disorder recurrence. Iran J Psychiatry. 2021;16(1):68.

Roediger E, Melli G, Marsigli N. Schema therapy, contextual schema therapy and case formulation: commentary on chapter "case formulation in process-based therapies". In: CBT case formulation as therapeutic process. Springer International Publishing; 2021. p. 139–42.

Roelofs J, Muris P, Lobbestael J. Acting and feeling like a vulnerable child, an internalized "bad" parent, or a healthy person: the assessment of schema modes in non-clinical adolescents. J Personal Disord. 2016;30(4):469–82.

Salgó E, Bajzát B, Unoka Z. Schema modes and their associations with emotion regulation, mindfulness, and self-compassion among patients with personality disorders. Bord Personal Disord Emot Dysregul. 2021;8(1):19.

Schaich A, Braakmann D, Richter A, Meine C, Assmann N, Köhne S, Arntz A, Schweiger U, Fassbinder E. Experiences of patients with borderline personality disorder with imagery rescripting in the context of schema therapy—a qualitative study. Front Psych. 2020;11:550833.

Schilder MB, van Der Borg JA, Vinke CM. Intraspecific killing in dogs: predation behavior or aggression? A study of aggressors, victims, possible causes, and motivations. J Vet Behav. 2019;34:52–9.

Selby EA, Harnedy LE, Hiner M, Kim J. Developmental and momentary dynamics in the onset and maintenance of nonsuicidal self-injurious behavior and borderline personality disorder. Curr Psychiatry Rep. 2022;24(12):897–909.

Semeniuc S, Sterie MC, Soponaru C, Butnaru S, Gavrilovici O. Therapists' problematic experiences when working with obsessive-compulsive disorder: a qualitative investigation of schema modes, mode cycles, and strategies to return to healthy adult mode. Front Psych. 2023;14:1157553.

Shorey RC, Elmquist J, Anderson S, Stuart GL. The relationship between early maladaptive schemas, depression, and generalized anxiety among adults seeking residential treatment for substance use disorders. J Psychoactive Drugs. 2015;47(3):230–8.
Simpson SG, Morrow E, van Vreeswijk M, Reid C. Group schema therapy for eating disorders: a pilot study. Front Psychol. 2010;1:182.
Skewes SA, Samson RA, Simpson SG, van Vreeswijk M. Short-term group schema therapy for mixed personality disorders: a pilot study. Front Psychol. 2015;5:124048.
Spirou D, Raman J, Leith M, Collison J, Bishay RH, Ahlenstiel G, Hay P, Smith E. The psychometric properties of the grazing questionnaire in an obesity sample with and without binge eating disorder. J Eat Disord. 2022a;10(1):82.
Spirou D, Raman J, Bishay RH, Ahlenstiel G, Smith E. Childhood trauma, posttraumatic stress disorder symptoms, early maladaptive schemas, and schema modes: a comparison of individuals with obesity and normal weight controls. BMC Psychiatry. 2022b;22(1):517.
Stavropoulos A, Haire M, Brockman R, Meade T. A schema mode model of repetitive negative thinking. Clin Psychol. 2020;24(2):99–113.
Streit H, Keinert M, Schindler-Gmelch L, Eskofier BM, Berking M. Disgust-based approach-avoidance modification training for individuals suffering from elevated stress: a randomized controlled pilot study. Stress Health. 2024;17:e3384.
Sunde T, Hummelen B, Himle JA, Walseth LT, Vogel PA, Launes G, Haaland VØ, Haaland ÅT. Early maladaptive schemas impact on long-term outcome in patients treated with group behavioral therapy for obsessive-compulsive disorder. BMC Psychiatry. 2019;19:1–3.
Talbot D, Smith E, Tomkins A, Brockman R, Simpson S. Schema modes in eating disorders compared to a community sample. J Eat Disord. 2015;3:1–4.
Tan YM, Lee CW, Averbeck LE, Brand-de Wilde O, Farrell J, Fassbinder E, Jacob GA, Martius D, Wastiaux S, Zarbock G, Arntz A. Schema therapy for borderline personality disorder: a qualitative study of patients' perceptions. PLoS One. 2018;13(11):e0206039.
Tariq A, Quayle E, Lawrie SM, Reid C, Chan SW. Relationship between early maladaptive schemas and anxiety in adolescence and young adulthood: a systematic review and meta-analysis. J Affect Disord. 2021;295:1462–73.
Taylor CD, Bee P, Haddock G. Does schema therapy change schemas and symptoms? A systematic review across mental health disorders. Psychol Psychother Theory Res Pract. 2017;90(3):456–79.
Unoka Z, Tölgyes T, Czobor P, Simon L. Eating disorder behavior and early maladaptive schemas in subgroups of eating disorders. J Nerv Ment Dis. 2010;198(6):425–31.
van den End A, Beekman AT, Dekker J, Thomaes K. Self-rated personality disorder symptoms do not predict treatment outcome for posttraumatic stress disorder in routine clinical care. Clin Psychol Psychother. 2023;30(6):1338–48.
van der Wijngaart R, Hayes C. Fine tuning imagery rescripting. 2018.
van der Linde RP, Huntjens RJ, Bachrach N, Rijkeboer MM. Personality disorder traits, maladaptive schemas, modes and coping styles in participants with complex dissociative disorders, borderline personality disorder and avoidant personality disorder. Clin Psychol Psychother. 2023a;30(6):1234–45.
van der Linde RP, Huntjens RJ, Bachrach N, Rijkeboer MM, de Jongh A, van Minnen A. The role of dissociation-related beliefs about memory in trauma-focused treatment. Eur J Psychotraumatol. 2023b;14(2):2265182.
Van Dijk SD, Veenstra MS, Bouman R, Peekel J, Veenstra DH, Van Dalen PJ, Van Asselt AD, Boshuisen ML, Van Alphen SP, Van den Brink RH, Oude Voshaar RC. Group schema-focused therapy enriched with psychomotor therapy versus treatment as usual for older adults with cluster B and/or C personality disorders: a randomized trial. BMC Psychiatry. 2019;19:1–4.
van Dijk SD, Veenstra MS, van den Brink RH, van Alphen SP, Oude Voshaar RC. A systematic review of the heterogeneity of schema therapy. J Personal Disord. 2023;37(2):233–62.

Van Donzel L, Ouwens MA, Van Alphen SP, Bouwmeester S, Videler AC. The effectiveness of adapted schema therapy for cluster C personality disorders in older adults–integrating positive schemas. Contemp Clin Trials Commun. 2021;21:100715.

Van Genderen H, Rijkeboer M, Arntz A. Theoretical model: schemas, coping styles, and modes. In: The Wiley-Blackwell handbook of schema therapy: theory, research, and practice. John Wiley & Sons; 2012. p. 27–40.

Van Vlierberghe L, Diamond G, Bosmans G. Middle childhood attachment-based family therapy: theory and model description. Fam Process. 2023;62(3):1040–54.

Van Wijk-Herbrink MF, Broers NJ, Roelofs J, Bernstein DP. Schema therapy in adolescents with disruptive behavior disorders. Int J Forensic Ment Health. 2017;16(3):261–79.

van Wijk-Herbrink MF, Bernstein DP, Broers NJ, Roelofs J, Rijkeboer MM, Arntz A. Internalizing and externalizing behaviors share a common predictor: the effects of early maladaptive schemas are mediated by coping responses and schema modes. J Abnorm Child Psychol. 2018;46:907–20.

Varmazyar A, Makvandi B, Seraj KN. Effectiveness of schema therapy in social anxiety, rumination, and psychological Well-being among depressed patients referred to health centers in Abadan, Iran. Razavi Int J Med. 2021;9(1):32–9.

Videler AC, Rossi G, Schoevaars M, Van Der Feltz-Cornelis CM, Van Alphen SP. Effects of schema group therapy in older outpatients: a proof of concept study. Int Psychogeriatr. 2014;26(10):1709–17.

Videler AC, Van Royen RJ, Heijnen-Kohl SM, Rossi G, Van Alphen SP, Van der Feltz-Cornelis CM. Adapting schema therapy for personality disorders in older adults. Int J Cogn Ther. 2017;10(1):62–78.

Videler AC, Hutsebaut J, Schulkens JE, Sobczak S, Van Alphen SP. A life span perspective on borderline personality disorder. Curr Psychiatry Rep. 2019;21:1–8.

Vonk R. Impression formation and impression management: motives, traits, and likeability inferred from self-promoting and self-deprecating behavior. Soc Cogn. 1999;17(4):390–412.

Wetzelaer P, Farrell J, Evers SM, Jacob GA, Lee CW, Brand O, van Breukelen G, Fassbinder E, Fretwell H, Harper RP, Lavender A. Design of an international multicentre RCT on group schema therapy for borderline personality disorder. BMC Psychiatry. 2014;14:1–5.

Wibbelink CJ, Arntz A, Grasman RP, Sinnaeve R, Boog M, Bremer OM, Dek EC, Alkan SG, James C, Koppeschaar AM, Kramer L. Towards optimal treatment selection for borderline personality disorder patients (BOOTS): a study protocol for a multicenter randomized clinical trial comparing schema therapy and dialectical behavior therapy. BMC Psychiatry. 2022;22(1):89.

Williams LH. Thinking through death and employment: the automatic yet temporary use of schemata in everyday reasoning. Eur J Cult Stud. 2019;22(1):110–27.

Yakın D, Arntz A. Understanding the reparative effects of schema modes: an in-depth analysis of the healthy adult mode. Front Psych. 2023;14:1204177.

Yakın D, Grasman R, Arntz A. Schema modes as a common mechanism of change in personality pathology and functioning: results from a randomized controlled trial. Behav Res Ther. 2020;126:103553.

Young JE, McGinn L, Salkovskis P. Schema-focused therapy. In: Springer series on comparative treatments for psychological disorders, vol. 291; 1996.

Young JE, Klosko JS, Weishaar ME. Schema therapy, vol. 254. New York: Guilford; 2003. p. 653–8.

Young JE, Brown G. Young schema questionnaire-short form; Version 3. Psychological Assessment, 2005.

Young JE, Klosko JS, Weishaar ME. Schema therapy: a practitioner's guide. Guilford press; 2006.

Young JE, Rygh JL, Weinberger AD, Beck AT. Cognitive therapy for depression. In: Clinical handbook of psychological disorders: a step-by-step treatment manual, vol. 4. Guilford press; 2008. p. 250–305.

Chapter 10
Dissociation in Borderline Personality Disorder

Introduction

Borderline personality disorder (BPD) is a heterogenous disorder (Garland and Miller 2020) which is considered as a significant issue in general psychiatry comprising 20% of psychiatric inpatients (American Psychiatric Association 2022). BPD affects nearly 1–6% of the population (Grant et al. 2008), with a high prevalence in psychiatric settings roughly 10% to 15% (Gunderson and Hoffman 2007). More than 80% of individuals with BPD experience dissociative symptoms which contribute to poor functional outcomes in pathological dissociation (Krause-Utz et al. 2017; Brand and Lanius 2014; Langeland et al. 2020). In this chapter, we will explore the association between dissociative symptoms in BPD.

Dissociation is a multifaceted transdiagnostic phenomena that is notably prevalent in dissociative disorders such as dissociative identity disorder (DID), posttraumatic stress disorder (PTSD), major depressive disorder (MDD) (Lyssenko et al. 2018), and BPD (APA 2022; Lyssenko et al. 2018; Ellickson-Larew et al. 2020; Özdemir et al. 2015). Dissociation has been presented as a process which provides protective mental containment and detachment from overwhelming experiences (Briere 2006; van der Hart et al. 2008, 2022), and even it is suggested as physical analgesia for intensely severe experiences, usually of a traumatic or stressful nature (Nijenhuis and den Boer 2010). Dissociation can be identified as the loss of control or awareness of cognitive and physical processes, which are normally controlled or involved in consciously awareness processes (Campbell et al. 2023), and is characterized by interruption of identity, thought, memory, emotion, perception, and consciousness (Nester et al. 2022). As mentioned by DSM-5, dissociation is defined as a disruption of integrated functions, encompassing considerable discontinuity in sense of self (depersonalization, feeling numbness, watching oneself from a distance like watching a movie), environment (derealization, feeling foggy-like world, experiencing familiar places and persons like strange, tunnel vision), consciousness

E. A. Selby, M. Salavati, *Theories of Borderline Personality Disorder*,
https://doi.org/10.1007/978-3-031-75503-3_10

(such as trance states, nonepileptic seizures, pseudo-delirium), memory (such as disturbances in autobiographical memory and dissociative amnesia), and identity (such as identity confusion, experiencing discrete and discordant senses of self and dissociated self-states) that are accompanied by changes in affect, behavior, perception, cognition, and/or sensory-motor functioning (APA 2022; Brand and Lanius 2014; Salmon et al. 2023).

Dissociative symptoms often happen during periods of experiencing extreme stress, intense emotions, mental conflict, or inescapable threat (Brand and Lanius 2014; Salmon et al. 2023), occur in response to a real or imagined abandonment (APA 2022), and can be chronic and severely disabling (Lyssenko et al. 2018). At a symptomatic level, dissociative symptoms are manifested as memory impairment, subjective disconnectedness from the self (depersonalization), or external stimuli (derealization), loss of bodily sensation and voluntary control, and changed sense of identity (Cardeña and Carlson 2011; Romero-López 2016). The dissociative spectrum is complicated: depersonalization and derealization, the most severe manifestations of dissociation, are considered as self-monitoring and identity. Moreover, there are a series of coincident domains and symptoms, including (a) *emotion* (withdrawal/detachment), (b) *memory* (amnesia, memory encoding shifting), (c) *sensory perception* (changed time, visual or contextual perception, proprioception, analgesia, alteration in olfaction, taste), and (d) *cognition* (limited attention, neglect, confusion, changed related capacity) (Vermetten and Spiegel 2014). Dissociative symptoms are exhibited in two distinct types of representations (van Dijke et al. 2010; Vermetten and Spiegel 2014), including *positive* ones comprising intrusive symptoms such as reexperiencing trauma memories, while *negative* ones are identified as apparent losses including not available experiences to one dissociative part of the personality in contrast be available actually to another part (van Dijke et al. 2010; Frewen and Lanius 2006). Furthermore, dissociative manifestations have been categorized into psycho-form (mental experiences such as memory impairment and depersonalization) (Maldonado and Spiegel 2024) and somatoform including sensory symptoms (i.e., pain, loss or change in sensory modalities), or motor (i.e., weakness, involuntary movement) (Nijenhuis et al. 1998, 2004; van der Boom et al. 2010). Based on investigations, pathological dissociation is a characteristic of several mental issues and psychiatric disorders (Lyssenko et al. 2018; Hendrickson et al. 2015; Roydeva and Reinders 2021; Yayla et al. 2015; Spiegel 2022), such as dissociative disorders, PTSD, BPD, and conversion disorder (Lyssenko et al. 2018), schizophrenia (Holowka et al. 2003), major depressive disorder (Parlar et al. 2017), bipolar disorder (Tuineag et al. 2020), and OCD (Rufer et al. 2005).

Several theoretical models have been proposed to elucidate and conceptualize dissociation, encompassing typological perspectives, dimensional perspectives, traits versus peritraumatic reactions, and conceptual mismatch (Indelli et al. 2018). The first conceptualization of dissociation conceptualizes the experience as existing along a continuum from normative to moderate and then severe. Normative experiences can be considered as an example of normative dissociation, while identity changes are example of most severe of pathological dissociation. In contrast to a continuum, the "taxon" viewpoint has been applied to discuss a discrete and categorical dissociative taxon where most people never experience dissociation, but for those that do have the experience, it is almost always connected with the most severe dissociative states and disorders (Brand and Frewen 2017). For instance, some researchers refer to individuals in dissociative subtypes of PTSD as belonging to a dissociative taxon (Lanius et al. 2014). In line with traditional *typological perspectives*, dissociative presentation is categorized based on the existence of two distinct forms including *categorical* model and *bipartite* model. The *categorical* model views dissociation as either nonpathological or pathological. The nonpathological view of dissociation originated from the idea that dissociative presentation can involve normal aspects of daily functioning, encompassing benign conditions with partially reduced awareness of internal states, such as absorption, daydreaming (Lynn and Rhue 1994), and is considered a natural response to specific triggers such as sleep deprivation and extreme fear (Medford et al. 2003; Hunter et al. 2003). The pathological view of dissociative presentation needs a persistent state involved in long-term interferences with an individual's experiences and the competence to sustain contact with others and the environment, such as amnesia, depersonalization, and identity diffusion (Putnam et al. 1996). *Bipartite* model proposes identifies detachment (*a changed state of consciousness featured by a sense of separation of one's body, emotional experience, a sense of self and its circumstances, and feeling of being disconnected or being in a dream*) and compartmentalization (*lack of intentional control of certain psychological processes, disturbing the ability to provide accessible information to conscious awareness*) as qualitatively differentiated and autonomous forms of dissociation (Holmes et al. 2005). According to the *dimensional model* of dissociative presentations, dissociative processes can impact four independent levels comprising (1) behavior, (2) affect, (3) sensation, and (4) knowledge. Continuous dimensional perspective declared that changed states of consciousness are associated with processing event-related information and behaviors, meaning making, affective experiences, and associated bodily sensations, and a preserved memory capacity is needed to provide a dynamic interaction between mentioned four levels (Braun 1988). The second conceptualizing of dissociation considers dissociation as state versus trait, providing that dissociation is a transient and noncurrent state which is experienced during or immediately after trauma exposure and dose not last more than few weeks, and also it is identified as a trait-like chronic dissociative experiences which usually continues long after trauma exposure (Brand and Frewen 2017; Lynn et al. 2012; Giesbrecht et al. 2008; Carlson et al. 2012). The traits versus peritraumatic reactions model differentiates dissociative traits (*remarkable effect of a person's identity which are more diffuse and prolonged expression in comparison to dissociative reactions*) or dissociative reactions (*a dissociative response that happens during or in the aftermath of a traumatic event which is associated with event-related memory declined, disintegrated or fragmented recollections, amnesia, depersonalization, and derealization*) (Marmar et al. 2007; Briere et al. 2005a, b; Murray et al. 2002). The *mismatch model* has been developed due to debate about the presence of a broad range of definitions of dissociative phenomena and lack of a coherent common ground to discuss dissociative presentations (Brown 2006; Van der Hart et al. 2004). The third conceptualization of dissociation refers to mechanism versus outcome. In the mechanism perspective, dissociation is considered as a psychological process of voluntary or involuntary attachment from one's environment, which is caused through narrowing the consciousness, such as a trance-like state (Dell 2009). In contrast, from an outcome perspective, dissociation refers to psychological consequences of experiencing events, such as having greater risk for high dissociation scores because of experience earlier onset of abuse. For example, detachment can be considered as a mechanism, while compartmentalization (lack of integration between psychological processes comprising identity and memory) can be viewed as an outcome of the process of detachment or structural dissociation (Holmes et al. 2005; Brand and Frewen 2017). Based on literature reviews, several categories have been suggested, including dissociation as the idea of nonconscious and disintegrated psychological modules or systems, which are subdivided into (1) dissociation as the nonexistence of the conscious awareness of disturbing stimuli or ongoing behaviors; (2) dissociation as the coexistence of differentiated psychological systems, which should be integrated in an individual's consciousness, memory, or identity; and (3) dissociation as current behavior or perception, which is inconsistent with individual's introspective verbal report (Cardefia 1994; Indelli et al. 2018).

According to defense-cascade models (Kozlowska et al. 2015; Lanius et al. 2018; Schauer and Elbert 2015) propose that dissociation is, "a part of an automatically activated, biologically grounded set of defense behaviors triggered in response to perceived threats" (Danböck et al. 2024, p. 77). In line with these models, there are positive associations between dissociation and defense responses at low, and negative associations at high dissociation levels. In other words, in the beginning threat contributes to active defense responses (fight-to-flight), manifested by behavioral, physiological, and experiential hyperarousal such as motoric and sympathetic activation, negative emotions, and pain. If active defense is no longer possible, it is assumed that a passive defense response (shutdown) happens, features by motoric, physiological, and experiential hyperarousal such as immobility, parasympathetic dominance, emotional numbing, and analgesia, which help the victim survive the threat. In critical situation, dissociation levels elevate all the way through the defense cascade, causing an inverted U-shaped, nonlinear correlation with behavioral, physiological, and experiential hyperarousal responses (Abrams et al. 2012; Danböck et al. 2024).

The Extent of Dissociation in BPD

A substantial body of empirical and clinical studies have indicated significant associations have been found between BPD and both exposure to psychological trauma and dissociative experiences (Vermetten and Spiegel 2014; Korzekwa et al. 2009a, b), and exacerbated role of dissociative symptoms in the symptomatology of BPD (Scognamiglio et al. 2024). Several documented findings have demonstrated that among a subgroup of BPD individuals with higher symptoms severity and more remarkable severe traumatic experiences, the dissociative symptoms are reported more severe (Jaeger et al. 2017; Bohus et al. 2021; Salmon et al. 2023). Zanarini et al. (2023) examined the severity of dissociative experiences of adolescents with BPD, and also the range of clinically meaningful predictors of the severity dissociation in 89 hospitalized adolescents and 290 adult inpatients with BPD. The findings indicated that BPD adolescents and adults showed nonsignificant differences of dissociative experiences. Further, temperament and childhood adversity revealed no significant predictor of severity of dissociative symptoms in adolescents. In adult BPD, childhood sexual abuse and co-occurring PTSD were significantly associated with the severity of dissociative symptoms (Zanarini et al. 2023). Based on two meta-analyses, substantially higher rates of dissociative symptoms have been reported among PTSD and dissociative disorders compared to BPD (Lyssenko et al. 2018; Scalabrini et al. 2017), although dissociation among individuals with BPD is related to greater level of BPD severity (Jaeger et al. 2017; Scherpiet et al. 2014). Expect patients with dissociative disorders who report high level of dissociative manifestations (Zanarini et al. 2000; Putnam et al. 1996), the level of dissociation is categorically greater in individuals with BPD compared to healthy controls, the general psychiatric population, and even patients with other types of personality disorders (Rodríguez-Delgado et al. 2019). In line with some theoretical models, dissociation is fundamental to BPD, happening on three various levels: primary, secondary, and tertiary. Each of these three levels contributes to different problems and are encompassing different phenomena (Meares 2013). Other theories keep similar viewpoint while proposing that association between primary and secondary levels, and defensive processes and subsequent division in the personality, contributing to long-term issues in integrating emotional experiences into everyday personality functioning (Van Der Hart et al. 2004). Zanarini and Frankenburg (2008) examined the severity if dissociation reported by 290 individuals with BPD and 72 axis II comparison subjects over 10 years of prospective follow-up. The results indicated the overall severity of dissociative experiences among both study groups reduced substantially over time but notably higher in BPD patients (61% vs. 43%), with subtypes of absorption, depersonalization, and amnesia (Zanarini and Frankenburg 2008). Stress-related dissociation is one of the major diagnostic features among individuals with BPD (APA 2022), and more than 80% of BPD patients have experienced transient dissociative symptoms (Krause-Utz et al. 2021). Graumann et al. (2023) studied the relation between baseline dissociation and stress-induced state dissociation in two patient samples: 65 BPD and/or PTSD, 84 MDD, and 44 nonclinical controls (NCC). The findings indicated significant increase in all state dissociation among patients with BPD and/or PTSD and patients with MDD, but not in NCCs. Heightened levels of somatoform dissociation and derealization were substantially related to greater levels of baseline dissociation among BPD and/or PTSD individuals, but not in MDD or NCCs (Graumann et al. 2023).

Despite high rates of comorbidity between BPD with dissociative disorders and PTSD (Chlebowski and Gregory 2012), distinguishing disorder-specific influences of dissociation is perplexing (Krause-Utz et al. 2021; Vermetten and Spiegel 2014). Significant overlap has been reported between BPD and DID; BPD is diagnosed in 30% to 70% of DID patients (e.g., Sar et al. 2014, 2017a, b; Korzekwa et al. 2009b), as well as dissociative disorders (DDs) are diagnosed in 41% to 72% of BPD patients (e.g., Sar et al. 2006, 2014, 2017a, b; Zittel Conklin and Westen 2005; Sack et al. 2013). DDS may be manifested by NSSI, suicidal behaviors, emotional dysregulation, intolerance to unpleasant emotional experiences, and identity issues, thus it may be diagnosed as BPD (Brand and Lanius 2014; Ross et al. 2014; Brand and Frewen 2017). Numerous comorbidities and similarities have been found in individuals with DDs and BPD (Ross 2014; Sar et al. 2006, 2014, 2017a, b; Zittel Conklin and Westen 2005; Ellason and Ross 1995), encompassing frequent experiences of identity and emotional fluctuations, and depersonalization derealization under experiencing stressful conditions, and also dispel great levels of NSSI and suicidal behaviors (Foote et al. 2008; Zanarini 2003).

Experienced dissociative symptoms reported in individuals with BPD are passive, breakdown-phenomena that are reflecting the episodic nature of disruptions in BPD patient's proneness, poor-integrated/disintegrated, perceptual/neurocognitive/affective frame reference. In contrast, the experienced dissociative manifestations in dissociative identity disorder (DID) are active, persuaded, high-hypnotizability-enabled, mental trials to escape pain, repetitively, and automatically (Korzekwa et al. 2009b). Three dissociative subgroups can be recognized among individuals with BPD. The first subgroup encompassing about one quarter to one-third of BPD with minimal abuse histories, who have minimal dissociative symptoms with mild severity. The second subgroup including about one-third to one half of BPD, probably with a history of disturbed attachment status and more remarkable abuse history. The third group comprising severe cases of DID and dissociative identity disorder not otherwise specified, and consisting of 30% to 40% of clinical samples of BPD with highly disturbed attachment and severe abuse histories (Classen et al. 2006; Holmes 2003; Stiglmayr et al. 2008; Ludäscher et al. 2010; Ebner-Priemer et al. 2009).

Experimental findings have indicated significant association between state and trait dissociation and BPD severity and severity of comorbid mental health symptoms. In line with investigations, the necessity of differentiating between state and trait dissociation in personality disorders were highlighted (Salmon et al. 2023), especially it has been found that state and trait dissociation differentially associated with functioning and outcomes in BPD (Bekrater-Bodmann et al. 2015; Kleindienst et al. 2016). State dissociation is defined as a transient symptom, which can be last from minutes to days, while trait dissociation is described as partially stable individual differences in dissociative experiences (Krause-Utz et al. 2021). Studies have shown that trait dissociation is intensified by stress and has notably prevalence in individuals with BPD compared to other psychiatric disorders (APA 2022), as well as state dissociation is associated with higher levels of severity in patients with BPD (Scherpiet et al. 2014). In line with empirical research, two main findings have been found: (1) preserving attention to a target task during the presentation of interfering emotional and neutral data is disturbed during dissociation, and (2) attention–emotion interactions during dissociative states may be featured by great recruitment of attentional and emotion regulation resources related to a blunted emotional response (Winter 2016). Salmon et al. (2023) examined the co-occurrence of state and trait dissociation among 51 individuals with BPD to identify whether state or trait dissociation was related to symptom severity in BPD patients. The results indicated a significant association between state and trait dissociation, as well as a strong association was found between state dissociation and PTSD symptom severity accompanied by a high association with BPD severity and severity of depressive and stress symptoms. No significant association was found between trait dissociation and BPD features and BPD symptoms severity (Salmon et al. 2023).

Despite the diagnostic role of dissociation in the BPD diagnosis and affected population, empirical findings seem to indicate that dissociation is not specifically a core characteristic symptom of BPD, but rather may highlight the existence of dissociation in a continuum of severity in other psychiatric issues such PTSD, substance use disorder, and dissociative disorders (Scalabrini et al. 2017). Furthermore, dissociation is accompanied by a large variety of mental disorders comprising acute stress disorder, panic disorder, mood disorder, and psychoses (Wolf et al. 2012; Steuwe et al. 2012; Lanius et al. 2010, 2012). In one meta-analytic review done to clarify the role of dissociation in BPD, investigators evaluated the extent of dissociation in BPD in comparison with other psychiatric disorders (Scalabrini et al. 2017). The results indicated moderately higher levels of dissociation in BPD compared to other psychiatric disorders, generally. The findings supported the role of dissociation as diagnostic criteria in BPD, and, the results postulated that dissociation may play a substantial role in individuals with BPD but not in all cases contribute to the assumption of heterogeneity within BPD population (Scalabrini et al. 2017). Aligned with prior systematic scoping reviews and meta-analysis, the extent of current research concerning the influence of dissociation on BPD and to explore knowledge gaps has also been analyzed (Al-Shamali et al. 2022). Overall, substantial association was found between dissociation and elevated BPD symptoms, self-harm, and diminished psychotherapeutic responses. Mixed findings were found regarding suicide risk. Additionally, dissociation was related to working memory and cognitive disturbances, reduced levels of pain perception, changed body ownership, no substance/sedative abuse, heightened fantasy proneness, personality fragmentation, dream anxiety, perceived stress and changed responses to stress, increased cumulative body mass index, various neurological correlates, and alterations in gene expression. In line with the association between BPD and considerable dissociative symptoms, it was concluded that this association may have contributed to severely serious and at-risk BPD patients (Al-Shamali et al. 2022; Waller et al. 1996). Severe dissociation is associated with more reports of traumatic experiences, post-traumatic symptoms, behavioral issues, and self-injurious behaviors, as well as lower levels of adaptive functioning comprising higher frequency and duration of inpatients' treatment (Korzekwa and Dell 2009). Three dissociative subgroups have been suggested among individuals with BPD: low dissociation, moderate dissociation, and severe dissociation. In addition, less than one-third of individuals with BPD indicated a great level of dissociation which provided the idea of that the severity of dissociation is associated with the severity of traumatic/abusive experiences and impaired attachment (Zanarini et al. 2000; Zanarini and Frankenburg 2008).

A body of empirical studies have demonstrated a substantially positive association between dissociative presentations and personality factors such as neuroticism, openness to experience (De Silva 2015; Ruiz et al. 1999), and self-transcendence (Grabe et al. 1999). Additionally, negative relations were indicated between dissociative phenomena and extraversion, agreeableness, conscientiousness (Ruiz et al. 1999), and self-directedness (Grabe et al. 1999). Several studies have demonstrated higher dissociation scores compared to normal controls or psychiatric controls among individuals with BPD (Zanarini et al. 2000). Rodríguez-Delgado et al. (2019) identified the most significant comorbid personality disorders to determine whether these comorbidities can predict severe dissociative experiences in individuals with BPD among 301 patients diagnosed BPD. The results indicated the most prevalent personality disorders comorbid to BPD include paranoid (83.2%), and depressive (81.3%). Also, schizotypal, obsessive-compulsive, and antisocial personality disorders showed higher risk for presence of severe dissociative experiences (Rodríguez-Delgado et al. 2019).

In line with the biosocial model of BPD (Linehan 1993), emotion regulation has been proposed as a core manifestation in patients with BPD (Wolke et al. 2012; Glenn and Klonsky 2009; Carpenter and Trull 2015). A substantial body of literature have shown that dissociative presentations are highly frequent in individuals with BPD which may impact psychophysiological reactions to emotional stimuli (Stiglmayr et al. 2008; Barnow et al. 2012; Ebner-Priemer et al. 2008). On the other hand, Briere (2006) explored that emotion dysregulation and high post-traumatic stress symptoms may have a determinant role in identifying whether traumatized individuals develop pathological dissociation or not. It was concluded that emotion regulation issues can be as a mediator for the association between trauma and dissociation (Briere 2006). Recent studies have proposed a new perspective to emotion dysregulation as derealization, depersonalization, and dissociative amnesia, which are considered as dissociative symptoms (Korzekwa et al. 2009a, b). Moreover, dissociation is associated with other BPD core clinical characteristics, especially emotion dysregulation (Bohus et al. 2021). Emotion regulation is a propensity to intensely emotional reactions, as well as maladaptive emotion regulation strategies such as suicidal behaviors, NSSI, risky behaviors, and substance abuse (Gunderson et al. 2018). Strong associations have been revealed between the strength, frequency, and intensity of dissociation and emotional distress (Stiglmayr et al. 2008), as well as impulsive decision-making (Kaplan et al. 2020). Emotion dysregulation is suggested to be a mechanism relating trauma to dissociation (Brand and Lanius 2014). Based on habituation studies, it was found the mediating role of dissociation on baseline startle reactivity among individuals with BPD (Barnow et al. 2012; Ebner-Priemer et al. 2005). Decreasing emotional distress and ending dissociation play a main role in elevating motivation for terminating NSSI in individuals with BPD (Perez et al. 2020), maybe due to declining levels of pain-processing analgesic, which occur during dissociative states (Ludäscher et al. 2007; Schmahl et al. 2004).

Dissociation has been demonstrated to be associated with more intense suicidal thoughts among adolescents with BPD characteristics; however, it did not lead to NSSI in adolescents (Sumlin et al. 2020; Zanarini et al. 2011; Wedig et al. 2012), as well as higher levels of dissociation are associated with NSSI, suicidal thoughts, and suicidal attempts (Brokke et al. 2022). The BPD manifestation prominently features both suicide and dissociation (Conway et al. 2018; Scalabrini et al. 2017). Recent investigations have demonstrated that dissociation can be recognized as a pertinent factor for suicide attempts, and can predict significantly those who attempted suicide over those who ideated (Levinger et al. 2015; Webermann et al. 2016), compared to controls (Mergler et al. 2017). In line with findings, patients with a dissociative disorder reported more self-injurious behaviors and suicidal attempts compared to other psychiatric disorders, as well as psychiatric in-patient populations with a history of attempted suicide have reported more severe dissociative symptoms in comparison to those without (Calati et al. 2017). Individuals with DDs are at high risk for being involved in self-destructive, dangerous behaviors, such as NSSI and suicidal attempts (Nester et al. 2022). Several theoretical models have attempted to elucidate the association between dissociation and suicidal thoughts and attempts. Schneiderman (1980) assumed that dissociation contributes to the development of a constriction of options and tunnel vision, causing suicidal processes. Additionally, Baumeister (1990) identified dissociation as cognitive deconstruction, reducing inhibition to suicidal behavior, and elevating the willingness to escape using suicide. Ultimately, Orbach (1994) cited that dissociation is associated with insensitivity to pain and indifference to body, rendering a suicide behavior as possible. Following experiencing a traumatic event, the interaction of detachment from the body and being exposed to physical pain contribute to considering suicide as an option (Orbach et al. 1996). Nester et al. (2022) assessed the reasons for NSSI among a clinical sample of 156 DDs patients. Six themes of reasons for NSSI were recognized in the qualitative data: (1) trauma-related cues, (2) emotion dysregulation, (3) stressors, (4) psychiatric and physical health symptoms, (5) dissociative experiences, and (6) ineffective coping attempts. The results showed that the substantial number of DID patients reported being unaware of themes contributed to NSSI (Nester et al. 2022). Vine et al. (2020) examined adolescents' dissociative experiences in daily life and assessed the relation between dissociative experiences and suicide risk comprising the independence of this relationship from related emotional and clinical states and demographic characteristics among 162 adolescents. The results indicated that suicide risk was associated with daily dissociative experiences, and this association was reported independent of daily negative and positive emotion and comorbid BP symptoms. Further, the association between daily dissociative experiences and suicide risk was significant in adolescent girls (Vine et al. 2020).

Identity diffusion is another major feature of BPD (Winter et al. 2018; Winter et al. 2015), including experiencing rapid switches in identity, which are reported as incoherent, inconsistent, vague, and fragmented accompanied by incoherencies in cognitions, emotion, and behavior (Wilkinson-Ryan and Westen 2000). These identity impairments display substantial overlap with features of identity disorders

(Campbell et al. 2020). In line with empirical studies and clinical observations, identity disturbances in individuals with BPD is less stable and more subtle compared to dissociative identity disorder (Sar et al. 2017a); however, deficiencies in subjective coherence accompanied with an objective incoherence in thoughts, emotions, and behaviors can contribute to differentiation between BPD and other psychiatric disorders (Wilkinson-Ryan and Westen 2000). Identity and sense of self are associated with low self-esteem and are substantially unstable under daily life situations (Winter et al. 2018), and also negative self-esteem leads to negative body perception (Winter et al. 2015; Borgmann 2014), which is in relation with child sexual abuse (Kleindienst et al. 2021). Identity changes have been shown to be identified among individuals with BPD compared to DDs (Sar et al. 2017a).

Interpersonal relationship difficulties such as rejection sensitivity, trust issues, fear of abandonment, and substantial ambitendency between a severe need for closeness and a need for autonomy are main features of BPD (Liebke et al. 2018; Thome et al. 2016; Seidl et al. 2020). The most considerable issues in relationships among BPD patients include being more sensitive to negative social cues such as angry faces (Kaiser et al. 2017) as well as difficulties in identifying and memorizing positive social signal and events (Liebke et al. 2018; van Schie et al. 2020). Marked association has been revealed between distractibility by social cues such as interpersonal scenes and acute dissociation among individuals with BPD (Krause-Utz and Elzinga 2018); however, the influence of dissociation on perception of social stimuli has been remained ambiguous (Krause-Utz et al. 2021).

Despite frequent reports of child abuse experiences in BPD patients, it has been suggested that not all individuals with BPD have experienced child abuse and adverse traumatic experiences, and also not all dissociative symptoms in BPD are trauma-related (Korzekwa et al. 2009b; Vermetten and Spiegel 2014). Dissociation is a common reaction to sexual abuse (Brokke et al. 2022). Bichescu-Burian et al. (2017) found that BPD individuals with high peritraumatic dissociation indicated a significant heart rate reduction during imagery of traumatic events compared to healthy controls. Also, heart rate responses were anticipated by peritraumatic dissociation, not by measures of state or trait dissociation. Through performing a cognitive reappraisal emotion regulation task with neutral positive and negative images, Krause-Utz and Elzinga (2018) showed both individuals with BPD and BPD with comorbid PTSD reported higher arousal, lower well-being, and more dissociation compared to healthy controls. Additionally, BPD+PTSD revealed significantly lower heart rate variability (HRV), and higher state dissociation at baseline predicted greater HRV (Krause-Utz and Elzinga 2018). Dissociation may lead to elevated risk of revictimization in individuals with a history of child sexual abuse experiences, and studies have shown that dissociation can mediate this relation along with maladaptive cognitive coping styles such as self-blame (Webermann and Brand 2017). Sar et al. (2006) examined the dissociative disorder comorbidity of BPD and its association with childhood trauma among 1301 female college students and 80 students with BPD. The findings indicated that most BPD patients (72.5%) had a dissociative disorder, while this rate was 18.0% for the comparison group. Additionally, childhood sexual and emotional abuse, physical neglect, and total childhood trauma scores showed significant effect for, while emotional neglect and reduced minimization of childhood trauma had significant effect for dissociative disorder (Sar et al. 2006). Childhood maltreatment is a considerable predictor of suicide attempts and dissociation is a mediator in this relation. Dissociation has a full mediator role in the impact of emotional abuse and physical abuse on suicidal behaviors, and also is a partial mediator in the influence of sexual abuse and physical neglect on suicidal attempts (Demirkol et al. 2020). In a naturalistic study, Brokke et al. (2022) examined the influence of sexual abuse and dissociation on suicide attempt among 97 acute psychiatric patients with suicidal thoughts, of whom 32 reported a history of sexual abuse. The findings indicated participants who experienced sexual abuse reported greater levels of dissociation, and were younger at onset of suicidal ideation, more probability to NSSI, and more likely for suicidal attempts. Additionally, dissociative experiences notably mediate a substantive proportion of the association between sexual abuse and number of suicide attempts. Dissociative experiences mediated the role of sexual abuse as a predictor of more than four suicidal attempts (Brokke et al. 2022). Based on providing a primary clinical characterization, Bateman et al. (2023) investigated the levels of clinical functioning, well-being, dissociation, and mentalizing, and they identified whether mentalizing mediates the symptoms of PTSD in the context of BPD among 72 patients with BPD (43 with and 29 without comorbid PTSD symptoms). In comparison with patients with only BPD, individuals with comorbid BPD+PTSD indicated higher severity in terms of BPD and dissociative symptoms, met a wider range of BPD diagnostic criteria, reported greater sense of personal worthlessness and self-evaluated their well-being as remarkably decreased. Additionally, BPD+PTSD group showed a higher tendency to recall escalated instances of childhood sexual abuse. Mediation analysis exhibited mentalizing acts as a partial mediator for the association between dissociative symptoms and complex PTSD, yet no mediating role was found for mentalizing in the relationship between childhood sexual abuse and complex PTSD (Bateman et al. 2023). Sexual risky behaviors in individuals with BPD are assumed to be related with traumatic experiences and dissociative symptoms. Mazinan et al. (2024) studied the association between dissociative symptoms (derealization, depersonalization, and conversion in sexual situations) and sexual issues in 114 individuals with BPD and 114 healthy controls (HC). The findings showed that individuals with BPD exhibited greater dissociative symptoms in sexual situations compared to HC. Further, depersonalization and conversion symptoms in sexual situations were elucidated by severity of BPD, whereas derealization was explained by symptoms of PTSD. Higher levels of impulsive and sexual behaviors with an uncommitted partner were revealed in BPD group elucidated by derealization (Mazinan et al. 2024). Kulacaoglu et al. (2017) investigated complicated association between childhood trauma, impulsivity, dissociative symptoms, and the influence of ADHD on this association in 165 BPD patients and 165 health controls (HC). The findings exhibited higher ADHD symptoms, impulsivity, childhood trauma, and dissociation in comparison with HC. Significant associations were reported between adult ADHD symptoms and impulsivity, childhood trauma, and dissociation scores. Additionally, logistic regression analysis revealed that gender, attentional and motor impulsiveness were the predictors of individuals with ADHD and BPD, as well as gender and emotional neglect were key predicators of dissociation in BPD (Kulacaoglu et al. 2017).

Clinical Implications

Mentalization or mentalizing is represented as a process by which individuals make sense of each other and themselves in terms of subjective states and mental processes, implicitly or explicitly. Mentalization is addressed as a deeply social construct in the sense which leads to being attentive to mental states of those we are with, physically or psychologically. Based on mentalization model, the majority of psychiatric disorders are inevitably engaging some issues with mentalization, which contributes to the mind misinterpreting our experiences of itself, and a disorder of mentalization (Bateman and Fonagy 2010). Mentalization is presented as a form of social cognition, which is considered to be dependent on positive social childhood experiences (Allen and Fonagy 2006; Bateman and Fonagy 2013).

The mentalization theory has been applied in various psychiatric disorders, such as post-traumatic stress disorder (Allen 2001), eating disorders (Skarderud 2007), and depression (Allen et al. 2003), in different clinical contexts, for example, inpatient, partial hospital, and outpatient settings, as well as various group of patients including adolescents and families (Bateman and Fonagy 2004a, 2004b). This treatment method is developed basically as a therapeutic approach for BPD and is considered as central to the BPD etiology (Bateman and Fonagy 2008, 2010, 2013), which have found several empirical supports with randomized controlled trials (Bateman and Fonagy 1999; Bateman and Fonagy 2001). As mentioned, individuals with BPD have shown to have more frequently report childhood maltreatment or other traumatic events compared to other personality disorders or healthy individuals (APA 2022; Ntshingila et al. 2016; Vogt and Norman 2019). In line with mentalization theory, these adversely traumatic childhood has been associated with impairments in the abilities of "mentalize" (e.g., Bateman and Fonagy 2010; Brüne et al. 2016; Peterson 2016). In a normal infant caregiver interaction, infants will be able to find a modulated version of their internal states mirrored by their significant others and caregivers, contributing to developing a representation of their internal states that help them to regulate emotions and affects in themselves and comprehend them in others (Fonagy et al. 2002; Gergely and Watson 1996). A disturbed mentalized response to the infant on the part of the caregivers may undermine the healthy normal development of child's social cognitive abilities, capacities of affecting regulation, and the functioning of focused attention (Fonagy and Target 1997). Attachment disturbances and aversive childhood experiences lead to several obstacles in the development of normal social functioning contributing to disturbances in the capacity of mentalize (Bartels and Zeki 2004).

Mentalization-based treatment (MBT) concentrates on what is thought to be BPD fundamental deficits (Bateman and Fonagy 2010). Mentalization theory originated from Bowlby's attachment theory and is expanded by contemporary developmental psychologist addressing to constitutional vulnerabilities (Bateman and Fonagy 2008, 2010; Laurenssen et al. 2014a, b), and integrates the point that aversive childhood experiences impact the quality of future interpersonal relationships (Brüne et al. 2013). According to Bateman and Fonagy (2009), there are three routes which cause disruption in mentalization. First, mental defenses can be habitually activated to support a person from thinking about the psychological states of caregivers who have hostile thoughts toward them, preventing the development of mentalization. Second, switches in the activity of brain can happen as a consequence of trauma that turn off mentalizing more readily in individuals who experienced trauma. Third, attachment trauma can be generated in a hypersensitivity of the attachment system which may contribute to accelerating pace of intimacy (Bateman and Fonagy 2009). The purpose of MBT is to elevate patients' mentalization skills to promote their functioning in daily social interactions and to achieve higher levels of life (Bateman and Fonagy 2010). The repair of mentalizing in the context of attachment relations can be addressed as a major mechanism of various psychological treatment for BPD. The core aim of MBT is to establish a therapeutic process in which the patient's perception of one's own mind and the mind of other people becomes the concentration of therapy. Therefore, patients will be able to explore how one thinks and feels about oneself and others, how that demonstrates one's responses, and how errors in comprehending oneself and others contribute to behaviors, which are efforts to main stability and make sense of incomprehensible emotions and feelings (Fonagy and Bateman 2006, 2008).

References

Abrams MP, Carleton RN, Asmundson GJ. Tonic immobility does not uniquely predict posttraumatic stress symptom severity. Psychol Trauma Theory Res Pract Policy. 2012;4(3):278.

Allen JG. Traumatic relationships and serious mental disorders. Chichester: Wiley; 2001.

Allen JG, Fonagy P, editors. The handbook of mentalization-based treatment. Wiley; 2006.

Allen J, Bleiberg E, Haslam-Hopwood T. Mentalizing as a compass for treatment. Bull Menn Clin. 2003;67:1–11.

Al-Shamali HF, Winkler O, Talarico F, Greenshaw AJ, Forner C, Zhang Y, Vermetten E, Burback L. A systematic scoping review of dissociation in borderline personality disorder and implications for research and clinical practice: exploring the fog. Aust New Zealand J Psychiatry. 2022;56(10):1252–64.

American Psychiatric Association. Diagnostic and statistical manual of mental disorders. 5th ed. Text Revised (DSM-5-TR); 2022.

Barnow S, Limberg A, Stopsack M, Spitzer C, Grabe HJ, Freyberger HJ, Hamm A. Dissociation and emotion regulation in borderline personality disorder. Psychol Med. 2012;42(4):783–94.

Bartels A, Zeki S. The neural correlates of maternal and romantic love. NeuroImage. 2004;21(3):1155–66.

Bateman A, Fonagy P. Effectiveness of partial hospitalization in the treatment of borderline personality disorder: a randomized controlled trial. Am J Psychiatry. 1999;156:1563–9.

Bateman A, Fonagy P. Treatment of borderline personality disorder with psychoanalytically oriented partial hospitalisation: an 18- month follow-up. Am J Psychiatry. 2001;158:36–42.

Bateman A, Fonagy P. Psychotherapy for borderline personality disorder: mentalisation based treatment. Oxford: Oxford University Press; 2004a.
Bateman AW, Fonagy P. Mentalization-based treatment of BPD. J Personal Disord. 2004b;18(1):36–51.
Bateman A, Fonagy P. 8-year follow-up of patients treated for borderline personality disorder: Mentalization-based treatment versus treatment as usual. Am J Psychiatry. 2008;165(5):631–8.
Bateman A, Fonagy P. Randomized controlled trial of outpatient mentalization-based treatment versus structured clinical management for borderline personality disorder. Am J Psychiatry. 2009;166(12):1355–64.
Bateman A, Fonagy P. Mentalization based treatment for borderline personality disorder. World Psychiatry. 2010;9(1):11.
Bateman A, Fonagy P. Impact of clinical severity on outcomes of mentalisation-based treatment for borderline personality disorder. Br J Psychiatry. 2013;203(3):221–7.
Bateman AW, Gunderson J, Mulder R. Treatment of personality disorder. Lancet. 2015;385: 735–43. https://doi.org/10.1016/s0140-6736(14)61394-5.
Bateman A, Rüfenacht E, Perroud N, Debbané M, Nolte T, Shaverin L, Fonagy P. Childhood maltreatment, dissociation and borderline personality disorder: preliminary data on the mediational role of mentalizing in complex post-traumatic stress disorder. Psychol Psychother Theory Res Pract; 2023.
Baumeister RF. Suicide as escape from self. Psychol Rev. 1990;97(1):90.
Bekrater-Bodmann R, Chung BY, Richter I, Wicking M, Foell J, Mancke F, Schmahl C, Flor H. Deficits in pain perception in borderline personality disorder: results from the thermal grill illusion. Pain. 2015;156(10):2084–92.
Bichescu-Burian D, Steyer J, Steinert T, Grieb B, Tschöke S. Trauma-related dissociation: psychological features and psychophysiological responses to script-driven imagery in borderline personality disorder. Psychophysiology. 2017;54(3):452–61. https://doi.org/10.1111/psyp.12795
Bohus M, Stoffers-Winterling J, Sharp C, Krause-Utz A, Schmahl C, Lieb K. Borderline personality disorder. Lancet. 2021;398(10310):1528–40.
Borgmann CE. The constitutionality of government-imposed bodily intrusions. U Ill L Rev. 2014:1059.
Brand BL, Frewen P. Dissociation as a trauma-related phenomenon. 2017.
Brand BL, Lanius RA. Chronic complex dissociative disorders and borderline personality disorder: disorders of emotion dysregulation? Borderline Personal Disord Emot Dysregul. 2014;1:1–2.
Braun BG. Dissociation: Vol. 1, No. 1. The BASK Model of Dissociation; 1988. p. 004–23.
Briere J. Dissociative symptoms and trauma exposure: specificity, affect dysregulation, and posttraumatic stress. J Nerv Ment Dis. 2006;194(2):78–82.
Briere J, Weathers FW, Runtz M. Is dissociation a multidimensional construct? Data from the multiscale dissociation inventory. J Trauma Stress. 2005a;18(3):221–31.
Briere J, Scott C, Weathers F. Peritraumatic and persistent dissociation in the presumed etiology of PTSD. Am J Psychiatry. 2005b;162(12):2295–301.
Brokke SS, Bertelsen TB, Landrø NI, Haaland VØ. The effect of sexual abuse and dissociation on suicide attempt. BMC Psychiatry. 2022;22:1–8.
Brown RJ. Different types of "dissociation" have different psychological mechanisms. J Trauma Dissociation. 2006;7(4):7–28.
Brüne M, Dimaggio G, Edel MA. Mentalization-based group therapy for inpatients with borderline personality disorder: preliminary findings. Clin Neuropsychiatry. 2013;10:196–201.
Brüne M, Walden S, Edel MA, Dimaggio G. Mentalization of complex emotions inborderline personality disorder: the impact of parenting and exposure to trauma on the performance in a novel cartoon-based task. Compr Psychiatry. 2016;64:29–37.
Calati R, Bensassi I, Courtet P. The link between dissociation and both suicide attempts and non-suicidal self-injury: meta-analyses. Psychiatry Res. 2017;251:103–14.
Campbell K, Clarke KA, Massey D, Lakeman R. Borderline personality disorder: to diagnose or not to diagnose? That is the question. Int J Ment Health Nurs. 2020;29(5):972–81.

Campbell MC, Smakowski A, Rojas-Aguiluz M, Goldstein LH, Cardeña E, Nicholson TR, Reinders AA, Pick S. Dissociation and its biological and clinical associations in functional neurological disorder: systematic review and meta-analysis. BJPsych Open. 2023;9(1):e2.

Carlson EB, Dalenberg C, McDade-Montez E. Dissociation in posttraumatic stress disorder. Part I: Definitions and review of research. Psychol Trauma Theory Res Pract Policy. 2012;4(5):479.

Carpenter RW, Trull TJ. The pain paradox: borderline personality disorder features, self-harm history, and the experience of pain. Personal Disord Theory Res Treat. 2015;6(2):141.

Cardeña E, Carlson E. Acute stress disorder revisited. Annu Rev Clin Psychol. 2011;7(1):245–67.

Cardefia E. The domain of dissociation. Dissociation: clinical and theoretical perspectives. 1994; pp. 15–31.

Chlebowski SM, Gregory RJ. Three cases of dissociative identity disorder and co-occurring borderline personality disorder treated with dynamic deconstructive psychotherapy. Am J Psychother. 2012;66(2):165–80.

Classen CC, Pain C, Field NP, Woods P. Posttraumatic personality disorder: A reformulation of complex posttraumatic stress disorder and borderline personality disorder. Psychiatr Clin. 2006;29(1):87–112.

Conway P, Goldstein-Greenwood J, Polacek D, Greene JD. Sacrificial utilitarian judgments do reflect concern for the greater good: clarification via process dissociation and the judgments of philosophers. Cognition. 2018;179:241–65.

Danböck SK, Duek O, Ben-Zion Z, Korem N, Amen SL, Kelmendi B, Wilhelm FH, Levy I, Harpaz-Rotem I. Effects of a dissociative drug on fronto-limbic resting-state functional connectivity in individuals with posttraumatic stress disorder: a randomized controlled pilot study. Psychopharmacology. 2024;241(2):243–52.

Demirkol ME, Uğur K, Tamam L. The mediating effects of psychache and dissociation in the relationship between childhood trauma and suicide attempts. Anadolu Psikiyatri Dergisi. 2020;21(5):453–60.

De Silva N. The relationship between childhood abuse and dissociation. Alliant International University; 2015.

Dell PF. Understanding dissociation. 2009.

Ebner-Priemer UW, Badeck S, Beckmann C, Wagner A, Feige B, Weiss I, Lieb K, Bohus M. Affective dysregulation and dissociative experience in female patients with borderline personality disorder: a startle response study. J Psychiatr Res. 2005;39(1):85–92.

Ebner-Priemer UW, Kuo J, Schlotz W, Kleindienst N, Rosenthal MZ, Detterer L, Linehan MM, Bohus M. Distress and affective dysregulation in patients with borderline personality disorder: a psychophysiological ambulatory monitoring study. J Nerv Ment Dis. 2008;196(4):314–20.

Ebner-Priemer UW, Mauchnik J, Kleindienst N, Schmahl C, Peper M, Rosenthal MZ, Flor H, Bohus M. Emotional learning during dissociative states in borderline personality disorder. J Psychiatry Neurosci. 2009;34(3):214–22.

Ellason JW, Ross CA. Positive and negative symptoms in dissociative identity disorder and schizophrenia: a comparative analysis. J Nerv Ment Dis. 1995;183(4):236–41.

Ellickson-Larew S, Stasik-O'Brien SM, Stanton K, Watson D. Dissociation as a multidimensional transdiagnostic symptom. Psychol Conscious Theory Res Pract. 2020;7(2):126.

Fonagy P, Bateman AW. Mechanisms of change in mentalisation-based therapy with BPD. J Clin Psychol. 2006;62(4):411–30.

Fonagy P, Bateman A. The development of borderline personality disorder – a mentalizing model. J Personal Disord. 2008;22(1):4–21.

Fonagy P, Target M. Attachment and reflective function: their role in self-organization. Dev Psychopathol. 1997;9(4):679–700.

Fonagy P, Gergely G, Jurist E, Target M. Affect regulation, mentalization, and the development of the self. New York: Other Press; 2002.

Foote B, Smolin Y, Neft DI, Lipschitz D. Dissociative disorders and suicidality in psychiatric outpatients. J Nerv Ment Dis. 2008;196(1):29–36.

Frewen PA, Lanius RA. Toward a psychobiology of posttraumatic self-dysregulation: Reexperiencing, hyperarousal, dissociation, and emotional numbing. Ann N Y Acad Sci. 2006;1071(1):110–24.

Garland J, Miller S. Borderline personality disorder: part 1–assessment and diagnosis. BJPsych Advances. 2020;26(3):159–72.

Gergely G, Watson JS. The social biofeedback theory of parental affect-mirroring: the development of emotional self-awareness and self-control in infancy. Int J Psychoanal. 1996;77(Pt 6):1181–212.

Giesbrecht T, Lynn SJ, Lilienfeld SO, Merckelbach H. Cognitive processes in dissociation: an analysis of core theoretical assumptions. Psychol Bull. 2008;134(5):617.

Glenn CR, Klonsky ED. Social context during nonsuicidal self-injury indicates suicide risk. Personal Individ Differ. 2009;46(1):25–9.

Grabe HJ, Spitzer C, Freyberger HJ. Relationship of dissociation to temperament and character in men and women. Am J Psychiatry. 1999;156(11):1811–3.

Grant BF, Chou SP, Goldstein RB, Huang B, Stinson FS, Saha TD, Smith SM, Dawson DA, Pulay AJ, Pickering RP, Ruan WJ. Prevalence, correlates, disability, and comorbidity of DSM-IV borderline personality disorder: results from the Wave 2 National Epidemiologic Survey on Alcohol and Related Conditions. J Clin Psychiatry. 2008;69(4):533.

Graumann L, Cho AB, Kulakova E, Deuter CE, Wolf OT, Roepke S, Hellmann-Regen J, Otte C, Wingenfeld K. Impact of social exclusion on empathy in women with borderline personality disorder. Eur Arch Psychiatry Clin Neurosci. 2023;273(4):865–74.

Gunderson JG, Hoffman PD, editors. Understanding and treating borderline personality disorder: a guide for professionals and families. American Psychiatric Pub; 2007.

Gunderson JG, Herpertz SC, Skodol AE, Torgersen S, Zanarini MC. Borderline personality disorder. Nat Rev Dis Primers. 2018;4(1):1–20.

Hendrickson R, Popescu A, Ghearing G, Bagic A. Thoughts, emotions, and dissociative features differentiate patients with epilepsy from patients with psychogenic nonepileptic spells (PNESs). Epilepsy Behav. 2015;51:158–62.

Holmes EA. Intrusive, emotional mental imagery and trauma: experimental and clinical clues. Imagin Cogn Pers. 2003;23(2):147–54.

Holmes EA, Brown RJ, Mansell W, Fearon RP, Hunter EC, Frasquilho F, Oakley DA. Are there two qualitatively distinct forms of dissociation? A review and some clinical implications. Clin Psychol Rev. 2005;25(1):1–23.

Holowka DW, King S, Saheb D, Pukall M, Brunet A. Childhood abuse and dissociative symptoms in adult schizophrenia. Schizophr Res. 2003;60(1):87–90.

Hunter EC, Phillips ML, Chalder T, Sierra M, David AS. Depersonalisation disorder: a cognitive–behavioural conceptualisation. Behav Res Ther. 2003;41(12):1451–67.

Indelli P, Fernandez JL, Mograbi DC. In search of connection: towards a transdiagnostic view of dissociative phenomena through research domain criteria (RDoC) framework. Psicologia Clínica. 2018;30(3):509–40.

Jaeger S, Steinert T, Uhlmann C, Flammer E, Bichescu-Burian D, Tschöke S. Dissociation in patients with borderline personality disorder in acute inpatient care – a latent profile analysis. Compr Psychiatry. 2017;78:67–75.

Kaiser D, Jacob GA, Domes G, Arntz A. Attentional bias for emotional stimuli in borderline personality disorder: a meta-analysis. Psychopathology. 2017;49(6):383–96.

Kaplan B, Yazici Gulec M, Gica S, Gulec H. The association between neurocognitive functioning and clinical features of borderline personality disorder. Braz J Psychiatry. 2020;42:503–9.

Kleindienst N, Priebe K, Görg N, Dyer A, Steil R, Lyssenko L, Winter D, Schmahl C, Bohus M. State dissociation moderates response to dialectical behavior therapy for posttraumatic stress disorder in women with and without borderline personality disorder. Eur J Psychotraumatol. 2016;7(1):30375.

Kleindienst N, Vonderlin R, Bohus M, Lis S. Childhood adversity and borderline personality disorder. Analyses complementing the meta-analysis by Porter et al. (2020). Acta Psychiatr Scand. 2021;143(2):183.

Korzekwa MI, Dell PF, Pain C. Dissociation and borderline personality disorder: an update for clinicians. Curr Psychiatry Rep. 2009a;11(1):82–8.

Korzekwa MI, Dell PF, Links PS, Thabane L, Fougere P. Dissociation in borderline personality disorder: a detailed look. J Trauma Dissociation. 2009b;10(3):346–67.

Kozlowska K, Walker P, McLean L, Carrive P. Fear and the defense cascade: clinical implications and management. Harv Rev Psychiatry. 2015;23(4):263–87.

Krause-Utz A, Elzinga B. Current understanding of the neural mechanisms of dissociation in borderline personality disorder. Curr Behav Neurosci Rep. 2018;5:113–23.

Krause-Utz A, Frost R, Chatzaki E, Winter D, Schmahl C, Elzinga BM. Dissociation in borderline personality disorder: recent experimental, neurobiological studies, and implications for future research and treatment. Curr Psychiatry Rep. 2021;23(6):37.

Krause-Utz A, Frost R, Winter D, Elzinga BM. Dissociation and alterations in brain function and structure: implications for borderline personality disorder. Curr Psychiatry Rep. 2017;19:1–22.

Kulacaoglu F, Solmaz M, Belli H, Ardic FC, Akin E, Kose S. The relationship between impulsivity and attention-deficit/hyperactivity symptoms in female patients with borderline personality disorder. Psychiatry Clin Psychopharmacol. 2017;27(3):249–55.

Langeland W, Jepsen EK, Brand BL, Kleven L, Loewenstein RJ, Putnam FW, Schielke HJ, Myrick A, Lanius RA, Heir T. The economic burden of dissociative disorders: a qualitative systematic review of empirical studies. Psychol Trauma Theory Res Pract Policy. 2020;12(7):730.

Lanius RA, Vermetten E, Loewenstein RJ, Brand B, Schmahl C, Bremner JD, Spiegel D. Emotion modulation in PTSD: clinical and neurobiological evidence for a dissociative subtype. Am J Psychiatry. 2010;167(6):640–7.

Lanius RA, Boyd JE, McKinnon MC, Nicholson AA, Frewen P, Vermetten E, Jetly R, Spiegel D. A review of the neurobiological basis of trauma-related dissociation and its relation to cannabinoid-and opioid-mediated stress response: a transdiagnostic, translational approach. Curr Psychiatry Rep. 2018;20:1–4.

Lanius RA, Brand B, Vermetten E, Frewen PA, Spiegel D. The dissociative subtype of posttraumatic stress disorder: rationale, clinical and neurobiological evidence, and implications. Depress Anxiety. 2012;29(8):701–8.

Lanius RA, Wolf EJ, Miller MW, Frewen PA, Vermetten E, Brand B, Spiegel D. The dissociative subtype of PTSD. Handbook of PTSD: Science and practice; 2014. p. 234–50.

Laurenssen EMP, Hutsebaut J, Feenstra DJ, Bales DL, Noom MJ, Busschbach JJV, Luyten P. Feasibility of mentalization-based treatment for adolescents with borderline symptoms: a pilot study. Psychotherapy (Chic). 2014a;51(1):159–66.

Laurenssen EMP, Smits ML, Bales DL, Feenstra DJ, Eeren HV, Noom MJ, Verheul R. Day hospital Mentalization-based treatment versus intensive outpatient Mentalizationbased treatment for patients with severe borderline personality disorder: protocol of a multicentre randomized clinical trial. BMC Psychiatry. 2014b;14

Levinger S, Somer E, Holden RR. The importance of mental pain and physical dissociation in youth suicidality. J Trauma Dissociation. 2015;16(3):322–39.

Linehan MM. Skills training manual for treating borderline personality disorder. Guilford Press; 1993.

Liebke L, Koppe G, Bungert M, Thome J, Hauschild S, Defiebre N, Izurieta Hidalgo NA, Schmahl C, Bohus M, Lis S. Difficulties with being socially accepted: an experimental study in borderline personality disorder. J Abnorm Psychol. 2018;127(7):670.

Ludäscher P, Bohus M, Lieb K, Philipsen A, Jochims A, Schmahl C. Elevated pain thresholds correlate with dissociation and aversive arousal in patients with borderline personality disorder. Psychiatry Res. 2007;149(1–3):291–6.

Ludäscher P, Valerius G, Stiglmayr C, Mauchnik J, Lanius RA, Bohus M, Schmahl C. Pain sensitivity and neural processing during dissociative states in patients with borderline personality

disorder with and without comorbid posttraumatic stress disorder: a pilot study. J Psychiatry Neurosci. 2010;35(3):177–84.
Lynn SJ, Rhue JW. Dissociation: clinical and theoretical perspectives. The Guilford Press; 1994.
Lynn SJ, Lilienfeld SO, Merckelbach H, Giesbrecht T, McNally RJ, Loftus EF, Bruck M, Garry M, Malaktaris A. The trauma model of dissociation: inconvenient truths and stubborn fictions. Comment on Dalenberg et al. (2012).
Lyssenko L, Schmahl C, Bockhacker L, Vonderlin R, Bohus M, Kleindienst N. Dissociation in psychiatric disorders: a meta-analysis of studies using the dissociative experiences scale. Am J Psychiatry. 2018;175(1):37–46.
Maldonado JR, Spiegel D. Dissociative disorders. In: Tasman's psychiatry. Cham: Springer; 2024. p. 1–46.
Marmar CR, Metzler TJ, Otte C, McCaslin S, Inslicht S, Haase CH. The peritraumatic dissociative experiences questionnaire an international perspective. In: Cross-cultural assessment of psychological trauma and PTSD. Boston: Springer; 2007. p. 197–217.
Mazinan RG, Dudek C, Warkentin H, Finkenstaedt M, Schröder J, Musil R, Kratzer L, Fuss J, Biedermann SV. Borderline personality disorder and sexuality: causes and consequences of dissociative symptoms. Borderline Personal Disord Emot Dysregul. 2024;11(1):8.
Meares R. A malady of representations: dysautonomic aspects of borderline personality disorder. Psychother Aust. 2013;19(2):58–65.
Medford N, Baker D, Hunter E, Sierra M, Lawrence E, Phillips ML, David AS. Chronic depersonalization following illicit drug use: a controlled analysis of 40 cases. Addiction. 2003;98(12):1731–6.
Mergler M, Driessen M, Lüdecke C, Ohlmeier M, Chodzinski C, Weirich S, Schläfke D, Wedekind D, Havemann-Reinecke U, Renner W, Schäfer I. Relationships between a dissociative subtype of PTSD and clinical characteristics in patients with substance use disorders. J Psychoactive Drugs. 2017;49(3):225–32.
Murray J, Ehlers A, Mayou RA. Dissociation and post-traumatic stress disorder: two prospective studies of road traffic accident survivors. Br J Psychiatry. 2002;180(4):363–8.
Nester MS, Brand BL, Schielke HJ, Kumar S. An examination of the relations between emotion dysregulation, dissociation, and self-injury among dissociative disorder patients. Eur J Psychotraumatol. 2022;13(1):2031592.
Nijenhuis ER, den Boer JA. 21 psychobiology of traumatization. Dissociation and the dissociative disorders: DSM-V and beyond; 2010. p. 337.
Nijenhuis ER, Spinhoven P, Van Dyck R, van der Hart O, Vanderlinden J. Degree of somatoform and psychological dissociation in dissociative disorder is correlated with reported trauma. J Trauma Stress. 1998;11:711–30.
Nijenhuis ER, Van Der Hart O, Kruger K, Steele K. Somatoform dissociation, reported abuse and animal defence-like reactions. Aust New Zealand J Psychiatry. 2004;38(9):678–86.
Ntshingila N, Poggenpoel M, Myburgh CPHPH, Temane A. Experiences of women living with borderline personality disorder. Health SA Gesondheid. 2016;21:110–9.
Orbach I, Stein D, Palgi Y, Asherov J, Har-Even D, Elizur A. Perception of physical pain in accident and suicide attempt patients: self-preservation vs self-destruction. J Psychiatr Res. 1996;30(4):307–20.
Orbach A. Psychotherapy in the third age. Br J Psychother. 1994;11(2):221–31.
Özdemir O, Özdemir PG, Boysan M, Yilmaz E. The relationships between dissociation, attention, and memory dysfunction. Nöro Psikiyatri Arşivi. 2015;52(1):36.
Parlar M, Densmore M, Hall GB, Frewen PA, Lanius RA, McKinnon MC. Relation between patterns of intrinsic network connectivity, cognitive functioning, and symptom presentation in trauma-exposed patients with major depressive disorder. Brain Behav. 2017;7(5):e00664.
Peterson A. Consilience, clinical validation, and global disorders of consciousness. Neurosci Conscious. 2016;2016(1):niw011.

Perez S, Lorca F, Marco JH. Dissociation, posttraumatic stress symptoms, emotional dysregulation, and invalidating environments as correlates of NSSI in borderline personality disorder patients. J Trauma Dissociation. 2020;21(5):520–35.

Putnam FW, Carlson EB, Ross CA, Anderson G, Clark P, Torem M, Bowman ES, Coons P, Chu JA, Dill DL, Loewenstein RJ. Patterns of dissociation in clinical and nonclinical samples. J Nerv Ment Dis. 1996;184(11):673–9.

Rodríguez-Delgado A, Fresán A, Miranda E, Garza-Villarreal E, Alcalá-Lozano R, Duque-Alarcón X, Balducci T, Arango de Montis I. Comorbid personality disorders and their impact on severe dissociative experiences in Mexican patients with borderline personality disorder. Nord J Psychiatry. 2019;73(8):509–14.

Romero-López MJ. A review of the dissociative disorders: from multiple personality disorder to the posttraumatic stress. Anales De Psicología. 2016;32(2):448.

Ross CA. Unresolved problems in the theory of structural dissociation. Psichiatria e Psicoterapia. 2014;33(3)

Ross CA, Ferrell L, Schroeder E. Co-occurrence of dissociative identity disorder and borderline personality disorder. J Trauma Dissociation. 2014;15(1):79–90.

Roydeva MI, Reinders AA. Biomarkers of pathological dissociation: a systematic review. Neurosci Biobehav Rev. 2021;123:120–202.

Rufer M, Held D, Cremer J, Fricke S, Moritz S, Peter H, Hand I. Dissociation as a predictor of cognitive behavior therapy outcome in patients with obsessive-compulsive disorder. Psychother Psychosom. 2005;75(1):40–6.

Ruiz MA, Pincus AL, Ray WJ. The relationship between dissociation and personality. Personal Individ Differ. 1999;27(2):239–49.

Salmon AP, Nicol K, Kaess M, Jovev M, Betts JK, Chanen AM. Associations of state or trait dissociation with severity of psychopathology in young people with borderline personality disorder. Borderline Personal Disord Emot Dysregul. 2023;10(1):20.

Sar V, Akyuz G, Kugu N, Ozturk E, Ertem-Vehid H. Axis I dissociative disorder comorbidity in borderline personality disorder and reports of childhood trauma. J Clin Psychiatry. 2006;67(10):1583–90.

Sar V, Alioğlu F, Akyuz G, Karabulut S. Dissociative amnesia in dissociative disorders and borderline personality disorder: self-rating assessment in a college population. J Trauma Dissociation. 2014;15(4):477–93.

Sar V, Alioğlu F, Akyuz G. Depersonalization and derealization in self-report and clinical interview: the spectrum of borderline personality disorder, dissociative disorders, and healthy controls. J Trauma Dissociation. 2017a;18(4):490–506.

Sar V, Alioğlu F, Akyuz G, Tayakısı E, Öğülmüş EF, Sönmez D. Awareness of identity alteration and diagnostic preference between borderline personality disorder and dissociative disorders. J Trauma Dissociation. 2017b;18(5):693–709.

Sack M, Sachsse U, Overkamp B, Dulz B. Trauma-related disorders in patients with borderline personality disorders: results of a multicenter study. Nervenarzt. 2013;84:608–14.

Scalabrini A, Cavicchioli M, Fossati A, Maffei C. The extent of dissociation in borderline personality disorder: a meta-analytic review. J Trauma Dissociation. 2017;18(4):522–43.

Schauer M, Elbert T. Dissociation following traumatic stress. Zeitschrift für Psychologie/J Psychol. 2015.

Scherpiet S, Brühl AB, Opialla S, Roth L, Jäncke L, Herwig U. Altered emotion processing circuits during the anticipation of emotional stimuli in women with borderline personality disorder. Eur Arch Psychiatry Clin Neurosci. 2014;264:45–60.

Schmahl CG, Vermetten E, Elzinga BM, Bremner JD. A positron emission tomography study of memories of childhood abuse in borderline personality disorder. Biol Psychiatry. 2004;55(7):759–65.

Schneiderman S, editor. Returning to Freud: clinical psychoanalysis in the school of Lacan. New Haven: Yale University Press; 1980.

Scognamiglio C, Sorge A, Borrelli G, Perrella R, Saita E. Exploring the connection between childhood trauma, dissociation, and borderline personality disorder in forensic psychiatry: a comprehensive case study. Front Psychol. 2024;15:1332914.
Seidl E, Padberg F, Bauriedl-Schmidt C, Albert A, Daltrozzo T, Hall J, Renneberg B, Seidl O, Jobst A. Response to ostracism in patients with chronic depression, episodic depression and borderline personality disorder a study using Cyberball. J Affect Disord. 2020;260:254–62.
Skarderud F. Eating one's words. Part III: Mentalisation-based psychotherapy for anorexia nervosa. An outline for a treatment and training manual. Eur Eat Disord Rev. 2007;15:323–39.
Spiegel D. Integrating dissociation. In: Dissociation and the dissociative disorders. Routledge; 2022. p. 811–5.
Steuwe C, Lanius RA, Frewen PA. Evidence for a dissociative subtype of PTSD by latent profile and confirmatory factor analyses in a civilian sample. Depress Anxiety. 2012;29(8):689–700.
Stiglmayr CE, Ebner-Priemer UW, Bretz J, Behm R, Mohse M, Lammers CH, Anghelescu IG, Schmahl C, Schlotz W, Kleindienst N, Bohus M. Dissociative symptoms are positively related to stress in borderline personality disorder. Acta Psychiatr Scand. 2008;117(2):139–47.
Sumlin E, Wall K, Sharp C. The moderating role of dissociation in the relation between borderline features and factors of self-injury in adolescents. Personal Ment Health. 2020;14(2):215–26.
Thome J, Liebke L, Bungert M, Schmahl C, Domes G, Bohus M, Lis S. Confidence in facial emotion recognition in borderline personality disorder. Personal Disord Theory Res Treat. 2016;7(2):159.
Tuineag M, Therman S, Lindgren M, Rouanet M, Nahon S, Bertrand L, Saury S, Renaud S, Beaulieu S, Linnaranta O. Dissociative symptoms as measured by the Cambridge Depersonalization Scale in patients with a bipolar disorder. J Affect Disord. 2020;263:187–92.
van der Boom KJ, van den Hout MA, Huntjens RJ. Psychoform and somatoform dissociation, traumatic experiences, and fantasy proneness in somatoform disorders. Personal Individ Differ. 2010;48(4):447–51.
van der Hart O, Steele K. The theory of trauma-related structural dissociation of the personality. In: Dissociation and the dissociative disorders. Routledge; 2022. p. 263–80.
Van der Hart O, Nijenhuis E, Steele K, Brown D. Trauma-related dissociation: conceptual clarity lost and found. Austr New Zealand J Psychiatry. 2004;38(11–12):906–14.
van der Hart O, van Ochten JM, van Son MJ, Steele K, Lensvelt-Mulders G. Relations among peritraumatic dissociation and posttraumatic stress: a critical review. J Trauma Dissociation. 2008;9(4):481–505.
van Dijke A, van der Hart O, Ford JD, van Son M, van der Heijden P, Bühring M. Affect dysregulation and dissociation in borderline personality disorder and somatoform disorder: differentiating inhibitory and excitatory experiencing states. J Trauma Dissociation. 2010;11(4):424–43.
van Schie CC, Chiu CD, Rombouts SA, Heiser WJ, Elzinga BM. Stuck in a negative me: fMRI study on the role of disturbed self-views in social feedback processing in borderline personality disorder. Psychol Med. 2020;50(4):625–35.
Vermetten E, Spiegel D. Trauma and dissociation: implications for borderline personality disorder. Curr Psychiatry Rep. 2014;16:1.
Vine V, Byrd AL, Mohr H, Scott LN, Beeney JE, Stepp SD. The structure of psychopathology in a sample of clinically referred, emotionally dysregulated early adolescents. J Abnorm Child Psychol. 2020;48:1379–93.
Vogt KS, Norman P. Is mentalization-based therapy effective in treating the symptoms of borderline personality disorder? A systematic review. Psychol Psychother Theory Res Pract. 2019;92(4):441–64.
Waller N, Putnam FW, Carlson EB. Types of dissociation and dissociative types: a taxometric analysis of dissociative experiences. Psychol Methods. 1996;1(3):300.
Webermann AR, Brand BL. Mental illness and violent behavior: the role of dissociation. Borderline Personal Disord Emot Dysregul. 2017;4:1–3.

Webermann AR, Myrick AC, Taylor CL, Chasson GS, Brand BL. Dissociative, depressive, and PTSD symptom severity as correlates of nonsuicidal self-injury and suicidality in dissociative disorder patients. J Trauma Dissociation. 2016;17(1):67–80.

Wedig MM, Silverman MH, Frankenburg FR, Reich DB, Fitzmaurice G, Zanarini MC. Predictors of suicide attempts in patients with borderline personality disorder over 16 years of prospective follow-up. Psychol Med. 2012;42(11):2395–404.

Wilkinson-Ryan T, Westen D. Identity disturbance in borderline personality disorder: an empirical investigation. Am J Psychiatry. 2000;157(4):528–41.

Winter D, Koplin K, Lis S. Can't stand the look in the mirror? Self-awareness avoidance in borderline personality disorder. Borderline Personal Disord Emot Dysregul. 2015;2:1–6.

Winter D. Attention to emotional stimuli in borderline personality disorder–a review of the influence of dissociation, self-reference, and psychotherapeutic interventions. Borderline Personal Disord Emot Dysregul. 2016;3(1):11.

Winter D, Steeb L, Herbert C, Sedikides C, Schmahl C, Bohus M, Lis S. Lower self-positivity and its association with self-esteem in women with borderline personality disorder. Behav Res Ther. 2018;109:84–93.

Wolf EJ, Lunney CA, Miller MW, Resick PA, Friedman MJ, Schnurr PP. The dissociative subtype of PTSD: a replication and extension. Depress Anxiety. 2012;29(8):679–88.

Wolke D, Schreier A, Zanarini MC, Winsper C. Bullied by peers in childhood and borderline personality symptoms at 11 years of age: a prospective study. J Child Psychol Psychiatry. 2012;53(8):846–55.

Yayla S, Bakım B, Tankaya O, Ozer OA, Karamustafalioglu O, Ertekin H, Tekin A. Psychiatric comorbidity in patients with conversion disorder and prevalence of dissociative symptoms. J Trauma Dissociation. 2015;16(1):29–38.

Zanarini MC. Zanarini Rating Scale for Borderline Personality Disorder (ZAN-BPD): a continuous measure of DSM-IV borderline psychopathology. J Personal Disord. 2003;17(3):233–42.

Zanarini MC, Frankenburg FR. A preliminary, randomized trial of psychoeducation for women with borderline personality disorder. J Personal Disord. 2008;22(3):284–90.

Zanarini MC, Ruser T, Frankenburg FR, Hennen J. The dissociative experiences of borderline patients. Compr Psychiatry. 2000;41(3):223–7.

Zanarini MC, Laudate CS, Frankenburg FR, Reich DB, Fitzmaurice G. Predictors of self-mutilation in patients with borderline personality disorder: a 10-year follow-up study. J Psychiatr Res. 2011;45(6):823–8.

Zanarini MC, Martinho E Jr, Temes CM, Glass IV, Aguirre BA, Goodman M, Fitzmaurice GM. Dissociative experiences of adolescents with borderline personality disorder: description and prediction. Borderline Personal Disord Emot Dysregul. 2023;10(1):9.

Zittel Conklin C, Westen D. Borderline personality disorder in clinical practice. Am J Psychiatry. 2005;162(5):867–75.

Chapter 11
Acceptance and Commitment Model of Borderline Personality Disorder

Introduction

Over the past three decades, behavioral interventions encompassing mindfulness and acceptance have evolved from traditional cognitive behavior therapy (Hayes et al. 2004, 2013; Zhang et al. 2021; Keulen et al. 2023; Ruiz 2010). Acceptance and commitment therapy (ACT; Hayes et al. 1999) is one of these novel modalities that was launched with the constitutional understanding of the inevitable nature of experiencing pain, grief, loss, disappointment, illness, fear, and anxiety in human life (Dindo et al. 2017; Hayes et al. 2011, 2013). ACT was developed as the third wave of cognitive and behavioral therapies, which was built on the traditional behavior analysis (Hayes et al. 2004, 2012), and is one of the most documented and experimentally supported psychotherapeutic approaches named contextual therapies (Ruiz 2010; Hayes 2004; Luciano et al. 2011; Hayes et al. 2013). ACT is focused on the role of individuals' psychological resources in stressful situations (Twohig et al. 2010; Twohig 2012), and has been defined as a therapeutic approach that utilizes acceptance and mindfulness processes, and commitment and behavior change processes, to create higher level of psychological flexibility (Hayes et al. 2004, 2013; Hayes 2016). The ACT model focuses on the interruption of destructive experiential avoidance, as well as elaborating psychological flexibility based on substantially experimental evidence account of the pertinent role of defusion and values elements (Hayes et al. 2012; Torneke 2010; Ruiz 2010; Luciano et al. 2011; Jiang et al. 2024). Additionally, ACT is an empirically documented approach based on traditional behavior therapy attempting to decrease psychological inflexibility and promoting individuals' involvement in valued behavior in spite of experiencing unpleasant private events (Houghton and Joinson 2014; Bajari et al. 2014). ACT refers to a psychological model which physiologically originated from *functional contextualism* (Hayes 1993, 2012; Ruiz 2010; Hayes et al. 2013), and theoretically rooted in *relational frame theory* (RFT; Hayes et al. 2001, 2012, 2013; Ruiz 2010).

M. Salavati, E. A. Selby, *Theories of Borderline Personality Disorder*,
https://doi.org/10.1007/978-3-031-75503-3_11

It should be mentioned that ACT is not merely a disorder-specific treatment; instead, it is considered as a general approach that can incite the development of a wide range of protocols, concentrated on specific issues, patients' populations, various contexts, and settings. ACT assimilates scientifically theoretical knowledge about contingency formed behavioral and verbal associations into a more effective therapeutic whole (Hayes et al. 2004; Ruiz 2010). The ACT interventions explicitly embrace acceptance instead of decreasing the primary somatic complaints that led the patient to engage in psychotherapy (Hayes et al. 2012, 2013). Hayes et al. (1999) nominated the development and methodology of ACT as a *contextual behavioral science* (CBS) approach, a core concept in ACT, based on specific philosophical assumptions, certain useful and reliable theories for clinicians, and desired methods of examining new clinical developments (Hayes et al. 2012, 2013; Ruiz 2010). ACT has been established on the language perspective in which language is considered as the core construct of various psychological disorders specifically, generally human suffering. ACT brings language to heal; therefore, it can be used whenever it is useful, rather than be such a covert process that assumes the humans that host it (Hayes et al. 2013).

Substantially growing body of empirical and clinical studies have shown considerable efficacy and effectiveness of acceptance and commitment therapy not only in a wide range of various psychiatric issues but also in mental health promotion (Hayes et al. 2006; Houghton et al. 2014; Baruch et al. 2009; Beygi et al. 2023), such as *obsessive-compulsive disorder* (Twohig et al. 2006; Woods et al. 2006), *depression and anxiety* (Shiri et al. 2022; Ravanbakhsh et al. 2023; Kelson et al. 2019; Reeve et al. 2021; Gloster et al. 2020; Bai et al. 2020; Coto-Lesmes et al. 2020; Harris and Samuel 2020; Haller et al. 2021; Ferreira et al. 2022; Sun et al. 2022; A-Tjak et al. 2015; Beygi et al. 2023), *impulse control disorder* (Houghton et al. 2014; Morrison et al. 2014), *motor neuron disease* (Gould et al. 2023), *cancer & breast cancer* (Sinclair et al. 2023; Fawson et al. 2023; Li et al. 2021; Mathew et al. 2021), *psychosis and psychotic disorders* (Morris et al. 2024; Yıldız 2020; Baruch et al. 2009), *mental health difficulties in cosmetic surgery applicants* (Mahmoudfakhe et al. 2023), *generalized anxiety disorder* (Shiri et al. 2022; Sharif Ara et al. 2023), *difficulties in emotion regulation* (Vaezi et al. 2023), *psychological inflexibility* (Zancan et al. 2023; Stokton et al. 2019), *mental health problems in children and adolescents* (Fan et al. 2020; Berger et al. 2021; Parmar et al. 2021; Chua and Shorey 2022; Knight and Samuel 2022), *somatic problems/undiagnosed issues* (Thompson et al. 2021; A-Tjak et al. 2015), *social anxiety* (Galletti et al. 2023), *different biological/physical disease* (Wang et al. 2022; Thompson et al. 2022), *nonresponsive patients with personality disorders* (Chakhssi et al. 2015), *substance use disorder* (A-Tjak et al. 2015; Twohig et al. 2018; Li et al. 2022), *chronic pain* (Vowles and McCracken 2008; Wicksell et al. 2007), *epilepsy* (Lundgren et al. 2008; Lundgren et al. 2006); *chronic skin picking* (Twohig et al. 2018), and *impulsivity* (Morrison et al. 2014).

Functional Contextualism

Basically, ACT is founded on a pragmatic philosophy of science named *functional contextualism* (Biglan and Hayes 1996; Hayes et al. 2006; Zhang et al. 2021). The main analytic unit of contextualism includes the ongoing act-in-context (Pepper 1942), and is a holistic approach in which the whole event (the context of event) is primary (Hayes et al. 2012). Functional contextualism perspective refers to psychological events as an interaction between whole organism and a context that are described historically including former learning history, and also, situationally consisting of current antecedents and consequences, verbal rules (Hayes et al. 2004, 2012, 2013). Functional contextualism concentrates on the current and ongoing action of an individual, as well as it focuses on the environment in which the action is happening (Bach and Moran 2008). Searching the "predict-and-influence" of these interactions is the most significant focus of functional contextualist (Hayes et al. 2012, 2013). In other words, functional contextualism is precise about goals searching the prediction-and-influence of psychological events, with precision, scope, and depth (Hayes and Brownstein 1986; Hayes et al. 2004). The conceptual standards used to assess the prediction and influences include precision (the specificity with which associated variables are recognized), scope (the degree to which the theory can be done with fewer concepts), and depth (the degree of coherence achievable with useful concepts established at other levels of analysis) (Hayes et al. 2012).

Relational Frame Theory

ACT originated from principles based on a naturalistic approach to human behavior that was set in traditional radical behaviorism (Ivancic and Belisle 2019; Belisle 2020; Zhang et al. 2021). It also emphasized the fundamental analysis of verbal behaviors originated directly from an integrated focus on both psychological well-being and applied work (Hayes et al. 2012, 2013). The preliminary foundation of ACT is based on a developing line of constitutionally behavioral investigations on human language and cognition named *relational frame theory* (RFT; Hayes et al. 2001; Enoch and Nicholson 2020; Zhang et al. 2021; Harte et al. 2023). ACT and RFT encompass an integrated approach, accordance to theoretical premises and a constellation of principles that are different in concentration and level of analysis, from the most fundamental to the most applied (Hayes et al. 2004, 2013; Harte et al. 2023). The fundamental assumption behind both ACT and RFT encompasses the evolution of human language contributed to the development of a unique form of psychological suffering for human beings. As mentioned, ACT concentrates on the significance of human language and cognition similar to previous schools of philosophy and psychology, such as narrative psychology and psycholinguistics. The majority of these approaches are not apparent practical connection; however, they are completely interesting. ACT is relevant to a core science account named relational frame theory (RFT; Hayes et al. 2001, 2013). RFT is a functional contextual theory of human language and cognition, which is the most active aspect of constitutional behavior analytic investigation on human behavior. Since RFT emphasizes on changeable contexts, it is readily associated to practical concerns (Hayes et al. 2012; Gross and Fox 2009). ACT principles and processes has been expanded based on relational frame theory (RFT), and it is considered as an approach explicitly established to change functional patterns of relational frame (Belisle and Dixon 2022; Enoch and Nicholson 2020; Zhang et al. 2021; Gross and Fox 2009; Harte et al. 2023). RFT states how relations appear when there is no direct reinforcement (Hayes et al. 2001). According to RFT, the crucial foundation of language and higher cognition is the capacity to learn and exert a "relational frame." According to Hayes et al. (2012), a relational frame involves "learned behavior that shows three main properties under arbitrary contextual control, namely, mutual entailment, combinatorial entailment, and transformation of stimulus function" (Hayes et al. 2012, p. 44). In line with an experimental study, when a person was asked to choose a stimulus B in the presence of A (A–B) and to choose a stimulus C in the presence of B (B–C), it was possible for the person to match A to C and C to A. For instance, a stimulus A involves participating in a test in the college. Related to student's history, this situation may provoke intensely negative emotions such as anxiety and fear which can contribute to avoidance or escape functions. In this condition, these unpleasant experiences can be elicited again not only in the next actual test-taking situations but also conditions encompassed similar stimuli such as hearing the word "test" or seeing the written word "TEST," which will be led to experiencing and functions consistent to previous real experiences (e.g., Dougher et al. 2007). In other words, the functions of test and TEST will be transformed in terms of their relative associations with test-taking situations, which will cause test anxiety in student contributing to significant avoidance behaviors like procrastination (Belisle and Dixon 2022). In behavior analysis models, these behaviors can be the explicit targets for behavioral interventions such as ACT. ACT proposes an understanding of associations between relational frames, transformation of stimulus function, and avoidant behaviors (Belisle and Dixon 2022). The process of stimulus equivalence contributed to two main related matters. First, the elucidation of this phenomenon in terms of direct reinforcement contingencies will be complicated due to previously unreinforced responses that "appeared" during testing. Second, there was an apparent association between stimulus equivalence and human language, because it was explored that during teaching fundamental reading skills, and nonhumans failed to show clear evidence of equivalence responding (Harte et al. 2023). RFT proposes an explanation for these equivalences according to considering equivalence responding as a class of generalized operant behavior and early language acquisition contributing to the development of equivalence and symbolic associations as functionally synonymous (Hayes 1991). The most fundamental relational network or frame is identified as generalized pattern of relational responding processing the properties of mutual entailment, combinational entailment, and the transformation of stimulus functions. During the period of early language learning, children are taught to answer based on relational frames, including opposite, difference, and comparison; subsequently, a wide range of derived relational responses would be possible (Harte et al. 2023; Hayes et al. 2013).

The ACT Theory of Change

ACT as a therapeutic approach tries to assist the clients to bring language and cognition under appropriate contextual control, applying logical, linear language when it is useful, as well as letting direct experience using as a guide when it is more effective (Hayes et al. 2004, 2013). The psychological flexibility model refers to an analogical nature which is associated with fundamental human processes. It is a model of psychopathology, as a model of psychological health, and a model of psychological intervention (Hayes et al. 2012, 2013; Pearson et al. 2010; Keulen et al. 2023). The ACT psychological flexibility model comprises of six subprocesses, including acceptance (learning to accept unpleasant emotions, cognitions, and situation rather than avoiding of them), defusion (altering the unwanted functions of thoughts, instead of changing their form, frequency, or sensitivity), flexible attention to the present moment (learning to concentrate on here-and-now, rather than rumination about past or worry about the future), self-as-context (establishing a flexible viewpoint of self which led to observing and accepting the content of self), values (deciding what is most significant for oneself), and committed action (altering behavior in the direction of one's value) (Hayes et al. 2012, 2013; Ong and Eustis 2023; Jiang et al. 2024; Pearson et al. 2010; Dindo et al. 2017; Keulen et al. 2023). Additionally, psychological flexibility can be considered based on three processes in ACT, consisting of (1) being open (acceptance, defusion); (2) being aware (present moment awareness, self-as-context); and (3) being active (values, committed action) (Hayes et al. 2011, 2013; Ong and Eustis 2023). The primary ACT model has been present in Fig. 11.1.

Psychological Flexibility Psychological flexibility refers to "the ability to contact the present moment more fully as a conscious human being, and to change or persist in behavior when doing so serves valued ends" (Hayes et al. 2006, p. 7). According to the psychological flexibility model, there are six core processes comprising: *accepting and defusion* from though inner experiences and manifest *in the present moment*, identifying that *self is the context* for these inner experiences, to continue personal *values* by *committing to actions* consistent with those values (Ong and Eustis 2023; Bach and Moran 2008; Hayes et al. 2013). Each of these processes assist the development of change processes associated with selected values (Hayes et al. 2004, 2013; Waltz and Hayes 2010). According to Hayes et al. (2012), there are six core *pathological* processes leading to the development of psychological inflexibility: inflexible attention, disruption of chosen values, inaction or impulsivity, attachment to conceptualized self, cognitive fusion, and experiential avoidance. In other words, the absence of one or more of these core processes may contribute

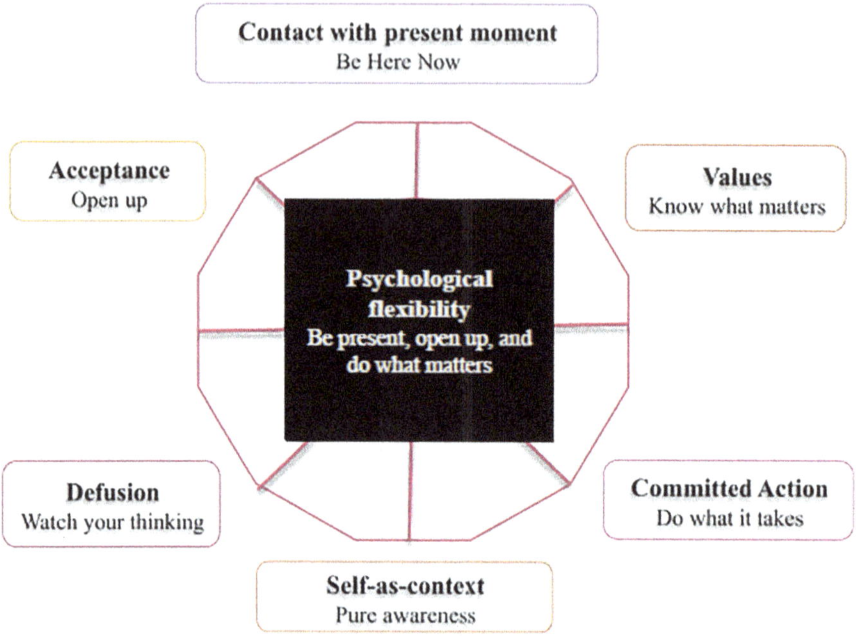

Fig. 11.1 The primary ACT model. (Source: adapted Hayes et al. 2012)

to the increased risks for the development of psychological rigidity, which is an origin resulting to human suffering and maladaptive functioning. In line with psychological flexibility, pain is a natural consequence of life, yet the overall level of psychological rigidity prevents adaptation with the internal or external context, they suffer unessentially pain. This unnecessary suffering happens when verbal and cognitive processes limit human repertoires in core aspects by cognitive entanglement and experiential avoidance. Whenever individuals over-recognize, or "fuse," with dysfunctional verbal regulations, their behavioral repertoire becomes limited and narrow, therefore, they lose efficient contact with the direct results of action. Consequently, this response restrains their competency to alter when current strategies are unworkable. Additionally, it can lead them to be more persistent to analyze and comprehend their problems and issues. In other words, being "right" about what is "wrong" may develop in their mind which is more significant than life in a vital and efficacious manner. Through being involved in experiential avoidance, individuals' behaviors would be under unfavorable control, so in most situations, they try to avoid, suppress, or escape from thoughts, emotions, memories, or bodily sensations. These avoidances contribute to further restricted behaviors which may be contribute to gradual loss of contact with the positive consequences of responding. To conclude, a vicious cycle of avoidance will be dominant, strengthening the need to avoid even as "collateral damage" mounts, such as reduction in the quality of interpersonal relationships, lost hopes, and desires (Hayes et al. 2004, 2012, 2013).

Acceptance Acceptance is a core component of change within ACT, and also it is one of the most significant aspects of the psychological flexibility model that underlies ACT (Hayes et al. 2012, 2013; Bordieri 2022; Blackledge and Barnes-Holmes 2009). Based on Hayes et al. (2004), acceptance means is "to take what is offered" (Hayes et al. 2004, p. 7). Acceptance is defined as "the voluntary adoption of an intentionally open, receptive, flexible, and non-judgmental posture with respect to moment-to-moment experience" (Hayes et al. 2012, p. 272). Acceptance refers to willingness and tendency to experience personal cognitions, thoughts, emotions, memories, body sensations, derives, and urges, with no attempt to alter their form or frequency, or expressed in different way. In other words, acceptance is a consciously opened hug of private events that occur in our previous and current life (Hayes et al. 2012, 2013; Marvin et al. 2023; Blackledge and Barnes-Holmes 2009; Bach and Moran 2008). Acceptance encompasses secondary alteration instead of primary change, such as changing in ways of a person associates to their private events rather than an alteration in the intensity and frequency of the events themselves events (Merwin et al. 2023; Waltz and Hayes 2010). Acceptance is associated with the reduction of emotional distress through relinquishing the suppression and avoidance from unwanted internal experiences which cause decreasing distress by circumventing paradoxical escalation in these aversive experiences due to deliberated suppression (Wegner 1994). In addition, whenever experiential avoidance interferes with behavioral flexibility and efficiency, acceptance is elicited to offer the demands of the situation, or consistently with deeply maintain personal values (Marvin et al. 2023; Bach and Moran 2008; Hayes et al. 2013).

Cognitive Defusion Defusion refers to an invented word defined as undoing fusion. Cognitive defusion encompasses creating a space between the individual and their private events (Bennett and Oliver 2019; Hayes et al. 2013; Waltz and Hayes 2010), or pulling an "individual" apart from the "mind" (Hayes et al. 2012). Therefore, a person is permitted to associate and consider alternative behaviors, specifically, those related to personal values and goals (Ruiz et al. 2018). Defusion can be thought of as a process of well-established verbal stimulus transformations that are troubled by the displacement of contextual states that control relational responding in general (Blackledge and Barnes-Holmes 2009; Hayes et al. 2013). Cognitive defusion involves being consciously aware of private events as current relational processes to diminish their immediate verbal functions and be in contact with various sources of stimulus control (Hayes et al. 2012; Luoma et al. 2007; Ruiz et al. 2018; Bach and Moran 2008). Based on Hayes et al. (2012), cognitive fusion includes learning to be consciously aware of one's thinking as it happens, which a person should be aware to separate current cognitive processes from the cognitive outputs. In other words, defusion decreases the automatic influences of verbal meaning on human behaviors so that other sources of behavioral management and regulation would be more effective take part in the moment (Hayes et al. 2012, 2013), contributing to facilitating being involved in verbal activity. This process will permit contacting values and the actions available in this context which advance toward values (Ruiz et al. 2018).

Present Moment Awareness Present moment awareness is a core strategy in ACT (Ruiz et al. 2018; Bach and Moran 2008), and refers to being observant and noticing what is present in one's ongoing environmental context and in private inner experience. In addition, awareness includes the ability to label and describe what is present with no judgment and evaluation (Hayes et al. 2004) and be voluntarily flexible (Hayes et al. 2012; Waltz and Hayes 2010). Being present contributes to a sense of "self as a process of ongoing awareness of events and experiences" (Hayes et al. 2004, p. 10). Individuals who have several difficulties in ability of being in contact with here-and-now, indicate numerous issues in altering their behavior to match the changing demands of their social-interpersonal context (Hayes et al. 2012, 2013). Furthermore, being present in the moment encompasses the discrimination of the contingencies ongoing exerting control over behavior (Blackledge and Barnes-Holmes 2009).

Values Values are defined as selected qualities of purposive actions and behaviors, which can merely be instantiated rather than processed as an object (Hayes et al. 2004, 2013). In the perspective of the ACT model, most people already own everything that is required to have a rich and meaningful life (Hayes et al. 2012, 2013; Bach and Moran 2008; Waltz and Hayes 2010). An accurate term in valuing refers to "freely chosen, verbally constructed consequences of ongoing, dynamic, evolving patterns of activity, which establish predominant reinforcers for that activity that are intrinsic in engagement in the valued behavioral pattern itself" (Wilson et al. 2012, p. 64).

Self-as-Context As has previously been mentioned, focusing on elevated contact with alternative types of self-experience is a crucial point in ACT model perspective (Blackledge and Barnes-Holmes 2009; Hayes et al. 2013). Having a place of sanctuary protecting individuals from being involved from toxic self-evaluations, mindless rules following, and self-destructive coping responses is a vital necessity in human life. This secure shelter is an experience of being aware which keep our private experience, including thoughts, emotions, memories, and bodily sensations (Hayes et al. 2004, 2012; Blackledge and Barnes-Holmes 2009; Bach and Moran 2008). In line with the ACT model, a transcendent sense of self is established in verbal elements of human experience, which may be accessed through defusion and mindfulness processes. Another point that should be considered is *self-as-context*, which supports acceptance (Hayes et al. 2004, 2013; Waltz and Hayes 2010). Self-as-context encompasses all stories, evaluations, and descriptions that individuals construct about "I", ongoing knowing self and current experience, included of every verbally known aspect of life which integrates self-knowledge of individual's ongoing and all of one's conscious experiences comprising historical emotions, bodily sensations, preferences, abilities, cognitions, interactions, and learning (McHugh and Stapleton 2023; Hayes et al. 2013; Waltz and Hayes 2010).

Committed Action Whenever the psychological obstacles of avoidance and fusion are more identified, recognizing and establishing certain commitments becomes helpful. Commitments in ACT model consisted of recognizing and defining goals while predicting and making psychological obstacles (Hayes et al. 2004, 2013; Waltz and Hayes 2010). Commitment is defined as a *done* action, which is meant to promise or pledge that a person will do a specific thing and maintain doing it (McCracken 2023), and it is not really about the future at all, rather it is about doing a certain action in a situation and situationally appropriate behaviors in the context of external and internal stimuli and forces (Hayes et al. 2012). According to Hayes et al. (2012), committed action refers to "a values-based action that occurs at a particular moment in time and that is deliberately linked to creating a pattern of action that serves the value" (Hayes et al. 2012, p. 328). The primary ACT model of psychopathology is presented in Fig. 11.2.

Experiential Avoidance Experiential avoidance refers to the attempt to avoid or escape from the form, frequency, and situation of unwanted private events, even when this attempt contributes to psychological harm (Marvin et al. 2023; Hayes et al. 2004, 2006). Experiential avoidance is defined experiential avoidance as happening when an individual is willing to stay in contact with private experiences, including bodily sensations, emotions, thoughts, memories, and behavioral predispositions (Pearson et al. 2010; Hayes et al. 2013; Dindo et al. 2017). Two main forms of experiential avoidance consist of suppression and situational escape/avoidance. In *suppression*, a person actively tries to control and/or remove the immediate

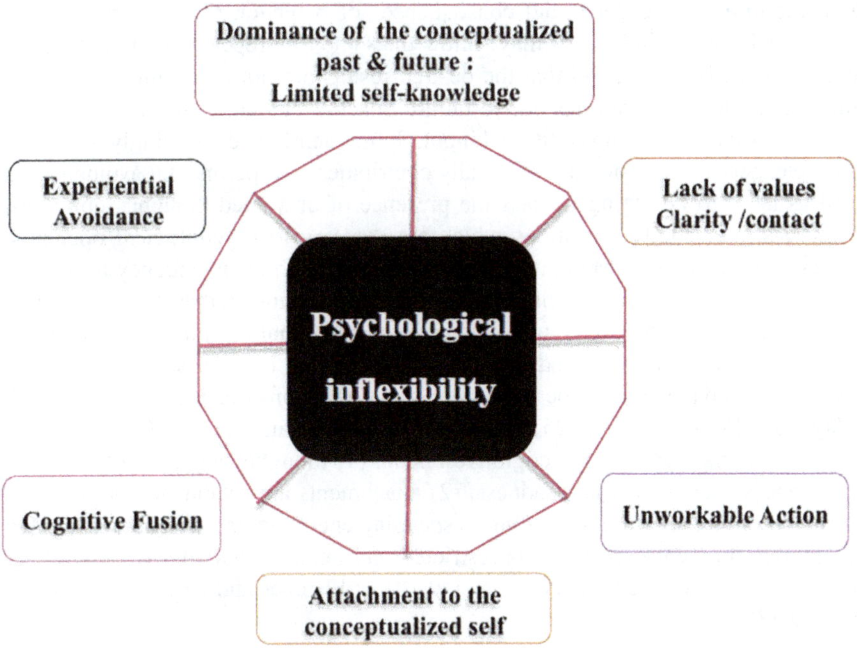

Fig. 11.2 The primary ACT model of psychopathology. (Source: adapted Hayes et al. 2012)

experience of an unpleasant negative private event including unwanted thoughts, emotions, memories, or bodily sensation. In *situational escape/avoidance*, an individual attempts to change the antecedent contextual characteristics that are related to the appearance of an unwanted private experience (Hayes et al. 2004; Marvin et al. 2023). There are three substantial negative consequences of experiential avoidance. First, decreasing contact with how the present is related to one's history contributed to the reduction in person's experiential intelligence, which causes an inability to understand what is working and what is not. Second, it contributes to low levels of awareness toward being avoidant, which means that individuals may not even be conscious that they are avoiding, which results in no opportunity to identify whether or not avoidance is what a person really wants. Third, since avoidance repeatedly thwarts the development of one's behaviors toward positively valued behavioral patterns, damaging several aspects of real life (Hayes et al. 2012, 2013).

Cognitive Fusion Cognitive fusion is another central construct in the ACT model of human suffering. One of the most basic challenging concepts in humans involves being aware of our mind during learning while attending to the here-and-now. Fusion refers to the pouring verbal and cognitive processes which contributes to an inability to discriminate between these two processes (Hayes et al. 2013). Therefore, fusion limits our response repertoire in some aspects of our life, leading to formulating situations symbolically and managing our behaviors to match our demands based on rules programmed to follow. These rules cause an overwhelmed contact with the direct antecedents and consequences of behavior. Consequently, in as-fused condition, an individual may follow the same rule repeatedly in all contexts and never really understand that the desired results are not happening because of eliciting more and more rules due to failure in achievement. In this state, thinking regulates behavior with no additional input. Subsequently in distressingly unwanted private experiences, fusion automatically contributes to experimental avoidance, as well as leads to not being witness the presence of unwanted thoughts, emotions, memories, and bodily sensations which are contrary to psychological openness. Hayes and Pierson (2005) defined cognitive fusion as "human tendency to interact with events on the basis of their verbally ascribed functions rather than their direct functions, while being oblivious to the ongoing relational framing that establishes these functions. The event and one's thinking about it become so fused as to be inseparable and that creates the impression that verbal construal is not present at all" (Hayes and Pierson 2005, p. 25). According to Fletcher and Hayes (2005), there are three issues that happen with cognitive fusion: (1) thoughts are related to internal experiences such as fear and sadness; (2) attachments are established on thoughts which describe the self, contributing to spending energy to prove right or alter; and (3) present-moment experience is restricted and being overwhelmed by thinking about the future or the past (Pearson et al. 2010; Fletcher and Hayes 2005; Hayes et al. 2013).

Acceptance and Commitment Approach of BPD

Because ACT is still a relatively newer treatment approach, less research has been done on its tenants and effectiveness in treating BPD. However, the work that has been done appears that ACT may be quite promising for ameliorating BPD symptoms. Individuals who are suffering from personality disorders and have a history of nonresponsive treatment are considered among the most challenging patients to treat (Verheul and Herbrink 2007; Chakhssi et al. 2015). ACT has revealed efficacy and effectiveness in treatment-resistant patients with chronic or recurrent depressive disorders with or without comorbid personality traits and disorders (Jacobs et al. 2013; Clarke et al. 2015). Despite a growing body of empirically and clinically documented findings on the ACT model, very few studies have examined treating BPD patients with ACT (Morgan and Aljabari 2019). It has been documented that the symptoms of BPD have shown similar functional analysis to other psychiatric disorders reported successful results of treatment with ACT (Twohig et al. 2010; Twohig 2012), contributing to increasing the probability of profit from psychotherapies based on a heightened level of present-moment awareness, increase acceptance of though emotions, promote recognition of values, and escalate committed action on values (Morton et al. 2012). As previously noted, ACT model proposes that experiential avoidance is a harmful strategy that arises when an individual is not willing to be in contact with certain private experiences, such as thoughts, emotions, bodily sensations, memories, and behavioral predispositions, while they try to change the form and frequency of these events and the contexts in which they occur (Hayes et al. 2013; Blackledge and Hayes 2001; Marvin et al. 2023). Based on clinical reports and empirical studies, a notoriously retarded process of change has been indicated in BPD patients over time, therefore, ACT is concentrated on (1) symptom management rather than symptom reduction; and (2) promoting functioning and valued living lead to a suitable match for helping patients' symptoms management which may not completely remit (Morgan and Aljabari 2019).

Experiential avoidance is presented to have a basic role in the course and development of psychopathology among patients diagnosed with personality disorder criteria (Jacobs et al. 2013). In line with a body of growing studies, it has been documented that many of the impairing symptoms observed in patients with BPD are driven by unworkable experiential avoidance strategies (Morgan and Aljabari 2019). Experiential avoidance strategies are applied by patients with BPD to change unpleasant internal experiences, encompassing self-injury, denial, distraction, substance or alcohol use, and thoughts and emotion suppression (Chapman et al. 2011; Bateman and Fonagy 2004; Linehan 1993). Patients with BPD involve in a wide range of avoidance-based behaviors, such as self-injury, repeatedly attempt suicide and substance use, contribute to decreasing the experiences of distress and unpleasant emotions at the moment, while escalating impairments and distress in the long run (Morgan and Aljabari 2019; Ostafin et al. 2012; Schellhas et al. 2016). In line with clinical findings, through increasing acceptance and decreasing experiential avoidance in DBT and ACT, patients with BPD revealed lower levels of depression and self-injurious behaviors, and also reduction in distress levels has been reported (Neacsiu et al. 2014a, 2014b; Berking et al. 2009; Krantz 2021; Krantz et al. 2018; Bond et al. 2011; Morton et al. 2012; Dixon-Gordon et al. 2017, 2021; Chapman et al. 2017; Chapman 2019). Morton et al. (2012) examined the efficacy of a 12-week ACT group therapy, compared to a treatment as usual (TAU) condition, for the symptoms of BPD through a public sector pilot study. The results showed a significant improvement in patients who received the combined of ACT and TAU. In addition, patients who received ACT group interventions revealed more positive changes in symptoms of anxiety and hopelessness, psychological flexibility, mindfulness, and emotional acceptance. Moreover, it was indicated that ACT processors can be considered as remarkable mediators of improvement in BPD symptoms, and targeting BPD symptoms and hopelessness instead of distress broadly. Furthermore, based on reports, a more sustained improvement was shown at three-month follow-up (Morton et al. 2012).

According to other findings, BPD symptom severity has significantly stronger association with experiential avoidance compared to emotion dysregulation and/or distress tolerance issues (Iverson et al. 2012); however, evidence emphasizes on the remarkable roles of both experiential avoidance and emotion dysregulation in the development of BPD (Schramm et al. 2013). Sloan (2004) examined the emotional reactions of individuals during the watching of pleasant, neutral, and unpleasant films. The findings showed that participants with high level of experiential avoidance displayed greater level of emotional experience and higher heart rate with the pleasant and unpleasant films in comparison to participants with lower levels (Sloan 2004). Gratz and Gunderson (2006) examined the efficacy of acceptance-based emotion regulation group intervention among self-harm women with BPD. The result demonstrated that the group intervention had positive influences on self-harm, emotion dysregulation, experiential avoidance, and BPD-specific symptoms, and also the symptoms of depression, anxiety, and stress. Additionally, the findings showed more normative levels of functioning generally (Grtaz and Gunderson 2006).

Defusion is associated with decreased avoidance-based coping and heightened approach-based coping in patients without BPD criteria (Donald et al. 2017). Defusion contributes to the development of abilities toward behaviors based on values even when painful or contradictory thoughts are being experienced by patients (Blackledge 2007). According to several investigations, patients with BPD experience high rates of cognitive distortions, such as dichotomous thinking and overgeneralization, due to their distress (Kramer et al. 2013, 2018, 2020), which learning defusion techniques assist them to answer more flexible to these distortions (Morgan and Aljabari 2019). Furthermore, present moment awareness (mindfulness) has a negative association with BPD symptomatology among clinical and nonclinical samples (Peters et al. 2013, 2017; O'Toole et al. 2012; Fossetti et al. 2012), and lack of mindfulness is a core feature of BPD pathology (Morgan and Aljabari 2019; Mitchell et al. 2019; Scheibner et al. 2016; Selby et al. 2016). In addition, based on theoretical studies, self-as-context skills are crucial for promoting perspective-taking, empathy, self-compassion, and compassion for others (Hayes et al. 2012; Yu et al. 2021), as well as allow for a non-driven sense of self-contributing to self-knowledge without judgment (Morgan and Aljabari 2019). Morton et al. (2012) reported changes in mindfulness through applying 12-week ACT group interventions among patients with BPD (Morton et al. 2012). Gratz and Gunderson (2006) reported that patients with BPD were influenced strongly by value discussions and pursued to apply values and committed action in their lives (Gratz and Gunderson 2006). Finally, Cameron et al. (2014, 2020) proposed rationale for considering values work in the psychotherapy of BPD which contributing to increased motivation for treatment, therapeutic adherence, and general quality of life (Cameron et al. 2014, 2020). Overall, ACT approaches appear promising in the future treatment of BPD and may inform the underlying mechanisms driving BPD emotional and behavioral problems, as well as key identity, interpersonal, and existential symptoms.

To conclude, the ACT model concentrates on the promotion of psychological flexibility and physiologically stemmed from *functional contextualism* and theoretically rooted in *relational frame theory*. ACT has revealed remarkable efficacy and effectiveness in the treatment of a notable range of different psychiatric disorders and in treatment-resistant patients, and also promotion in mental health well-being. The ACT psychological flexibility model consists of six subprocesses, comprising acceptance, defusion, flexible attention to the present moment, self-as-context, values, and committed action, which are based on three processes in ACT: being open, being aware, and being active. Furthermore, six core pathological processes contributing to the development of psychological inflexibility include inflexible attention, disruption of chosen values, inaction or impulsivity, attachment to conceptualized self, cognitive fusion, and experiential avoidance. As mentioned, individuals with BPD uses experiential avoidance strategies to avoid negative internal experiences, including self-injurious behaviors, denial, distraction, substance or alcohol use, and thoughts and emotion suppression, while increasing distress. Therefore, ACT focuses on the elaboration of present moment awareness (mindfulness), self-as-context skills, perspective-taking, empathy, self-compassion, and compassion for others, as well as allow for a non-driven sense of self and applying values and committed action in their lives in the treatment of individuals with BPD.

References

Ara BS, Khosropour F, Zarandi HM. Effectiveness of acceptance and commitment therapy (ACT) on emotional processing, irrational beliefs and rumination in patients with generalized anxiety disorder. J Adolesc Youth Psychol Stud (JAYPS). 2023;4(4):34–44.

A-Tjak JG, Davis ML, Morina N, Powers MB, Smits JA, Emmelkamp PM. A meta-analysis of the efficacy of acceptance and commitment therapy for clinically relevant mental and physical health problems. Psychother Psychosom. 2015;84(1):30–6.

Bach PA, Moran DJ. ACT in practice: case conceptualization in acceptance & commitment therapy. New Harbinger Publications; 2008.

Bai Z, Luo S, Zhang L, Wu S, Chi I. Acceptance and commitment therapy (ACT) to reduce depression: A systematic review and meta-analysis. J Affect Disord. 2020;260:728–37.

Baruch DE, Kanter JW, Busch AM, Juskiewicz KL. Enhancing the therapy relationship in acceptance and commitment therapy for psychotic symptoms. Clin Case Stud. 2009;8(3):241–57.

Bateman AW, Fonagy P. Mentalization-based treatment of BPD. J Personal Disord. 2004;18(1):36–51.
Bajari P, Houghton S, Tadelis S. Bidding for incomplete contracts: an empirical analysis of adaptation costs. Am Econ Rev. 2014;104(4):1288–319.
Belisle J. Model dependent realism and the rule-governed behavior of behavior analysts: applications to derived relational responding. Perspect Behav Sci. 2020;43:321–42.
Belisle J, Dixon MR. Relational behavior and ACT: a dynamic relationship. Behav Anal Pract. 2022;15:1–2.
Bennett R, Oliver J. Acceptance and commitment therapy: 100 key points and techniques. Routledge; 2019.
Berger JH, Chen F, Faerber JA, O'Byrne ML, Brothers JA. Adherence with lipid screening guidelines in standard-and high-risk children and adolescents. Am Heart J. 2021;232:39–46.
Berking M, Neacsiu A, Comtois KA, Linehan MM. The impact of experiential avoidance on the reduction of depression in treatment for borderline personality disorder. Behav Res Ther. 2009;47(8):663–70.
Beygi Z, Jangali RT, Derakhshan N, Alidadi M, Javanbakhsh F, Mahboobizadeh M. An overview of reviews on the effects of acceptance and commitment therapy (ACT) on depression and anxiety. Iran J Psychiatry. 2023;18(2):248.
Biglan A, Hayes SC. Should the behavioral sciences become more pragmatic? The case for functional contextualism in research on human behavior. Appl Prev Psychol. 1996;5(1):47–57.
Blackledge JT, Hayes SC. Emotion regulation in acceptance and commitment therapy. J Clin Psychol. 2001;57(2):243–55.
Blackledge JT. Disrupting verbal processes: cognitive defusion in acceptance and commitment therapy and other mindfulness-based psychotherapies. Psychol Rec. 2007;57:555–76.
Blackledge JT, Barnes-Holmes D. Core processes in acceptance and commitment therapy. Accept Commit Ther Contemp Theory Res Pract. 2009;1:41–58.
Bond FW, Hayes SC, Baer RA, Carpenter KM, Guenole N, Orcutt HK, Waltz T, Zettle RD. Preliminary psychometric properties of the acceptance and action questionnaire–II: a revised measure of psychological inflexibility and experiential avoidance. Behav Ther. 2011;42(4):676–88.
Bordieri MJ. Acceptance: a research overview and application of this core ACT process in ABA. Behav Anal Pract. 2022;15(1):90–103.
Cameron AY, Palm Reed K, Gaudiano BA. Addressing treatment motivation in borderline personality disorder: rationale for incorporating values-based exercises into dialectical behavior therapy. J Contemp Psychother. 2014;44:109–16.
Cameron AY, Erisman S, Palm RK. The relationship among shame, nonsuicidal self-injury, and suicidal behaviors in borderline personality disorder. Psychol Rep. 2020;123(3):648–59.
Chakhssi F, Janssen W, Pol SM, Van Dreumel M, Westerhof GJ. Acceptance and commitment therapy group-treatment for non-responsive patients with personality disorders: an exploratory study. Personal Ment Health. 2015;9(4):345–56.
Chapman AL. Borderline personality disorder and emotion dysregulation. Dev Psychopathol. 2019;31(3):1143–56.
Chapman AL, Dixon-Gordon KL, Walters KN. Experiential avoidance and emotion regulation in borderline personality disorder. J Ration Emot Cogn Behav Ther. 2011;29:35–52.
Chapman AL, Rosenthal MZ, Dixon-Gordon KL, Turner BJ, Kuppens P. Borderline personality disorder and the effects of instructed emotional avoidance or acceptance in daily life. J Personal Disord. 2017;31(4):483–502.
Chua JY, Shorey S. The effect of mindfulness-based and acceptance commitment therapy-based interventions to improve the mental Well-being among parents of children with developmental disabilities: a systematic review and meta-analysis. J Autism Dev Disord. 2022;52(6):2770–83.
Clarke IE, Karlov L, Neale NJ. The many faces of narcissism: narcissism factors and their predictive utility. Personal Individ Differ. 2015;81:90–5.

Coto-Lesmes R, Fernández-Rodríguez C, González-Fernández S. Acceptance and commitment therapy in group format for anxiety and depression. A systematic review. J Affect Disord. 2020;263:107–20.

Dindo L, Van Liew JR, Arch JJ. Acceptance and commitment therapy: a transdiagnostic behavioral intervention for mental health and medical conditions. Neurotherapeutics. 2017;14(3):546–53.

Dixon-Gordon KL, Peters JR, Fertuck EA, Yen S. Emotional processes in borderline personality disorder: an update for clinical practice. J Psychother Integr. 2017;27(4):425.

Dixon-Gordon KL, Fitzpatrick S, Haliczer LA. Emotion regulation and borderline personality features in daily life: the role of social context. J Affect Disord. 2021;282:677–85.

Donald JN, Atkins PW, Parker PD, Christie AM, Guo J. Cognitive defusion predicts more approach and less avoidance coping with stress, independent of threat and self-efficacy appraisals. J Pers. 2017;85(5):716–29.

Dougher MJ, Hamilton DA, Fink BC, Harrington J. Transformation of the discriminative and eliciting functions of generalized relational stimuli. J Exp Anal Behav. 2007;88(2):179–97.

Enoch MR, Nicholson SL. Acceptance and commitment therapy and relational frame theory in the field of applied behavior analysis: the acceptability and perspective of the practicing BCBA. Behav Anal Pract. 2020;13:609–17.

Fan J, Ding C, Gong W, Yuan F, Zhang Y, Feng G, Song C, Liu A. Association of sleep duration and overweight/obesity among children in China. Int J Environ Res Public Health. 2020;17(6):1962.

Fawson S, Moon Z, Novogrudsky K, Moxham F, Forster K, Tribe I, Moss-Morris R, Johnson C, Hughes LD. Acceptance and commitment therapy processes and their association with distress in cancer: a systematic review and meta-analysis. Health Psychol Rev. 2023:1–22.

Ferreira MG, Mariano LI, de Rezende JV, Caramelli P, Kishita N. Effects of group acceptance and commitment therapy (ACT) on anxiety and depressive symptoms in adults: a meta-analysis. J Affect Disord. 2022;309:297–308.

Fletcher L, Hayes SC. Relational frame theory, acceptance and commitment therapy, and a functional analytic definition of mindfulness. J Ration Emot Cogn Behav Ther. 2005;23:315–36.

Galletti C, Ciodaro F, Freni F, Bruno G. Pneumoparotid and subcutaneous emphysema in a man with psychiatric disorders. Int J Otorhinolaryngol Clin. 2023;14(3):110–3.

Gloster AT, Walder N, Levin ME, Twohig MP, Karekla M. The empirical status of acceptance and commitment therapy: a review of meta-analyses. J Contextual Behav Sci. 2020;18:181–92.

Gould RL, Rawlinson C, Thompson B, Weeks K, Gossage-Worrall R, Cantrill H, Serfaty MA, Graham CD, McCracken LM, White D, Howard RJ. Acceptance and commitment therapy for people living with motor neuron disease: an uncontrolled feasibility study. Pilot Feasib Stud. 2023;9(1):116.

Gratz KL, Gunderson JG. Preliminary data on an acceptance-based emotion regulation group intervention for deliberate self-harm among women with borderline personality disorder. Behav Ther. 2006;37(1):25–35.

Gross AC, Fox EJ. Relational frame theory: an overview of the controversy. Anal Verbal Behav. 2009;25:87–98.

Haller H, Breilmann P, Schröter M, Dobos G, Cramer H. A systematic review and meta-analysis of acceptance-and mindfulness-based interventions for DSM-5 anxiety disorders. Sci Rep. 2021;11(1):20385.

Harris E, Samuel V. Acceptance and commitment therapy: a systematic literature review of prevention and intervention programs for mental health difficulties in children and young people. J Cogn Psychother. 2020;34(4):280–305.

Harte C, Barnes-Holmes D, de Rose JC, Perez WF, de Almeida JH. Grappling with the complexity of behavioral processes in human psychological suffering: some potential insights from relational frame theory. Perspect Behav Sci. 2023;46(1):237–59.

Hayes SC, Pierson H. Acceptance and commitment therapy. Springer US; 2005.

Hayes SC. A relational control theory of stimulus equivalence. In: Dialogues on verbal behavior; 1991. p. 1.
Hayes SC. Acceptance and commitment therapy, relational frame theory, and the third wave of behavioral and cognitive therapies. Behav Ther. 2004;35(4):639–65.
Hayes SC. The ACT in context. Routledge; 2016.
Hayes SC, Brownstein AJ. Mentalism, behavior-behavior relations, and a behavior-analytic view of the purposes of science. Behav Anal. 1986;9:175–90.
Hayes SC, Strosahl KD, Wilson KG. Acceptance and commitment therapy. New York: Guilford Press; 1999.
Hayes SC, Barnes-Holmes D, Roche B, editors. Relational frame theory: a post-Skinnerian account of human language and cognition. Springer; 2001. p. 141–54.
Hayes SC, Strosahl KD, Strosahl K, editors. A practical guide to acceptance and commitment therapy. Springer; 2004.
Hayes SC, Luoma JB, Bond FW, Masuda A, Lillis J. Acceptance and commitment therapy: model, processes and outcomes. Behav Res Ther. 2006;44(1):1–25.
Hayes SC, Strosahl KD, Wilson KG. Acceptance and commitment therapy: the process and practice of mindful change. Guilford Press; 2011.
Hayes SC, Barnes-Holmes D, Wilson KG. Contextual behavioral science: creating a science more adequate to the challenge of the human condition. J Contextual Behav Sci. 2012;1(1–2):1–6.
Hayes SC, Levin ME, Plumb-Vilardaga J, Villatte JL, Pistorello J. Acceptance and commitment therapy and contextual behavioral science: examining the progress of a distinctive model of behavioral and cognitive therapy. Behav Ther. 2013;44(2):180–98.
Houghton DJ, Joinson AN. Privacy, social network sites, and social relations. In: Human services in the network society. Routledge; 2014. p. 77–97.
Houghton DC, Compton SN, Twohig MP, Saunders SM, Franklin ME, Neal-Barnett AM, Ely L, Capriotti MR, Woods DW. Measuring the role of psychological inflexibility in trichotillomania. Psychiatry Res. 2014;220(1–2):356–61.
Ivancic M, Belisle J. Resolving barriers to an applied science of the human condition: rule governance and the verbal behavior of applied scientists. Anal Verbal Behav. 2019;35:196–220.
Iverson KM, Follette VM, Pistorello J, Fruzzetti AE. An investigation of experiential avoidance, emotion dysregulation, and distress tolerance in young adult outpatients with borderline personality disorder symptoms. Personal Disord Theory Res Treat. 2012;3(4):415.
Jacobs HI, Radua J, Lückmann HC, Sack AT. Meta-analysis of functional network alterations in Alzheimer's disease: toward a network biomarker. Neurosci Biobehav Rev. 2013;37(5):753–65.
Jiang X, Sun J, Song R, Wang Y, Li J, Shi R. Acceptance and commitment therapy reduces psychological distress in patients with cancer: a systematic review and meta-analysis of randomized controlled trials. Front Psychol. 2024;14:1253266.
Kelson J, Rollin A, Ridout B, Campbell A. Internet-delivered acceptance and commitment therapy for anxiety treatment: systematic review. J Med Internet Res. 2019;21(1):e12530.
Keulen J, Matthijssen D, Schraven J, Deković M, Bodden D. The effectiveness and cost-effectiveness of acceptance and commitment therapy as a transdiagnostic intervention for transitional-age youth: study protocol of a randomized controlled trial. BMC Psychiatry. 2023;23(1):51.
Knight L, Samuel V. Acceptance and commitment therapy interventions in secondary schools and their impact on students' mental health and well-being: a systematic review. J Contextual Behav Sci. 2022;25:90–105.
Kramer U, de Roten Y, Perry JC, Despland JN. Beyond splitting: observer-rated defense mechanisms in borderline personality disorder. Psychoanal Psychol. 2013;30(1):3.
Kramer U, Kolly S, Maillard P, Pascual-Leone A, Samson AC, Schmitt R, Bernini A, Allenbach G, Charbon P, de Roten Y, Conus P. Change in emotional and theory of mind processing in borderline personality disorder: a pilot study. J Nerv Ment Dis. 2018;206(12):935–43.
Kramer U, Grandjean L, Beuchat H, Kolly S, Conus P, de Roten Y, Draganski B, Despland JN. Mechanisms of change in brief treatments for borderline personality disorder: a protocol of a randomized controlled trial. Trials. 2020;21:1–3.

Krantz DJ. Emotion regulation through multiple customer mistreatment episodes: distinguishing the immediate and downstream effects of reappraisal and acceptance. Doctoral dissertation, The University of Akron; 2021

Krantz LH, McMain S, Kuo JR. The unique contribution of acceptance without judgment in predicting nonsuicidal self-injury after 20-weeks of dialectical behaviour therapy group skills training. Behav Res Ther. 2018;104:44–50.

Li H, Wong CL, Jin X, Chen J, Chong YY, Bai Y. Effects of acceptance and commitment therapy on health-related outcomes for patients with advanced cancer: a systematic review. Int J Nurs Stud. 2021;115:103876.

Li Z, Shang W, Yang K. Characteristics and trends in acceptance and commitment therapy research: a bibliometric analysis. Front Psychol. 2022;13:980848.

Linehan MM. Skills training manual for treating borderline personality disorder. Guilford Press; 1993.

Luciano C, Ruiz FJ, Torres RM, Martín VS, Martínez OG, López JC. A relational frame analysis of defusion interactions in acceptance and commitment therapy. A preliminary and quasi-experimental study with at-risk adolescents. Int J Psychol Psychol Ther. 2011;11(2):165–82.

Lundgren T, Dahl J, Melin L, Kies B. Evaluation of acceptance and commitment therapy for drug refractory epilepsy: a randomized controlled trial in South Africa – a pilot study. Epilepsia. 2006;47(12):2173–9.

Lundgren T, Dahl J, Hayes SC. Evaluation of mediators of change in the treatment of epilepsy with acceptance and commitment therapy. J Behav Med. 2008;31:225–35.

Luoma JB, Hayes SC, Walser RD. Learning ACT: an acceptance & commitment therapy skills-training manual for therapists. New Harbinger Publications; 2007.

Mahmoudfakhe H, Hasanzadeh N, Shiri H. The effectiveness of acceptance and commitment therapy on feelings of inferiority, fear of body image, and feeling of self-worth in cosmetic surgery applicants. J Res Psychopathol. 2023;4(12):31–8.

Marvin W, Harvey J, Ruth N. Barriers and facilitators to achieving well-being in pediatric providers. J Wellness. 2023;5(1):6.

Mathew A, Doorenbos AZ, Jang MK, Hershberger PE. Acceptance and commitment therapy in adult cancer survivors: a systematic review and conceptual model. J Cancer Surviv. 2021;15:427–51.

McCracken LM, Gould RL, Rawlinson C, Thompson B, Weeks K, Gossage-Worrall R, Cantrill H, Serfaty MA, Graham CD, White D, Howard RJ. Acceptance and commitment therapy for people living with motor neuron disease: an uncontrolled feasibility study. Pilot Feasib Stud. 2023;9(1):116.

McCracken LM. Personalized pain management: is it time for process-based therapy for particular people with chronic pain? Eur J Pain. 2023;27(9):1044–55.

McHugh L, Stapleton A. Self-as-context 11. The Oxford handbook of acceptance and commitment therapy; 2023. p. 249.

Mitchell R, Roberts R, Bartsch D, Sullivan T. Changes in mindfulness facets in a dialectical behaviour therapy skills training group program for borderline personality disorder. J Clin Psychol. 2019;75(6):958–69.

Morgan RE, Truman JL. Criminal victimization, 2018. Bureau Justice Stat. 2019;845:11–8.

Morgan TA, Aljabari R. Using acceptance and commitment therapy in the treatment of borderline personality disorder: rationale, preliminary evidence, and future directions. Curr Treat Options Psychiatry. 2019;6:271–83.

Morris EM, Johns LC, Gaudiano BA. Acceptance and commitment therapy for psychosis: current status, lingering questions and future directions. Psychol Psychother Theory Res Pract. 2024;97(1):41–58.

Morrison KL, Madden GJ, Odum AL, Friedel JE, Twohig MP. Altering impulsive decision making with an acceptance-based procedure. Behav Ther. 2014;45(5):630–9.

Morton J, Snowdon S, Gopold M, Guymer E. Acceptance and commitment therapy group treatment for symptoms of borderline personality disorder: a public sector pilot study. Cogn Behav Pract. 2012;19(4):527–44.
Neacsiu AD, Lungu A, Harned MS, Rizvi SL, Linehan MM. Impact of dialectical behavior therapy versus community treatment by experts on emotional experience, expression, and acceptance in borderline personality disorder. Behav Res Ther. 2014a;53:47–54.
Neacsiu AD, Bohus M, Linehan MM. Dialectical behavior therapy: an intervention for emotion dysregulation. Handb Emot Regul. 2014b;2:491–507.
O'Toole SK, Diddy E, Kent M. Mindfulness and emotional well-being in women with borderline personality disorder. Mindfulness. 2012;3:117–23.
Ong CW, Eustis EH. Psychological flexibility. The oxford handbook of acceptance and commitment therapy; 2023. p. 169–81.
Ostafin BD, Bauer C, Myxter P. Mindfulness decouples the relation between automatic alcohol motivation and heavy drinking. J Soc Clin Psychol. 2012;31(7):729–45.
Parmar A, Esser K, Barreira L, Miller D, Morinis L, Chong YY, Smith W, Major N, Church P, Cohen E, Orkin J. Acceptance and commitment therapy for children with special health care needs and their parents: a systematic review and meta-analysis. Int J Environ Res Public Health. 2021;18(15):8205.
Pearson A, Macera MH, Follette V. Acceptance and commitment therapy for body image dissatisfaction: a practitioner's guide to using mindfulness, acceptance, and values-based behavior change strategies. New Harbinger Publications; 2010.
Pepper SC. World hypotheses: a study in evidence. University of California Press; 1942.
Peters JR, Upton BT, Baer RA. Brief report: relationships between facets of impulsivity and borderline personality features. J Personal Disord. 2013;27(4):547–52.
Peters JR, Eisenlohr-Moul TA, Upton BT, Talavera NA, Folsom JJ, Baer RA. Characteristics of repetitive thought associated with borderline personality features: A multimodal investigation of ruminative content and style. J Psychopathol Behav Assess. 2017;39(3):456–66.
Ravanbakhsh L, Ebrahimi MI, Haddadi A, Yazdi-Ravandi S. Effects of the acceptance and commitment therapy on resiliency, self-compassion, and Corona disease anxiety on medical staff involved in COVID-19 pandemic. Iran J Psychiatry Behav Sci. 2023; (in press)
Reeve A, Moghaddam N, Tickle A, Young D. A brief acceptance and commitment intervention for work-related stress and burnout amongst frontline homelessness staff: a single case experimental design series. Clin Psychol Psychother. 2021;28(5):1001–19.
Roche B, Barnes-Holmes Y, Barnes-Holmes D, Stewart I, O'Hora D. Relational frame theory: a new paradigm for the analysis of social behavior. Behav Anal. 2001;25:75–91.
Ruiz FJ. A review of acceptance and commitment therapy (ACT) empirical evidence: correlational, experimental psychopathology, component and outcome studies. Int J Psychol Psychol Ther. 2010;10(1):125–62.
Ruiz FJ, Flórez CL, García-Martín MB, Monroy-Cifuentes A, Barreto-Montero K, García-Beltrán DM, Riaño-Hernández D, Sierra MA, Suárez-Falcón JC, Cardona-Betancourt V, Gil-Luciano B. A multiple-baseline evaluation of a brief acceptance and commitment therapy protocol focused on repetitive negative thinking for moderate emotional disorders. J Contextual Behav Sci. 2018;9:1–4.
Scheibner HJ, Spengler S, Kanske P, Roepke S, Bermpohl F. Behavioral assessment of mindfulness difficulties in borderline personality disorder. Mindfulness. 2016;7:1316–26.
Schellhas L, Ostafin BD, Palfai TP, de Jong PJ. How to think about your drink: action-identification and the relation between mindfulness and dyscontrolled drinking. Addict Behav. 2016;56:51–6.
Schramm AT, Venta A, Sharp C. The role of experiential avoidance in the association between borderline features and emotion regulation in adolescents. Personal Disord Theory Res Treat. 2013;4(2):138.
Selby EA, Fehling KB, Panza EA, Kranzler A. Rumination, mindfulness, and borderline personality disorder symptoms. Mindfulness. 2016;7:228–35.

Shiri S, Farshbaf-Khalili A, Esmaeilpour K, Sattarzadeh N. The effect of counseling based on acceptance and commitment therapy on anxiety, depression, and quality of life among female adolescent students. J Educ Health Promot. 2022;11(1):66.

Sinclair F, Gillanders D, Rooney N, Bonathan C, Hendry K, McLoone P, Hewitt C. Real-world evaluation of an acceptance and commitment therapy–based group programme for breast cancer survivors with fear of cancer recurrence. Support Care Cancer. 2023;31(12):700.

Sloan DM. Emotion regulation in action: emotional reactivity in experiential avoidance. Behav Res Ther. 2004;42(11):1257–70.

Stockton D, Kellett S, Berrios R, Sirois F, Wilkinson N, Miles G. Identifying the underlying mechanisms of change during acceptance and commitment therapy (ACT): a systematic review of contemporary mediation studies. Behav Cogn Psychother. 2019;47(3):332–62.

Sun Y, Ji M, Zhang X, Chen J, Wang Y, Wang Z. Comparative effectiveness and acceptability of different ACT delivery formats to treat depression: a systematic review and network meta-analysis of randomized controlled trials. J Affect Disord. 2022;313:196–203.

Thompson EM, Destree L, Albertella L, Fontenelle LF. Internet-based acceptance and commitment therapy: a transdiagnostic systematic review and meta-analysis for mental health outcomes. Behav Ther. 2021;52(2):492–507.

Thompson B, Moghaddam N, Evangelou N, Baufeldt A, Das NR. Effectiveness of acceptance and commitment therapy for improving quality of life and mood in individuals with multiple sclerosis: a systematic review and meta-analysis. Mult Scler Relat Disord. 2022;63:103862.

Torneke N. Learning RFT: an introduction to relational frame theory and its clinical application. New Harbinger Publications; 2010.

Twohig MP. Acceptance and commitment therapy: introduction. Cogn Behav Pract. 2012;19(4):499–507.

Twohig MP, Hayes SC, Masuda A. Increasing willingness to experience obsessions: acceptance and commitment therapy as a treatment for obsessive-compulsive disorder. Behav Ther. 2006;37(1):3–13.

Twohig MP, Hayes SC, Plumb JC, Pruitt LD, Collins AB, Hazlett-Stevens H, Woidneck MR. A randomized clinical trial of acceptance and commitment therapy versus progressive relaxation training for obsessive-compulsive disorder. J Consult Clin Psychol. 2010;78(5):705.

Twohig MP, Abramowitz JS, Smith BM, Fabricant LE, Jacoby RJ, Morrison KL, Bluett EJ, Reuman L, Blakey SM, Ledermann T. Adding acceptance and commitment therapy to exposure and response prevention for obsessive-compulsive disorder: a randomized controlled trial. Behav Res Ther. 2018;108:1–9.

Vaezi S, Bisheh KA, Fakhri MK. Comparing of the effectiveness of group acceptance and commitment therapy and group cognitive behavioral therapy on emotion regulation, psychological capital and coping strategies of students. J Adolesc Youth Psychol Stud (JAYPS). 2023;4(7):31–40.

Verheul R, Herbrink M. The efficacy of various modalities of psychotherapy for personality disorders: a systematic review of the evidence and clinical recommendations. Int Rev Psychiatry. 2007;19(1):25–38.

Vowles KE, McCracken LM. Acceptance and values-based action in chronic pain: a study of treatment effectiveness and process. J Consult Clin Psychol. 2008;76(3):397.

Waltz TJ, Hayes SC. Acceptance and commitment therapy. In: Cognitive and behavioral theories in clinical practice; 2010. p. 148–92.

Wang X, Chen J, Liu YE, Wu Y. The effect of acceptance and commitment therapy on psychological nursing of acute cerebral infarction with insomnia, anxiety, and depression. Comput Math Methods Med. 2022;2022(1):8538656.

Wegner DM. Ironic processes of mental control. Psychol Rev. 1994;101(1):34.

Wicksell RK, Melin L, Olsson GL. Exposure and acceptance in the rehabilitation of adolescents with idiopathic chronic pain – a pilot study. Eur J Pain. 2007;11(3):267–74.

Wilson KG, Flynn MK, Bordieri M, Nassar S, Lucas N, Whiteman K. Acceptance and cognitive behavior therapy. Cognitive behavior therapy: core principles for practice; 2012. p. 377–98.

Woods DW, Wetterneck CT, Flessner CA. A controlled evaluation of acceptance and commitment therapy plus habit reversal for trichotillomania. Behav Res Ther. 2006;44(5):639–56.

Yıldız E. The effects of acceptance and commitment therapy in psychosis treatment: a systematic review of randomized controlled trials. Perspect Psychiatr Care. 2020;56(1):149–67.

Yu H, Qiao A, Gui L. Predictors of compassion fatigue, burnout, and compassion satisfaction among emergency nurses: A cross-sectional survey. Int Emerg Nurs. 2021;55:100961.

Zancan RK, Constantinopolos LB, Pankowski BE, Bellini BD, Oliveira MD. Acceptance and commitment therapy for university students: perception of a pilot program. Psicologia: Teoria e Prática. 2023;25(1)

Zhang D, Lee EK, Mak EC, Ho CY, Wong SY. Mindfulness-based interventions: an overall review. Br Med Bull. 2021;138(1):41–57.

Chapter 12
Nonsuicidal Self-Harm and Suicide in Borderline Personality Disorder

Introduction

This chapter is focused on nonsuicidal self-harm (NSSH) and suicidal behaviors, as well as attempting to explore the theories of the development of suicide and NSSH. To reach these aims, first of all, an expanded definition through various theoretical and experimental perspectives of nonsuicidal self-harm (NSSH) and suicidal behaviors will be presented, including definitions used in modern research, as well as the distinction between suicidal behaviors and NSSH will be discussed. After providing an expanded overview of definitions of and differences between suicidal behaviors and NSSH, we will review the evidence-based models in the development of NSSH and suicidal behaviors.

Nonsuicidal Self-Injury (NSSI): Definition and Conceptualization

Nonsuicidal self-injury (NSSI) is one form of NSSH and involves a clinically substantial behavior reported frequently in adolescents and young adults across the world (Swannell et al. 2014; Brunner et al. 2014; Rausch et al. 2021), and an important public mental health concern among adolescents and adults in clinical settings, which are associated with psychological distress and impairment (Mendez et al. 2022; Klonsky and Moyer 2008; Wilkinson et al. 2022; Gardner et al. 2021a, b; Selby et al. 2012; Lu et al. 2024), and aggravated prevalence (Glenn and Klonsky 2013; Kiekens et al. 2018; Wilkinson et al. 2022). NSSI not only is a clinical concern, but also imposes a remarkable economic impact worldwide (Tsiachristas et al. 2020; Doran and Kinchin 2020; Kinchin et al. 2017; Gardner et al. 2021a, b; Shepard et al. 2016). Nonsuicidal self-injury (NSSI) is defined as an intentional and

M. Salavati, E. A. Selby, *Theories of Borderline Personality Disorder*,
https://doi.org/10.1007/978-3-031-75503-3_12

self-inflicted damage of body tissue, which has been assumed having emotion regulation function (Slabbert et al. 2022). NSSI has received growing recognition as a clinically significant mental health problem (Liu et al. 2017; Lu et al. 2024). NSSI is a common issue but in many cases, it is considered as a hidden behavioral problem, especially among adolescents (Hauber et al. 2019; Lockwood et al. 2018, 2020a, b; Lu et al. 2024). In comparison to suicide, less empirically attention has been proposed to NSSI traditionally (Muehlenkamp et al. 2005; Deng et al. 2023). This neglect has been stemmed from various views about the severity. In other words, based on the existence of a continuum of severity and mortality risk, NSSI refers to less severe form of self-injurious behavior (Brent 2015; Liu et al. 2016, 2017). It should be accentuated that in spite of several studies considered NSSI as an essential feature of borderline personality disorder (BPD), a growing body of investigations revealed NSSI comorbid a wide range of psychiatric disorders, such as depression, PTSD, substance use disorder, eating disorders, and other personality disorders (Gratz et al. 2015; Wilkinson 2013; Hauber et al. 2019; Lu et al. 2024; Deng et al. 2023). Klonsky et al. (2003) posited that that NSSI is associated with psychiatric morbidity and in several cases contributed to death even in nonclinical populations (Klonsky and May 2014). Claes et al. (2010) realized a greater level of psychopathology and a declined levels of adaptive personality traits and coping skills in patients with both NSSI and suicide attempts (Claes et al. 2010). Based on the growing empirical and clinical findings, NSSI contributes to the development of *mental disorders* (e.g., Nock et al. 2006, 2018; Brunner et al. 2022; Whitlock et al. 2008), such as heightened *risk for suicide and further suicide attempts* (Ribeiro et al. 2016; Gardener et al. 2022; Gratz et al. 2014; Crowell et al. 2014; Liu et al. 2017; Asarnow et al. 2011; Wilkinson et al. 2011; Skegg 2005; Sapyta et al. 2012; Burke et al. 2021; Turner et al. 2022, 2021), *completed suicide* (Gratz et al. 2014; Shafii 1985), *anxiety, mood disorder, and PTSD* (Klonsky and Olino 2008; Hamza and Willoughby 2016; Kiekens et al. 2018; Cipriano et al. 2017; Niu et al. 2024; Deng et al. 2023), *eating disorders* (e.g., Whitlock et al. 2008; Cipriano et al. 2017; Buelens et al. 2020a, b; Krug et al. 2021; Selby et al. 2010; Cucchi et al. 2016), *BPD* (e.g., Klonsky and Olino 2008; Møhl 2019; Cipriano et al. 2017; Niu et al. 2024; Deng et al. 2023), *internalizing and externalizing psychopathology and social problem solving deficits* (Hawton et al. 1999, 2002; Muehlenkamp et al. 2013; Bentley et al. 2015; Meszaros et al. 2017), and *serious harm* (e.g., Bergen et al. 2012). Moreover, NSSI has a predictive function for further suicidal ideation and suicide attempts (Brunner et al. 2022; Glenn and Klonsky 2013; Crowell et al. 2014; Grandclerc et al. 2016). Furthermore, self-injurious behaviors (SIB) and NSSI may contribute to several school, occupation, and interpersonal dysfunctions (e.g., Lewinsohn et al. 1993), low self-esteem, emotional and behavioral problems, and experiencing distress (e.g., Hilt et al. 2018; Bjärehed and Lundh 2008), and intensified risk of unacceptable outcomes, such as academic underperformance (Kiekens et al. 2016). Moreover, rumination, experiencing feelings of embarrassment, fear of stigma, and as a result low levels of seeking help (Buelens et al. 2019, 2020a, b; Burke et al. 2021; Moran et al. 2012).

During the past decades, different terminology has been utilized to define and describe self-injury (Brunner et al. 2022). Based on literature, various terminology is applied to provide a clear definition for self-injury, such *nonsuicidal self-injury* (NSSI), *self-inflicted injuries* (SII), *nonsuicidal self-harm* (NSSH), *nonsuicidal self-directed behaviors* (NSSDB), *deliberate self-harm* (DSH), and *self-injurious thoughts and behaviors* (SITBs). The most significant factors leading to various terms are on the basis of being direct or indirect self-injury, existence of intention to die, and being included suicide behaviors or not. These definitions will be covered in the following pages. Recently, theoretical and empirical investigations have emphasized on the differences in these terms based on the intent to die (e.g., Gratz 2003; Chapman et al. 2006; Nock and Kessler 2006; Jacobson and Gould 2007), as well as the functions of these behaviors. Regardless of various definitions, in clinical settings, distinguishing whether there are intentions to die or not has a significant role in assessing suicide risk and selecting appropriate therapeutic interventions. In addition, Kaufman et al. (2020a, b) suggested a series of terms to define self-inflicted injury behaviors, including ambivalent self-inflicted injury, self-inflicted self-harm, thwarted suicide attempt, suicide threat, suicide gesture, parasuicide, suicide-related ideation, passive suicide-related ideation, and suicide-related communications (Kaufman et al. 2020a, b; Silverman et al. 2007a, b; Selby et al. 2013a, b, c).

Based on the definition provided by the International Society for the Study of Self-injury (ISSS; 2018), ***nonsuicidal self-injury*** (NSSI) is defined as an intentional and self-directed act, injuring one's body tissue with no intention of suicide, which is socially unacceptable (international society for the study of self-injury, 2018; Buelens et al. 2020a, b, Møhl 2019; Hooley et al. 2020a, b), with a substantial emphasize on intentional and deliberate in nature (Hooley et al. 2020a, b). NSSI refers to the nonfatal, deliberate behavior contributed to the destruction or changes in bodily tissue, which occurs in the absence of conscious suicidal intent (American Psychiatric Association 2013; Klonsky et al. 2015; Mendez et al. 2022; Nock 2010; Vega et al. 2018; Hooley et al. 2020a, b; Turner et al. 2018; Niu et al. 2024; Deng et al. 2023), and is a ubiquitous mental health issue among teenagers and youth in age of 18–25 years (Swannell et al. 2014; Hamza et al. 2021; Gillies et al. 2018; Niu et al. 2024; Deng et al. 2023; Chen et al. 2023; Lu et al. 2024). NSSI is defined as direct and intentional destruction of one's own body tissue with no intention for death and suicidal intention (e.g., Liu et al. 2017; Nock 2010; Allen and Hooley 2019; Zelkowitz and Cole 2016; Klonsky and Muehlenkamp 2007; Gratz and Roemer 2008; Hooley et al. 2020a, b; Bentley et al. 2021; Kerr et al. 2010), which is not socially sanctioned (Valencia and Sinambela 2020; Paul et al. 2015; Nock 2010; Bentley et al. 2021), and has been recently recognized as a clinically notable phenomenon (e.g., Liu et al. 2017), with potentially detrimental consequences and a wide range of destruction in a wide range of functions, such as interpersonal, academic, and daily functions and can contribute to high risk of suicide (Mendez et al. 2022; Daukantaitė et al. 2020). Most often, NSSI is associated with BPD, although it can occur in individuals with no BPD diagnosis (Selby et al. 2010; Klonsky 2007). Based on the DSM-5-TR (2022), NSSI has been highlighted in clinical conditions and behavioral problems that may be a focus of clinical attention and was described "as intentional self-inflicted damage to the body in the absence of suicidal intent." (DSM-5-TR 2022, p.822). It means NSSI is a deliberate self-directed or intentional self-inflicted damage to the body in a way to lead to bleeding, bruising, or pain (e.g., cutting, burning, stabbing, hitting, excessive rubbing; e.g., Hooley et al. 2020a, b) in the absence of suicidal intent (DSM-5-TR 2022). Although NSSI has a strong association with suicide (e.g., Allen and Hooley 2019; Klonsky et al. 2013, 2016; Wilkinson et al. 2011; Niu et al. 2024; Chen et al. 2023; Lu et al. 2024), and is a significant predictor for future suicidal behavior (Ribeiro et al. 2016; Turner et al. 2018), NSSI has higher prevalence, more frequency, greater various methods, higher severity, and more functionality (temporarily alleviate intense negative emotions) compared to suicide attempts (Klonsky et al. 2016). To confirm, some investigations indicated that individuals may engage in NSSI behaviors to alleviate their intense negative emotions and cope with them, and also, as an inhibitory strategy against acting out on their suicidal thoughts (Nixon et al. 2002, 2008; Laye-Gindhu 2011; Klonsky 2007; Klonsky et al. 2016; Klonsky and Muehlenkamp 2007; Muehlenkamp et al. 2005; Muehlenkamp and Gutierrez 2004).

According to estimated reports in 2014, the lifetime prevalence of NSSI varied from 5.5% in adults to 17.2% in adolescents (Liu et al. 2017; Swannell et al. 2014). In line with Rockett et al. (2023), suicides together with nonsuicide mortality due to drug-intoxication (undetermined and accidental deaths), demonstrate self-injury mortality (SIM). They emphasized these fatalities as deaths due to mental disorders and distress (Rockett et al. 2023). Through an ecological perspective, these deaths are rooted in various factors such as detrimental life circumstances and personal distress (Caine 2013, 2020). According to CDC (2015), NSSI have virtually 16–18% prevalence in adolescents who report suicidal ideation experiences each year (CDC 2015; Ivey-Stephenson 2020; Lu et al. 2024) and approaching one-third of adolescents with suicidal thoughts pursue to attempt suicide (Nock et al. 2013; Hamza et al. 2021). NSSI is a major concern among adolescent populations (Brown and Plener 2017) reported 14–15% of adolescents in community samples (Laye-Gindhu 2011; Ross et al. 2009), and 40% or more in psychiatric populations (Kumar 2010). The prevalence in adolescents has been estimated 17–38% in community samples (Brunner et al. 2014; Niu et al. 2024; Deng et al. 2023), and 50–60% in clinical samples (Kaess et al. 2013). Based on epidemiological findings depending on various methodological variations and dissimilar definitions, the prevalence rates of NSSI among inpatient adolescents is different from almost 35% to 80% (Koenig et al. 2017; Hauber et al. 2019). Epidemiological studies represent high prevalence of NSSI (Selby et al. 2015a, b), for instance, 13% to 45% among adolescents (e.g., Bentley et al. 2014; Muehlenkamp et al. 2012, 2018; Selby et al. 2015a, b; Reinhardt et al. 2022), and 4% to 28% among adults (Bentley et al. 2014, Shaffer and Jacobson 2009; Selby et al. 2015a, b). McManus and Gunnell (2020) cited colleague students and non-colleague students of the same age do not display any differences in rates of NSSI (McManus and Gunnell 2020). NSSI can be considered as a remarkable indicator of suicide risk (Andrews and Hanna 2020; Selby et al. 2015a, b; Hooley et al. 2020a, b; Ribeiro et al. 2015), and further suicidal behaviors (Ribeiro et al. 2015; Gardner et al. 2021b; Hamza et al. 2012; Ribeiro et al. 2016; Castellví et al. 2017; Selby et al. 2015a, b; Cox et al. 2012; Guan et al. 2012; Wilkinson et al. 2011). In one recent research which assessed the lifetime prevalence of NSSI, it was reported more than 50% of the young sample engaged at least one time in NSSI behaviors. It should be accentuated that due to cultural dissimilarities and traditional matters among different countries, the prevalence of NSSI may be influenced, and as a consequence the prevalence rates of NSSI may be realized different. This happens because cultural differences can influence on different NSSI risk factors like family integrity and dynamic, childhood family adversity, being rejected from peers, victimization, and socioeconomic status (Cassels et al. 2018; Giletta et al. 2013; Brunner et al. 2014). It should be noted since these self-directed injury behaviors are significantly frequent in BPD, recognizing them as a predictor of suicide risk may be limited (Andrews and Hanna et al. 2020; Selby et al. 2015a, b). Through a meta-analysis systematic review of well-established 62 articles published from 1st of January 2010 to 30th of June 2021, Xiao et al. (2022a, b) perused the global prevalence and characteristics of NSSI among nonclinical adolescents, especially repetition of NSSI (Martin et al. 2016; Hawton et al. 2012). As reported, among 264,638 included adolescents, an aggravated lifetime prevalence was recognized, including of a lifetime prevalence 22.0%- and 12-months prevalence 23.2%, which were consistent with former findings reported from a meta-analysis between 1989 and 2018 (lim et al. 2019). Higher levels of repetitive NSSI (20.3% vs 8.3%) were more common and a parallel frequency of mild injury (12.6%) to moderate injury (11.6%) was detected. Additionally, findings indicated that three types of NSSI among adolescents, including banging/hitting, pinching, and pulling hair. Swallowing drugs and toxic substances and chemical substances were seemed to be lower the other types of NSSI (Xiao et al. 2022a, b). Turner et al. (2018) examined NSSI prevalence, course, and its relationship with suicidal thoughts and suicide attempts among 21,449 active-duty soldiers and 38,507 newly enlisted soldiers. The findings revealed NSSI has a high prevalence among US Army soldiers, and is related to substantial escalation likelihood of further suicidal ideation and suicide attempts, even after recovery of NSSI (Turner et al. 2018).

In line with research on patient populations, age onset of NSSI is 13–14 (e.g., Klonsky and Muehlenkamp 2007; Nock et al. 2006, 2018; Faura-Garcia et al. 2021; Muehlenkamp et al. 2018; Glenn and Klonsky 2009; Deng et al. 2023; Lu et al. 2024). Growing findings have indicated that high prevalence of engaging in NSSI among adolescents (e.g., Swannell et al. 2014; Niu et al. 2024; Deng et al. 2023; Chen et al. 2023; Lu et al. 2024). Based on estimations, nearly 4% of general population engages in NSSI (Selby et al. 2010), and this rate has increased in colleague students' samples (Gratz 2006; Gratz et al. 2015), which can be considered as a challenging problem in academic situations (Selby et al. 2010, 2015a, b), being stigmatized by peer groups, interpersonal difficulties, and emotional sufferings

(Selby et al. 2015a, b; Asarnow et al. 2011; Klonsky 2009; Daukantaitė et al. 2020; Chen et al. 2023). Based on investigations, NSSI appears to be more prevalent among college populations, rated from 7% to 38% (Gollust et al. 2008; Whitlock et al. 2011; Anderson et al. 2018), whereas 4% among adult nonclinical populations (Klonsky et al. 2003). Research has indicated that higher levels of engaging in SIB in young women due to greater levels of psychological distress; however, under the same conditions of psychological distress, emotion dysregulation, and impulsivity, both women and men reported parallel experiences of NSSI (Lutz et al. 2022).

Hooley et al. (2020a, b) challenged these definitions of NSSI and suggested a significant aspect of NSSI is being intentional and deliberate, if an individual engages during dissociative episodes and in state of detachment from reality, can be claimed that NSSI it is intentional, and person's motivation is to feel something? NSSI's intention is self-injury with no intention for death, and also does not consist of socially sanctioned behaviors. Furthermore, as defined, NSSI should be direct with no intervention between the action and the injury such as poisoning (e.g., Nock and Favazza 2009). Nevertheless, based on different cultures and contexts, some specific behaviors including piercing and tattoos are excluded from NSSI behaviors which propose the influence of culture and context in the definition of NSSI (e.g., Favazza 2009). In NSSI, the extent of bodily and tissues damage includes a moderately intense harm (Favazza 2009). The word "moderate" can be misleading and induce a little clinical problem to mind, while NSSI is a globally problematic mental health concern. Hooley et al. (2020a, b) posited that that that there some types of more minor and highly normative behaviors like lip-biting, scab-picking, and nail-biting are not included as NSSI, as well as skin-picking and hair pulling are excluded. Whereas skin-picking and hair pulling are mild, they contribute to little damage, and in their severe forms, they are considered as distinct disorders named excoriation and trichotillomania, which both are destructive behaviors and can be considered as NSSI. Finally, NSSI is differentiated from Stereotypic self-injury because it occurs at a very high frequencies with a fixed and rhythmic in nature, with no guilt and shame (e.g., Nock and Favazza 2009). Some researchers pursue to utilize terms including nonlethal SIB and considered these behaviors as "self-harm." On the other hand, some researchers purported that the term "NSSI" is imprecise, and posited that NSSI behaviors are highly comorbid with suicidal acts. In addition, they mentioned it is common that individuals who engage in NSSI behaviors report some feeling of ambivalence about living or death (e.g., Kapur et al. 2013), which questions the range to which NSSI is nonsuicidal (Hooley et al. 2020a, b). Hooley et al. (2020a, b) suggested it is necessary to keep NSSI and suicidal behaviors in two distinct categories in spite of their overlaps. Based on several reports, many people who attempt suicide have no history of engaging in SIB (e.g., Taylor et al. 2017), and also many individuals engaged in NSSI deny any suicidal thoughts and behaviors (e.g., Fox et al. 2020). In conclusion, Hooley et al. (2020a, b) emphasized on the importance of using a precise definition of NSSI to prevent from inflated rates of NSSI (Hooley et al. 2020a, b).

Based on Gardener et al. (2022), ***self-harm*** is a term which embraces both nonsuicidal and suicidal behaviors, is considered as a main risk factor for subsequent suicide attempts (see, Gellen and Klonsky 2013; Crowell et al. 2014; Gardner et al. 2016, 2021a, b; Ribeiro et al. 2016; Mars et al. 2019), and based on growing evidence, is a major factor for impaired mental health/well-being (Gardner et al. 2021a, b; Jacobson and Gould 2007; Mars et al. 2014; Brunner et al. 2022). In other words, self-harm is like as umbrella included NSSI and suicidal behaviors (Shafti et al. 2021). Gardner et al. (2021a, b) posit self-harm is defined as a socially unacceptable and deliberate destructive action against body tissues (e.g., cutting) and self-poisoning with no suicidal intention (American Psychiatric Association 2013), and encompasses a wide spectrum of directed self-damaging behaviors, including NSSI and suicidal ideation irrespective of the degree of suicidal intent (Hawton et al. 2003a, b) with high incidence in teenagers (Geulayov et al. 2019). Consistent with this definition, there is no distinctive border between suicidal and nonsuicidal self-harm (NSSH). In other words, ***nonsuicidal self-harm*** (NSSH) consists of not only direct self-injury (a destructive action against one's body tissue), but also self-poisoning (an action that does not damage body tissue) without suicidal intent, both are not socially sanctioned (American Psychiatric Association 2013). Gardner et al. (2021a) suggested the term "HSSH" is more precise to utilize in describing and investigations about self-damaging behaviors, specifically based on findings revealed NSSH is as prevalent as NSSI (international pooled prevalence of 17.2% compared to 13.4% for youth and 5.5% for adults; Swannell et al. 2014) (Gardner et al. 2021a, b, p.142).

Deliberate self-harm (DSH) has been assumed as NSSI and is conceptualized as contradictory to suicidal behaviors (Gratz et al. 2019a, b, 2022; Gratz 2003), with different functions and correlates (Brown et al. 2014, 2016, 2017; Nock and Kessler 2006). A growing body of empirical studies have provided evidence about the association between deliberate self-harm and emotional and behavioral problems, and difficulties in various areas of interpersonal and intrapersonal functions in adolescents (e.g., Jacobson and Gould 2007). Several investigations have distinguished adolescents who engage in self-deliberate self-injury and suicidal behaviors suffer from higher levels of depression, anger, loneliness, and tendency to take high-risk behaviors, such as substance use than adolescents with only suicidal behaviors (Gratz et al. 2019a, b, 2022; Guertin et al. 2001). Moreover, these adolescents with both DSH and suicidal behaviors are prone to experience higher levels of MDD, suicidal ideation, and PTSD in comparison to adolescents with only deliberate self-harm (Jacobson et al. 2008).

Self-injurious thoughts and behaviors (STIBs) are with an intention to die (e.g., suicidal thoughts and acts) or with no intention to die (e.g., NSSI). STIBs consist of suicidal thoughts and ideation, suicidal plan, suicide attempts, and suicide death (Bentley et al. 2021; Nock 2010).

Self-injurious behaviors (SIB) include both deliberate self-harm (DSH) and suicidal behaviors, and is defined as an intentional, self-directed destructive behavior which damages the tissues of body without any intention for suicide (Gratz et al. 2019a, b, 2022). Based on Gratz et al. (2014), there is wide range in the intention of engaging in self-injury behaviors in an individual from a clear or ambivalent intent to die (e.g., Crowell et al. 2009), to no purpose for death (e.g., Chapman et al. 2006; Fliege et al. 2009).

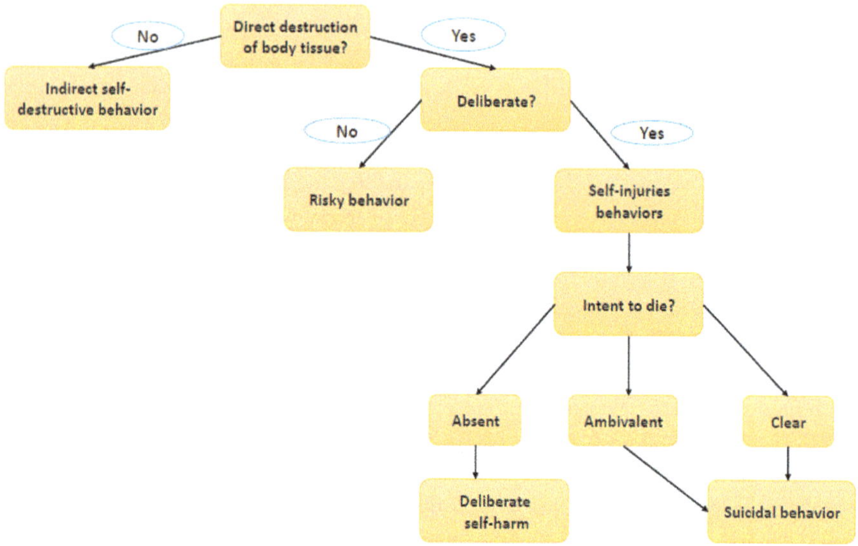

Source: adapted from Gratz et al. (2014), p. 196

Self-injurious behaviors (SIB) can be categorized into two classes: *direct self-injury* and *indirect self-injury* (Møhl 2019). **Direct self-injury** refers to the self-inflicted harm which is obvious and generally easy to detect. Direct and deliberate infliction of harm is a requirement for NSSI, and self-harm should take place with no hesitation after the behavior itself, such as a wound appearing immediately after self-cutting (Nock and Favazza 2009). A wealthy body of investigations have demonstrated self-directed NSSH compasses injurious behaviors, such as cutting, scratching, self-hitting, and burning (e.g., Mettler et al. 2023; Nock and Favazza 2009; Klonsky and May 2014; Gratz and Gunderson 2006; Kaufman et al. 2020a, b; Gratz 2007), including *cutting* (50–90%; Klonsky 2007), *hitting* (64% in male and 39% in female; Rubæk and Møhl 2023), *scratching* (21% in male and 31% in female; Bresin and Schoenleber 2015), *burning* (20% in male and 18% in female; Bresin and Schoenleber 2015), *compulsive headbanging* (28% in male 24% in female; Bresin and Schoenleber 2015), *trichotillomania* (12% in male and 35% in female; Bresin and Schoenleber 2015), *skin picking* (1.4%, DSM-5, 2022), *self-inflicted fractures*, *biting* (27% in female and 16% in male), *inserting needles under the skin* (20% in male and 24% in female), *carving the skin* (18% in male and 27% in female), *sewing the skin with threat, rubbing the skin violently, pouring acid on the skin, and self-inflicted tattoos* (Bresin and Schoenleber 2015; Møhl 2019; Lloyd-Richardson et al. 2007; Madge et al. 2008; Hawton et al. 2012; Hawton and Harriss 2008, 2003a, b). Prevalent modes of NSSI consist of cutting, burning, or carving the skin (Klonsky and May 2014; Buelens et al. 2020a, b). In sum, NSSI encompasses a wide range of behaviors, including cutting, burning, scratching the skin, self-hitting, head banging, bone breaking, interfering with wound healing, hair pulling, and nail biting resulting bleeding (McKenzie and Gross 2014). The most common types of NSSI consist of skin-cutting, burning, and severe scratching (Glenn and Klonsky 2013; Nock and Prinstien 2004; Whitlock et al. 2006).

Indirect self-injury refers to an action which contributes to escalating the risk of unintended long-term consequences, rather than leading to a straightforward or apparent injury, including heavy drinking or smoking, being eating and purging, alcohol-related blackout, substance use problems, unprotected safe, reckless driving, and gambling. In other words, the most remarkable characteristic of indirect self-injury is an elevation in the harmful and nonfatal consequences of these behaviors for an individual (Møhl 2019). Most of the time, in indirect harmful behaviors, a prompt personal harm is not a primitive motivator of self-injurious behavior, and physical pain and suffering happens downstream of the behavior itself (Hooley et al. 2020a, b). It should be mentioned in the case of direct self-injury, the damage is predictable and as soon as it occurs, its negative effects will appear. Yet, identifying the indirect self-injury precisely is difficult and challenging because of its implicit nature. In addition, studies have shown that individuals who engage in direct self-injury, have a more considerable history of suicidal ideation and attempted suicide, in comparison with individuals engaged in indirect self-injury (Germain and Hooley 2012; Møhl 2019).

Yet, it should be mentioned often direct and indirect of NSSI are comorbid (Hooley et al. 2020a, b), such as eating disorders (e.g., Gollust et al. 2008) and anorexia nervosa or bulimia (e.g., Cucchi et al. 2016). Krug et al. (2021) examined the high co-occurrence of NSSI and eating disorder symptoms based on a new integrative model, among 123 members of a clinical sample with eating disorder and 531 nonclinical individuals. The results indicated that the comorbidity between NSSI and eating disorder can be attributed to both common factors, such as attachment and maladaptive schema, and specific factors like impulsivity (Krug et al. 2021; Niu et al. 2024; Deng et al. 2023; Chen et al. 2023; Lu et al. 2024). Despite sharing many similarities (Germain and Hooley 2012, 2013), there are some core differences (Germain and Hooley 2012; Hooley et al. 2020a, b). Germain and Hooley (2012) demonstrated individuals who engage in both NSSI (as a direct self-harm) and indirectly detrimental behaviors experienced greater levels of self-criticism and higher levels of elevated suicidal tendencies (Germain and Hooley 2012).

Møhl (2019) suggested a new feature of self-injury encountered by many clinicians working in clinical settings and is not typically mentioned in literature, referring to this experience as *self-injury by proxy*, which refers to "*a situation where the person enlists the cooperation of another person to inflict the injury*" (Møhl 2019, p. 7). Møhl (2019) emphasized on the distinction between *Munchausen's syndrome by proxy*, where children undergo harm and injury by their parents rather than others. Instead, in self-injury by proxy, there is an active persuasion or provoking by patient to encourage another person to inflict the injury on the patient, deliberately of subconsciously. The purpose of these encouragements may be emotion regulation or as form of self-punishment. There are various manifestations of self-injury by proxy, such as piercing the tongue, nipples, or genitals, with no anesthetic procedures, or plastic surgery without medically indication, like penis extension or cosmetic changes in labia. Møhl (2019) posited that that that "by ***enlisting*** others to inflict the injury, the person (1) has an opportunity to engage with others, (2) is able to absolve him/herself of responsibility for the self-injurious behavior and take on the role of victim ('others are doing this to me'), (3) is able to legitimize and act out his or her anger, which may in self-injury by proxy but also in the kind of close and intense engagement with others that many patients with BPD lack due to a feeling of inner emptiness" (Møhl 2019, p. 8).

Crowell et al. (2014) proposed ***self-inflicted injury*** (SII) as any deliberate action of self-injury with the purpose of creating bodily harm and tissue damages, including NSSI, suicide attempts, and committing suicide (Crowell et al. 2014; Nock 2008). Kaufman et al. (2020a, b) considered that SII like an umbrella to encompasses a full-blown spectrum of all intentional behaviors of self-harm, from NSSI to die from suicide. In other words, as stated by Kaufman et al. (2020a, b), ***self-inflicted injury*** (SII) consists of both NSSH and suicide attempts, with various etiological influences (Kaufman et al. 2020; Crowell et al. 2014). The most distinctive feature is based on the existence intention for death or not (e.g., Zlotnick et al. 1999), which have in distinguishing suicidal behavior from NSSI, especially their functionality and operative impacts (see, Kaufman et al. 2020a, b; Crowell et al. 2014).

Møhl (2019) listed expanded risk factors for developing NSSI, including a history of sexual abuse and childhood maltreatment (e.g., Liu et al. 2017), raising in an invalidating environment, experiencing a hostile and critical family relationship, loss of parents, emotion dysregulation (Niu et al. 2024; Deng et al. 2023; Chen et al. 2023; Lu et al. 2024; Wolff et al. 2019; Valencia-Agudo et al. 2018), alexithymia, attachment matters and mental capacity issues, low self-esteem and self-confidence, self-criticism and perfectionism, body image dissatisfaction (Muehlenkamp et al. 2013), mental disorders, substance use disorders, interpersonal problems with peers, bullying, withdrawal and isolation, fear of perceived abandonment, being a member of sexual minority group and LGBTQ, and sleep issues (Møhl 2019).

Risk factors associated with NSSH have overlap among children, adolescents and adult populations who engage in NSSH. Genetic factors, having a history of childhood maltreatment and sexual abuse, lack of parental support and communication, experiencing stressful and traumatic events, exposure to peer NSSI, suffering from mental problems such as anxiety and eating disorder, and bullying are considered as significant risk factors for NSSH (e.g., Emelianchik-Key and La Guardia 2019; Martorana 2015; Deng et al. 2023). Baetens et al. (2014) proposed that parental warmth and supporting behavior have a considerable interaction effect to NSSI to contribute to escalated risk of NSSI among adolescents (Baetens et al. 2014). In an experimental study among 1238 students, Bureau et al. (2010) demonstrated poor quality of child–parent relationship can contribute to increasing rate of NSSI (Bureau et al. 2010). In addition, based on Guvendeger Doksat et al. (2017), parental separation/divorce escalate the risk of self-inflicted injurious behavior and suicide attempts (Guvendeger Doksat et al. 2017). Through a meta-analysis study, Wang et al. (2022) identified and categorized NSSI risk factors into 7 groups, including mental disorders, bullying, low health literacy, behavioral issues, adverse childhood experiences, physical symptoms, and the female gender (Wang et al. 2022). Studies have indicated that adverse childhood experiences have a distinguished role as risk factors of BPD, especially the effect of the quality of parental relationship associated with negative childhood experiences (Hessels et al. 2018, 2022), whereas the role of interpersonal relationships seems more complicated (Hessels et al. 2018, 2022; Bifulco et al. 1994).

In order to clarify the etiology and psychopathology that contributed to NSSI, a large body of empirical and clinical investigations have been done. A very important field that has attracted the attention of many researchers is emotion regulation difficulties. Tang et al. (2020) perused the effect of the internet addiction as a risk factor for NSSI among adolescents aged 11–20 and pointed out the internet addiction may lead to more frequent SIB compared to non-NSSI group (Tang et al. 2020). Since cyberbullying is a documented risk factor for suicidal thoughts and behavior in adolescents, Lanzillo et al. (2023) investigated the relationship between cyberbullying and self-injurious thoughts and behaviors separately, through focusing on the effect of being the subject of online rumors, illicit photographs, and threatening messages related to NSSI, suicidal ideation, and suicide attempt among 64 adolescent psychiatric samples. The results indicated that endorsement of any form of cyberbullying was significantly related NSSI. In addition, individuals who were the victims of online rumors were more than fifteen times as likely to engage in NSSI, and all participants who reported involvement in illicit photographs showed SIB, as well as almost seventeen times more likely to report suicide attempts history. There were recognized no significant relationship between the forms of cyberbullying and suicidal ideation (Lanzillo et al. 2023). Xie et al. (2024) demonstrated opioid and sedative misuse may be a considerable risk factors for engaging in NSSI behaviors among adolescents aged 10–20 (Xie et al. 2024). In a recent study, Berghoff et al. (2022) studied the relationship between interpersonal and emotional experiences and subsequent stressful events among 101 youth engaged in NSSI and without NSSI. The results revealed no diversities in positive or negative interpersonal levels beyond and behind stressful events. Individuals who reported engaging in NSSI showed higher levels of negative emotion following stressful events in comparison with individuals without NSSI behaviors. Furthermore, in the NSSI group, some levels of positive emotions were reported by individuals who experienced lower level of negative emotional responses. Overall, it was concluded that negative emotions subsequent to stressful events may be downregulated by positive interpersonal experiences among individuals with NSSI behaviors, which provide the assumption of interpersonal emotion regulation importance among NSSI individuals (Berghoff et al. 2022). Houben et al. (2017) indicated a significant contingency between the occurrence of an aversive emotional state and following self-injurious behavior. Furthermore, he posited that not only does negative reinforcement of NSSI contribute to decrease of emotional suffering, but also NSSI predicts the subsequent aversive emotion and following NSSI behaviors in the case of experiencing this aversive emotion, which lead to the development of a vicious circle overtime (Houben et al. 2017). In growing of clinical studies, researchers have pointed put NSSI as a coping strategy for regulating intensely negative emotion, coping with trauma and memories related to trauma, solving interpersonal conflicts in communicative contexts (Yakeley and Burbridge-James 2018; Turp 2003; Motz 2010; Brady et al. 2014; Stänicke et al. 2018).

Self-harm behaviors are considered as an individual's strategy to cope with a dissociated state of mind and experiencing positive emotions and removing negative emotions (Paul et al. 2015; Valencia and Sinambela 2020). In several investigations, it has been demonstrated adolescents engage in SIB to manage their anger and pain in intimate relationships and cope with communicative conflicted contexts due to difficulties with family and friends (Wadman et al. 2018; Gelinas and Wright 2013; McAndrew and Warne 2014). Pursuant to Stanicke (2018), adolescents and youth reported engaging in NSSI to release their negative emotion, take control on unpleasant and painful emotion, display unaccepted emotion, and make connections with people. It can be assumed self-harm behaviors not only have emotion regulation function (e.g., Paul et al. 2015), but also may be considered as an attempt to express or share significant conflicted emotional and relational knowledge from the adolescent's intrapsychic life (Stänicke et al. 2018). Bježančević et al. (2019) identified the features of NSSI among 105 with a history of NSSI, and identified an association between NSSI with female gender, alcohol consumption, and a wide range of psychiatric comorbidities (Bježančević et al. 2019). Moreover, several investigations have recognized that fluctuations and turbulence in negative and positive emotion are associated with SIB (e.g., Arbuthnott et al. 2015; Selby et al. 2013a, b, c). Through a systematic meta-analytic review about the association between NSSI and emotion dysregulation on 48 publications, Wolff et al. (2019) concluded higher levels of emotion dysregulation is related to greater risk of nonsuicidal injurious behaviors, regardless of age or sex. Moreover, based on findings, it was indicated that unique aspects of dysregulation may have implications for NSSI (Wolff et al. 2019). Noticeably, Franklin et al. (2014) pointed out the former NSSI frequency and number of how individuals engaged in NSSI were significant predictors of following NSSI (Franklin et al. 2014). Through a systematic review of the literature, a longitudinal study was done to assess the course of NSSI and deliberate self-harm based on 32 studies. In line with results, an escalation in rates of NSSI and DSH in adolescents with a decrease in youth and young adults were identified. Findings revealed female gender, a history of previous NSSI and suicidal attempts, NSSI thoughts, and also low implicit and explicit aversion to NSSI stimuli can be considered as predictive factors for future NSSI. Furthermore, psychiatric disorders such as depressive symptoms, anxiety, substance use disorders, persistent psychotic experiences, as well as familial and social factors, constituting parental depression, low reprieved family support, problems with peers and modeling from friends with NSSI can predict the following NSSI among adolescents and young adults over time (Plener et al. 2015).

Taken together, based on studies, it can be concluded: (1) former NSSI is a strong predictor of NSSI; and (2) some specific factors such as emotion dysregulation and implicit identification with self-cutting can distinguish NSSI from non-NSSI individuals, whereas may not be able to have an active role maintaining and continuing NSSI behaviors (Franklin et al. 2014; Glenn and Klonsky 2011). Glenn and Klonsky

(2010) highlighted the role of seeing blood in NSSI and indicated that seeing blood during NSSI is a significant reinforcing factor in SIB. They cited among individuals with NSSI, spending five minutes or less looking at the blood after doing NSSI, have a function of "relieving tension" which contribute to "feeling of calmness." In addition, greater lifetime frequency of skin-cutting and higher relief in interpersonal functions of NSSI, such as emotion regulation and self-punishment. Furthermore, it was revealed that the higher urge to see blood during NSSI, the more likely to report BPD symptoms (Glenn and Klonsky 2010). Hamza et al. (2012) indicated that an association between recent exposure to stressful experiences and perceived escalated emotional reactivity contributes to aggravated risk of NSSI (Hamza et al. 2012). Fox et al. (2015) reported that a history of previous NSSI, hopelessness, cluster B features, female gender, depression, history of suicide ideation and suicide attempt, peer NSSI, feeding and eating disorder and childhood maltreatment as prominent risk factors for subsequent NSSI (Fox et al. 2015). Mettler et al. (2021) compared perceived vs. actual emotion reactivity and regulation among 36 women with a recent history of NSSI within 2 years and 34 individuals with no NSSI behaviors to clarify the differences between individuals with and without NSSI on the experience of positive and negative emotion in terms of personal emotional reactivity, personal emotion regulation, and subjective experience of emotion in response to positive and negative mood induction. According to the findings, likewise previous studies, individuals engaged in NSSI displayed higher difficulties in negative emotion reactivity (e.g., Gratz 2006; Jenkins and Schmitz 2012), as well as reported greater problems in regulating negative emotion compared to non-NSSI participants (e.g., Gratz and Roemer 2008; Peh et al. 2017). In addition, there were no significant differences in reactivity or regulating of positive emotion among two groups, in contrast to prior research shown experiencing less positive emotion in individuals with a history of NSSI (e.g., Arbuthnott et al. 2015; Santangelo et al. 2017) and less rumination on positive emotion (e.g., Burke et al. 2019). Andover and Morris (2014) posited that NSSI both reduces intense negative emotion and increases the levels of positive emotion, which reinforces an individual to utilize NSSI repeatedly (Andover and Morris 2014).

Several investigations have pointed out the co-occurrence of psychiatric problems may be an explanation for the association between dispositional emotional reactivity and NSSI (e.g., Claes et al. 2014; Glenn and Klonsky 2011; Smith and Reidy 2021), contrary to investigations proposed that positive emotion can be considered as protective factors against NSSI (e.g., Burke et al. 2019; Hasking et al. 2019). In addition, repeated constant negative emotional condition can contribute to an accumulation over time which led to a greater subjective experience of being overwhelming and an emotional cascade by negative emotion, which may escalate the risk of engaging in NSSI to relieve intense and unpleasant negative emotion (e.g., Selby and Joiner Jr 2009; Slabbert et al. 2018). Muehlenkamp et al. (2013) studied body regard as a moderator of the association between emotional dysregulation and NSSI among 398 individuals engaged in NSSI to clarify the interactive effect of emotion dysregulation and body regard on the frequency of NSSI. Based on the findings, it was demonstrated that emotion dysregulation and NSSI were related only when there were low levels of body regards. It meant that attention to body has a significant role in identifying who engages in NSSI within the emotion dysregulation context. Through making interactive model of emotion dysregulation and body regard, they tried to elucidate the influence of this model on NSSI, and illustrated that body regard may be a vital factor to facilitate the onset and repetition of NSSI (Muehlenkamp et al. 2013). Kruzan et al. (2022) perused a moderated-mediation study to test whether body regard moderated the mediational influence of self-blame coping strategy on the association between impaired self-concept and NSSI, among 1906 university students who engaged in NSSI behaviors over the last year. Based on their findings, positive body regard can be considered as a protective factor and may strengthen the relationship between poor self-concept and self-blame coping on NSSI mitigated. In addition, in the condition of low or average body regard, poor self-concept is related to escalated NSSI because of self-blaming coping (Kruzan et al. 2022). These findings were consistent with a growing literature supporting the significance of positive body regard and attitude towards body in understanding NSSI (e.g., van Dijk et al. 2014; Vartanian 2009; Vartanian et al. 2018).

Suicide: Definition and Conceptualization

Suicide is mentioned as a public mental health problem worldwide (Moselli et al. 2021a, b; Gold 2020; Silvers et al. 2016; Silver et al. 2023; McClelland et al. 2023; Chapman-Hilliard et al. 2024; Watt-McMahon et al. 2023), in which its reduction is considered as a primary goal at the global level by World Health Organization (WHO 2014; Moselli et al. 2021a, b; McClelland et al. 2023; Chapma-Hilliard et al. 2024; Watt-McMahon et al. 2023). Suicide has been the center of several investigations during recent decades. Suicidal behaviors, which comprise ideation, attempts, and deaths are remarkable mental health concerns with an increased trend over the past decade (McClelland et al. 2023; Chapman-Hilliard et al. 2024; Watt-McMahon et al. 2023; Yen et al. 2020; Martinez-Ales et al. 2020). In other words, it can be claimed that that suicide is a global concern posing dramatic load to society (Keefner and Stenvig 2020). Death caused by suicide is a considerable public mental health problem firmly related to psychiatric disorders (Gold 2020). Every year 703,000 people die due to death by suicide and even more engage in suicide attempts (World Health Organization 2022), and approximately 800,000 persons die from suicide every year, with an expected increase of 2.4% by 2020 (WHO 2019). According to the Centers for Disease Control and Prevention (CDC), it is the second leading cause of death in individuals aged 12–34 (CDC 2020; Cha et al. 2018). Suicide is the fourth leading cause of death among 15–29-year-old in 2019 (World Health Organization 2022). In addition, in 2020, suicide was among the 9 top leading causes of death for people ages 19–64, as well as the second leading cause of death for people ages 10–14 and 25–34. Surprisingly, based on CDC (2022), suicide rates in 2020 were 30% higher than in 2000, nearly 46,000 people died by suicide in 2020, and also, in adults, it has been estimated that 12.2 million experience serious thoughts about suicide, 3.2 million made a plan for suicide, and 1.2 million attempted suicides. In addition, suicide can contribute to severe emotional, physical, and financial consequences (e.g., CDC 2022; Gardner et al. 2021b). In line with Bachmann (2018), suicide is the second leading reason to premature death among individuals aged 15–29 years, third reason in people aged 15–44, and is more prevalent, almost 78%, in low to middle-income countries (Bachmann 2018). Not only a person may be affected by suicide and suicidal attempts, such as a variety range of physical and psychiatric problems and associated with clinically remarkable psychopathology (e.g., Crowell et al. 2014; Gardner et al. 2021b), but also their families, friends, and community can suffer from serious negative consequences of a suicidal family member, like experiencing shock, anger, and even thoughts of suicide themselves (CDC 2022). In addition, these malignant mental health problems contribute to substantial economic impact worldwide (e.g., Gardner et al. 2021b; Doran and Kinchin 2020; Kinchin et al. 2017; Shepard et al. 2016). In 2020, suicide was reported as the 12th leading cause of death in all age groups, as well as the second leading cause for death in age group of 10–34 and the fifth in people aged 35–54 (National Center for Health Statistics 2021). In 2018, 1.4 million American adults had suicide attempts while nearly 47,000 died from suicide across all ages (Drapeau et al. 2018). Adolescence is period of life in which many outstanding changes have occurred, and maturation developments contribute to substantial impacts on adolescents' psychological health, emotion regulation, and behavioral control (Reinhardt et al. 2022). Due to many reasons, suicide is a social concern (Keefner and Stenvig 2020). First, when suicidal thoughts and suicide attempts begin for the first time in adolescence, they may continue to adulthood and compound the risk of death by suicide (Miller and Prinstein 2019). Second, the more death wishes increases, the more suicide attempts escalate (Chung and Joung 2012). Third, since most of the suicidal tendencies are stigmatized in different society, a significant number of suicidal cases are underestimated (Nock and Banaji 2007). Ultimately, die from suicide can be prevented if suicidal thoughts and suicide attempts are assessed once they appear (Keefner and Stenvig 2020).

There are various definitions of suicide and suicidal behavior. Suicidality is described as a continuum ranging from suicidal thoughts and plan to suicidal behaviors and in severe cases refers to death by suicide (Lönnqvist 2021). The subset of psychopathological issues ranging from suicidal thoughts and ideation to ambivalent suicide attempt, suicide attempt and death by suicide have been presented (Linehan 1987; Klonsky et al. 2016). According to Stone (2017), suicide is a part of a wider group of behaviors: namely *self-directed violence*, intentionally directed behaviors at oneself contributed to injury, or the potential for injury. In line with Stone (2017), self-directed behaviors consist of **nonsuicidal behaviors** and **suicidal behaviors** including suicide *(a death caused by self-directed injurious behaviors with the intention of death)*, and **suicide attempt** *(nonfatal self-directed injurious behaviors which may or may not result in injury, such as intentional self-inflicted poisoning, injury, or self-harm)* (Stone 2017; Vijayakumar and Phillips 2016). According to the CDC (2015), suicidal self-directed violence is defined as death effected by *self-directed injurious behaviors* with an intent for death due to these behaviors. *Suicide attempt* is described as a nonlethally self-directed injurious behavior with an intention for death because of this behavior even if it does not contribute to death. A set of alterations have been made by CDC (2017) to offer a uniform language and improving a communicative definition to remove the negative social judgments from current various terminology of suicide behaviors and make them more understandable and precise. For this purpose, the CDC (2017) replaced specific terms used for suicide by appropriate suggested terms (see, Table 12.1). Gold and Frierson (2020) cited CDC attempted to omit some terms associated to suicide, such as failed suicide, successful suicide, suicide gesture or threat, and suicidality, because they assumed that these terms have negative social implications (Crosby et al. 2011; Gold and Frierson 2020). Furthermore, the CDC's terminology attempts to propose a nonjudgmental with minimal stigmatization, such as *suicide death, death from suicide*, or *died from suicide* which are more neuter, precise, and accurate rather than problematic terms, like *committed suicide* or *death by suicide* (see, Table 12.2; Gold and Frierson 2020).

Suicidal ideation has been defined as thoughts, images, and wish to die and/or death by suicide, contribute to aggravated risks for later suicide attempts (Selby et al. 2013a, b, c; Lewinsohn et al. 1996; Spirito and Esposito-Smythers 2006), and death from suicide (Beck et al. 1999; Selby et al. 2013a, b, c). In other words, suicidal ideation defined as experiencing cognitions and thoughts about engaging in suicide associated behaviors (Grosby 2011; Gold and Frierson 2020). Aligned with suggestions made by the CDC (2017) and US National Strategy for Suicide Prevention, suicide ideation is defined as thoughts of engaging in suicide-related behaviors (Grosby 2011). As per CDC (2015), suicidal ideation is presented as any thinking about suicide, taking into consideration and making a suicidal plan in mind (CDC 2015). This definition has a wide range of various aspects from specific plans for death to explicit intention to die which can be an impending death (Jobes and Joiner 2019). As has been described by Klonsky et al. (2016), growing advances have been made in the field of suicide research and theory, continuing to elaborate our knowledge about this debilitating global phenomenon. One of the most significant developments is the ideation-to-action framework, including the formation of suicidal ideation and providing distinguishing elucidations and predictors for the progression of suicide ideation and suicide attempts as two distinct phenomena. Furthermore, proposing a growing body of investigations about separated factors

Table 12.1 CDC suggestion for uniform terminology and definition for suicide and self-directed injury

Unacceptable term	Suggested replacement
Completed suicide or successful suicide	Suicide
Failed attempt or failed suicide	Suicide attempt or suicidal self-directed violence
Nonfatal suicide	Suicide attempt
Suicidality	Suicidal thoughts and suicidal behavior
Suicide gesture, manipulative act, or suicide threat	Nonsuicidal self-directed violence or suicidal self-directed violence

Source: Grosby (2011, pp. 21,23,90) (Gold and Frierson 2020)

Table 12.2 CDC suggestion for uniform terminology and definition for suicide

Term	Definition
Suicidal ideation	*Experiencing cognitions and thoughts about engaging in suicide-associated behaviors*
Suicidal intent	*Explicit or implicit evidence reveals that in the time of self-harm the person wished to die or intended to kill her/himself, and the person is aware of likelihood consequences of his/her leading to death actions*
Suicidal plan	*An associated thought contributed to facilitating self-harm by leading to self-initiated action, including organized way of involvement in suicidal behaviors, such as time frame and method*
Suicidal attempt	*A deliberately nonlethal potentially harmful behaviors with the aim of death which can contribute to death or not as a result of injury*
Suicide	*Death caused by deliberately self-directed harmful behaviors with the intent of death*

source: Grosby (2011) (Gold and Frierson 2020)

and predictors of suicidal ideation and suicide attempts. Moreover, the proliferation of theories of suicide have been developed to provide various perspective for explanations the ideation-to-action framework (Klonsky et al. 2016), such as emotional cascade model (Selby et al. 2009), interpersonal theory (Joiner 2005), biosocial model (Linehan 1993), the integrated motivational-volitional model (Rory O'connor 2011), and the three-step theory (Klonsky et al. 2016).

Suicidal behaviors are intentional and potentially harmful SIB with at least some desire to die (DSM-5-TR, APA 2022). Suicidal behavior has no single determining causal factor, rather a broad spectrum of elements and multiple factors interact with each other to contribute to suicide, including biological, interpersonal, environmental, and societal factors which interact with each other over time (e.g., Mars et al. 2015; O'Connor et al. 2018; Selby et al. 2014a, b, c; Macintyre et al. 2021). As per Klonsky et al. (2016), the term suicidal behaviors are a general word to describe suicide, including suicidal thoughts or actions, with no guide to distinguish thoughts from plans, from nonlethal attempts, and from attempts lead to death, as well as NSSH is described as any deliberate SIB without intention to die. Providing distinct definition of these terms and distinguishing them from each other are vitally important to understand their prevalence rates, functional aspects, clinical associations, and consequences (Klonsky et al. 2016). Pursuant to Moutier (2021a, b), there are several myths and much misinformation about suicide throughout past decade which contributes to a multitude of negative influences, strongly stigmatizing the experiences where this health issue is considered. Therefore, without scientific investigations, myths and untruths continued to thrive.

Based on various investigations about health factors associated to suicide including mental and physical health, brain structure and functioning, genetic, psychological components and aspects, and the role of life stressors, many strong individuals have taken their lives and people who die by suicide have often fought to survive very hard in spite of suffering from psychological pain. Therefore, it can be claimed these people are weak or having deficiencies. A growing body of studies have demonstrated that suicide is a multifactorial phenomenon that encompasses a broad range of biological, genetic, psychological, social, in which these factors are interwoven and have interactional associations with each other (Cavanagh et al. 2003; Dombrovski and Hallquist 2021; Oquendo et al. 2014; McClelland et al. 2023; Chapma-Hilliard et al. 2024; Watt-McMahon et al. 2023). Furthermore, suicidal individuals are not "bent on suicide" because suicide risk is dynamic. The human mind has a dynamic nature and tries constantly to find hope and be resilient in spite of suffering from psychological pain and suicide is a solution for a painful problem. Therefore, ambivalence is a part of suicide leading to endeavor for seeking hope and recovery despite mental pain. Moreover, in line with several findings, many individuals with history of suicide attempts (85–95%) continue to live. Although history of suicidal behaviors can be considered as a strong predictor for further suicide attempts, it cannot be claimed that these individuals will die certainly by next suicide (Hawton et al. 2003a, b). Self-injurious and suicidal behaviors are assumed as signs of experiencing psychological suffering and these self-destructive behaviors are "Cry for Help." Suicidal behaviors stem from a wide array of psychopathology, genetic, and environmental impacts, and people show suicidal behaviors due to many behaviors and characterological reasons which propose signals of distress needed to urgent and immediate intervention. In keeping with several research, more than 50% of individuals with suicidal thoughts and behaviors talk with a friend, a family member, or healthcare provider about the intention to take their lives weeks before committing suicide. Suicidal individuals are different in expressing their thoughts and emotions about suicide, with some groups prefer to be silent about their suicidal ideation and plan, and others trying to talk about their psychological suffering and how it pushes them toward suicidal behaviors. Therefore, it is a wrong conclusion that individuals who express suicidal ideation are less at risk for suicidal attempts (Pompili et al. 2016). Due to fear of being stigmatized and cultural ethics, many suicidal people prefer to be isolated or withdrawn when they are suffering mental distress and try to hide their internal experiences which lead to an "out of the blue" perception of much suicidal behavior. It should be mentioned that suicidal behaviors are not generally impulsive acts rather suicide has an actual build up which can be traced cautiously by health providers and even family members and friends. Moreover, a growing number of studies have indicated that when using of an identified lethal mean become restricted and out of access, the rate of suicidal behaviors for the whole population will be diminished, even when other means are available. Additionally, following switching to a different suicide method, the rate of suicide shows 35–40% decrease (Gunnell and Miller 2010). Providing a sense of connection, establishing empathetic communication, supportive relationships, and a caring conversation are necessary to help an individual with suicide attempts (Gould et al. 2005). Finally, based on several empirical investigations, suicide crisis can cause changes in health components and brain structures and functions which contribute to cognitive constriction and a temporary but considerably inability to access adaptive coping strategies (Moutier 2021a, b).

A growing body of experimental and clinical investigations have been done to elucidate the various risk factors of suicide including biological, genetic, psychological, and socio-environmental components. Suicide attempts can be considered as a single trigger issue. In line with WHO (2014), the risk factors of suicidal tendencies and suicide attempts are categorized into five macro-areas based on socio-ecological models. These areas consist of the context determines; the cultural, religious and legal aspects; the relational areas; an individual level; and low serotonin levels or developmental changes (de Leo and Giannotti 2022). However, based on various definitions, the most significant motivation for suicide attempts is the desire to die, several empirical and clinical investigations have revealed individuals are motivated to attempt suicide by a set of numerous causes like escaping, communicating, changing environment, and dealing with an intolerable mind suffering (May and Klonsky 2013; Klonsky et al. 2016; Chapman and Dixon-Gordon 2007; Brown et al. 2014, 2016, 2017). In addition, the role of internal motivators in contributing to increase intent for death and escalated suicide attempts have been studied, such as significantly overwhelming mental pain and hopelessness (May and Klonsky 2013; May and Klonsky 2016), as well as communication motivations (May and Klonsky 2013; Hjelmeland et al. 2002). Several risk factors have been proposed by various empirical and clinical investigations for suicidal behaviors, such as childhood maltreatment, NSSI, and a history of previous suicide attempts (Hennings 2020; Franklin et al. 2017; Huang and Ribeiro 2020; Klonsky et al. 2013). Childhood adversity, especially childhood sexual abuse has been shown as a significant risk factor for NSSI and suicide attempts (Maniglio 2011; Ystgaard et al. 2004), depending on the age of victim at the time of experiencing abuse (Bruffaerts et al. 2010). Several meta-analyses have tested the associations between suicidal ideation and behaviors with psychiatric disorders (McClelland et al. 2023; Chapma-Hilliard et al. 2024; Watt-McMahon et al. 2023; Caves 2021; Harris and Barraclough 1997; Chesney et al. 2021; San Too et al. 2019; Conner et al. 2019; Boggs et al. 2018). Mood and anxiety disorders have been presented as common risk factors for suicidal behaviors. Due to several functional impairments which contribute to increasing various competency-efficiency issues in all areas such as occupation, home, and social roles among people who suffered from mood and anxiety disorders, many external problems usually escalate subjective negative inner feelings. Somatic complaints, depressed and anxious mood, helplessness, and hopelessness contribute to a chaotic state of mind, in which suicidal behaviors can be recruited to avoid experiencing these unpleasant conditions (Lönnqvist 2021). Hopelessness, guilt feeling, loss of interest, low self-esteem, previous suicide attempt, severity of depression, comorbidity with anxiety, and substance use are significantly associated with suicidal behaviors (Hawton et al. 2012; Lönnqvist 2021; Aaltonen et al. 2018). Family history of death by suicide is an important risk factor for suicide attempts in patients with bipolar disorder (Romero et al. 2007). In addition, individuals who suffer from anxiety disorders reported about 3 times more often suicidal thoughts, suicide attempts, and death by suicide compared to individuals with no anxiety disorder (Kanwar et al. 2013). Based on meta-analysis studies, considerable relationship between OCD and suicide was identified. Severity of suicidality is associated with unacceptable obsessive thoughts, comorbidity with other mental disorders such as anxiety and depression, hopelessness, and history of previous suicidal behaviors (Lönnqvist 2021; Angelakis et al. 2015; Albert et al. 2019). Suicidal thoughts and behaviors are prevalent among individuals who are traumatized and suffer from PTSD (Teismann et al. 2024; Angelakis et al. 2020; Panagioti et al. 2015; Nock 2012). Based on several studies, in individuals who met PTSD demonstrated different functional impairments displayed such as disrupted sleep patterns, inadequate social support, escalated likelihood of marital matters, and PTSD hyperarousal symptoms (Dell'Osso et al. 2014; Kotler et al. 2001; Costa-Maia et al. 2021; Stanley et al. 2019). These functional impairments are associated with high level of risk for suicide (Ribeiro et al. 2018). Greater levels of social support have revealed a relationship with lower PTSD severity (Zalta et al. 2021), and lower risk of suicidal thoughts and behaviors. Teismann et al. (2021) demonstrated that positive mental health and social support can moderate the influence of PTSD symptoms on suicidal ideation and behaviors in Iranian and German students (Teismann et al. 2021). Suicidality is associated with personality disorders and substance use which contribute to increasing risk for suicide (Rönnqvist et al. 2021). Alcohol use disorder, heavy drinking, and substance use disorder can lead to escalating significantly the risk of suicidal behaviors (Maes and Dom 2021; Roche et al. 2018; Norström and Ramstedt 2018; Xuan et al. 2016; Borges et al. 2017). Aggression, impulsivity, and hopelessness with the severity of alcohol use disorder may lead to high levels of suicide attempts and death (Van Heeringen and Mann 2014). Overall, in line with investigation, it has been indicated that 85–95% of individuals who die by suicide met a diagnosable psychiatric disorder at the time of attempting suicide (Moutier 2021a, b; Cavanagh et al. 2003), including major depression (50–60%), bipolar disorder (10%), substance use disorders (25%9), psychosis (15%), BPD (10%), anxiety disorders and PTSD (6%), impulse control disorders and eating disorders (Bertolote and Fleischmann 2002; Cavanagh et al. 2003; Harris and Barraclough 1997; Nordentoft et al. 2011; Moutier 2021a, b; Stanley et al. 2021).

Moreover, numerous psychological factors may contribute to aggravating the risk for suicidal ideation and behaviors, including distorted negative perceptions, intensified negative emotions, inflexible and rigid problem-solving style, impulsive personality traits, and deficits in executive functioning. As well as, proximal risk factors comprised of hopelessness, burdensomeness, worthlessness, experiencing negative emotion provoked events such as educational and occupational transitions, sense of failure and loss, sense of rejection and lack of social support, history of childhood maltreatment are proposed as risk factors for suicidal thoughts and behaviors. In addition, several socio-environmental factors may lead to increasing the risk of suicide, including the availability to fatal means, interpersonal conflicts, legal issues, financial crisis, exposure to peer suicide, and cultural and religious beliefs (William et al. 2018; Carli et al. 2022; Barber and Miller 2014; Moutier 2021a, b; McClelland et al. 2023; Chapma-Hilliard et al. 2024; Watt-McMahon et al. 2023). Jeon et al. (2022) examined the association between behavioral, psychological, and economic impacts of COVID-19 on suicidal thoughts' severity among 90 undergraduate students. Based on findings, alterations in loneliness experiences, loneliness due to social withdrawal, and problems in social connection, concerns about pandemic issues, anxiety of COVID contagion showed a significant correlation with pre-pandemic suicidal thoughts severity (Jeon et al. 2022).

Personality Traits as Prospective Predictors of NSSH and Suicide

Personality Traits are important to understand in contributing suicidality, and these traits can be considered as common correlates of suicide outcomes (Brezo et al. 2006; McClelland et al. 2023; Chapma-Hilliard et al. 2024; Watt-McMahon et al. 2023), predictors (Fergusson et al. 2003), endophenotypes (Turecki 2005; Baud 2005), and targets in mental health strategies (Krueger 2022; Brezo et al. 2008). A large body of research about why individuals attempt suicide and do self-harm behaviors have been done in recent decades, and almost most of them have suggested several risk factors belonged to specific categories, including biological, psychological, and social/environmental. Yet, it should be emphasized that these groups of risk and protective factors are somewhat overlapping with each other, and they are not just distinct categories. Moreover, even risk and protective factors have multidirectional interaction with each other (Moutier 2021a, b). Recognizing these elements as key factors related to self-inflicted injury and suicide is crucial for clinicians to manage these issues, especially in individuals with high rate of risk factors. Noticeably, studies have illuminated there are strong relationship between personality traits and suicidal tendency (Misra and Ghanekar 2017). Several investigations have suggested personality traits as prospective predictors of suicide attempts. It has been indicated that BPD and history of prior suicide attempts are strong predictors for subsequent suicide (Aouidad et al. 2020a, b). The onset of NSSH behaviors in adolescents may have an association with impulsivity and negative urgency (Riley et al. 2015), and are related to psychological distress and maladaptive coping styles with stressful situation (Wilcox et al. 2012), such as negative stress coping or dysfunctional emotional-based coping strategies (Kharsati and Bhola 2015). Hauber et al. (2019) examined various aspects of NSSI among 140 inpatients adolescents to study the association between NSSI and personality disorders. Longitudinal investigations have demonstrated psychological issues consisting of psychological distress, hopelessness, emotional problems, low self-esteem, higher internalizing difficulties, behavioral impulsivity, negative emotions, attachment issues, and negative attribution and cognitive style have shown crucial role in predicting further NSSI (Plener et al. 2015). Pursuant to the findings, it has been demonstrated that NSSI was associated to several personality disorders not just to a specific one. In addition, adolescents with NSSI behaviors showed more symptoms and self-blame as a negative coping strategy, as well as lower levels of positive coping strategy of refocusing and reappraisal (Hauber et al. 2019). One of the most prominent emotions which is associated with NSSI is shame (Brown et al. 2009), which lead to negative self-evaluation and consequently self-hatred and self-punishment especially among individuals with BPD (Brown et al. 2002, 2014). This self-punishment can be a strategy to distinguish BPD patients from other mental problems such as depression (Rosenthal et al. 2006), and is an important motivation for individuals with BPD engaged in NSSH (Brown et al. 2002, 2014; Kleindienst et al. 2008). Shame interferes with functional behaviors to regulate emotions and contribute to maladaptive and dysfunctional behaviors such as NSSI among individuals with BPD (Kleindienst et al. 2008; Brown et al. 2009). Several investigations have indicated that individuals engaged in NSSI frequently have reported more severe psychological impairments, such as depression, history of childhood abuse, and BPD (e.g., Klonsky and Olino 2008; Whitlock et al. 2008). NSSI and suicidal behaviors can be differentiated based on the severity of psycho-social impairments (Hamza and Willoughby 2013). Victor et al. (2015) suggested individuals who engage in NSSH behaviors have a desire to avoid suicide in comparison to people who being involved in suicidal behaviors (Victor et al. 2015). Furthermore, diminished self-esteem, self-hate, loathed self-image, self-minimization, highly self-criticism, and lack of emotional regulation strategies can be as personality characteristics of individuals who do NSSH (Møhl 2019; Forrester et al. 2017; Emelianchik-Key and La Guardia 2019; Nock et al. 2009; Ferrara et al. 2012). In line with Klonsky (2009), people are motivated to do NSSH because they consider themselves worthy to harm and injury. Moreover, high levels of emotional pain, shame, guilt, embarrassment, sadness, and self-directed anger after practicing NSSI have been reported (Klonsky 2009). Shame is a significant emotional precursor for suicidal behaviors and NSSH among individuals with BPD (Brown et al. 2009), and the 5th grade predicted subsequent suicide attempts by youth (Tangney and Dearing 2003). It has been indicated that women with BPD showed greater levels of shame-proneness compared to social phobia sample (Rüsch et al. 2007). Based on an investigation, women with BPD and PTSD did not reveal higher shame proneness in comparison with BPD women with no PTSD criteria, which provide this assumption that escalated shame-proneness is more specific to BPD than other disorders (Rüsch et al. 2007); therefore, some researchers have conceptualized BPD as a chronic shame response (Crowe 2004). Spitzen et al. (2020) demonstrated the pathology of BPD and its significant association with self-conscious emotion can contribute to high rates of NSSI occurrence. Furthermore, they posited highly motivated BPD patients to be engaged in SIB are prone to greater risk of repeated self-harm behaviors in the future (Spitzen et al. 2020). In addition, their low self-esteem and hated self-image originated from an irrational and inexcusable guilt feeling and shame, as well as, bullying and psychological distress (National Council for Children 2016; Møhl 2019). It has been that revealed individuals who engage in both NSSI and suicidal acts manifest more severe symptoms of psychopathology and report more impairment in psychosocial functions in comparison to individuals who merely engage in NSSI behaviors (e.g., Muehlenkamp et al. 2011; Asarnow et al. 2011; Csorba et al. 2009; Brausch and Gutierrez 2010; Jacobson et al. 2008). More severe anhedonia and negative self-evaluations were reported among youth who had a history of NSSI and at least one suicide attempt in comparison to individuals who had just a history of NSSI (Muehlenkamp and Gutierrez 2007; Brausch and Gutierrez 2010). Andrewes et al. (2017) found that the prevalence of NSSI may be greater in the early course of BPD, which proposes the underlying normative increase in rates of NSSI at puberty, which is a rising trend in adolescence and decreasing in adulthood (Andrewes et al. 2017). Higher rates of self-punishment, greater levels of self-critical, more negative self-image, and more perfectionism have been revealed in individuals who engage in NSSI behaviors (Hooley and Franklin 2018).

Neuroticism, a tendency to experience severe negative emotions (Gratz et al. 2020a, b), is the most significant personality trait which is associated with suicidal ideation and NSSI and is considered a consistent candidate that play a considerable role in suicide attempts (Gratz et al. 2020a, b; Misra and Ghanekar 2017; Perlman et al. 2018; Peters et al. 2018; Chioqueta and Stiles 2005; Ormel et al. 2017; Rappaport et al. 2017; Brezo et al. 2006; Tsoh et al. 2005; Sarchiapone and Zeppegno 2022; Bi et al. 2017; Weintraub et al. 2017; Valencia and Sinambela 2020). Neuroticism is a dimension of temperament recognized by escalated stress reactivity resulting in the frequent experience of negative emotions (Barlow et al. 2019), which contains features such as negative affectivity (Eysenck 1997; McCrae and Costa 1987) which has an association with NSSI, and heightened emotional reactivity and instability (e.g., Larson et al. 2002; Anthony et al. 2002). Neuroticism can be considered a common personality dimension underlying many psychological disorders, such as mood and anxiety disorders (Ormel et al. 2017), increasing suicide risk (Sareen et al. 2005; Beautrais et al. 1999; Fergusson et al. 2000), and also is associated with BPD (Möller-Leimkühler 2003; Distel et al. 2009). Generally, individuals with high neuroticism are more introverted and sensitive. Whenever they experience adverse events in their life, they misinterpret the information of stimuli and show deviation in information processing; therefore, the stimuli will be perceived as threat, so they tend to answer it through self-inflicted behaviors (Liao et al. 2022; Kendler et al. 2023; Pickles et al. 2010). It has been found in some studies that neuroticism proposes a response system of negative emotions and elicits intensely biological and emotional response in these situations where negative emotions are evoked (Lear et al. 2019). The results of various investigations have indicated that when highly neurotic individuals constantly feel under harassment, slander, or exposure to violation of privacy, and they display negative emotions, such as depression, anxiety, and guilt. Since they have several problems in dealing with these emotions, they tend to punish themselves and alleviate these intense negative emotions through NSSI. It can be concluded that negative emotions, especially depressive mood, is a significant risk factor that contributed to engaging in NSSI behaviors in high neurotic individuals (Marshall et al. 2013; Başgöze et al. 2023). Neuroticism has revealed a great association with self-harm behaviors (Pennel et al. 2018; Bi et al. 2017; Lin et al. 2017, 2018; Weintraub et al. 2017; Mullins-Sweatt et al. 2013; MacLaren and Best 2010). In a recent study, the relationship between neuroticism and NSSI behaviors among college students was assessed and the finding demonstrated neuroticism is a strong predictor of NSSI behaviors, and also has an effect on NSSI via mediating effect of emotion regulation and depression. In addition, neuroticism negatively predicts emotion regulation strategies (Liao et al. 2022). Peters et al. (2018) found neuroticism exacerbates the risk of suicide in both men and women, as well as is a strong predictor of suicide attempt for women (Peters et al. 2018). Rappaport et al. (2017) concluded there is a complicated association between neuroticism and suicidality than previously explained. They cited neuroticism escalates risk for suicidal ideation, whereas elevated neuroticism is associated with decline risk for suicide attempt among individuals who reported suicidal thoughts. It can be deduced that despite decrease in suicidal ideation through elevated neuroticism, a decrease occurs by high neuroticism, which proposes this idea that elevated neuroticism has a protective effect on suicide attempt following the onset of suicidal thoughts (Rappaport et al. 2017). In a multicenter study of Italian and Austrian psychiatric patients and students, Stefa-Missagli et al. (2020) found out personality traits, including neuroticism, anxiety, extraversion, and depression, are associated with the intensity of suicidal ideation. They proposed that elevated suicidal risk has a relationship with neuroticism and depressive symptoms, and extraversion is found as a protective factor in geographically and regionally different populations (Sarchiapone and Zeppegno 2022). Tonta et al. (2020) demonstrated perfectionism had a direct relationship with escalated odds of NSSI, as well as an indirect association with odds through rumination and negative affect, consistent to previous research (Vaartstra et al. 2023). In addition, it was found that the association between rumination and perfectionism can be moderated by focused attention (Tonta et al. 2020). Several investigations have indicated that the perfectionism trait increased the levels of perfectionism can heighten the risk for NSSI in adolescents and adults and general population (Gyori and Balazs 2021; Claes et al. 2014; Hoff and Muehlenkamp 2009). Nicolai et al. (2016) highlighted that the interaction between high negative affectivity and high levels of rumination may predict both probability and frequency of engagement in NSSI behaviors (Nicolai et al. 2016). Several experimental and clinical theories have proposed how various intrapersonal (e.g., biological, emotional, and cognitive vulnerabilities), interpersonal (e.g., adverse experiences), and social and cultural elements (e.g., gender inequality, social media negative effects) have multiple interactions with depression and psychological distress and even contribute to greater levels of these issues in female populations (e.g., Hyde and Mezulis 2020). Various evidence has demonstrated higher levels of rumination concurrent with adverse experience are associated and remarkably modifying women' mental distress (Nolen-Hoeksema 2012; Nurullah 2010), and subsequently lead to SIB (Voon et al. 2014). Based on Matera et al. (2021), no clear evidence has been found about which emotional and behavioral components are specifically related to NSSI, they assessed internal and external emotion regulation, craving, non-planning, and total impulsivity in order to identify the specified associated elements in nonsuicidal SIB among 54 individuals with NSSI. Significant differences in craving were found among individuals with multiple NSSI episodes, suicide attempters, and multiple injurious behaviors. As well as, remarkable differences were shown in internal emotion regulation, sensation seeking, and motor impulsivity between NSSI individuals with and without a history of suicide attempts, besides significant differences in cognitive impulsivity between NSSI patients with multiple injurious behaviors and single-NSSI group (Matera et al. 2021). Other personality traits are associated with increasing risk of NSSI, suicidal ideation, and suicide attempts including high levels of depression (Lee et al. 2009; Bramness et al. 2007; Emelianchik-Key and La Guardia 2019), especially less self-conscientiousness (Brezo et al. 2006; Tsoh et al. 2005), low levels of extroversion (Brezo et al. 2006; Duberstein et al. 2003), Psychoticism (Lolas et al.

1991; Roy 2003), agreeableness (Soto and John 2014; Duberstein et al. 2000; McCann 2011), conscientiousness (Farmer et al. 2003), introversion and perfectionism (Brezo et al. 2006), and less openness (Duberstein et al. 1994). Based on a cross-sectional investigation among 505 adolescents aged 12–17, Oliveria Costa et al. (2021) perused the profile of NSSI and the association between NSSI and impulsiveness and loneliness, likewise previous studies (e.g., Giletta et al. 2012), the score of loneliness, as well as greater levels of impulsiveness were substantially aggregated compared to non-NSSI participants. The most common reasons of NSSI, which were reported by individuals engaged in NSSI, were to get an immediate relief from SIB and lower rate of concerns about long-term consequences. Oliveria Costa et al. (2021) suggested a "NSSI cycle" to clarify and elaborate understanding of NSSI evoked from intense negative emotional states (Fig. 12.1).

Several studies have indicated that repetitive self-harm and suicide with low fatality rate in individuals with suicide attempts, which are major manifestations of BPD, are associated with disturbed decision-making skill and cognitive inflexibility (LeGris and van Reekum 2006). Research has also shown some symptoms of BPD such as impulsivity, aggression, and emotion dysregulation are associated with NSSI (Cloutier et al. 2010; Dougherty et al. 2009). Suicide attempters can be distinguished from non-attempters based on the level of impulsivity and aggression in adolescents (Renaud et al. 2008), whereas there are little knowing about the differences between adolescents with NSSI and suicide attempts based on these variables (Muehlenkamp et al. 2011). Most individuals who engage in suicidal acts experience a strong ambivalent decision-making to end their lives, and a significant variable for acting out to attempt suicide is impulsiveness (de Leo and Giannotti 2022). Moreover, it has been revealed, cognitive rigidity, which leads to interpersonal conflicts, is one of the primary features of rejection and is an underlying trait of compulsivity factor. All these three factors, including impaired decision-making, cognitive inflexibility, and compulsivity, are personality constructs that are associated with suicide attempts in different populations (e.g., Kaslow et al. 2004; Brezo et al. 2008). Overall, several former investigations have highlighted levels of greater neuroticism (Allroggen et al. 2014; Kiekens et al. 2015; Mullins-Sweatt et al. 2013), higher levels of depressive symptoms (Muehlenkamp and Gutierrez 2007; Hankin and Abela 2011), higher rates of alexithymia (Cerutti et al. 2018; Garisch and Wilson 2015; Lüdtke et al. 2016; Gatta et al. 2016), lower levels of self-esteem and self-confidence (Garisch and Wilson 2015; Cawood and Huprich 2011), greater levels of impulsivity and impulsive behaviors (Claes and Muehlenkamp 2013; Hamza et al. 2015), lower levels of perceived well-being (Vansteenkiste and Ryan 2013), lower levels of actual social support (Andrews et al. 2014), lower levels of familiar functionality (Baetens et al. 2014), and poor academic function (Mortier et al. 2015) are associated with engaging in SIB (Tang et al. 2021).

Theoretical and empirical models have posited distress tolerance is another significant factor that contributed to SIB. Distress tolerance is defined as a personal perceived and actual capability to tolerate adverse physical and emotional states (Leyro et al. 2010; Slabbert et al. 2022, 2021). Pursuant to several documented studies, low levels of distress tolerance are associated with NSSI and suicide attempts (e.g., Anestis et al. 2013; Lin et al. 2018; Hasking et al. 2019; Slabbert et al. 2021). Several studies have been focused on the association between trait negative affectivity and aggravated risk of self-injury (e.g., Horgan and Martin 2016; Boyes et al. 2020; Hasking et al. 2019). The higher levels of experiencing negative emotion, the greater likelihood of existing history of NSSI have been found (Slabbert et al. 2022). Slabbert et al. (2021) examined the role of distress tolerance in the association between emotion and NSSI. Based on studies' result, a direct association was found between figures of distress tolerance, including negative and positive affectivity, appraisal (negative perceptions of distress) and absorption (allotting of attention to distress) with NSSI. Furthermore, an interaction has been shown between positive affectivity and appraisal to distinguish individuals based on a history of NSSI, as well as an interaction between positive affectivity and absorption to identify individuals with NSS and non-NSSI individuals. Finally, a negative association has been revealed between positive affectivity and NSSI among individuals who allotted less attention to distress. Hence, it was concluded that to enhance our understanding of NSSI, it is crucial to assume the independent roles of positive and negative affectivity besides peculiar figures of distress tolerance and their interactions with emotional experience (Slabbert et al. 2022).

A growing experimental and clinical investigation has demonstrated the association between negative emotionality and emotional reactivity with SIB (e.g., Hill et al. 2020; Claes et al. 2014; Smith et al. 2014). Additionally, a recall bias has been figured out among individuals engaged in NSSI toward emotional experiences (Hasking et al. 2019). Conforming to previous studies, emotional intensity has a crucial role in onset and maintenance of NSSI (e.g., Selby and Joiner Jr 2009; Chapman et al. 2006). However, based on daily diary and experimental research, individuals with a history of NSSI respond less intensely to emotional stimuli (e.g., Bresin 2014; Tatnell et al. 2018), they display escalated perseveration of this negative emotion over time (Boyes et al. 2020). Structural and functional neuroimaging studies in BPD and depression have proposed that there are different brain regions implicated in emotional processing and decision-making in individuals with suicide attempts and non-attempters (Soloff et al. 2014; Sublette et al. 2013; Du et al. 2014; Pan et al. 2013; Gujral et al. 2014). Boyes et al. (2020) investigated NSSI-related differences based on experiencing of positive and negative emotion among 214 undergraduate students with and without history of NSSI. In keeping with the findings, individuals with a history of NSSI revealed aggregated levels of reactivity, intensity, and perseveration of dispositional negative emotionality compared to individuals without a history of NSSI. As well as, individuals engaged in NSSI reported experiencing of less intense but greater persistent negative emotion over time (Boyes et al. 2020).

Recent research revealed emotional context in which NSSI occurs is significantly important. In other words, emotional experiences have crucial roles in determining who engage in NSSI and who not. In keeping with theoretical viewpoints, individuals engaged in SIB revealed higher levels of predisposition to experience emotions more severely (Chapman et al. 2006; Houben et al. 2017; Chen et al. 2023), show more sensitivity to emotional stimuli (Nock 2008; Chen et al. 2023), and report greater experiencing emotion for longer periods of time (Boyes et al. 2020; Chen et al. 2023). It seems self-inflicted injuries are more likely to occur under the experience of more frequent, intense, and dysregulated negative emotions in daily life compared to individuals who do not engage in these SIB (Andover et al. 2018; Gratz and Roemer 2008; Nock 2008; Klonsky et al. 2003). Overall, as mentioned, emotion regulation, distress tolerance, experiential avoidance, and positive and negative emotions have been associated to NSSI (e.g., Weis et al. 2015; Preece et al. 2021; Boyes et al. 2020). In a large body of investigations, there are significant overlaps between these constructs (Chapman et al. 2006; Hasking 2017). Juarascio et al. (2020a, b) detected constructs, including anxiety sensitivity, negative urgency, distress tolerance, emotional dysregulation, avoidance, have association with emotional states encompassed under "negative emotion." In other words, the centrality of emotional constructs in the majority of theoretical models (e.g., Selby and Joiner Jr 2009; Nock 2009, Chapman et al. 2006; Klonsky and Glenn 2009; Hasking 2017) were emphasized (Juarascio et al. 2020a, b). As stated, emotional experiences are in association with SIB, as well as, considering the overlap and complementary quality of emotion-related constructs are crucial (Gross 2008, 2014). Emotion-related constructs consist of multiple processes and skills that are simultaneously distinct and, in some levels, have interrelatedness (Haywood et al. 2022; Gross 1998). Haywood et al. (2024) investigated whether emotion-related constructs associated to the experiencing and emotion regulation are significant in initiating and continuing NSSI. Through analyzing emotion regulation, distress tolerance, experiential avoidance, and positive and negative emotions demonstrated moderate to large associations between all these constructs and substantial overlap, and all these emotion-related constructs, except lack of awareness, showed a great load onto a single factor. The findings pointed out although most of the models and theories assume multiple emotion-related constructs as risk factors and main elements for onset and continuing NSSI, these results suggested these assumptions can be explanatory for NSSI in the case these constructs are considered individually. Yet, under the situation in which we considered emotion-related constructs collectively, it seems for the majority of these constructs such as alexithymia, negative emotion, emotional reactivity, and emotion regulation issues, the shared variance with other associated constructs should be accounted for the relationship with SIB (Haywood et al. 2024).

As mentioned, several experimental systematic investigations have been done to elucidate and identify personality patterns and traits regarded to nature, severity, and cognitive-emotional correlations of NSSI. One of the most outstanding theories in the field of SIB is the *Big Five Model* of personality (Costa and McCare 1992), a typological approach to personality (Widiger and Costa Jr 2013; Goddard et al. 2021). Based on a body of empirical investigations, individuals with a history of engagement in NSSI reported greater levels of Neuroticism and Openness, in contrast lower scores of Agreeableness and Conscientiousness in comparison to individuals without NSSI history (e.g., MacLaren and Best 2010; Hasking et al. 2010; Bijttebier et al. 2015; Baetens et al. 2011). McCann (2011) reported that lower neuroticism and lower agreeableness showed a great association with higher levels of suicide attempts. Based on their findings, lower neuroticism and lower agreeableness can be assumed as important risk factors for death by suicide but not suicidal thoughts or attempted suicide (McCann 2011). A great body of studies have demonstrated among individuals with completed suicide higher levels of neuroticism (Useda et al. 2007; Tsoh et al. 2005), lesser levels of conscientiousness (Tsoh et al. 2005), lower degrees of openness (Tsoh et al. 2005), and lesser levels of extraversion (Tsoh et al. 2003). Research has showed that individuals with suicide attempts reported higher levels of neuroticism (Useda et al. 2007), rather individuals with death by suicide revealed lower in neuroticism (Tsoh et al. 2005). As well as, studies have indicated that individuals with repeated suicide reported significantly higher level of neuroticism (Beautrais 2004). In addition, more conscientious (Useda et al. 2007; Tsoh et al. 2005), and less openness and more agreeableness (Tsoh et al. 2005) were found among the reports of individuals with death by suicide (McCann 2011). Overall, distal psychological factors including neuroticism, perfectionism, inflexible and rigid cognitive style, innate pessimism, and sensitivity to experience are considered as enduring personality risk factors for suicide (Moutier 2021a, b). Goddard et al. (2021) attempted to investigate whether the traits-based Big Five Model exists among individuals who engaged in NSSI, and also to explore systematic disparities considering gender, age, emotional avoidance, alexithymia, psychological distress, emotion regulation strategies, and severity and functions of NSSI among 236 university students with a history of NSSI. On the word of the findings, resilient and dysregulated profiles were revealed at an extreme opposite of a spectrum related to severity of NSSI, less adaptive emotion regulation strategies, alexithymia, and psychological distress. In addition, dysregulated features were related to emotion regulation and self-punishment functions of NSSI, as well as, disagreeable characteristics showed a great association with high alexithymia and psychological distress (Goddard et al. 2021). Among a sample of 185 BPD patients, Sleuwaegen et al. (2017) examined whether there is an association between NSSI and alexithymia, as well as whether by controlling gender and depression, this association would be continued. Findings demonstrated as association between NSSI and alexithymia, and also problems in identifying emotions can contribute to be engaged in NSSI regardless of depression in BPD cases. In addition, the more PBD patients report difficulties in identifying and naming their emotions, the more frequent NSSI is reported. It indicated that experiencing difficulties in verbalization and communication about emotions have greater association with NSSI in comparison to identification and distinguishing of emotions (Sleuwaegen et al. 2017). Through a longitudinal qualitative and quantitative investigation on broad and narrow personality traits between one-time and frequent suicide attempts, Brezo et al. (2008) indicated that emotional and cognitive dysregulation and related behavioral matters may have associations with suicide attempts of various severity. Also, they found anxiousness and compulsivity can make distinction between one-time and frequent suicide attempters. In addition, anxiousness and emotional instability may differentiate individuals with no suicide attempts and one-time suicide attempters. Consistent with previous studies (e.g., Rudd et al. 1996), they cited emotion dysregulation, a trait related to neuroticism and harm avoidance, may contribute to frequent suicide attempts, due to related individual's inability to tolerate and express frustration (Sarfati et al. 2003; Brezo et al. 2008). It has been demonstrated that college students with NSSI have stronger emotion dysregulation than control group (Heath et al. 2009), similar to adults with suicide attempts (Slee et al. 2008). Emotional instability compared to emotional intensity is a core characteristic of individuals who engage in NSSI (Santangelo et al. 2017). Noticeably, adolescents are considered as a high-risk group for engaging in SIB due to immature mind and instability in emotional control (Xiao et al. 2022a, b). Furthermore, it has been proposed that anxiousness and emotional instability are two significant correlates traits of suicide attempts and complete suicide (Neeleman et al. 1998), and BPD (Bagge and Trull 2003). Brezo et al. (2008) reported that emotional instability levels were remarkably higher in individuals with one-time suicide attempts in comparison to nonsuicide attempters. Although anxiousness was associated with lower probability of one-time suicide attempts, is was also linked to higher levels of repeated suicide attempts. In addition, anxiousness is more frequent in repeated suicide attempts rather than one-time suicide attempts (Brezo et al. 2008), which brings up the effect of childhood anxiety as a predisposition to several suicide attempts (Rudd et al. 2004). As a conclusion, it has been suggested that compulsivity and emotion dysregulation are two important personality correlates associated with suicide attempts (Brezo et al. 2008). It has been demonstrated that adults who engage in both NSSI and suicidal behaviors report considerably greater levels of depression feeling of hopelessness and lower extroversion (Claes et al. 2010; Baetens et al. 2011), as well as, more maladjusted personality characteristics in comparison to individuals with only NSSI (Andover and Gibb 2010), and more help-seeking following self-harm behaviors (Maddock et al. 2010; Baetens et al. 2011). Individuals who engage in both NSSI and suicide attempt are more likely to report high-fatality suicide attempts (Andover and Gibb 2010), higher courage, and competency to attempt suicide (Stanley et al. 2021), and greater levels of aggressive behaviors, feeling of anxiousness, hopelessness, and physical punishment (Claes et al. 2010), in comparison to individuals with suicide attempts and without NSSI (Hamza et al. 2012). Recently, research was done to analyze impulsivity and neuroticism among psychiatric and nonclinical populations, it has been revealed that some personality traits are different among suicide attempters based on the existence of psychiatric disorders. Psychiatric disorders as well as personality disorders have been viewed as prominent risk factors for suicidal behaviors (Holma et al. 2014; De Crescenzo et al. 2017; Giner et al. 2013), especially cluster B personality disorders (Tyrer et al. 2015; Kongerslev et al. 2015; McGirr et al. 2008). Furthermore, it has been indicated that neuroticism is a significant risk factor for suicidal tendencies in individuals suffering from psychiatric disorders. Whereas, among nonclinical individuals, impulsivity plays a considerable role in suicide attempts (Bi et al. 2017), and impulsivity has been assumed as a potential construct in NSSI (Glenn and Klonsky 2010). Impulsivity is described as a disposition to behave quickly with no thinking about its consequences and any analysis about whether that behavior is actually a suitable one (Gratz et al. 2020a, b). McGirr et al. (2008) proposed that higher levels of impulsive-aggressive traits have a significant role in occurring suicidal tendencies among younger people, with a declining trend in increasing age (McGirr et al.

2008). Lynam et al. (2011) claimed despite impulsivity is one of the most significant predisposing factors for self-harm behaviors (e.g., Glenn and Klonsky (2010), the relations between impulsivity and suicidal behaviors and NSSI have been ambiguous yet due to the heterogeneous nature of impulsivity construct. In other words, it is unknown which of the traits underlying impulsive behavior are associated with suicidal behavior and NSSI. Therefore, they attempted to utilize a comprehensive model to examine the associations between impulsivity-related traits, suicidality, and NSSI above and beyond BPD symptoms based on UPPS model (Lynam et al. 2006; Cyders et al. 2007; Lynam et al. 2011; Dougherty et al. 2009). Based on Big Five theory, personality constitutes of five dimensions including openness, consciousness, agreeableness, extraversion, and neuroticism (Valencia and Sinambela 2020; Klonsky et al. 2011; Watson and Clark 1997). UPPS model of personality disorder is a prominent model of impulsive personality originated from Five Factor Model of Personality that consists of Negative Urgency, lack of Premeditation, lack of Perseveration, and Sensation Seeking (UPPS). This model emphasizes on the vital role of distinctive multidimensional traits due to specificity of these traits regarding to various risk behaviors (Lynam et al. 2006; Cyder et al. 2007; Um et al. 2018; Lutz et al. 2022). Lynam et al. (2011) tested the associations among 4 impulsivity-related traits, including Negative Urgency, lack of Premeditation, lack of Perseveration, and Sensation Seeking with suicide and NSSI in BPD based on UPPS model. Their findings revealed that Negative Urgency, lack of Premeditation, and lack of Perseveration domains were relatively associated with suicidal behavior and NSSI, with more consistent effect size in Negative Urgency. Furthermore, Negative Urgency, lack of Premeditation, and lack of Perseveration indicated that considerable relations with BPD scores, which propose a substantial overlap among these three of UPPS domain of impulsivity-related traits, BPD, and both suicidal behavior and NSSI. In line with the interactions among these 4 impulsivity-related traits, it has been revealed these interactions worked among individuals with high Negative Urgency and Lack of Premeditation were at significant risk for suicidal tendencies and NSSI. Negative Urgency, lack of Premeditation, and lack of Perseveration were significantly associated with BPD and impulsivity-related traits. Overall, this study proposes that impulsivity-related traits from two discrete personality domains, including Neuroticism (Negative Urgency) and Conspicuousness (Lack of Premeditation) are significant to comprehend suicidal behavior and NSSI. Furthermore, BPD was associated with suicidal behavior and NSSI when considered alone, whereas there was no incremental validity above and beyond impulsivity-related traits, yet these impulsivity-related traits were significantly important for obtaining information about suicidal behaviors and NSSI even after bringing up BPD (Lynam et al. 2011). Conforming to Glenn and Klonsky (2010), Urgency is a tendency to be involved in hasty acts in the exposure to negative emotion. Based on investigations, Elevated Urgency has been found in individuals engaged in NSSI compared to individuals without SIB, which may be interpreted as greater emotion dysregulation, more likelihood to be involved in hasty decisions in negative emotion conditions, and choose to engage in SIB to reduce negative experiences in people with NSSI in comparison to non-NSSI individuals (Glenn and

Klonsky 2010; Klonsky et al. 2003; Nock and Prinstien 2004; Klonsky 2007). Lack of premeditation such as being unable to pause an action to make a plan, contribute to poor planning in individuals with NSSI (Glenn and Kolnsky 2010; Hawton et al. 2003a, b, 2012; Hawton and Harriss 2008). In line with previous studies, NSSI individuals were not differentiated based on high sensation seeking such as a tendency to seek for exciting and adventure and low perseverance like the ability to keep doing a task to completion. In addition, less premeditation indicates a declined ability to predict the consequences of dysfunctional behaviors, which reveals a rising trend in acting on self-injurious urge. Overall, based on the UPPS model, NSSI can be differentiated by Urgency, lack of Premeditation, Sensation Seeking, and lack of Perseverance (Glenn and Klonsky 2010). Lutz et al. (2022) pointed out since in contrast to women, men report aggregated positive urgency associated with NSSI (Lutz et al. 2022; Cyders 2013) and escalated levels of high-risk acts (Cyders and Smith 2010); therefore, they posited that maybe positive urgency attenuate the entirely relationship between gender and NSSI (Lutz et al. 2022). Pursuant to theory of Urgency (Cyders and Smith 2008), some individuals are prone to impulsive behaviors under experiencing intense negative emotions which lead them to be involved in self-inflicted injurious behaviors to obtain the immediate short-term relief (Cyders and Smith 2008). Moreover, compared to women, men revealed substantially greater levels of sensation seeking as a psychological trait (Argyriou et al. 2020). Lutz et al. (2022) found a considerable association between NSSI and lower levels of sensation seeking (Lutz et al. 2022), consistent with studies suggested a direct relationship between sensation seeking and NSSI (e.g., Edmondson et al. 2016). Furthermore, based on their results, no gender differences were reported between emotion dysregulation and negative urgency, as well as both women and men engage in NSSI in the same conditions of mental distress, emotion dysregulation, and impulsivity. As per previous studies, UPPS-P subscales are associated with NSSI and suicidal behaviors in both genders, and the gender factor does not play any modifying role in the relationships between emotion dysregulation, positive urgency, and NSSI (Peckham et al. 2020; Wolff et al. 2019).

According to ongoing research, there is a profound relationship between impulsivity and self-inflicted injurious behaviors (e.g., Lin et al. 2017, 2018; Lin and Lee, 2022; Bi et al. 2017; Pennel et al. 2018; Guvendeger Doksat et al. 2017) and leads to exacerbation of vulnerability to be engaged in NSSI and other dysfunctional self-destructive behaviors to relive negative emotional state and perceived effective function of NSSI contribute to negative reinforcement of self-inflicted behaviors (Matera et al. 2021). Impulsivity is considered as a multifaceted construct that consists of urgency, sensation seeking, inattentiveness, lack of perseverance and premeditation, disinhibition, and distractibility (e.g., Carver et al. 2011; Cyders et al. 2007; Dillahunt et al. 2022). Consistent with various experimental and clinical investigations, these self-destructive behaviors are characterized by being dependent, loss of control, and a great tendency to engage in NSSI repeatedly despite harmful consequences (e.g., Nixon et al. 2002, 2008).

Nonsuicidal Self-Injury (NSSI) and Suicide in Borderline Personality Disorder

Borderline personality disorder (BPD) is presented as a severely debilitating mental disorder characterized by considerable problematic behaviors, especially deliberate self-harm and suicidal behaviors, patterns of dysfunctional instability across emotional, behavioral, cognitive, and interpersonal domains (e.g., Gratz and Gunderson 2006; Stead et al. 2019; Skodol et al. 2002; Sharp and Wall 2018; Reichl and Kaess 2021; McClelland et al. 2023; Chapman-Hilliard et al. 2024; Watt-McMahon et al. 2023). BPD is well known as a disorder with a remarkable frequent engagement in NSSI and suicide attempts (Kaplan et al. 2016; Nock et al. 2006, 2018; Muehlenkamp et al. 2011; Howard et al. 2021; Brickman et al. 2014; Selby and Gardner 2015; Sitton et al. 2021; Oldham 2006; Pompili et al. 2005; Turner et al. 2021; McClelland et al. 2023; Chapman-Hilliard et al. 2024; Watt-McMahon et al. 2023), and one of the mental disorders which is strongly associated with deliberate self-harm (DSH) is BPD (Selby et al. 2012; Reichl and Kaess 2021; Turner et al. 2021; McClelland et al. 2023; Chapman-Hilliard et al. 2024; Watt-McMahon et al. 2023). Studies have shown that BPD is one of the main predictors of suicide attempts (e.g., Barak-Corren et al. 2020; Witt et al. 2019; Turner et al. 2021; Aouidad et al. 2020a, b). As mentioned, BPD is a serious psychological condition in which an individual suffers from severely mental illness (DSM-5-TR, APA 2022), and associated with a great mortality rate (e.g., Paris et al. 2004; Van den Broeck et al. 2015). Self-harm behaviors and BPD are associated (Gunderson and Ridolfi 2001; Linehan 1987; Paris 2019), and is referred to as the borderline individual's "behavioral specialty" (Gunderson 2009; Gunderson and Ridolfi 2001). These SIB consist of impulsive behaviors that are potentially harmful such as high-risk sexual behaviors, self-destructive behaviors, intentional self-inflicted injurious behavior, and suicide attempts and death by suicide (Oldham 2006; Brodsky and Stanley 2013; Valencia and Sinambela 2020; MacLaren and Best 2010). Individuals who met BPD diagnosis are at escalated risk factor for engaging in self-inflicted injurious and behaviors, including NSSI, suicidal thoughts, and suicide attempts. In line with Gardner et al. (2021b), not only NSSI but also suicide are main public mental health problems that are related to psychological distress and disturbances (e.g., Selby et al. 2012, 2014a, b, c, 2015a, b, 2022; Victor and Klonsky 2014a, b; Eskin et al. 2016; Gratz et al. 2019a, b, 2022; Crowell et al. 2014; Brunner et al. 2014). Approximately 50–80% of individuals with BPD are involved in deliberate self-harm (DSH) (Oumaya et al. 2008), and patients with BPD are prone to suicide attempts 3.3 times and up to 10% died by suicide (Zanarini et al. 2008; McMain et al. 2018; Stokke Westad et al. 2021). Patients with BPD showed 9–33% of all suicides (Runeson and Beskow 1991; Kullgren 1986). Based on Temes et al. (2019) proposed that nearly 5.9% to 14.0% of individuals with BPD die as a result of suicide or nonsuicidal-related causes, parallel to 1.4% to 5.5% of individuals with other personality disorders (Reichl and Kaess 2021). A meta-analytic study indicated a 52-fold increase in suicide rates among individuals with BPD in comparison to the general population

(Pompili et al. 2005). Based on Paris (2019), up to 10% of individuals with BPD will die because of death by suicide (Paris 2019).

However, studies have demonstrated the high prevalence of NSSH and suicidal behaviors in BPD (McClelland et al. 2023; Chapman-Hilliard et al. 2024; Watt-McMahon et al. 2023; Somma et al. 2017; Colle et al. 2020), and NSSI and suicide are neither vital nor sufficient for BPD diagnosis (McClelland et al. 2023; Chapman-Hilliard et al. 2024; Glenn and Klonsky 2013), it should be noticed that self-inflicted injuries are not restricted to the diagnosis of BPD (Selby et al. 2012). Gratz et al. (2012) cited despite a reliable association between BPD features and NSSI status, there are various rates of NSSI based on gender, racial/ethnic background, and academic levels. They posited that NSSI have association with a set of various factors, including social and ethical elements, rather than a unique relationship with BPD (Gratz et al. 2012). Through a cross-sectional study among 825 adolescent patients, Muehlenkamp et al. (2017) indicated that adolescents with high-NSSI displayed greater level of depressive, borderline personality, and substance use symptoms proposing that these groups are experiencing increased levels of psychological and psychiatric distress (Muehlenkamp et al. 2010, 2017, 2023). Geissbühler (2013) proposed that the strongest predictors for suicide attempts among individuals with BPD consist of a history of suicide attempts, childhood sexual abuse, and history of psychiatric hospitalization (Geissbühler 2013). Sitton et al. (2021) examined psychological predictions of SIB among 116 individuals with BPD traits and colleague students. The findings posited that BPD can predict SIB, as well as they indicated that a considerable interaction in which psychological distress had an escalated association with SIB with characteristics of BPD (Sitton et al. 2021). A growing body of studies have demonstrated the role of BPD in suicidal behaviors, as well as predicating role overtime. BPD symptoms including emotional instability, impulsivity, and identity diffusion have a predictive association with suicidal behaviors (Moselli et al. 2021a, b). In a multisite, longitudinal study, Yen et al. (2020) examined related factors that are associated with prospectively suicide attempts among 733 BPD youth and adults who were referred for psychotherapy over 10 years of follow-up. The results showed that identity disturbance, chronic feelings of emptiness, and frantic efforts to avoid abandonment were considerably in association with suicide attempts. Furthermore, they concluded BPD symptoms including identity disturbance, chronic feelings of emptiness, and frantic efforts to avoid abandonment were clinically overemphasized characteristics of BPD in predicting of suicide attempts (Yen et al. 2020).

The prevalence of NSSH and suicide attempts are high in BPD adolescents (e.g., Andrewes et al. 2017). A total of 8% of adult people with BPD have complete suicide (Pompili et al. 2005; McClelland et al. 2023). A notable attention has been dedicated to BPD as a predictor of NSSI and suicidal behaviors (Lynam et al. 2011; McClelland et al. 2023), a strong association between NSSI and BPD (e.g., Stead et al. 2019), and also, NSSI, a type of behavioral dysregulation, is considered as a main feature of BPD (e.g., Leichsenring et al. 2011; Chen et al. 2023). Self-harm behaviors can be considered as a risk marker in the early detection of BPD (Pompili et al. 2010; Chen et al. 2023; Deng et al. 2023; Lu et al. 2024). Studies have shown that the most prominent motivation among individuals who are engaged in SIB consists of intrapersonal functions, emotion regulation strategies for escaping from intense negative emotions, and experiencing positive emotions (Taylor et al. 2018; Paris 2019; Linehan 1993; Chen et al. 2023; Deng et al. 2023; Lu et al. 2024), as well as reducing dissociative experiences and self-punishment functions (Pompili 2021; Colle et al. 2020). The only mental disorder in DSM-5-TR criteria in which NISS and suicide are included is BPD (DSM-5-TR, APA 2022; Stead et al. 2019). Consistent with criterion five in DSM-5-TR, individuals with BPD demonstrate recurrent suicidal thoughts or behaviors, or/and NSSI behaviors. These self-destructive behaviors are usually triggered by threats of separation, rejection, or abandonment. Self-mutilation behaviors, such as cutting or burning, are remarkably frequent in BPD, which contribute to decreasing or escaping from intense negative emotional states (DSM-5-TR, APA 2022). Therefore, it is not surprising if it is claimed that there are strong associations among NSSI, suicidal tendencies, and BPD (Chen et al. 2023; Deng et al. 2023; Lu et al. 2024; McClelland et al. 2023; Glenn and Klonsky 2009; Saffer et al. 2015; Buelens et al. 2020a, b; Zanarini et al. 2011; Somma et al. 2017). Buelens et al. (2020a, b) examined the comorbidity of NSSI-D and BPD symptoms among 347 adolescents with a history of at least one NSSI. In line with findings, NSSI-D has been pointed out as a distinct disorder, as well as, loneliness, impulsivity, separation anxiety, repeated thinking about NSSI, and intense negative emotions that are experienced before engaging in NSSI were found as outstanding linking symptoms between NSSI-D and BPD (Buelens et al. 2020a, b). According to previous research, a broad range of differences in the phenomenology and functions of NSSI have been reported among BPD individuals; with NSSI and patients with NSSI without BPD. Based on these findings, individuals with BPD and NSSI demonstrate frequent and severe NSSI, aggregated comorbidity with other psychiatric disorders, greater depressive symptoms, frequent suicidal ideation, and emotion dysregulation in comparison to individuals with NSSI and without BPD (Glenn and Klonsky 2013; Turner et al. 2021; Chen et al. 2023; McClelland et al. 2023). Emotion dysregulation is assumed to have significant role in leading to NSSH and suicidal behaviors (Van Heeringen and Mann 2014; Nock et al. 2006, 2018; Chen et al. 2023), as a useful marker for detection of individuals who are at high risk for development of BPD (Pompili 2021; Groschwitz et al. 2015), impulsivity (Wilson et al. 2012), substance use (Reichl and Kaess 2021), depressive disorders (Gunderson et al. 2011), and problematic interpersonal relationships (Davis et al. 2017). In addition, individuals with BPD revealed engaging in NSSI more recently with a larger variety of methods, which contributed to more physically severe injuries needed medical interventions, in comparison to individuals who engage in NSSI but were not met BPD traits (Turner et al. 2021). Moreover, more frequent self-punishment, anti-suicide, and anti-dissociation functions were revealed among adolescent BPD patients with NSSI compared to patients with NSSI and without BPD (Bracken-Minor and McDevitt-Murphy 2014; Chen et al. 2023; McClelland et al. 2023; Chapman-Hilliard et al. 2024). In addition to the relationship between insufficient ability to regulate emotion and vulnerability for being engaged in self-inflicted injurious behaviors, dissociative features such as derealization, depersonalization, and psychogenic amnesia have been assumed to play a considerable role in NSSI (Yates 2004). Based on a body of investigation, dissociative experiences like distorted perceptions of feelings and behaviors have been related to several forms of self-harm behaviors. NSSI is considered as a method for producing emotional and physical sensations which contribute to gaining a real sense of self (Klonsky 2007; Gratz et al. 2002). Colle et al. (2020) investigated dissociative experiences individuals with BPD to clarify whether these experiences are correlated to an altered sense of agency and whether self-inflicted injuries can be assumed as a coping strategy for the decrease of the distress related to dissociative experiences among 20 individuals with BPD. Based on these results, BPD patients with high levels of NSSI revealed greater dissociative symptoms compared to individuals with no NSSI behaviors. Also, BPD patients who reported self-harm behaviors demonstrated similar degree of attenuation with nonclinical sample, which showed NSSI can be assumed as a coping strategy for diminishing the sense of agency. Various studies have shown the physiological effects due to the relationship between dissociation and NSSH. First, investigations have indicated an association between dissociation and pain reduction and decreasing sensitivity to pain (e.g., Schmahl et al. 2004; Magerl et al. 2012; Ludäscher et al. 2009, 2010; Russ et al. 1999). The second physiological phenomena due to the relationship between dissociation and self-harm consist of two elements of awareness including the sense of body ownership (related feelings that distinguish body parts of a unitary body (Bekrater-Bodmann et al. 2016; Löffler et al. 2018, 2022), and the sense of agency (the feeling of having ability to control and lead one's own behaviors which contribute to influence the events in external world (Haggard 2017).

Somma et al. (2017) assessed the association among BPD features, NSSI, and emotion dysregulation in 122 community-dwelling Italian adolescents, and suggested despite considerable relationship between BPD features and NSSI, emotion dysregulation did not remarkably account for the association between BPD characteristics and NSSI (Somma et al. 2017). Several clinical researchers have identified problems in regulating emotions as being related to suicidality (Yen et al. 2004; Gratz and Gunderson 2006; Hasking et al. 2010; Chen et al. 2023; McClelland et al. 2023). Moreover, nonclinically investigations have demonstrated an association between issues in emotion regulation and suicidal behaviors (Weinberg and Klonsky 2009; Bradley et al. 2011). According to Yen et al. (2004), the existence of predictive association of BPD features for suicidal attempts is not simply due to criterion overlap (Yen et al. 2004). Mirkovic et al. (2021) examined the associative contributions of emotion dysregulation to suicidal attempts among 85 adolescents with BPD. The results indicated that emotional dysregulation has a mediator role in suicide attempts among BPD adolescents (Mirkovic et al. 2021).

Tschan et al. (2017) investigated temperament and character traits based on *Cloninger's personality model* (Cloninger et al. 1998) focused on comparison impulsivity among adolescents with NSSI disorder and BPD (NSSI+BPD) and without BPD (NSSI-BPD) to clinical and nonclinical control groups. The results showed distinctive personality profiles among groups, and a remarkable difference in temperament and personality traits between adolescents with NSSI+BPD and adolescents with NSSI-BPD. Adolescents with NSSI-BPD indicated that escalated novelty seeking and harm avoidance, lower self-directedness in comparison to patients with NSSI+BPD, which propose that adolescents with NSSI-BPD are more careful, fearful and negative that adolescents with NSSI+BPD and control groups. In addition, adolescents with NSSI-BPD displayed differences regarding psychopathology and borderline symptomatology, in spite of similar personality pattern to adolescents with NSSI+BPD. Tschan et al. (2015) concluded personality patterns including novelty seeking and harm avoidance in adolescents with NSSI+BPD were consistent with Cloninger (2008) and Kaess et al. (2013). In addition, they cited that the approach-avoidance conflict stemming from this pattern can elucidate the emotional turbulence in individuals with BPD (see Cloninger 1994). Moreover, lower levels of directedness were found among adolescents with NSSI+BPD in comparison to control groups, similar to Hefti (2013) and Joyce et al. (2010). Finally, they reported lower levels of cooperativeness among both adolescents with NSSI+BPD and NSSI-BPD in comparison to control groups, which can explain more interpersonal problems and distress and aggregated rate of destructive conflict behaviors in social interactions (Tschan et al. 2017).

As mentioned, several empirical data have revealed a strong association between self-harm behaviors, including NSSH and suicide with BPD, both in adults (e.g., Lereya et al. 2017; Somma et al. 2017; Selby et al. 2015a, b; Chen et al. 2023; McClelland et al. 2023; Deng et al. 2023), and adolescents (Deng et al. 2023; Lu et al. 2024; Stepp et al. 2014). Furthermore, NSSI often appears prior to a full-blown BPD diagnosis (Hessels et al. 2018, 2022). Through a literature search using Embase, MEDLINE, and PsycINFO, Stead et al. (2019) found significant longitudinal associations between NSSI and later BPD and BPD symptoms (Stead et al. 2019). Recurrent and high frequency of self-inflicted injuries and suicidal behaviors in BPD contribute to a greater rate of fatality and high costly demand for psychiatric and psychological services (Solof et al. 2000; Zanarini 2000; Kaplan et al. 2016). Several psychiatric disorders are associated with an exacerbated rate of suicidal risk factors, yet based on investigations, it has been revealed 73% of individuals with BPD will have nearly 3 suicide attempts in their lifetime (Solof et al. 2000; Yen et al. 2020), and approximately 9% of these patients commit suicide (Brickman et al. 2014; Yen et al. 2020). In addition, studies have shown more than 30% of adult individuals with BPD reported their first self-inflicted injurious behavior occurred before the age of 12, and some of them did SIB between the age of 13–17, which raise that self-harm can be noticed as a key precursor for BPD (Hessels et al. 2018, 2022; Chanen and Kaess 2012; Chanen and Thompson 2014). Although it should be mentioned approximately 50% of individuals with NSSH, both adults and adolescents, do not meet the diagnostic criteria for BPD (e.g., Ayodeji et al. 2015), especially in adolescents (Nakar et al. 2016). Aouidad et al. (2020a, b) suggested that young age at first attempts, NSSI and anxiety disorders are related to the greater degree of clinical severity of BPD, as well as adolescents with suicide attempts are at high risk of BPD. In addition, adolescents with BPD who attempted suicide showed greater comorbidity with both externalizing and internalizing disorders (Aouidad et al. 2020a, b; Ha et al. 2014; Shah and Zanarini 2018).

As stated, over 90% of individuals who commit suicide suffer from at least one mental disorder (Klonsky et al. 2016; Bertolote and Fleischmann 2002), although more than 98% of individuals with psychiatric disorders do not die by suicide (Nordentoft et al. 2011). In line with studies, in developed countries, bipolar disorder, PTSD, and major depression strongly predict further suicide attempts, rather in developing countries, the most considerable predictors are PTSD, conduct disorder, and substance use disorder (Nock et al. 2009; Deng et al. 2023). It has been revealed that psychiatric comorbidity can be considered as prominent risk factors of suicide attempts in individuals diagnosed with BPD, such as escalated risk of suicide due to BPD and major depressive disorder comorbidity (Soloff et al. 2000), and higher level of impulsive traits comorbid antisocial personality disorder and depressive symptoms among BPD individuals with suicide attempts (Barbe et al. 2005). Psychiatric disorders play as secondary or coexisting factors which lead to escalating the level of suicidal attempts in individuals with BPD (Pompili et al. 2005). Some studies have indicated an increased mortality rate of suicidal behaviors in the cases of comorbidity between major depressive episodes and BPD (McGlashan 1986; Stone 2004, 2013), but not all of suicide attempts (Paris 2018; Kjelsberg et al. 1991). Several investigations have demonstrated that self-inflicted injury leads to increasing rate of suicide attempts, death by suicide, and adult psychopathology in adolescents, as well as high rates of depression in adolescents who engage in NSSI have been reported (Crowell and Kaufman et al. 2016).

Several studies have illustrated the role of impulsivity in suicide and conceptualized impulsivity as a key risk factor for suicide attempts (Anestis et al. 2014; Klonsky et al. 2016; Bryan and Rudd 2016; Yen et al. 2020; Chesin et al. 2010; Gunderson 2011); however, other studies did find no association between trait of impulsivity and impulsive suicide attempts (e.g., Wyder and De Leo 2007). In addition, Klonsky and May (2010) demonstrated there are differences between the measures of impulsivity in individuals with suicide attempts and individuals with just suicide ideation (Klonsky and May 2010), in spite of other finding which have shown aggregated levels of impulsivity in individuals who have either suicide ideation or attempts in comparison to individuals with no history of suicidality (Klonsky et al. 2016). Based on Yen et al. (2020), in consistence with the results of a follow-up intervals of the Collaborative Longitudinal Study of Personality Disorders (CLPS), in spite of prospective associations between emotional instability, impulsivity, and identity disturbance with suicidal behavior; merely the BPD emotional instability criterion was associated with suicidal attempts (Yen et al. 2004), as well as, suicide attempts were associated with negative affectivity after 7 years of follow-up (Yen et al. 2015). Selby and Gardner (2015) examined BPD symptoms and dysregulated behaviors, including NSSI, eating problems and substance use among 128 nonclinical students. Their findings revealed five profiles based on suicidality and NSSI in BPD, including a low BPD profile with low dysregulated behavior, a low BPD profile with great suicidality, a low BPD profile with escalated NSSI, a high BPD profile with low NSSI and relatively high suicidality, and a high BPD profile with high NSSI and low suicidality. According to results, it can be concluded high suicidality and NSSI may appear in severe cases of BPD, as well as in individuals with high levels of BPD severity may engage in NSSI behaviors with no suicide attempts. In addition, they proposed NSSI may have a function like the "anti-suicide," in which NSSI is recruited as a compromise to play a role like suicide without the risk of death. Moreover, greater levels of suicidal ideation have been found in high BPD with high NSSI profile, and relatively elevated levels of suicidality have been displayed in individuals with low BPD with high NSSI profile (Selby et al. 2015a, b). Through an ecological momentary assessment study, it has been revealed that negative affectivity can predict the urge for NSSI among individuals with low levels of self-concept (Scala et al. 2018). In addition, Santangelo et al. (2017) demonstrated youth with NSSI reported considerably higher levels of emotional and interpersonal instability (Santangelo et al. 2017). Several investigations have demonstrated the associations among emotional instability, aggression, impulsivity, NSSI, suicidal ideation, and dysregulated behaviors in BPD (e.g., Yen et al. 2020; Selby et al. 2013a, b, c, 2015a, b). Previous research showed difficulties in regulating emotion which may lead to self-inflicted injuries (Niedtfeld et al. 2010; Gratz 2003, 2007; Brown et al. 2002, 2014), and emotion dysregulation is related to self-harm behaviors in individuals with BPD (Sadeh et al. 2014; Selby et al. 2015a, b).

However, engaging in repetitive NSSI behaviors or suicide attempts is a diagnostic feature of BPD, there is little data to clarify whether other symptoms of BPD manifest various patterns of relation among single or repeat self-harm behaviors, which propose the necessity of identifying key BPD symptoms (Muehlenkamp et al. 2011). Muehlenkamp et al. (2011) studied about how specific BPD symptoms are associated with suicide attempts and NSSI among 441 adolescents, and identifying whether specific BPD symptoms differentiate NSSI from suicide attempts. Findings showed the probability of a full-blown BPD diagnosis escalates among individuals who engage in SIB, including NSSI and suicide attempts. Moreover, it has been indicated that the presence of both NSSI and suicide attempts can be considered as a common marker of growing distress and dysfunction, as well as to implicating an escalated probability of meeting a number of diagnostic criteria for BPD. Furthermore, it has been detected there is a positive association between the severity of BPD symptoms and increased engagement in both NSSI and suicide attempts. More importantly, a lack of specificity between NSSI and suicide attempt regarded to BPD symptoms were reported. This point proposed identifying whether or not there are different forms of self-harm happening, including NSSI and suicide, is a crucial point to understanding the association between self-harm and BPD symptoms, due to the indistinguishable nature of NSSI and suicide association with BPD, when each of them occurs singularly (Muehlenkamp et al. 2011). Negative affectivity, neuroticism, negative temperament, and disinhibition are personality traits which have shown strong association with the frequency of suicide attempts (Brezo et al. 2006; Yen et al. 2009), as well as cluster B personality traits can contribute to increasing the rate of suicidal behaviors (Trull et al. 2005, 2008, 2010). Several studies have indicated that heightened impulsivity and affective instability in BPD can be considered as potential risk factors for self-inflicted injury and suicidal behaviors (Morgan et al. 2013, 2022; Peckham et al. 2020; Zanarini and

Frankenburg 2007; Soloff 2018; Glenn and Klonsky 2009, 2013b; Silvers et al. 2016; Silver et al. 2023). Yen et al. (2013) found adolescents with more BPD Criteria reported higher levels of negative affectivity, depression, anxiety, and higher emotional instability (Yen et al. 2013). According to studies, suicidal behaviors are associated to emotions connected with interpersonal relationships (Wedig et al. 2013; Hawton et al. 2012; Glenn and Klonsky 2013b). You et al. (2012) examined the associations between NSSI and four main BPD features, including affective instability, disturbed interpersonal relationship, unstable sense of self, and behavioral impulsivity among 4782 Chinese adolescents. The results showed these four major symptoms can differentiate adolescents with and without NSSI. The findings indicated that three features consisting of affective instability, disturbed interpersonal relationships, and behavioral impulsivity were remarkably related to the presence of NSSI both concurrently and longitudinally, and these features contributed to subsequent initiation of NSSI. Behavioral impulsivity was the only symptom which significantly contributed to the repetition of NSSI, and lower levels of affective instability was related to stopping NSSI. In addition, behavioral impulsivity had an important effect on the repetition of NSSI in adolescents. Based on You et al. (2012), unstable sense of self does not have significant role in elucidating NSSI presence and initiation (You et al. 2012). The quality of interpersonal relationships is a crucial element in psychopathology of BPD, especially insecure and disorganized attachment patterns (Moscoso et al. 2019; Sharp et al. 2018). In addition, difficulties in interpersonal relationships can be the origin of hopelessness and helplessness which contribute to suicidal behaviors (Soloff et al. 2019).

Links et al. (2008) identified components of affective instability related to elevated probability of impulsivity, as well as resolved whether these components portray individuals with BPD and suicidal behavior among 82 patients with BPD and a history of recurrent suicidal behavior. According to findings, there was a correlation between mood domain and impulsivity, as well as based on mood domain and negative mood intensity, BPD individuals revealed higher levels of suicidal behavior risk. To sum, two components of affective instability were found to be related the increased likelihood of suicidal behavior in individuals with BPD, including negative mood intensity and mood amplitude. Negative mood intensity catches the patient's internalizing amplitude and increased level of neuroticism, and also, alterations in mood amplitude from high to low level may associated with the dimension of trait impulsivity. A combined state of these two components may lead to development of a subgroup of BPD with escalated risk for suicidal behavior and suicide attempts (Links et al. 2008). It has been assumed that two core features of BPD, including interpersonal difficulties and experiential disturbances, have a strong association with the traits of affective instability among individuals with personality disorders (Koenigsberg et al. 2001).

Theoretical reconsiderations have revealed that emotional, behavioral, and interpersonal factors may have influences on thoughts of death and suicidal ideation. Selby et al. (2013c) assessed the dynamic influence of these factors in association with suicidal ideation and death thoughts. Their findings revealed emotional sensitivity, behavioral dysregulation, peer invalidation, and suicidal ideation were exceedingly related to chronically and acutely SI levels, whilst depression, negative emotional intensity, and family invalidation have been shown more acutely predictive of suicidal ideation. In addition, they suggest exacerbated levels of SI reciprocally increase all these factors (Selby et al. 2013a, b, c). Previous research results have indicated that cognitive deficits in BPD are related to hyperarousal which leads to the progression of the suicide process. Due to hypersensitivity to emotional stimulus and emotion dysregulation, BPD individuals have several difficulties when negative life events trigger episodes of emotional instability and behavioral disinhibition. These issues lead to impulsive aggression and self-inflicted injuries and suicidal behaviors in BPD cases which contribute to high-fatality suicide attempts by them (Rutter et al. 2021; Cackowski et al. 2014; Soloff et al. 2017). In addition, due to behavioral disinhibition (inability to manage impulsive behaviors), individuals with BPD may be more vulnerable to aggressive self-destructive behaviors, especially in interpersonal relationships (Cackowski et al. 2017). Under stressful life experiences, emotion dysregulation in BPD individuals interferes with cognitive abilities contribute the development of maladaptive strategies, such as response disinhibition, impaired decision-making, distracted attention, disturbed planning, and non-goal-directed behaviors (Soloff et al. 2017). Furthermore, emotion dysregulation may be facilitated due to emotional interference with executive function. Finally, accumulation of emotion dysregulation and lack of behavioral control leads to SIB and suicidal thoughts and attempts in individuals with BPD (Soloff et al. 2017; Rutter et al. 2020). Moreover, several executive functions impairments have been acquired in BPD individuals resembling individuals who attempt suicide, such as difficulties in attention, cognitive inflexibility, learning and memory issues, problems in planning, processing speed matters, and difficulties in visual-spatial abilities (Howard et al. 2021; Fincham et al. 2002; Lezak 2004).

Through an investigation on 228 adolescents in clinical settings based on BPD-traits, current psychological distress and maintenance of NSSI, it was indicated adolescents with low perceived social support have more vulnerability for developing NSSI related to high BPD traits. Furthermore, it has been documented that borderline traits have a mediation role in the association between perceived social support and NSSI. To conclude, the results showed the relation among long-lasting traits vis-a-vis state symptoms in the association between perceived social support and NSSI (Mendez et al. 2022). Blasczyk-Schiep et al. (2018) studied various mediators of self-harm behaviors and suicidal acts, and the results indicated that experiencing childhood adversities and emotional neglect contribute to difficulties in self-regulation of emotion and lead to the development of BPD and exacerbate the risk of self-harm behaviors and suicide attempts (Blasczyk-Schiep et al. 2018; Tresno et al. 2012). In line with growing documents, NSSI has exhibited interpersonal and interpersonal functions in individuals with BPD (Klonsky and Glenn 2009; Brown et al. 2002, 2014; Klonsky 2007). Based on Nock (2008), some individuals with BPD engage in NSSI due to social excuses because it is believed that "actions speak louder than words" in order to evoke caregiver's attention to provide care, as well as in BPD individuals, the act of NSSI can be postulated as "a signal of distress hypothesis" whenever low intensity signals of distress such as excessive reassurance-seeking cannot be effective for evoking caregiver responses (Nock et al. 2008). Therefore, Selby et al. (2009) suggested the likelihood of a subgroup of BPD cases for which interpersonal and social functions of NSSI are significant, and suggest that BPD is associated with greater levels of excessive reassurance seeking (Selby et al. 2009). Lu et al. (2024) investigated the risk factors associated with NSSI influencing secondary vocational school students, and also, analyzing the role of BPD tendencies in improving the occurrence of NSSI among 1848 students with depressive mood. The results showed that female, drinking history, history of suicidal death exposure, depressive mood, and BPD tendencies were independent risk factors for NSSI. Moreover, BPD tendencies moderated the association between depressive mood and NSSI. Based on findings, the stronger the BPD tendencies, the more NSSI behavior happened when they were depressed (Lu et al. 2024).

Tang et al. (2021) investigated the prevalence of NSSI pending COVID-19 prevalence to assess the psychological risk factors among adolescents engaged in NSSI, and based on the results, greater rates of neuroticism, depression, impulsivity, alexithymia, virtual social support, dissatisfaction with academic performance, and also, lower scores in perceived well-being, self-esteem, social support, and family function were found out in NSSI individuals in comparison to non-NSSI group (Tang et al. 2021). Valencia and Sinambela (2020) suggested that there are an association between self-harm behavior, neuroticism personality, and parental separation. Impulsivity is one of the main features of neuroticism which can lead to difficulties in impulse control, highlighting why neuroticism personality traits are often involved in self-inflicted injurious behaviors. Finally, parental separation can be considered as a childhood traumatic experience that may cause self-harm behaviors (Valencia and Sinambela 2020).

Comprehensive Theories of the Development of Nonsuicidal Self-Injuries (NSSI) and Suicide Behaviors in BPD

Several contemporary psychological theories elucidate the development of nonsuicidal self-injuries and suicide in BPD during recent decades. Affect regulation, self-punishment, interpersonal influence, anti-dissociation, anti-suicide, sensation seeking, interpersonal boundaries, attachment matters, and implications of different functions are proposed as reasons of involving in NSSI (Klonsky and Muehlenkamp 2007; Møhl 2019; Klonsky 2007). Over the few decades, there have been a considerate great deal of investigations and debates, empirical and clinical, to elucidate and propose a clearer picture of two common and frequent public mental health issues, including NSSI and suicide. Historically, studies delineated NSSI and suicide in BPD have been illustrated from abundantly independent investigations, as well as it seems that no specified borders have been represented between suicide and NSSI (Kaufman et al. 2020a, b; Linehan 1997). Furthermore, causal factors of NSSI and suicide have been debated for centuries (e.g., Durkheim 1897). In fact, we have seen a growing stream of nonsuicidal self-injuries and suicide studies during past decade that lead to deeper understanding of NSSI and suicide (nonfatal suicidal thoughts and behaviors, as well as the distinctions between these two issues (Gardner et al. 2021b). In other words, several investigations have been conducted to elucidate the predisposition and risk factors for NSSH, through heritability biological-genetic, psychological, and social lenses (e.g., Crowell et al. 2014; Selby et al. 2008, 2009; Kaufman et al. 2020a, b; Chapman et al. 2006; Nock and Prinstien 2004; Klonsky 2007). Moreover, there are a growing publication which have been cited in hundreds of studies to argue and propose answers for the nature of NSSI and related issues of this problem (Klonsky and May 2014). A group of these investigations suggest a distinction between NSSI and other SIB, and several studies argued about the necessity of distinction between NSSI and suicide attempts, and even distinguishing NSSI from other types of SIBs, and regarded them as an independent clinical symptom (e.g., Claes et al. 2010; Muehlenkamp et al. 2005; Muehlenkamp and Gutierrez 2004). A body of studies are constantly moving toward multi-facet, interactive approaches that are based on multiple-levels-of-analysis perspectives to propose an expanded explanation about the predisposition and tendency to develop psychopathology, as well as underlying mechanisms for stability and alterations of different types of psychological problems, such as NSSH and suicide (e.g., Beauchaine and McNulty 2013; Kaufman et al. 2020a, b; Crowell and Kaufman 2016; Crowell et al. 2009; Selby 2007; Selby et al. 2009; Linehan 1993; Mann 2003; Gibb et al. 2006). In line with Klonsky et al. (2015), in spite of some significant exceptions (Pattison and Kahan 1983; Walsh and Rosen 1988), studies focused on NSSI and its nature and etiology were few until the early 2000s, when can be referred as a turning point for identifying this issue (Klonsky and May 2014).

Through reviewing various articles in the field of psychopathology and theoretical perspective of SIB, including NSSH and suicide attempts, we distinguished the different point of views to elucidate SIBs, especially the synchronicity of these issues with BPD. While the interpersonal-psychological theory of suicide provides an explanation for understanding various aspects of suicide, such as belongingness, perceived burdensomeness, acquired capability, and ability to act; theories based on bio-psycho-social components propose a conceptualization about the internal and external conditions which may contribute to shifting from suicidal thoughts to suicidal attempts (Emelianchik-Key and La Guardia 2019). As mentioned, several theories try to provide various explanations about different reasons for engaging NSSI and attempting suicide from bio-psycho-social views in BPD, including emotional cascade model (Selby et al. 2008, 2009), biosocial theory (Linehan 1993), biosocial developmental model (Crowell et al. 2009, 2014; Kaufman et al. 2020a, b), and emotion dysregulation theory (Gratz 2007).

An Emotion Regulation Perspective of NSSI and Suicide in BPD

Emotion regulation concept involves a set of neurobiological and physiological processes, for example, emotion recognition, emotion reactivity, and cognitive control (Gross 2015; Ochsner et al. 2009; Phillips et al. 2008; Wolff et al. 2019). During years, emotion regulation issues and the concept of emotion dysregulation have been concentrated by several studies and many researches have attempted to clarify and identify the role this matter in the development of NSSI and suicidal thoughts and behaviors (e.g., Aldao et al. 2010, 2016), and also proposed theoretical models based on emotion regulation theory to suggest evidence-based frameworks to recognize different aspects of NSSI and suicide (e.g., Linehan 1993; Brown et al. 2002, 2014; Chapman et al. 2006; Selby et al. 2008, 2009, 2014a, b, c; Klonsky 2007; Crowell et al. 2009, 2014). The majority of these models have focused on emotion regulation skills deficiencies, which contribute to difficulties in experiencing and tolerance of unwanted negative emotion and create an urge for escaping or avoiding from these intense unpleasant emotion (e.g., Linehan 1993; Chapman et al. 2006). NSSI is widely noticed to propose an emotion-regulatory function. It should be mentioned just by simply naming NSSI as "emotion regulatory" does not provide precise information about the process and nature of NSSI, because in various ways NSSI plays a role as emotion regulatory at any moment. This problem suggests we should clarify the exact and precise functions of an individual in a particular context (McKenzie and Gross 2014). One of the most significant factors that not only leads to formation of self-injury but also contributes to maintenance of SIB is emotion dysregulation (Gratz 2007; Chapman et al. 2017; Chapman 2019). Pursuant to Linehan (1993), emotion dysregulation is the crucial feature of BPD and underlies the majority of BPD features, compromising self-injury which is referred to as an emotion regulation function (Linehan 1993). Several investigators have conceptualized self-injury as an emotion regulation strategy, such as Gratz (2003) and Klonsky (2007).

In line with emotion regulation models, individuals engage in SIB to reduce or avoid negative emotional states, self-punishment, escape from interpersonal conflicts, and to enhance feelings or to release anger (Brown et al. 2002, 2014, 2016; Matel-Anderson et al. 2019). Klonsky (2007) indicated that negative emotion precedes SIB, NSSI has relationship with the aim of mitigating negative emotion, reducing negative affect (Klonsky 2007). In addition, Klonsky (2009) demonstrated an association between NSSI and the enhancement of emotional valence, including reducing negative emotion and escalating positive emotion, as well as emotional arousal among individuals with NSSI (Klonsky 2009). Based on research findings, feeling of emptiness, a BPD symptom, may be an antecedent for engaging in NSSI among adolescents (Klonsky 2009), and, there is an association between identity diffusion and a history of self-harm behaviors (Claes et al. 2014). Spitzen et al. (2020) reported that NSSI was related to emotional regulation function in BPD individuals, as well as fear, inner emptiness, and aggression lead the person to be engaged in self-inflicted injuries (Spitzen et al. 2020). Brickman et al. (2014)

studied the relationship between NSSI and BPD symptoms to identify individuals with BPD symptoms and escalated order BPD factors which contribute to escalation of individual vulnerability of NSSI among 720 college students. The findings indicated that partial support for the significance of emotion dysregulation in the association between NSSI and BPD symptoms. Overall, this study suggested a set of BPD symptoms and related factors may play a remarkable role in the vulnerability for NSSI, aside from symptoms which were directly related to ability to regulate emotion. They claimed that these contrast findings are due to nonclinical samples in comparison to other studies which clinical samples were recruited for investigations. Furthermore, they suggested among BPD individuals with milder forms of emotion dysregulation, individuals engage in NSSI when emotional turbulence is reinforced by intense anger and aggression and/or fear of abandonment. In addition, Brickman et al. (2014) detected that the BPD intrapersonal matters such as identity confusion and feeling of emptiness can be considered prior to the beginning of NSSI among their sample (Brickman et al. 2014). Sadeh et al. (2014) indicated that BPD affect regulation have a strong relationship with intrapersonal function of NSSI, as well as difficulties in emotion regulation and self-punishment contribute to maintenance of SIB (Sadeh et al. 2014).

Biosocial Developmental Model of Self-Injuries and Suicidal Behaviors and BPD (Crowell et al. 2009, 2014)

As mentioned in the prior chapter related to biosocial developmental model of BPD (Crowell et al. 2009), emotion dysregulation and impulsivity were two main components contributed to the development of BPD (Crowell et al. 2009, 2014). Based on the biosocial developmental model, NSSI is claimed that to be a developmental precursor of BPD pathology (Crowell et al. 2008, 2012, 2014; Homan et al. 2017; Grazt et al. 2014). Emotion dysregulation is considered as a core feature of BPD which contributes to maladaptive strategies of emotion regulation and suicidal behaviors (e.g., Mirkovic et al. 2021). Crowell et al. (2014) conceptualized self-injurious thoughts and behaviors (SITBs) as a wider classification, and suicide attempts were categorized just as subset. They suggested *self-inflicted injury* can be divided into (1) *nonsuicidal self-injury* (NSSI), a wide spectrum of deliberate behaviors with the purpose of damaging body tissue without intention of death; and (2) *suicidal behaviors* (SBs), with an ambivalent or remarked intention for death. Furthermore, they posited that since suicidal ideation is a cognitive process rather than a behavior, they formalized it a separate category. Therefore, in their attempt to propose a biosocial developmental model for BPD and self-injury and suicidal behaviors, they just considered SB and repetitive NSSI (Crowell et al. 2014). The body of empirical investigations have demonstrated emotion dysregulation can be considered as a core etiological factor in the emergence and perpetuation of SITBs (e.g., Kaufman et al. 2020a, b; Anestis et al. 2011; Ammerman et al. 2015; Law et al. 2015; Klonsky and Glenn 2009; Linehan 1993). In line with several studies, emotion dysregulation has been illustrated being a crucial developmental precursor for engaging in NSSI (e.g., Linehan 1993; Klonsky and Muehlenkamp 2007), and a well-perpetuated factor to maintain further NSSI (e.g., Klonsky 2007, 2009; Klonsky and Muehlenkamp 2007), and has been found as a proximal risk factor for initiating suicide attempts (Ammerman et al. 2015; Andover and Morris 2014; Kaufman et al. 2020a, b). A growing body of studies have attempted to display various features of emotion dysregulation in initiating and maintenance of SITBs, including mood swings, emotional turbulence, high emotional sensitivity, escalated emotional intensity, irritability, and slow return to baseline (e.g., Linehan 1993; Brezo et al. 2008; Perez-Rodriguez et al. 2012; Gratz and Roemer 2008; Crowell et al. 2005, 2012; Houben et al. 2017; Gratz and Trull 2010). In contrast to this large volume of studies, several investigations have demonstrated ameliorating emotion regulation contributes to SITBs cease (e.g., Gratz et al. 2015; Whitlock et al. 2015; Kaufman et al. 2020a, b). These findings have been contributed to conceptualize SITBs as a manifestation of a wide range of problematic emotion regulation strategies (e.g., Chapman et al. 2006; Linehan 1993; Gratz and Roemer 2004; Howard et al. 2021). However, emotion dysregulation has been pointed out as a key risk factor for SII and suicide attempts (SITBs), Crowell et al. (2009) reformulated this model and cited emotion dysregulation and impulsivity display simultaneously transactional roles which contribute to the development of SITBs (Crowell et al. 2009, 2014).

In line with this model, *Biology X Environmental* interactions lead to a complex of specified difficulties and maladaptive coping strategies. In other words, trait impulsivity and emotional instability have an interactive relationship with each other across the developmental stages of life, as well as interact with the problematic environmental and contextual risk factors. This process provides vulnerable predisposition for more extreme behaviors and emotion dysregulation, chaotic interpersonal relationships, and a wide range of difficulties in individual's functions. Therefore, an individual may be more vulnerable and the risk for developing BPD criteria will be exasperated (Crowell et al. 2009, 2014; Kaufman et al. 2020a, b). Figure 12.2 proposes a description of developmental biosocial model of BPD and SII (Kaufman et al. 2017a, b, 2023).

As has been shown in Fig. 12.1, biological-based heritable vulnerabilities are a key precursor in development of SII. In other words, various investigations have proposed that biological underpinnings have significant impact on the development of BPD and SITBs (Kaufman et al. 2020a, b; Crowell et al. 2014). In line with Crowell et al. (2009), differences in temperament, such as emotional sensitivity, experiencing intense negative emotions, irritability, and trait impulsivity, various genetically and epigenetically in monoamine neurotransmitter function, and, neuroanatomical and psychophysiological differences are the most significant biologically based heritable vulnerabilities contribute to BPD and SITBs. As stated, Crowell et al. (2009) conceptualized impulsivity as a key feature contributed to BPD and SITBs in association with emotion dysregulation. They emphasized the heritable aspect of trait impulsivity associated with suicidal behaviors based on

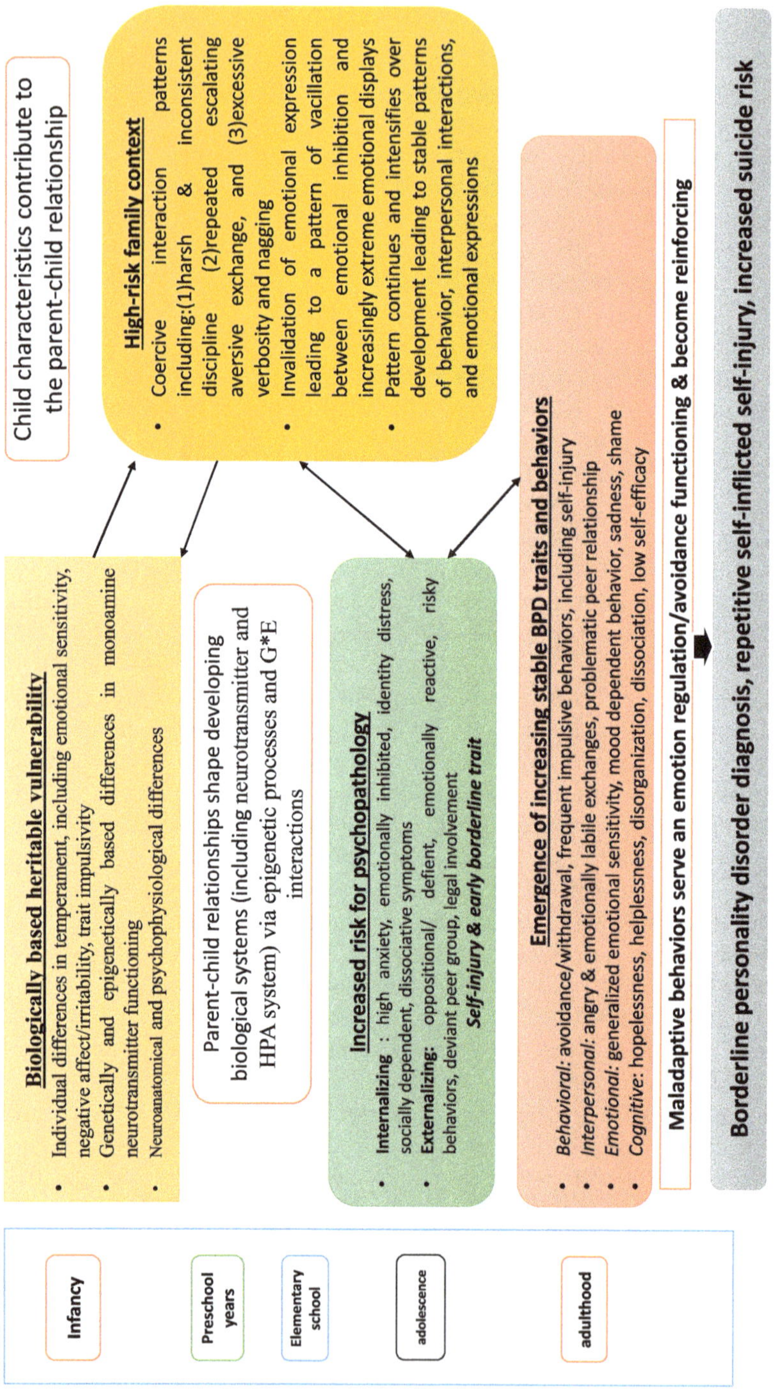

Fig. 12.1 Biosocial Developmental of BPD and SII. (Source: adapted Kaufman et al. (2017a, b), p.649)

family and twin studies. Convergent findings collected from multitude of research projects, including adoption, family, genome scan, molecular genetics, surname and twin studies of suicide, propose that genetic contributions to suicide risk. Based on empirical findings, impulsivity is associated with a wide range of suicidal acts. Voracek and Loibl (2007) conducted a comprehensive review of the twins' studies (19 case reports, 5 twin-register-based studies, 4 population-based epidemiological studies, 4 studies of surviving co-twins) which were published between 1812 and 2006 in six languages from 13 countries to demonstrate the role of genetics of suicide (Voracek et al. 2007). Marco et al. (2015) found individuals with BPD who reported low meaning of life revealed more depression, hopelessness, more frequent NSSI in comparison with people who felt high level of life meaning (Marco et al. 2015). Through empirical observational research with an analytical perspective based on a cross-sectional design, Arango-Tobón et al. (2021) examined the relationship among hopelessness, depression, and impulsivity with respect to suicidal thoughts and behaviors, and also, to identify the role of impulsivity as a mediator mechanism in the hopelessness and depression association among 228 university students. The results showed a high variance ranged from 57% to 67% the risk of suicidal thoughts and behaviors can be explained by depression, impulsivity, and hopelessness. This means these three factors significantly elevate the risk of suicidal thoughts and behaviors. In addition, based on a structural equation modeling, three models were distinguished suggesting that impulsivity mediates the association between depression and suicidal thoughts and behaviors, and this kind of mediator roles can exacerbate the effect of impulsivity on suicidal thoughts and behaviors. As well as impulsivity plays a role similar to a mediator of depressive symptoms, and indirectly effect on the prediction of suicidal thoughts and behaviors (Arango-Tobón et al. 2021). Impulsivity acts like a risk factor for providing the transition from ideation to suicide attempt, as well as emotional factors contribute to negative thoughts about self and future lead had a relationship with suicidal thoughts while impulsive reactions to intense negative emotional factors were associated with suicide attempts (Auerbach et al. 2017). Impulsivity responses exacerbate the frequency of suicide attempts (Bagge et al. 2013; Kasen et al. 2011). It has been pointed out impulsive behaviors can be understood as a trigger which can act like a determinant for suicide attempts in youth with depressive symptoms (Gómez et al. 2020; Gómez 2019).

The Experiential Avoidance Model (EAM) (Chapman et al. 2006)

According to several studies, emotional functioning is broadly impaired in BPD (e.g., Linehan 1993; Selby et al. 2008; Nock 2009; Klonsky 2007; Chapman et al. 2017; Chapman 2019; Gratz 2003; Crowell et al. 2009). In comparison with non-BPD individuals, people with BPD indicate more intense and frequent negative emotions (e.g., Rosenthal et al. 2015), as well as higher rate of problems in regulating negative emotion (e.g., Putnam and Silk 2005). A growing body of studies have demonstrated the association between BDP features and experiential avoidance and avoidant coping strategies (e.g., Chapman et al. 2017; Chapman 2019; Dillahunt et al. 2022; Bijttebier and Vertommen 1999). Experiential avoidance refers to individuals' endeavors or desire to escape, avoid, or suppress unpleasant and unwanted internal experiences, such as emotions, thoughts, body sensations, memories, and urges (Hayes et al. 1996; Shepherd-McMullen et al. 2015). In line with various investigation, experiential avoidance plays a main role in initiation and maintenance of a broad range of maladaptive, dysfunctional behaviors and psychopathologies, such as BPD (Chapman et al. 2005), self-harm (Chapman et al. 2006), PTSD (Orcutt et al. 2005), and GAD (Roemer et al. 2005). Individuals with BPD and BPD symptoms report increased inclination toward avoidant emotion regulation (Rosenthal et al. 2006; Chapman et al. 2005; Cheavens et al. 2005), as well as controlling for symptoms of other mental problems (Aldao and Dixon-Gordon 2014). Furthermore, individuals with BPD show greater avoidance from emotional state and indicate avoiding responses to intense negative emotions compared with other strategies such as cognitive reappraisal (Sheppes and Levin 2013; Sheppes et al. 2011). Since these emotional avoidances contribute to the reduction of intense negative affect in short-term, avoidance behaviors are reinforced over time due to decreasing in emotional distress (Chapman et al. 2017; Chapman 2019; Farmer and Chapman 2016), as well as escalating the reinforcing impacts of avoidance or escape behavior (Chapman et al. 2017; Chapman 2019). Through standardized negative emotion induction investigations, it has been realized that directed suppression of emotional manifestations contribute to higher levels of negative emotion (Xie et al. 2021).

Deliberate self-harm (DSH) has self-defeating and self-destructive nature and is difficult to understand why people intentionally injure their body and are engaged in self-inflict tissue damage (Chapman et al. 2006). According to Chapman et al. (2006), deliberate self-harm can be considered as "express, concretize, and or effect regulation function" (Chapman et al. 2006, p.374). Linehan's biosocial theory (1993) posited the core feature of BPD in emotion dysregulation which originated from the transaction between environmental invalidation and biological vulnerabilities which contribute to poor emotion regulation skills and emotion dysregulation. Environmental invalidation leads to disruptions in the process of learning adaptive emotion regulation to manage intense emotional reactions, which subsequently contribute to impulsivity and short-term strategies to regulate unwanted painful emotions. In line with this perspective, self-harm is considered as an emotion regulation strategy to decrease or avoid aversive emotions which lead to be reinforced due to escaping from experiencing unpleasant negative affect (Chapman et al. 2005; Linehan 1993). Figure 12.2 illustrates an association between the biosocial theory of BPD to experiential avoidance and self-harm.

The core element emphasized in Linehan's biosocial theory (1993) is the significance of *experiential avoidance* or behavior with the function of avoidance or escape from unwanted emotion, thoughts, or somatic sensation (Chapman et al. 2005; Hayes et al. 1996). Thought suppression, alcohol/drug abuse, impulsive

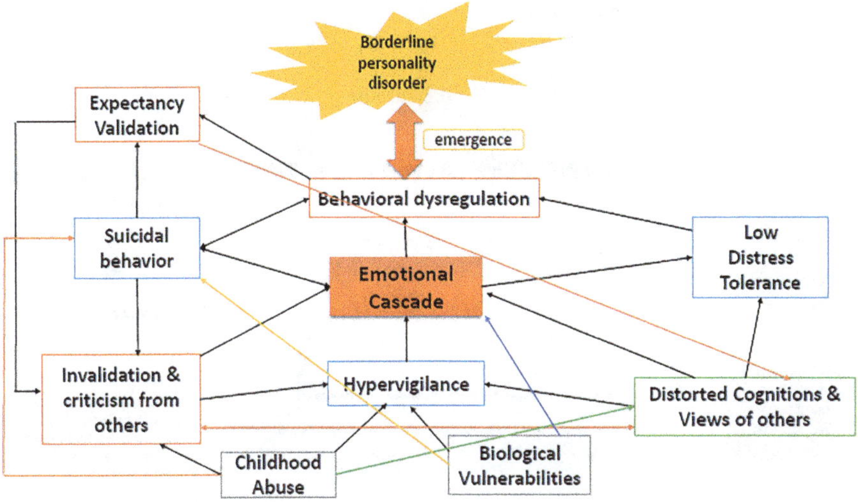

Fig. 12.2 Emotional cascade model and the emergence of BPD. (Source: adapted Selby et al. (2014a), p.161)

eating, impulsive spending, suicide attempts, self-harm, dissociation, and avoidant coping are considered as powerful experiential avoidance created by poor emotion regulation skills and emotion dysregulation in individuals with BPD. Additionally, an emotional stimulus can cause unwanted negative emotional states which contribute to self-harm. Since the function of these SIB are escaping from emotional arousal and contribute to reduction of intense emotional experiencing, consequently, negative reinforcement for self-harm occurs which leads to maintenance of deliberate self-harm (Chapman et al. 2005; Linehan 1993; Turner et al. 2013). A growing body of investigations have revealed that individuals who experience higher levels of emotional intensity or greater sensitivity report more difficulties in controlling or regulating their emotions, hence engaging in NSSI as a strategy for avoiding negative emotions and obtaining control over their internal states (e.g., Hilt et al. 2018; Weierich and Nock 2008; Zettle et al. 2005; Chapman et al. 2005; Kashdan and Steger 2006; Chawla and Ostafin 2007; Anderson et al. 2018).

The Experiential Avoidance Model (EAM, Chapman et al. 2006) is one of the most prominent models to understand the role of NSSI in regulating emotion (Møhl 2019). Chapman et al. (2006) proposed a theoretical model of deliberate self-harm (DSH) to provide a comprehensive understanding of this self-injurious behavior based on a behavioral theory of DSH, which was applied to DSH at a general level among different population, such as personality disorders, PTSD, and depression (Chapman et al. 2006). Figure 12.3 illustrates the Experiential Avoidance Model (EAM) of deliberate self-harm (DSH).

According to the Experiential Avoidance Model (Chapman et al. 2006), deliberate self-harm is considered as a negatively reinforce strategy used for decreasing or finishing unwanted emotional arousal. In other words, NSSI is an avoidant behavior

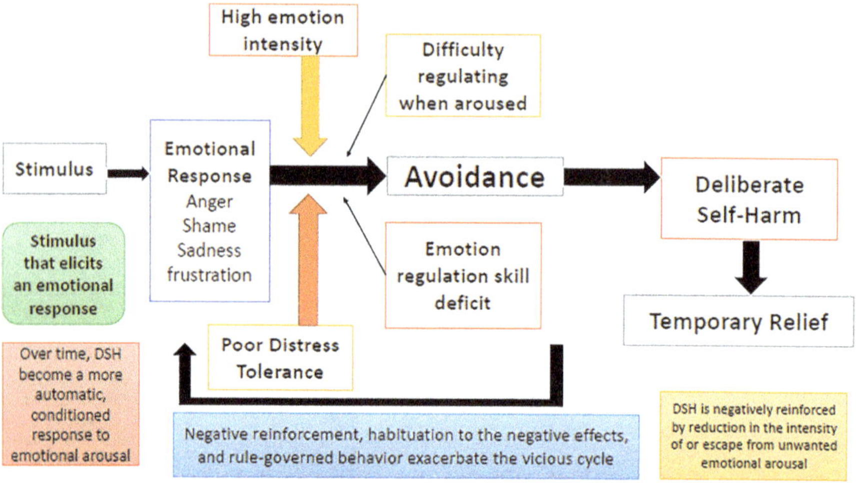

Fig. 12.3 The Experiential Avoidance Model (EAM) of Deliberate Self-Harm (DSH). (Source: adapted Chapman et al. (2006), p. 373)

that makes an individual capable to avoid unwanted and unpleasant emotions, thoughts, memories, and/or somatic sensations (Chapman et al. 2006). Therefore, due to being negatively reinforced, NSSI becomes an automatic escape response (Anderson et al. 2018). As illustrated in Fig. 12.3, the sequence initiates from a stimulant that elicits an intense negative emotional response, such as anger, shame, and sadness. High emotion intensity and difficulties in regulating unwanted emotions when aroused, as well as deficits in emotion regulation skill that leads to an inability in enduring distress and impaired distress tolerance result to a heightened tendency toward avoidance or escaping from unpleasant negative emotions via involving in deliberate self-harm. Subsequently, a temporary relief and short-term reduction occurs in the intensity of negative emotions and unwanted emotional arousal. Therefore, negative reinforcement, habituation to the negative influences, and rule-governed behavior worsen the repetitive vicious cycle of DSH. Continually, deliberate self-harm is strengthened, and becomes more automatic through reinforcement and conditioning process (Chapman et al. 2006). Chapman et al. (2005) examined the experiential avoidance and the mediating role of experiential avoidance in the relationship between BPD and DSH, among 105 female BPD cases. Results demonstrated that BPD severity was associated with higher levels of DSH frequency and greater experiential avoidance. In addition, they suggested that no mediating role was found for experiential avoidance in the relationship between BPD and DSH, except suppression which indicated an association with self-harm frequency (Chapman et al. 2005). Chapman et al. (2017) tested the influence of avoidance versus acceptance-oriented emotion regulation instructions among patients with BPD using ecological momentary assessment. Based on such findings, avoidance instructions contributed to reducing in negative emotion and urges for being engaged in dysfunctional and maladaptive behaviors in BPD, which propose that avoidance of negative emotions provides short-term advantages for individuals with BPD (Chapman et al. 2017; Chapman 2019). Gratz and Roemer (2004) demonstrated an association between greater levels of emotional nonacceptance with self-harm behavior among male undergraduate students (Gratz and Roemer 2004). Hulbert and Thomas (2010) found that experiential avoidance model can predict the frequency of SIB among BPD individuals, due to emotional relief (Hulbert and Thomas 2010). Kingston et al. (2010) indicated that experiential avoidance can be considered as a mediator in the association between risk factors and difficult behaviors. Weierich and Nock (2008) tested the role of childhood adversity and PTSD in SIB. Results indicated that avoidance strategies as well as issues in experiencing positive emotions can mediate the association between child abuse and self-injury (Weierich and Nock 2008).

Emotional Cascade Model of Self-Injuries and Suicidal Behaviors and BPD (Selby et al. 2009)

Emotional cascade model, discussed in a previous chapter, has been established by Selby and Joiner Jr (2009) to elucidate dysregulated behaviors in BPD. Based on Selby et al. (2010), growing evidence has shown the linking between NSSI and affect regulation. It means individual may choose NSSI to regulate emotion over other behaviors to decline their psychological pain. Yet, the most challenging unclear question is why people select NSSI to lessen their painful emotional experiences, instead of choosing adaptive and functional behavior. Selby et al. (2010) hypothesized two factors as explanation for this question: (1) intense rumination contributes to the emotion dysregulation which initiates NSSI, and (2) due to NSSI, fearlessness of pain may occur. They posit when these two factors co-occur simultaneously, since individuals experience intense negative emotion and do not afraid of pain at the same time, a strong wish to engage in SIB as a distraction from rumination and emotional cascade (Selby et al. 2010). Through a cross-sectional study among 127 BPD patients, Perez et al. (2020) demonstrated NSSI may be considered as a strategy to regulate intense emotions (Perez et al. 2020). Zaki et al. (2013a, b) indicated that rumination and emotion differentiation can be considered as a predictor for engaging in self-injurious behavior in individuals with BPD who has a history of NSSI (Zaki et al. 2013a, b).

Buelens et al. (2019) pointed out NSSI behaviors may exacerbate distress and rumination which assumed NSSI encompassed by broader network of cognitive-emotional antecedents and consequences; moreover, a long-term maladaptive cycle will be developed among emotion, cognition, and NSSI (Buelens et al. 2019, 2020a, b).

The preliminary hypotheses mentioned by Selby et al. (2009, 2010) was the impact of rumination as a factor which contributes to the initial emotional turbulence that consequently leads to NSSI (Selby 2007, 2011; Selby et al. 2009, 2010,

2014a, b, c). Rumination is a cognitive process which characterized with repetitive focus of attention on one's thoughts and emotions (Nolen-Hoeksema and Morrow 1991; Selby et al. 2010). According to several studies, it has been shown rumination aggravates and lengthens the effect of negative emotion (Moberly and Watkins 2008).

To sum, NSSI and suicidal thoughts and attempts are substantially pathological mental health issues which are highly prevalent and common among adolescents and adults. These problems are found in a wide range of clinical population, especially among individuals with BPD. Furthermore, it was discussed that the presence of NSSI and suicidal behaviors have been proposed as major risk factors for the development of BPD pathology, and numerous theoretical and empirical elucidations were suggested to conceptualize these associations. Emotion regulation issues, emotion dysregulation, neuroticism, distress tolerance difficulties, biological-genetic factors, emotional and cognitive avoidances, and impulsivity are prominent factors which can explain the development and maintenance of the associations between NSSI and suicide and BPD. Finally, various theories have tried to elucidate the relations between NSSI and suicide and BPD pathology, such as emotion regulation perspective, biosocial developmental of BPD and SII, experiential avoidance model, and emotional cascade theory.

References

Aaltonen KI, Isometsä E, Sund R, Pirkola S. Decline in suicide mortality after psychiatric hospitalization for depression in Finland between 1991 and 2014. World Psychiatry. 2018;17(1):110.

Albert U, Pellegrini L, Maina G, Atti AR, De Ronchi D, Rhimer Z. Suicide in obsessive-compulsive related disorders: prevalence rates and psychopathological risk factors. J Psychopathol. 2019;25(3):139–48.

Aldao A, Gee DG, De Los RA, Seager I. Emotion regulation as a transdiagnostic factor in the development of internalizing and externalizing psychopathology: current and future directions. Dev Psychopathol. 2016;28(4pt1):927–46.

Aldao A, Nolen-Hoeksema S, Schweizer S. Emotion-regulation strategies across psychopathology: a meta-analytic review. Clin Psychol Rev. 2010;30(2):217–37.

Aldao A, Dixon-Gordon KL. Broadening the scope of research on emotion regulation strategies and psychopathology. Cogn Behav Ther. 2014;43(1):22–33.

Allen KJ, Hooley JM. Negative Emotional Action Termination (NEAT): support for a cognitive mechanism underlying negative urgency in nonsuicidal self-injury. Behav Ther. 2019;50(5):924–37.

Allroggen M, Kleinrahm R, Rau TA, Weninger L, Ludolph AG, Plener PL. Nonsuicidal self-injury and its relation to personality traits in medical students. J Nerv Ment Dis. 2014;202(4):300–4.

American Psychiatric Association. Diagnostic and statistical manual of mental disorders. 5th ed, Text Revised (DSM-5-TR); 2022.

American Psychiatric Association DS. Diagnostic and statistical manual of mental disorders: DSM-5. Washington, DC: American Psychiatric Association; 2013.

Ammerman BA, Kleiman EM, Uyeji LL, Knorr AC, McCloskey MS. Suicidal and violent behavior: the role of anger, emotion dysregulation, and impulsivity. Personal Individ Differ. 2015;79:57–62.

Anderson NL, Smith KE, Mason TB, Crowther JH. Testing an integrative model of affect regulation and avoidance in non-suicidal self-injury and disordered eating. Arch Suicide Res. 2018;22(2):295–310.

Andover MS, Gibb BE. Nonsuicidal self-injury, attempted suicide, and suicidal intent among psychiatric inpatients. Psychiatry Res. 2010;178(1):101–5.

Andover MS, Morris BW. Expanding and clarifying the role of emotion regulation in nonsuicidal self-injury. Can J Psychiatry. 2014;59(11):569–75.

Andover MS, Schatten HT, Morris BW. Suicidal and nonsuicidal self-injury in borderline personality disorder. Borderline personality disorder. 2018:129–48.

Andrews T, Martin G, Hasking P, Page A. Predictors of onset for non-suicidal self-injury within a school-based sample of adolescents. Prev Sci. 2014;15:850–9.

Andrews S, Hanna P. Investigating the psychological mechanisms underlying the relationship between nightmares, suicide and self-harm. Sleep Med Rev. 2020;54:101352.

Andrewes HE, Hulbert C, Cotton SM, Betts J, Chanen AM. Ecological momentary assessment of nonsuicidal self-injury in youth with borderline personality disorder. Personal Disord Theory Res Treat. 2017;8(4):357.

Anestis MD, Coffey SF, Schumacher JA, Tull MT. Affective vulnerabilities and self-injury in suicide. Arch Suicide Res. 2011;15(4):291–303.

Anestis MD, Knorr AC, Tull MT, Lavender JM, Gratz KL. The importance of high distress tolerance in the relationship between nonsuicidal self-injury and suicide potential. Suicide Life Threat Behav. 2013;43(6):663–75.

Anestis MD, Tull MT, Lavender JM, Gratz KL. The mediating role of nonsuicidal self-injury in the relationship between impulsivity and suicidal behavior among inpatients receiving treatment for substance use disorders. Psychiatry Res. 2014;218(1–2):166–73.

Angelakis I, Gooding P, Tarrier N, Panagioti M. Suicidality in obsessive compulsive disorder (OCD): a systematic review and meta-analysis. Clin Psychol Rev. 2015;39:1–5.

Angelakis I, Austin JL, Gooding P. Association of childhood maltreatment with suicide behaviors among young people: a systematic review and meta-analysis. JAMA Netw Open. 2020;3(8):e2012563.

Anthony JL, Lonigan CJ, Hooe ES, Phillips BM. An affect-based, hierarchical model of temperament and its relations with internalizing symptomatology. J Clin Child Adolesc Psychol. 2002;31(4):480–90.

Aouidad A, Cohen D, Mirkovic B, Pellerin H, Garny de La Rivière S, Consoli A, et al. Borderline personality disorder and prior suicide attempts define a severity gradient among hospitalized adolescent suicide attempters. BMC Psychiatry. 2020a;20(1):525.

Aouidad A, Cohen D, Mirkovic B, Pellerin H, Garny de La Rivière S, Consoli A, Gérardin P, Guilé JM. Borderline personality disorder and prior suicide attempts define a severity gradient among hospitalized adolescent suicide attempters. BMC Psychiatry. 2020b;20:1–3.

Arbuthnott AE, Lewis SP, Bailey HN. Rumination and emotions in nonsuicidal self-injury and eating disorder behaviors: a preliminary test of the emotional cascade model. J Clin Psychol. 2015;71(1):62–71.

Arango-Tobón OE, Tabares AS, Serrano SJ. Structural model of suicidal ideation and behavior: mediating effect of impulsivity. Anais Da Academia Brasileira de Ciencias. 2021;93(suppl 4):e20210680.

Argyriou E, Um M, Wu W, Cyders MA. Measurement invariance of the UPPS-P impulsive behavior scale across age and sex across the adult life span. Assessment. 2020;27(3):432–53.

Asarnow JR, Porta G, Spirito A, Emslie G, Clarke G, Wagner KD, Vitiello B, Keller M, Birmaher B, McCracken J, Mayes T. Suicide attempts and nonsuicidal self-injury in the treatment of resistant depression in adolescents: findings from the TORDIA study. J Am Acad Child Adolesc Psychiatry. 2011;50(8):772–81.

Auerbach RP, Stewart JG, Johnson SL. Impulsivity and suicidality in adolescent inpatients. J Abnorm Child Psychol. 2017;45:91–103.

Ayodeji E, Green J, Roberts C, Trainor G, Rothwell J, Woodham A, Wood A. The influence of personality disorder on outcome in adolescent self-harm. Br J Psychiatry. 2015;207(4):313–9.

Bachmann S. Epidemiology of suicide and the psychiatric perspective. Int J Environ Res Public Health. 2018;15(7):1425.

Baetens I, Claes L, Onghena P, Grietens H, Van Leeuwen K, Pieters C, Wiersema JR, Griffith JW. Nonsuicidal self-injury in adolescence: a longitudinal study of the relationship between NSSI, psychological distress and perceived parenting. J Adolesc. 2014;37(6):817–26.
Bagge CL, Trull TJ. DAPP-BQ: factor structure and relations to personality disorder symptoms in a non-clinical sample. J Personal Disord. 2003;17(1):19–32.
Bagge CL, Glenn CR, Lee HJ. Quantifying the impact of recent negative life events on suicide attempts. J Abnorm Psychol. 2013;122(2):359.
Barak-Corren Y, Castro VM, Nock MK, Mandl KD, Madsen EM, Seiger A, Adams WG, Applegate RJ, Bernstam EV, Klann JG, McCarthy EP. Validation of an electronic health record–based suicide risk prediction modeling approach across multiple health care systems. JAMA Netw Open. 2020;3(3):e201262.
Barbe RP, Rubovszky G, Venturini-Andreoli A, Andreoli A. The treatment of borderline personality disorder patients with current suicidal behaviour. Clin Neuropsychiatr J Treat Eval. 2005;2(5):283–91.
Barber CW, Miller MJ. Reducing a suicidal person's access to lethal means of suicide: a research agenda. Am J Prev Med. 2014;47(3):S264–72.
Barlow DH, Bullis JR, Boettcher H, Sauer-Zavala S, Farchione TJ. What is an emotional disorder? A transdiagnostic mechanistic definition with implications for assessment, treatment, and prevention. Clin Psychol Sci Pract. 2019;26(2):20.
Başgöze Z, Demers L, Thai M, Falke CA, Mueller BA, Fiecas MB, Roediger DJ, Thomas KM, Klimes-Dougan B, Cullen KR. A multilevel examination of cognitive control in adolescents with nonsuicidal self-injury. Biol Psychiatr Global Open Sci. 2023;3(4):855–66.
Baud P. Personality traits as intermediary phenotypes in suicidal behavior: genetic issues. Am J Med Genet C: Semin Med Genet. 2005;133(1):34–42. Hoboken: Wiley Subscription Services, Inc., A Wiley Company
Baetens I, Claes L, Muehlenkamp J, Grietens H, Onghena P. Non-suicidal and suicidal self-injurious behaviour among Flemish adolescents: a web-survey. Arch Suicide Res. 2011;15(1):56–67.
Beauchaine TP, McNulty T. Comorbidities and continuities as ontogenic processes: toward a developmental spectrum model of externalizing psychopathology. Dev Psychopathol. 2013;25(4pt2):1505–28.
Beautrais AL. Further suicidal behavior among medically serious suicide attempters. Suicide Life Threat Behav. 2004;34(1):1.
Beautrais AL, Joyce PR, Mulder RT. Cannabis abuse and serious suicide attempts. Addiction. 1999;94(8):1155–64.
Beck AT, Brown GK, Steer RA, Dahlsgaard KK, Grisham JR. Suicide ideation at its worst point: a predictor of eventual suicide in psychiatric outpatients. Suicide Life Threat Behav. 1999;29(1):1–9.
Bekrater-Bodmann R, Chung BY, Foell J, Gescher DM, Bohus M, Flor H. Body plasticity in borderline personality disorder: a link to dissociation. Compr Psychiatry. 2016;69:36–44.
Bentley KH, Nock MK, Barlow DH. The four-function model of nonsuicidal self-injury: key directions for future research. Clin Psychol Sci. 2014;2(5):638–56.
Bentley KH, Cassiello-Robbins CF, Vittorio L, Sauer-Zavala S, Barlow DH. The association between nonsuicidal self-injury and the emotional disorders: a meta-analytic review. Clin Psychol Rev. 2015;37:72–88.
Bentley KH, Maimone JS, Kilbury EN, Tate MS, Wisniewski H, Levine MT, Roberg R, Torous JB, Nock MK, Kleiman EM. Practices for monitoring and responding to incoming data on self-injurious thoughts and behaviors in intensive longitudinal studies: a systematic review. Clin Psychol Rev. 2021;90:102098.
Bergen H, Hawton K, Waters K, Ness J, Cooper J, Steeg S, Kapur N. Premature death after self-harm: a multicentre cohort study. Lancet. 2012;380(9853):1568–74.
Berghoff CR, Dixon-Gordon KL, Chapman AL, Baer MM, Turner BJ, Tull MT, Gratz KL. Daily associations of interpersonal and emotional experiences following stressful events among young adults with and without nonsuicidal self-injury. J Clin Psychol. 2022;78(11):2329–40.
Bertolote JM, Fleischmann A. Suicide and psychiatric diagnosis: a worldwide perspective. World Psychiatry. 2002;1(3):181.

Bi B, Liu W, Zhou D, Fu X, Qin X, Wu J. Personality traits and suicide attempts with and without psychiatric disorders: analysis of impulsivity and neuroticism. BMC Psychiatry. 2017;17:1–9.

Bifulco A, Brown GW, Harris TO. Childhood Experience of Care and Abuse (CECA): a retrospective interview measure. J Child Psychol Psychiatry. 1994;35(8):1419–35.

Bijttebier S, Caeyenberghs K, Van den Ameele H, Achten E, Rujescu D, Titeca K, Van Heeringen C. The vulnerability to suicidal behavior is associated with reduced connectivity strength. Front Hum Neurosci. 2015;9:632.

Bijttebier P, Vertommen H. Coping strategies in relation to personality disorders. Personal Individ Differ. 1999;26(5):847–56.

Bjärehed J, Lundh LG. Deliberate self-harm in 14-year-old adolescents: how frequent is it, and how is it associated with psychopathology, relationship variables, and styles of emotional regulation? Cogn Behav Ther. 2008;37(1):26–37.

Bježančević M, Groznica Hržić I, Dodig-Ćurković K. Self-injury in adolescents: a five-year study of characteristics and trends. Psychiatr Danub. 2019;31(4):413–20.

Blasczyk-Schiep S, Kazen M, Jaworska-Andryszewska P, Kuhl J. Volitional determinants of self-harm behaviour and suicidal risk in persons with borderline personality disorder. Eur J Psychiatr. 2018;32(2):77–86.

Boggs JM, Beck A, Hubley S, Peterson EL, Hu Y, Williams LK, Prabhakar D, Rossom RC, Lynch FL, Lu CY, Waitzfelder BE. General medical, mental health, and demographic risk factors associated with suicide by firearm compared with other means. Psychiatr Serv. 2018;69(6):677–84.

Borges G, Bagge CL, Cherpitel CJ, Conner KR, Orozco R, Rossow I. A meta-analysis of acute use of alcohol and the risk of suicide attempt. Psychol Med. 2017;47(5):949–57.

Borne Radet, National Council for Children 2016.

Boyes ME, Wilmot A, Hasking PA. Nonsuicidal self-injury-related differences in the experience of negative and positive emotion. Suicide Life Threat Behav. 2020;50(2):437–48.

Bracken-Minor KL, McDevitt-Murphy ME. Differences in features of nonsuicidal self-injury according to borderline personality disorder screening status. Arch Suicide Res. 2014;18(1):88–103.

Brady KT, Carrà G, Bartoli F, Crocamo C, Clerici M. Attempted suicide in people with co-occurring bipolar and substance use disorders: systematic review and meta-analysis. J Affect Disord. 2014;167:125–35.

Bradley B, DeFife JA, Guarnaccia C, Phifer J, Fani N, Ressler KJ, Westen D. Emotion dysregulation and negative affect: association with psychiatric symptoms. J Clin Psychiatry. 2011;72(5):6427.

Bramness JG, Walby FA, Tverdal A. The sales of antidepressants and suicide rates in Norway and its counties 1980–2004. J Affect Disord. 2007;102(1–3):1–9.

Brausch AM, Gutierrez PM. Differences in nonsuicidal self-injury and suicide attempts in adolescents. J Youth Adolesc. 2010;39:233–42.

Brent D. Some promising news about psychosocial interventions for adolescent self-harm. BMJ Ment Health. 2015;18(3):93.

Bresin K. Five indices of emotion regulation in participants with a history of nonsuicidal self-injury: a daily diary study. Behav Ther. 2014;45(1):56–66.

Bresin K, Schoenleber M. Gender differences in the prevalence of nonsuicidal self-injury: a meta-analysis. Clin Psychol Rev. 2015;38:55–64.

Brezo J, Paris J, Turecki G. Personality traits as correlates of suicidal ideation, suicide attempts, and suicide completions: a systematic review. Acta Psychiatr Scand. 2006;113(3):180–206.

Brickman LJ, Ammerman BA, Look AE, Berman ME, McCloskey MS. The relationship between nonsuicidal self-injury and borderline personality disorder symptoms in a college sample. Borderline Personal Disord Emot Dysregul. 2014;1:1–8.

Brezo J, Paris J, Hébert M, Vitaro F, Tremblay R, Turecki G. Broad and narrow personality traits as markers of onetime and repeated suicide attempts: a population-based study. BMC Psychiatry. 2008a;8:1–1.

Brezo J, Paris J, Vitaro F, Hebert M, Tremblay RE, Turecki G. Predicting suicide attempts in young adults with histories of childhood abuse. Br J Psychiatry. 2008b;193(2):134–9.

Brown LA, Armey MA, Sejourne C, Miller IW, Weinstock LM. Trauma history is associated with prior suicide attempt history in hospitalized patients with major depressive disorder. Psychiatry Res. 2016;243:191–7.

Brown GK, Jager-Hyman S. Evidence-based psychotherapies for suicide prevention: future directions. Am J Prev Med. 2014;47(3):S186–94.

Brown RC, Plener PL. Nonsuicidal self-injury in adolescence. Curr Psychiatry Rep. 2017;19:1–8.

Brown MZ, Comtois KA, Linehan MM. Reasons for suicide attempts and nonsuicidal self-injury in women with borderline personality disorder. J Abnorm Psychol. 2002;111(1):198.

Brown MZ, Linehan MM, Comtois KA, Murray A, Chapman AL. Shame as a prospective predictor of self-inflicted injury in borderline personality disorder: a multi-modal analysis. Behav Res Ther. 2009;47(10):815–22.

Brown RC, Plener PL, Groen G, Neff D, Bonenberger M, Abler B. Differential neural processing of social exclusion and inclusion in adolescents with non-suicidal self-injury and young adults with borderline personality disorder. Front Psych. 2017;8:267.

Brown WC, Tragesser SL, Tomko RL, Mehl MR, Trull TJ. Recall of expressed affect during naturalistically observed interpersonal events in those with borderline personality disorder or depressive disorder. Assessment. 2014;21(1):73–81.

Brodsky BS, Stanley B. The dialectical behavior therapy primer: how DBT can inform clinical practice. Wiley; 2013.

Bruffaerts R, Demyttenaere K, Borges G, Haro JM, Chiu WT, Hwang I, Karam EG, Kessler RC, Sampson N, Alonso J, Andrade LH. Childhood adversities as risk factors for onset and persistence of suicidal behaviour. Br J Psychiatry. 2010;197(1):20–7.

Brunner R, Kaess M, Parzer P, Fischer G, Carli V, Hoven CW, Wasserman C, Sarchiapone M, Resch F, Apter A, Balazs J. Life-time prevalence and psychosocial correlates of adolescent direct self-injurious behavior: a comparative study of findings in 11 European countries. J Child Psychol Psychiatry. 2014;55(4):337–48.

Brunner G, Gajwani R, Gross J, Gumley AI, Krishnadas R, Lawrie SM, Schwannauer M, Schultze-Lutter F, Fracasso A, Uhlhaas PJ. Hippocampal structural alterations in early-stage psychosis: Specificity and relationship to clinical outcomes. NeuroImage Clin. 2022 1;35:103087.

Bryan CJ, Rudd MD. The importance of temporal dynamics in the transition from suicidal thought to behavior. Clin Psychol Sci Pract. 2016;23(1):21–5.

Buelens T, Luyckx K, Gandhi A, Kiekens G, Claes L. Non-suicidal self-injury in adolescence: longitudinal associations with psychological distress and rumination. J Abnorm Child Psychol. 2019;47:1569–81.

Buelens T, Luyckx K, Kiekens G, Gandhi A, Muehlenkamp JJ, Claes L. Investigating the DSM-5 criteria for nonsuicidal self-injury disorder in a community sample of adolescents. J Affect Disord. 2020a;260:314–22.

Buelens T, Luyckx K, Verschueren M, Schoevaerts K, Dierckx E, Depestele L, Claes L. Temperament and character traits of female eating disorder patients with (out) nonsuicidal self-injury. J Clin Med. 2020b;9(4):1207.

Bureau JF, Martin J, Freynet N, Poirier AA, Lafontaine MF, Cloutier P. Perceived dimensions of parenting and nonsuicidal self-injury in young adults. J Youth Adolesc. 2010;39:484–94.

Burke TA, Ammerman BA, Jacobucci R. The use of machine learning in the study of suicidal and nonsuicidal self-injurious thoughts and behaviors: a systematic review. J Affect Disord. 2019;245:869–84.

Burke TA, Allen KJ, Carpenter RW, Siegel DM, Kautz MM, Liu RT, Alloy LB. Emotional response inhibition to selfharm stimuli interacts with momentary negative affect to predict nonsuicidal self-injury urges. Behav Res Ther. 2021;142:103865.

Cackowski S, Krause-Utz A, Van Eijk J, Klohr K, Daffner S, Sobanski E, Ende G. Anger and aggression in borderline personality disorder and attention deficit hyperactivity disorder–does stress matter? Borderline Personal Disord Emot Dysregul. 2017;4:1–3.

Cackowski S, Reitz AC, Ende G, Kleindienst N, Bohus M, Schmahl C, Krause-Utz A. Impact of stress on different components of impulsivity in borderline personality disorder. Psychol Med. 2014;44(15):3329–40.

Caine ED. Forging an agenda for suicide prevention in the United States. Am J Public Health. 2013;103(5):822–9.
Caine ED. Building the foundation for comprehensive suicide prevention–based on intention and planning in a social–ecological context. Epidemiol Psychiatr Sci. 2020;29:e69.
Carli V, Hadlaczky G, Petros NG, Iosue M, Zeppegno P, Gramaglia C, Amore M, Baca-Garcia E, Batra A, Cosman D, Courtet P. A naturalistic, European multi-center clinical study of electrodermal reactivity and suicide risk among patients with depression. Front Psych. 2022;12:765128.
Carver CS, Johnson SL, Joormann J, Kim Y, Nam JY. Serotonin transporter polymorphism interacts with childhood adversity to predict aspects of impulsivity. Psychol Sci. 2011;22(5):589–95.
Cassels M, van Harmelen AL, Neufeld S, Goodyer I, Jones PB, Wilkinson P. Poor family functioning mediates the link between childhood adversity and adolescent nonsuicidal self-injury. J Child Psychol Psychiatry. 2018;59(8):881–7.
Castellví P, Lucas-Romero E, Miranda-Mendizábal A, Parés-Badell O, Almenara J, Alonso I, Blasco MJ, Cebrià A, Gabilondo A, Gili M, Lagares C. Longitudinal association between self-injurious thoughts and behaviors and suicidal behavior in adolescents and young adults: a systematic review with meta-analysis. J Affect Disord. 2017;215:37–48.
Cavanagh JT, Carson AJ, Sharpe M, Lawrie SM. Psychological autopsy studies of suicide: a systematic review. Psychol Med. 2003;33(3):395–405.
Caves Sivaraman J. The association between mental health/substance use disorders and suicide in the North Carolina Medicaid population, 2021.
Cawood CD, Huprich SK. Late adolescent nonsuicidal self-injury: the roles of coping style, self-esteem, and personality pathology. J Personal Disord. 2011;25(6):765–81.
Centers for Disease Control and Prevention (CDC) (2020, 2022).
Centers for Disease and Prevention (CDC). 2015, 2017.
Center for Disease Control and Prevention, 2017.
Center for Disease Control and prevention, National Center for Health Statistics 2021.
Cerutti R, Zuffianò A, Spensieri V. The role of difficulty in identifying and describing feelings in non-suicidal selfinjury behavior (NSSI): associations with perceived attachment quality, stressful life events, and suicidal ideation. Front Psychol. 2018;9:318.
Cha CB, Franz PJM, Guzmán E, Glenn CR, Kleiman EM, Nock MK. Annual research review: suicide among youth–epidemiology,(potential) etiology, and treatment. J Child Psychol Psychiatry. 2018;59(4):460–82.
Chanen AM, Kaess M. Developmental pathways to borderline personality disorder. Curr Psychiatry Rep. 2012;14(1):45–53.
Chanen AM, Thompson K. Preventive strategies for borderline personality disorder in adolescents. Curr Treat Options Psychiatry. 2014;1:358–68.
Chapman AL. Borderline personality disorder and emotion dysregulation. Dev Psychopathol. 2019;31(3):1143–56.
Chapman AL, Dixon-Gordon KL. Emotional antecedents and consequences of deliberate self-harm and suicide attempts. Suicide Life Threat Behav. 2007;37(5):543–52.
Chapman AL, Specht MW, Cellucci T. Borderline personality disorder and deliberate self-harm: does experiential avoidance play a role? Suicide Life Threat Behav. 2005;35(4):388–99.
Chapman AL, Gratz KL, Brown MZ. Solving the puzzle of deliberate self-harm: the experiential avoidance model. Behav Res Ther. 2006;44(3):371–94.
Chapman AL, Rosenthal MZ, Dixon-Gordon KL, Turner BJ, Kuppens P. Borderline personality disorder and the effects of instructed emotional avoidance or acceptance in daily life. J Personal Disord. 2017;31(4):483–502.
Chapman-Hilliard C, Pelham T, Mollo V, Henry P, Miller B, Yankura J, Denton EG. Clinical utility of depression measures and symptoms: implications for suicide risk assessment in high risk, resource limited youth populations. Suicide Life Threat Behav. 2024;
Chawla N, Ostafin B. Experiential avoidance as a functional dimensional approach to psychopathology: an empirical review. J Clin Psychol. 2007;63(9):871–90.
Cheavens JS, Rosenthal MZ, Daughters SB, Nowak J, Kosson D, Lynch TR, Lejuez CW. An analogue investigation of the relationships among perceived parental criticism, negative affect,

and borderline personality disorder features: the role of thought suppression. Behav Res Ther. 2005;43(2):257–68.

Chen Y, Hu R, Xu X, Hong B, Zhang J, Jia P, Zhao L. The effect of mental health status and family function on nonsuicidal self-injury: a longitudinal analysis of Chinese children and adolescents. Psychol Res Behav Manag. 2023;Volume 16:4491–500.

Chesney E, Rogers JP, Oliver D, Begum N, Saini A, Wang S, McGuire P, Fusar-Poli P, Lewis G, David AS. Suicide, self-harm and thoughts of suicide or self-harm in infectious disease epidemics: a systematic review and meta-analysis. Epidemiol Psychiatr Sci. 2021;30:e32.

Chesin MS, Jeglic EL, Stanley B. Pathways to high-lethality suicide attempts in individuals with borderline personality disorder. Arch Suicide Res. 2010;14(4):342–62.

Chioqueta AP, Stiles TC. Personality traits and the development of depression, hopelessness, and suicide ideation. Personal Individ Differ. 2005;38(6):1283–91.

Chung SS, Joung KH. Risk factors related to suicidal ideation and attempted suicide: comparative study of Korean and American youth. J Sch Nurs. 2012;28(6):448–58.

Cipriano A, Cella S, Cotrufo P. Nonsuicidal self-injury: a systematic review. Front Psychol. 2017;8:1946.

Claes L, Muehlenkamp J. The relationship between the UPPS-P impulsivity dimensions and nonsuicidal self-injury characteristics in male and female high-school students. Psychiatry J. 2013;2013(1):654847.

Claes L, Houben A, Vandereycken W, Bijttebier P, Muehlenkamp J. Brief report: the association between nonsuicidal self-injury, self-concept and acquaintance with self-injurious peers in a sample of adolescents. J Adolesc. 2010;33(5):775–8.

Claes L, Luyckx K, Bijttebier P. Nonsuicidal self-injury in adolescents: prevalence and associations with identity formation above and beyond depression. Personal Individ Differ. 2014;61:101–4.

Cloninger CR. Temperament and personality. Curr Opin Neurobiol. 1994;4(2):266–73.

Cloninger CR. The psychobiological theory of temperament and character: comment on Farmer and Goldberg, vol. 20; 2008. p. 292.

Cloninger CR, Bayon C, Svrakic DM. Measurement of temperament and character in mood disorders: a model of fundamental states as personality types. J Affect Disord. 1998;51(1):21–32.

Cloutier P, Martin J, Kennedy A, Nixon MK, Muehlenkamp JJ. Characteristics and co-occurrence of adolescent nonsuicidal self-injury and suicidal behaviours in pediatric emergency crisis services. J Youth Adolesc. 2010;39:259–69.

Colle L, Hilviu D, Rossi R, Garbarini F, Fossataro C. Self-harming and sense of agency in patients with borderline personality disorder. Front Psych. 2020;11:449.

Conner A, Azrael D, Miller M. Suicide case-fatality rates in the United States, 2007 to 2014: a nationwide population-based study. Ann Intern Med. 2019;171(12):885–95.

Costa PT, McCrae RR. Normal personality assessment in clinical practice: the NEO personality inventory. Psychol Assess. 1992;4(1):5.

Costa-Maia I, Marina S, Ricou M. Wish to die: suicide and its link to euthanasia. OMEGA-J Death Dy. 2021;83(4):927–43.

Costa RP, Peixoto AL, Lucas CC, Falcão DN, Farias JT, Viana LF, Pereira MA, Sandes ML, Lopes TB, Mousinho KC, Trindade-Filho EM. Profile of nonsuicidal self-injury in adolescents: interface with impulsiveness and loneliness. J Pediatr. 2021;97(2):184–90.

Cox GR, Robinson J, Williamson M, Lockley A, Cheung YT, Pirkis J. Suicide clusters in young people. Crisis. 2012;33:208.

Crosby A, Gfroerer J, Han B, Ortega L, Parks SE. Suicidal thoughts and behaviors among adults aged>_18 years—United States, 2008–2009. Atlanta: US Department of Health and Human Services, Centers for Disease Control and Prevention; 2011.

Crowe M. Never good enough–part 1: shame or borderline personality disorder? J Psychiatr Ment Health Nurs. 2004;11(3):327–34.

Crowell SE, Beauchaine TP, McCauley EL, Smith CJ, Stevens AL, Sylvers P. Psychological, autonomic, and serotonergic correlates of parasuicide among adolescent girls. Dev Psychopathol. 2005;17(4):1105–27.

Crowell SE, Beauchaine TP, Hsiao RC, Vasilev CA, Yaptangco M, Linehan MM, McCauley E. Differentiating adolescent self-injury from adolescent depression: possible implications for borderline personality development. J Abnorm Child Psychol. 2012;40:45–57.

Crowell SE, Beauchaine TP, McCauley E, Smith CJ, Vasilev CA, Stevens AL. Parent-child interactions, peripheral serotonin, and self-inflicted injury in adolescents. J Consult Clin Psychol. 2008;76(1):15.

Crowell SE, Beauchaine TP, Linehan MM. A biosocial developmental model of borderline personality: elaborating and extending Linehan's theory. Psychol Bull. 2009;135(3):495.

Crowell SE, Kaufman EA. Borderline personality disorder and the emerging field of developmental neuroscience. Personal Disord Theory Res Treat. 2016;7(4):324.

Crowell SE, Kaufman EA. Development of self-inflicted injury: comorbidities and continuities with borderline and antisocial personality traits. Dev Psychopathol. 2016;28(4pt1):1071–88.

Crowell SE, Derbidge CM, Beauchaine TP. 10 developmental approaches to understanding suicidal and self-injurious behaviors. In: The Oxford handbook of suicide and self-injury; 2014. p. 183.

Csorba J, Dinya E, Plener P, Nagy E, Páli E. Clinical diagnoses, characteristics of risk behaviour, differences between suicidal and nonsuicidal subgroups of Hungarian adolescent outpatients practising self-injury. Eur Child Adolesc Psychiatry. 2009;18:309–20.

Cucchi A, Ryan D, Konstantakopoulos G, Stroumpa S, Kaçar AŞ, Renshaw S, Landau S, Kravariti E. Lifetime prevalence of nonsuicidal self-injury in patients with eating disorders: a systematic review and meta-analysis. Psychol Med. 2016;46(7):1345–58.

Cyders MA, Smith GT. Longitudinal validation of the urgency traits over the first year of college. J Pers Assess. 2010;92(1):63–9.

Cyders MA, Smith GT, Spillane NS, Fischer S, Annus AM, Peterson C. Integration of impulsivity and positive mood to predict risky behavior: development and validation of a measure of positive urgency. Psychol Assess. 2007;19(1):107.

Cyders MA. Impulsivity and the sexes: measurement and structural invariance of the UPPS-P Impulsive Behavior Scale. Assessment. 2013;20(1):86–97.

Cyders MA, Smith GT. Clarifying the role of personality dispositions in risk for increased gambling behavior. Personal Individ Differ. 2008;45(6):503–8.

Daukantaitė D, Lantto R, Liljedahl SI, Helleman M, Westling S. One-year consistency in lifetime frequency estimates and functions of nonsuicidal self-injury in a clinical sample. Front Psych. 2020;11:538.

Davis LT, Weiss NH, Tull MT, Gratz KL. The relation of protective factors to deliberate self-harm among African-American adults: moderating roles of gender and sexual orientation identity. J Ment Health. 2017;26(4):351–8.

De Crescenzo F, Serra G, Maisto F, Uchida M, Woodworth H, Casini MP, Baldessarini RJ, Vicari S. Suicide attempts in juvenile bipolar versus major depressive disorders: systematic review and meta-analysis. J Am Acad Child Adolesc Psychiatry. 2017;56(10):825–31.

de Leo D, Giannotti AV. A contemporary view of suicide. In: Oxford textbook of social psychiatry; 2022. p. 447.

Dell'Osso L, Massimetti G, Conversano C, Bertelloni CA, Carta MG, Ricca V, Carmassi C. Alterations in circadian/seasonal rhythms and vegetative functions are related to suicidality in DSM-5 PTSD. BMC Psychiatry. 2014;14:1–8.

Deng W, Yan S, Xu Y, Lu Z, Liu L, Zhou Y, Chen M. Effects of BPD tendencies and subjective well-being on NSSI in adolescents with PTSD. Front Psych. 2023;14:1152352.

Dillahunt AK, Feldman DA, Thomas LR, Farstead BW, Frandsen SB, Lee S, Pazdera M, Galloway J, Bessette KL, Roberts H, Crowell SE. Self-injury in adolescence is associated with greater behavioral risk avoidance, not risk-taking. J Clin Med. 2022;11(5):1288.

Distel MA, Rebollo-Mesa I, Willemsen G, Derom CA, Trull TJ, Martin NG, Boomsma DI. Familial resemblance of borderline personality disorder features: genetic or cultural transmission? PLoS One. 2009;4(4):e5334.

Doran CM, Kinchin I. Economic and epidemiological impact of youth suicide in countries with the highest human development index. PLoS One. 2020;15(5):e0232940.

Dougherty DM, Mathias CW, Marsh-Richard DM, Prevette KN, Dawes MA, Hatzis ES, Palmes G, Nouvion SO. Impulsivity and clinical symptoms among adolescents with nonsuicidal self-injury with or without attempted suicide. Psychiatry Res. 2009;169(1):22–7.
Dombrovski AY, Hallquist MN. Search for solutions, learning, simulation, and choice processes in suicidal behavior. Wiley Interdiscip Rev Cogn Sci. 2021;13(1):e1561.
Drapeau CW, Lockman JD, Moore MM, Cerel J. Predictors of posttraumatic growth in adults bereaved by suicide. Crisis. 2018;40:196.
Du L, Merali Z, Poulter MO, Palkovits M, Faludi G, Anisman H. Catechol-O-methyltransferase Val158Met polymorphism and altered COMT gene expression in the prefrontal cortex of suicide brains. Prog Neuro-Psychopharmacol Biol Psychiatry. 2014;50:178–83.
Duberstein PR, Conwell Y, Conner KR, Eberly S, Caine ED. Suicide at 50 years of age and older: perceived physical illness, family discord and financial strain. Psychol Med. 2003;34(1):137–46.
Duberstein PR, Conwell Y, Seidlitz L, Denning DG, Dox C, Caine ED. Personality traits and suicidal behavior and ideation in depressed inpatients 50 years of age and older. J Gerontol Ser B Psychol Sci Soc Sci. 2000;55(1):P18.
Duberstein PR, Conwell Y, Caine ED. Age differences in the personality characteristics of suicide completers: preliminary findings from a psychological autopsy study. Psychiatry. 1994;57(3):213–24.
Durkheim E. Study of sociology. Paris: Alcan; 1897.
Edmondson AJ, Brennan CA, House AO. Nonsuicidal reasons for self-harm: a systematic review of self-reported accounts. J Affect Disord. 2016;191:109–17.
Emelianchik-Key K, La Guardia A. Nonsuicidal self-injury throughout the lifespan. Routledge; 2019.
Eskin M, Sun JM, Abuidhail J, Yoshimasu K, Kujan O, Janghorbani M, Flood C, Carta MG, Tran US, Mechri A, Hamdan M. Suicidal behavior and psychological distress in university students: a 12-nation study. Arch Suicide Res. 2016;20(3):369–88.
Eysenck HJ. Personality and experimental psychology: the unification of psychology and the possibility of a paradigm. J Pers Soc Psychol. 1997;73(6):1224.
Farmer RF, Chapman AL. Exposure-based interventions, 2016.
Farmer A, Mahmood A, Redman K, Harris T, Sadler S, McGuffin P. A sib-pair study of the temperament and character inventory scales in major depression. Arch Gen Psychiatry. 2003;60(5):490–6.
Faura-Garcia J, Orue I, Calvete E. Clinical assessment of non-suicidal self-injury: a systematic review of instruments. Clin Psychol Psychother. 2021;28(4):739–65.
Favazza AR. A cultural understanding of nonsuicidal self-injury, 2009.
Fergusson DM, Woodward LJ, Horwood LJ. Risk factors and life processes associated with the onset of suicidal behaviour during adolescence and early adulthood. Psychol Med. 2000;30(1):23–39.
Fergusson DM, Beautrais AL, Horwood LJ. Vulnerability and resiliency to suicidal behaviours in young people. Psychol Med. 2003;33(1):61–73.
Ferrara M, Terrinoni A, Williams R. Nonsuicidal self-injury (Nssi) in adolescent inpatients: assessing personality features and attitude toward death. Child Adolesc Psychiatry Ment Health. 2012;6:1–8.
Fincham JM, Carter CS, van Veen V, Stenger VA, Anderson JR. Neural mechanisms of planning: a computational analysis using event-related fMRI. Proc Natl Acad Sci. 2002;99(5):3346–51.
Fliege H, Lee JR, Grimm A, Klapp BF. Risk factors and correlates of deliberate self-harm behavior: a systematic review. J Psychosom Res. 2009;66(6):477–93.
Forrester RL, Slater H, Jomar K, Mitzman S, Taylor PJ. Self-esteem and nonsuicidal self-injury in adulthood: a systematic review. J Affect Disord. 2017;221:172–83.
Fox E, Krawczyk K, Staniford J, Dickens GL. A service evaluation of a 1-year dialectical behaviour therapy programme for women with borderline personality disorder in a low secure unit. Behav Cogn Psychother. 2015;43(6):676–91.
Fox KR, Huang X, Guzmán EM, Funsch KM, Cha CB, Ribeiro JD, Franklin JC. Interventions for suicide and self-injury: a meta-analysis of randomized controlled trials across nearly 50 years of research. Psychol Bull. 2020;146(12):1117.

Franklin JC, Lee KM, Puzia ME, Prinstein MJ. Recent and frequent nonsuicidal self-injury is associated with diminished implicit and explicit aversion toward self-cutting stimuli. Clin Psychol Sci. 2014;2(3):306–18.

Franklin JC, Ribeiro JD, Fox KR, Bentley KH, Kleiman EM, Huang X, Musacchio KM, Jaroszewski AC, Chang BP, Nock MK. Risk factors for suicidal thoughts and behaviors: a meta-analysis of 50 years of research. Psychol Bull. 2017;143(2):187.

Gardener AD, Hick EJ, Jacklin C, Tan G, Cashin AG, Lee H, Nunan D, Toomey EC, Richards GC. Open science and conflict of interest policies of medical and health sciences journals before and during the COVID-19 pandemic: a repeat cross-sectional study: open science policies of medical journals. JRSM Open. 2022;13(11):20542704221132139.

Gardner KJ, Paul E, Selby EA, Klonsky ED, Mars B. Intrapersonal and interpersonal functions as pathways to future self-harm repetition and suicide attempts. Front Psychol. 2021a;12:688472.

Gardner KJ, Klonsky ED, Selby EA. Advancing theory of suicide and nonsuicidal self-injury. Front Psychol. 2021b;12:780029.

Garisch JA, Wilson MS. Prevalence, correlates, and prospective predictors of nonsuicidal self-injury among New Zealand adolescents: cross-sectional and longitudinal survey data. Child Adolesc Psychiatry Ment Health. 2015;9:1–1.

Gatta M, Dal Santo F, Rago A, Spoto A, Battistella PA. Alexithymia, impulsiveness, and psychopathology in nonsuicidal self-injured adolescents. Neuropsychiatr Dis Treat. 2016;Volume 12:2307–17.

Geissbühler S. The rape of Jewish women and girls during the first phase of the Romanian offensive in the East, July 1941: a research agenda and preliminary findings. Holocaust Stud. 2013;19(1):59–80.

Gelinas BL, Wright KD. The cessation of deliberate self-harm in a university sample: the reasons, barriers, and strategies involved. Arch Suicide Res. 2013;17(4):373–86.

Germain SA, Hooley JM. Direct and indirect forms of nonsuicidal self-injury: evidence for a distinction. Psychiatry Res. 2012;197(1–2):78–84.

Germain SA, Hooley JM. Aberrant pain perception in direct and indirect nonsuicidal self-injury: an empirical test of Joiner's interpersonal theory. Compr Psychiatry. 2013;54(6):694–701.

Geulayov G, Casey D, Bale L, Brand F, Clements C, Farooq B, Kapur N, Ness J, Waters K, Tsiachristas A, Hawton K. Suicide following presentation to hospital for non-fatal self-harm in the Multicentre Study of Self-harm: a long-term follow-up study. Lancet Psychiatry. 2019;6(12):1021–30.

Gibb BE, Andover MS, Beach SR. Suicidal ideation and attitudes toward suicide. Suicide Life Threat Behav. 2006;36(1):12–8.

Giletta M, Scholte RH, Engels RC, Ciairano S, Prinstein MJ. Adolescent nonsuicidal self-injury: a cross-national study of community samples from Italy, The Netherlands and the United States. Psychiatry Res. 2012;197(1–2):66–72.

Giletta M, Burk WJ, Scholte RH, Engels RC, Prinstein MJ. Direct and indirect peer socialization of adolescent nonsuicidal self-injury. J Res Adolesc. 2013;23(3):450–63.

Gillies D, Christou MA, Dixon AC, Featherston OJ, Rapti I, Garcia-Anguita A, Villasis-Keever M, Reebye P, Christou E, Al Kabir N, Christou PA. Prevalence and characteristics of self-harm in adolescents: meta-analyses of community-based studies 1990–2015. J Am Acad Child Adolesc Psychiatry. 2018;57(10):733–41.

Giner L, Blasco-Fontecilla H, Perez-Rodriguez MM, Garcia-Nieto R, Giner J, Guija JA, Rico A, Barrero E, Luna MA, De Leon J, Oquendo MA. Personality disorders and health problems distinguish suicide attempters from completers in a direct comparison. J Affect Disord. 2013;151(2):474–83.

Glenn CR, Klonsky ED. A multimethod analysis of impulsivity in nonsuicidal self-injury. Personal Disord Theory Res Treat. 2010;1(1):67.

Glenn CR, Klonsky ED. Nonsuicidal self-injury disorder: an empirical investigation in adolescent psychiatric patients. J Clin Child Adolesc Psychol. 2013a;42(4):496–507.

Glenn CR, Klonsky ED. Social context during non-suicidal self-injury indicates suicide risk. Personal Individ Differ. 2009;46(1):25–9.

Glenn CR, Klonsky ED. Prospective prediction of nonsuicidal self-injury: a 1-year longitudinal study in young adults. Behav Ther. 2011;42(4):751–62.
Glenn CR, Klonsky ED. One-year test-retest reliability of the Inventory of Statements about Self-Injury (ISAS). Assessment. 2011;18(3):375–8.
Glenn CR, Klonsky ED. Nonsuicidal self-injury disorder: an empirical investigation in adolescent psychiatric patients. J Clin Child Adolesc Psychol. 2013;42(4):496–507.
Glenn CR, Klonsky ED. Reliability and validity of borderline personality disorder in hospitalized adolescents. J Can Acad Child Adolesc Psychiatry. 2013b;22(3):206.
Goddard A, Hasking P, Claes L, McEvoy P. Big five personality clusters in relation to nonsuicidal self-injury. Arch Suicide Res. 2021;25(3):390–405.
Gold LH. Suicide and firearms. In: The American Psychiatric Association publishing textbook of suicide risk assessment and management, vol. 8; 2020. p. 379.
Gold LH, Frierson RL, editors. The American Psychiatric Association publishing textbook of suicide risk assessment and management. American Psychiatric Pub; 2020.
Gollust SE, Eisenberg D, Golberstein E. Prevalence and correlates of self-injury among university students. J Am Coll Heal. 2008;56(5):491–8.
Gould MS, Marrocco FA, Kleinman M, Thomas JG, Mostkoff K, Cote J, Davies M. Evaluating iatrogenic risk of youth suicide screening programs: a randomized controlled trial. JAMA. 2005;293(13):1635–43.
Gómez SN, Frías Á, Palma C. Clinical differences and associations between women with borderline personality and their partners: an exploratory study. Cited in: EMBASE-Excerpta Medica Database• Index Copernicus• PsycINFO• SCOPUS• Google Scholar• Emerging Sources Citation Index (ESCI), a new edition of Web of Science, 2020. p. 264.
Gómez JM. High betrayal adolescent sexual abuse and nonsuicidal self-injury: the role of depersonalization in emerging adults. J Child Sex Abus. 2019;28(3):318–32.
Grandclerc S, De Labrouhe D, Spodenkiewicz M, Lachal J, Moro MR. Relations between nonsuicidal self-injury and suicidal behavior in adolescence: a systematic review. PLoS One. 2016;11(4):e0153760.
Gratz KL, Roemer L. Multidimensional assessment of emotion regulation and dysregulation: development, factor structure, and initial validation of the difficulties in emotion regulation scale. J Psychopathol Behav Assess. 2004;26:41–54.
Gratz KL, Conrad SD, Roemer L. Risk factors for deliberate self-harm among college students. Am J Orthopsychiatry. 2002;72(1):128–40.
Gratz KL. Risk factors for deliberate self-harm among female college students: the role and interaction of childhood maltreatment, emotional inexpressivity, and affect intensity/reactivity. Am J Orthopsychiatry. 2006;76(2):238–50.
Gratz KL. Risk factors for and functions of deliberate self-harm: an empirical and conceptual review. Clin Psychol Sci Pract. 2003;10(2):192.
Gratz KL. Targeting emotion dysregulation in the treatment of self-injury. J Clin Psychol. 2007;63(11):1091–103.
Gratz KL, Gunderson JG. Preliminary data on an acceptance-based emotion regulation group intervention for deliberate self-harm among women with borderline personality disorder. Behav Ther. 2006;37(1):25–35.
Gratz KL, Roemer L. The relationship between emotion dysregulation and deliberate self-harm among female undergraduate students at an urban commuter university. Cogn Behav Ther. 2008;37(1):14–25.
Gratz KL, Tull MT. The relationship between emotion dysregulation and deliberate self-harm among inpatients with substance use disorders. Cogn Ther Res. 2010;34:544–53.
Gratz KL, Dixon-Gordon KL, Tull MT. Predictors of treatment response to an adjunctive emotion regulation group therapy for deliberate self-harm among women with borderline personality disorder. Personal Disord Theory Res Treat. 2014;5(1):97.
Gratz KL, Latzman RD, Young J, Heiden LJ, Damon J, Hight T, Tull MT. Deliberate self-harm among underserved adolescents: the moderating roles of gender, race, and school-level and association with borderline personality features. Pers Disord Theory Res Treat 2012;3(1),39–54. https://doi.org/10.1037/a0022107

Gratz KL, Dixon-Gordon KL, Chapman AL, Tull MT. Diagnosis and characterization of DSM-5 nonsuicidal self-injury disorder using the clinician-administered nonsuicidal self-injury disorder index. Assessment. 2015;22(5):527–39.

Gratz KL, Kiel EJ, Mann AJ, Tull MT. The prospective relation between borderline personality disorder symptoms and suicide risk: the mediating roles of emotion regulation difficulties and perceived burdensomeness. J Affect Disord. 2022;313:186–95.

Gratz KL, Richmond JR, Dixon-Gordon KL, Chapman AL, Tull MT. Multimodal assessment of emotional reactivity and regulation in response to social rejection among self-harming adults with and without borderline personality disorder. Personal Disord Theory Res Treat. 2019a;10(5):395.

Gratz KL, Bjureberg J, Sahlin H, Tull MT. Emotion regulation group therapy for nonsuicidal self-injury. In: Nonsuicidal self-injury; 2019b. p. 148–63.

Gratz KL, Spitzen TL, Tull MT. Expanding our understanding of the relationship between nonsuicidal self-injury and suicide attempts: the roles of emotion regulation self-efficacy and the acquired capability for suicide. J Clin Psychol. 2020a;76(9):1653–67.

Gratz KL, Forbes CN, Wheeless LE, Richmond JR, Tull MT. Self-report assessment of emotion dysregulation. In: The Oxford handbook of emotion dysregulation; 2020b. p. 395–409.

Groschwitz RC, Plener PL, Kaess M, Schumacher T, Stoehr R, Boege I. The situation of former adolescent self-injurers as young adults: a follow-up study. BMC Psychiatry. 2015;15:1–9.

Gross JJ. Emotion regulation: current status and future prospects. Psychol Inq. 2015;26(1):1–26.

Gross JJ. The emerging field of emotion regulation: an integrative review. Rev Gen Psychol. 1998;2(3):271–99.

Gross JJ. Emotion and emotion regulation: personality processes and individual differences, 2008.

Gross JJ. Emotion regulation: conceptual and empirical foundations. In: Handbook of emotion regulation, vol. 2; 2014. p. 3–20.

Grosby S. Nationalism and social theory. In: Routledge international handbook of contemporary social and political theory; 2011. p. 280.

Guan K, Fox KR, Prinstein MJ. Nonsuicidal self-injury as a time-invariant predictor of adolescent suicide ideation and attempts in a diverse community sample. J Consult Clin Psychol. 2012;80(5):842.

Guertin T, Lloyd-Richardson E, Spirito A, Donaldson D, Boergers J. Self-mutilative behavior in adolescents who attempt suicide by overdose. J Am Acad Child Adolesc Psychiatry. 2001;40(9):1062–9.

Gujral S, Dombrovski AY, Butters M, Clark L, Reynolds CF III, Szanto K. Impaired executive function in contemplated and attempted suicide in late life. Am J Geriatr Psychiatry. 2014;22(8):811–9.

Gunderson JG, Stout RL, McGlashan TH, Shea MT, Morey LC, Grilo CM, Zanarini MC, Yen S, Markowitz JC, Sanislow C, Ansell E. Ten-year course of borderline personality disorder: psychopathology and function from the Collaborative Longitudinal Personality Disorders study. Arch Gen Psychiatry. 2011;68(8):827–37.

Gunderson JG. Borderline personality disorder: a clinical guide. American Psychiatric Pub; 2009.

Gunderson JG, Ridolfi ME. Borderline personality disorder: suicidality and self-mutilation. Ann N Y Acad Sci. 2001;932(1):61–77.

Gunderson JG. A BPD BRIEF. NEABPD (National Education Alliance Borderline Personality Disorder), 2011.

Gunnell D, Miller M. Strategies to prevent suicide. BMJ. 2010;6:341.

Guvendeger Doksat N, Zahmacioglu O, Ciftci Demirci A, Kocaman GM, Erdogan A. Association of suicide attempts and nonsuicidal self-injury behaviors with substance use and family characteristics among children and adolescents seeking treatment for substance use disorder. Subst Use Misuse. 2017;52(5):604–13.

Gyori D, Balazs J. Nonsuicidal self-injury and perfectionism: a systematic review. Front Psych. 2021;12:691147.

Ha C, Balderas JC, Zanarini MC, Oldham J, Sharp C. Psychiatric comorbidity in hospitalized adolescents with borderline personality disorder. J Clin Psychiatry. 2014;75(5):15864.

Hankin BL, Abela JR. Nonsuicidal self-injury in adolescence: prospective rates and risk factors in a 2 ½ year longitudinal study. Psychiatry Res. 2011;186(1):65–70.
Hamza CA, Stewart SL, Willoughby T. Examining the link between nonsuicidal self-injury and suicidal behavior: a review of the literature and an integrated model. Clin Psychol Rev. 2012;32(6):482–95.
Hamza CA, Willoughby T. Nonsuicidal self-injury and suicidal risk among emerging adults. J Adolesc Health. 2016;59(4):411–5.
Hawton K, Harriss L. Deliberate self-harm by under-15-year-olds: characteristics, trends and outcome. J Child Psychol Psychiatry. 2008;49(4):441–8.
Hawton K, Kingsbury S, Steinhardt K, James A, Fagg J. Repetition of deliberate self-harm by adolescents: the role of psychological factors. J Adolesc. 1999;22(3):369–78.
Hawton K, Rodham K, Evans E, Weatherall R. Deliberate self harm in adolescents: self report survey in schools in England. BMJ. 2002;325(7374):1207–11.
Haggard P. Sense of agency in the human brain. Nat Rev Neurosci. 2017;18(4):196–207.
Hamza CA, Willoughby T. Nonsuicidal self-injury and suicidal behavior: a latent class analysis among young adults. PLoS One. 2013;8(3):e59955.
Hamza CA, Willoughby T, Heffer T. Impulsivity and nonsuicidal self-injury: a review and meta-analysis. Clin Psychol Rev. 2015;38:13–24.
Hamza CA, Goldstein AL, Heath NL, Ewing L. Stressful experiences in university predict nonsuicidal self-injury through emotional reactivity. Front Psychol. 2021;12:610670.
Harris EC, Barraclough B. Suicide as an outcome for mental disorders. A meta-analysis. Br J Psychiatry. 1997;170(3):205–28.
Hasking PA, Coric SJ, Swannell S, Martin G, Thompson HK, Frost AD. Brief report: emotion regulation and coping as moderators in the relationship between personality and self-injury. J Adolesc. 2010;33(5):767–73.
Hasking P, Boyes ME, Finlay-Jones A, McEvoy PM, Rees CS. Common pathways to NSSI and suicide ideation: the roles of rumination and self-compassion. Arch Suicide Res. 2019;23(2):247–60.
Hasking P. Differentiating non-suicidal self-injury and risky drinking: a role for outcome expectancies and selfefficacy beliefs. Prev Sci. 2017;18(6):694–703.
Hauber K, Boon A, Vermeiren R. Nonsuicidal self-injury in clinical practice. Front Psychol. 2019;10:502.
Hawton K, Harriss L, Hall S, Simkin S, Bale E, Bond A. Deliberate self-harm in Oxford, 1990–2000: a time of change in patient characteristics. Psychol Med. 2003a;33(6):987–95.
Hawton K, Zahl D, Weatherall R. Suicide following deliberate self-harm: long-term follow-up of patients who presented to a general hospital. Br J Psychiatry. 2003b;182(6):537–42.
Hawton K, Bergen H, Kapur N, Cooper J, Steeg S, Ness J, Waters K. Repetition of self-harm and suicide following self-harm in children and adolescents: findings from the Multicentre Study of Self-harm in England. J Child Psychol Psychiatry. 2012;53(12):1212–9.
Hayes SC, Wilson KG, Gifford EV, Follette VM, Strosahl K. Experiential avoidance and behavioral disorders: a functional dimensional approach to diagnosis and treatment. J Consult Clin Psychol. 1996;64(6):1152.
Haywood SB, Hasking P, Boyes ME. We have so much in common: does shared variance between emotion-related constructs account for relationships with self-injury? J Affect Disord Rep. 2022;8:100332.
Haywood SB, Hasking P, Boyes ME. Untangling the link between experiential avoidance and nonsuicidal self-injury: a multidimensional approach. Aust J Psychol. 2024;76(1):2315951.
Heath NL, Ross S, Toste JR, Charlebois A, Nedecheva T. Retrospective analysis of social factors and nonsuicidal self-injury among young adults. Canad J Behav Sci/Revue canadienne des sciences du comportement. 2009;41(3):180.
Hefti F. Pathogenesis and biomechanics of adolescent idiopathic scoliosis (AIS). J Child Orthop. 2013;7(1):17–24.
Hessels CJ, van den Berg T, Lucassen SA, Laceulle OM, van Aken MA. Borderline personality disorder in young people: associations with support and negative interactions in relationships with mothers and a best friend. Borderline Personal Disord Emot Dysregula. 2022;9:1–1.

Hessels CJ, Laceulle OM, van Aken MA, Resch F, Kaess M. Differentiating BPD in adolescents with NSSI disorder: the role of adverse childhood experiences and current social relationships. Borderline Personal Disord Emot Dysregul. 2018;5:1–1.

Hennings JM. Function and psychotherapy of chronic suicidality in borderline personality disorder: using the reinforcement model of suicidality. Front Psych. 2020;11:199.

Huang X, Ribeiro JD. The differences between individuals engaging in nonsuicidal self-injury and suicide attempt are complex (vs. complicated or simple). Front Psych. 2020;11:239.

Hill NT, Robinson J, Pirkis J, Andriessen K, Krysinska K, Payne A, Boland A, Clarke A, Milner A, Witt K, Krohn S. Association of suicidal behavior with exposure to suicide and suicide attempt: a systematic review and multilevel meta-analysis. PLoS Med. 2020;17(3):e1003074.

Hilt LM, Tuschner RF, Salentine C, Torcasso G, Nelson KR. Development and initial psychometrics of a schoolbased screening program to prevent adolescent suicide. Pract Innov. 2018;3(1):1.

Hjelmeland H, Hawton K, Nordvik H, Bille-Brahe U, Leo DD, Fekete S, Grad O, Haring C, Kerkhof AJ, Lönnqvist J, Michel K. Why people engage in parasuicide: a cross-cultural study of intentions. Suicide Life Threat Behav. 2002;32(4):380–93.

Hoff ER, Muehlenkamp JJ. Nonsuicidal self-injury in college students: the role of perfectionism and rumination. Suicide Life Threat Behav. 2009;39(6):576–87.

Holma KM, Haukka J, Suominen K, Valtonen HM, Mantere O, Melartin TK, Sokero TP, Oquendo MA, Isometsä ET. Differences in incidence of suicide attempts between bipolar I and II disorders and major depressive disorder. Bipolar Disord. 2014;16(6):652–61.

Homan KJ, Sim LA, Fargo JD, Twohig MP. Five-year prospective investigation of self-harm/suicide-related behaviors in the development of borderline personality disorder. Personal Disord Theory Res Treat. 2017;8(2):183.

Hooley JM, Franklin JC. Why do people hurt themselves? A new conceptual model of nonsuicidal self-injury. Clin Psychol Sci. 2018;6(3):428–51.

Hooley JM, Fox KR, Boccagno C. Nonsuicidal self-injury: diagnostic challenges and current perspectives. Neuropsychiatr Dis Treat. 2020a;10:101–12.

Hooley JM, Dahlgren MK, Best SG, Gonenc A, Gruber SA. Decreased amygdalar activation to NSSI-stimuli in people who engage in NSSI: a neuroimaging pilot study. Front Psych. 2020b;11:238.

Horgan M, Martin G. Differences between current and past self-injurers: how and why do people stop? Arch Suicide Res. 2016;20(2):142–52.

Houben M, Claes L, Vansteelandt K, Berens A, Sleuwaegen E, Kuppens P. The emotion regulation function of nonsuicidal self-injury: a momentary assessment study in inpatients with borderline personality disorder features. J Abnorm Psychol. 2017;126(1):89.

Howard J, De Jesus-Romero R, Peipert A, Riley T, Rutter LA, Lorenzo-Luaces L. The significance of anxiety symptoms in predicting psychosocial functioning across borderline personality traits. PLoS One. 2021;16(1):e0245099.

Hulbert C, Thomas R. Predicting self-injury in BPD: an investigation of the experiential avoidance model. J Personal Disord. 2010;24(5):651–63.

Hyde JS, Mezulis AH. Gender differences in depression: biological, affective, cognitive, and sociocultural factors. Harv Rev Psychiatry. 2020;28(1):4–13.

Ivey-Stephenson AZ. Suicidal ideation and behaviors among high school students—youth risk behavior survey, United States, 2019. MMWR Suppl. 2020;69(1):47–55. https://doi.org/10.15585/mmwr.su6901a6.

Ivey-Stephenson AZ. Suicidal ideation and behaviors among high school students—youth risk behavior survey, United States, 2019. MMWR Suppl. 2020;69

International Society of the Study of Self-injury, 2018.

Jacobson CM, Gould M. The epidemiology and phenomenology of nonsuicidal self-injurious behavior among adolescents: a critical review of the literature. Arch Suicide Res. 2007;11(2):129–47.

Jacobson CM, Muehlenkamp JJ, Miller AL, Turner JB. Psychiatric impairment among adolescents engaging in different types of deliberate self-harm. J Clin Child Adolesc Psychol. 2008;37(2):363–75.

Jenkins AL, Schmitz MF. The roles of affect dysregulation and positive affect in nonsuicidal self-injury. Arch Suicide Res. 2012;16(3):212–25.
Jeon ME, Gomez MM, Gai AR, Ringer FB, Schafer KM, Joiner TE. Suicide risk during COVID-19: correlates of peri-pandemic suicidal ideation controlling for pre-pandemic ideation. Int J Cogn Ther. 2022;15(3):321–35.
Jobes DA, Joiner TE. Reflections on suicidal ideation, vol. 40; 2019. p. 227.
Joiner T. Why people die by suicide. Harvard University Press; 2005.
Joyce KE, Laurienti PJ, Burdette JH, Hayasaka S. A new measure of centrality for brain networks. PLoS One. 2010;5(8):e12200.
Juarascio A, Manasse S, Clark KE, Schaumberg K, Kerrigan S, Goldstein SP, Evans BC, Wyckoff E, Murray HB, Felonis CR, Forman E. Understanding the overlap and differences in terms describing patterns of maladaptive avoidance and intolerance of negative emotional states. Personal Individ Differ. 2020a;158:109859.
Juarascio AS, Parker MN, Manasse SM, Barney JL, Wyckoff EP, Dochat C. An exploratory component analysis of emotion regulation strategies for improving emotion regulation and emotional eating. Appetite. 2020b;150:104634.
Kaess M, Parzer P, Mattern M, Plener PL, Bifulco A, Resch F, Brunner R. Adverse childhood experiences and their impact on frequency, severity, and the individual function of nonsuicidal self-injury in youth. Psychiatry Res. 2013;206(2–3):265–72.
Kanwar A, Malik S, Prokop LJ, Sim LA, Feldstein D, Wang Z, Murad MH. The association between anxiety disorders and suicidal behaviors: a systematic review and meta-analysis. Depress Anxiety. 2013;30(10):917–29.
Kaplan C, Tarlow N, Stewart JG, Aguirre B, Galen G, Auerbach RP. Borderline personality disorder in youth: the prospective impact of child abuse on nonsuicidal self-injury and suicidality. Compr Psychiatry. 2016;71:86–94.
Kapur N, Hunt IM, Windfuhr K, Rodway C, Webb R, Rahman MS, Shaw J, Appleby L. Psychiatric in-patient care and suicide in England, 1997 to 2008: a longitudinal study. Psychol Med. 2013;43(1):61–71.
Kasen S, Cohen P, Chen H. Developmental course of impulsivity and capability from age 10 to age 25 as related to trajectory of suicide attempt in a community cohort. Suicide Life Threat Behav. 2011;41(2):180–92.
Kashdan TB, Steger MF. Expanding the topography of social anxiety: an experience-sampling assessment of positive emotions, positive events, and emotion suppression. Psychol Sci. 2006;17(2):120–8.
Kaslow NJ, Webb Price A, Wyckoff S, Bender Grall M, Sherry A, Young S, Scholl L, Millington Upshaw V, Rashid A, Jackson EB, Bethea K. Person factors associated with suicidal behavior among African American women and men. Cult Divers Ethn Minor Psychol. 2004;10(1):5.
Kaufman EA, Beeney JE, Stepp SD. Self-report response style bias and borderline personality features. Curr Psychol. 2023;42(24):20443–51.
Kaufman EA, Puzia ME, Mead HK, Crowell SE, McEachern A, Beauchaine TP. Children's emotion regulation difficulties mediate the association between maternal borderline and antisocial symptoms and youth behaviour problems over 1 year. J Personal Disord. 2017a;31(2):170–92.
Kaufman EA, Crowell SE, Lenzenweger MF. The development of borderline personality and self-inflicted injury. Child and adolescent psychopathology. 3rd ed; 2017b. p. 642–79.
Kaufman EA, Victor SE, Hipwell AE, Stepp SD. Reciprocal influences of parent and adolescent borderline personality symptoms over 3 years. J Personal Disord. 2020;34(Supplement B):130–45.
Kaufman EA, Puzia ME, Godfrey DA, Crowell SE. Physiological and behavioral effects of interpersonal validation: a multilevel approach to examining a core intervention strategy among self-injuring adolescents and their mothers. J Clin Psychol. 2020a;76(3):559–80.
Kaufman JA, Livingston MD, Komro KA. Unemployment insurance program accessibility and suicide rates in the United States. Prev Med. 2020b;141:106318.
Keefner TP, Stenvig T. Rethinking suicide risk with a new generation of suicide theories. Res Theory Nurs Pract. 2020;34(4):389.

Kendler KS, Ohlsson H, Mościcki EK, Sundquist J, Edwards AC, Sundquist K. Genetic liability to suicide attempt, suicide death, and psychiatric and substance use disorders on the risk for suicide attempt and suicide death: a Swedish national study. Psychol Med. 2023;53(4):1639–48.

Kerr PL, Muehlenkamp JJ, Turner JM. Nonsuicidal self-injury: a review of current research for family medicine and primary care physicians. J Am Board Fam Med. 2010;23(2):240–59.

Kharsati N, Bhola P. Patterns of nonsuicidal self-injurious behaviours among college students in India. Int J Soc Psychiatry. 2015;61(1):39–49.

Kiekens G, Bruffaerts R, Nock MK, Van de Ven M, Witteman C, Mortier P, Demyttenaere K, Claes L. Nonsuicidal self-injury among Dutch and Belgian adolescents: personality, stress and coping. Eur Psychiatry. 2015;30(6):743–9.

Kiekens G, Claes L, Demyttenaere K, Auerbach RP, Green JG, Kessler RC, Mortier P, Nock MK, Bruffaerts R. Lifetime and 12-month nonsuicidal self-injury and academic performance in college freshmen. Suicide Life Threat Behav. 2016;46(5):563–76.

Kiekens GH, Hasking P, Boyes M, Claes L, Mortier P, Auerbach RP, Cuijpers P, Demyttenaere K, Green JG, Kessler RC, Myin-Germeys I. The associations between nonsuicidal self-injury and first onset suicidal thoughts and behaviors. J Affect Disord. 2018;239:171–9.

Kinchin I, Mccalman J, Bainbridge R, Tsey K, Lui FW. Does indigenous health research have impact? A systematic review of reviews. Int J Equity Health. 2017;16:1–6.

Kingston J, Clarke S, Remington B. Experiential avoidance and problem behavior: a mediational analysis. Behav Modif. 2010;34(2):145–63.

Kjelsberg E, Eikeseth PH, Dahl AA. Suicide in borderline patients—predictive factors. Acta Psychiatr Scand. 1991;84(3):283–7.

Kleindienst N, Bohus M, Ludäscher P, Limberger MF, Kuenkele K, Ebner-Priemer UW, Chapman AL, Reicherzer M, Stieglitz RD, Schmahl C. Motives for nonsuicidal self-injury among women with borderline personality disorder. J Nerv Ment Dis. 2008;196(3):230–6.

Klonsky ED. The functions of deliberate self-injury: a review of the evidence. Clin Psychol Rev. 2007;27(2):226–39.

Klonsky ED. The functions of self-injury in young adults who cut themselves: clarifying the evidence for affect-regulation. Psychiatry Res. 2009;166(2–3):260–8.

Klonsky ED, Glenn CR. Assessing the functions of nonsuicidal self-injury: psychometric properties of the Inventory of Statements About Self-injury (ISAS). J Psychopathol Behav Assess. 2009;31:215–9.

Klonsky ED, May A. Rethinking impulsivity in suicide. Suicide Life Threat Behav. 2010;40(6):612–9.

Klonsky ED, Moyer A. Childhood sexual abuse and nonsuicidal self-injury: meta-analysis. Br J Psychiatry. 2008;192(3):166–70.

Klonsky ED, Muehlenkamp JJ. Self-injury: a research review for the practitioner. J Clin Psychol. 2007;63(11):1045–56.

Klonsky ED, Olino TM. Identifying clinically distinct subgroups of self-injurers among young adults: a latent class analysis. J Consult Clin Psychol. 2008;76(1):22.

Klonsky ED, Oltmanns TF, Turkheimer E. Deliberate self-harm in a nonclinical population: prevalence and psychological correlates. Am J Psychiatry. 2003;160(8):1501–8.

Klonsky ED, Muehlenkamp J, Lewis SP, Walsh B. Nonsuicidal self-injury. Hogrefe Publishing GmbH; 2011.

Klonsky ED, May AM, Glenn CR. The relationship between nonsuicidal self-injury and attempted suicide: converging evidence from four samples. J Abnorm Psychol. 2013;122(1):231.

Klonsky ED, May AM. Differentiating suicide attempters from suicide ideators: a critical frontier for suicidology research. Suicide Life Threat Behav. 2014;44(1):1–5.

Klonsky ED, Glenn CR, Styer DM, Olino TM, Washburn JJ. The functions of nonsuicidal self-injury: converging evidence for a two-factor structure. Child Adolesc Psychiatry Ment Health. 2015;9:1–9.

Klonsky ED, May AM, Saffer BY. Suicide, suicide attempts, and suicidal ideation. Annu Rev Clin Psychol. 2016;12(1):307–30.

Koenig J, Rinnewitz L, Niederbäumer M, Strozyk T, Parzer P, Resch F, Kaess M. Longitudinal development of pain sensitivity in adolescent nonsuicidal self-injury. J Psychiatr Res. 2017;89:81–4.

Koenigsberg HW, Harvey PD, Mitropoulou V, New AS, Goodman M, Silverman J, Serby M, Schopick F, Siever LJ. Are the interpersonal and identity disturbances in the borderline personality disorder criteria linked to the traits of affective instability and impulsivity? J Personal Disord. 2001;15(4):358–70.

Kongerslev MT, Chanen AM, Simonsen E. Personality disorder in childhood and adolescence comes of age: a review of the current evidence and prospects for future research. Scandinavian J Child Adolesc Psychiatr Psychol. 2015;3(1):31–48.

Kotler M, Iancu I, Efroni R, Amir M. Anger, impulsivity, social support, and suicide risk in patients with posttraumatic stress disorder. J Nerv Ment Dis. 2001;189(3):162–7.

Krueger NT. Racial homelessness, racial identity invalidation, family discrimination, and suicidal ideation in college-aged multiracial Americans: using path analysis to test the interpersonal-psychological theory of suicide (Doctoral dissertation), 2022.

Krug I, Arroyo MD, Giles S, Dang AB, Kiropoulos L, De Paoli T, Buck K, Treasure J, Fuller-Tyszkiewicz M. A new integrative model for the co-occurrence of nonsuicidal self-injury behaviours and eating disorder symptoms. J Eat Disord. 2021;9:1–7.

Kruzan KP, Muehlenkamp JJ, Claes L. Identity, self-blame, and body regard in NSSI: a test of moderated-mediation. Compr Psychiatry. 2022;116:152322.

Kullgren G. An empirical comparison of three different borderline concepts. Acta Psychiatr Scand. 1986;76(3):246–55.

Kumar SS. Understanding nonsuicidal self-injury in college populations, 2010.

Lanzillo EC, Zhang I, Jobes DA, Brausch AM. The influence of cyberbullying on nonsuicidal self-injury and suicidal thoughts and behavior in a psychiatric adolescent sample. Arch Suicide Res. 2023;27(1):156–63.

Larson RW, Moneta G, Richards MH, Wilson S. Continuity, stability, and change in daily emotional experience across adolescence. Child Dev. 2002;73(4):1151–65.

Law KC, Khazem LR, Anestis MD. The role of emotion dysregulation in suicide as considered through the ideation to action framework. Curr Opin Psychol. 2015;3:30–5.

Laye-Gindhu AM. Nonsuicidal self-injury in street-involved adolescents: identification of risk and protective factors (Doctoral dissertation, University of British Columbia). 2011.

Lear MK, Kozina RM, Stacy SE, Clapp JD, Pepper CM. Interpersonal needs and suicide risk: the moderating roles of sex and brooding. J Clin Psychol. 2019;75(9):1572–84.

Lee S, Tsang A, Huang YQ, He YL, Liu ZR, Zhang MY, Shen YC, Kessler RC. The epidemiology of depression in metropolitan China. Psychol Med. 2009;39(5):735–47.

Leichsenring F, Leibing E, Kruse J, New AS, Leweke F. Borderline personality disorder. Lancet. 2011;377(9759):74–84.

Lereya ST, Winsper C, Tang NK, Wolke D. Sleep problems in childhood and borderline personality disorder symptoms in early adolescence. J Abnorm Child Psychol. 2017;45:193–206.

LeGris J, van Reekum R. The neuropsychological correlates of borderline personality disorder and suicidal behaviour. Can J Psychiatry. 2006;51(3):131–42.

Lewinsohn PM, Rohde P, Seeley JR. Psychosocial characteristics of adolescents with a history of suicide attempt. J Am Acad Child Adolesc Psychiatry. 1993;32(1):60–8.

Lewinsohn PM, Rohde P, Seeley JR. Adolescent suicidal ideation and attempts: prevalence, risk factors, and clinical implications. Clin Psychol Sci Pract. 1996;3(1):25.

Leyro TM, Zvolensky MJ, Bernstein A. Distress tolerance and psychopathological symptoms and disorders: a review of the empirical literature among adults. Psychol Bull. 2010;136(4):576.

Lezak MD. Neuropsychological assessment. Oxford: Oxford University Press; 2004.

Liao S, Wang Y, Zhou X, Zhao Q, Li X, Guo W, Ji X, Lv Q, Zhang Y, Zhang Y, Deng W. Prediction of suicidal ideation among Chinese college students based on radial basis function neural network. Front Public Health. 2022;10:1042218.

Lim KS, Wong CH, McIntyre RS, Wang J, Zhang Z, Tran BX, Tan W, Ho CS, Ho RC. Global lifetime and 12-month prevalence of suicidal behavior, deliberate self-harm and nonsuicidal self-injury in children and adolescents between 1989 and 2018: a meta-analysis. Int J Environ Res Public Health. 2019;16(22):4581.

Lin LN, Lee MB. Recent advances in understanding non-suicidal self-injury in adolescents. J Suicidol. 2022;1;17(4):308–18.

Lin MP, You J, Ren Y, Wu JY, Hu WH, Yen CF, Zhang X. Prevalence of nonsuicidal self-injury and its risk and protective factors among adolescents in Taiwan. Psychiatry Res. 2017;255:119–27.

Lin HT, Lai CH, Perng HJ, Chung CH, Wang CC, Chen WL, Chien WC. Insomnia as an independent predictor of suicide attempts: a nationwide population-based retrospective cohort study. BMC Psychiatry. 2018;18:1–1.

Linehan MM. Dialectical behavior therapy for borderline personality disorder: theory and method. Bull Menn Clin. 1987;51(3):261.

Linehan M. Cognitive-behavioral treatment of borderline personality disorder. Guilford Press; 1993.

Linehan MM. Behavioral treatments of suicidal behaviors. Definitional obfuscation and treatment outcomes a. Ann N Y Acad Sci. 1997;836(1):302–28.

Links PS, Eynan R, Heisel MJ, Nisenbaum R. Elements of affective instability associated with suicidal behaviour in patients with borderline personality disorder. Can J Psychiatry. 2008;53(2):112–6.

Liu RT, Cheek SM, Nestor BA. Non-suicidal self-injury and life stress: a systematic meta-analysis and theoretical elaboration. Clin Psychol Rev. 2016;47:1–4.

Liu Y, Zhong M, Xi C, Jin X, Zhu X, Yao S, Yi J. Event-related potentials altered in patients with borderline personality disorder during working memory tasks. Front Behav Neurosci. 2017;11:67.

Li X, Mu F, Liu D, Zhu J, Yue S, Liu M, Liu Y, Wang J. Predictors of suicidal ideation, suicide attempt and suicide death among people with major depressive disorder: a systematic review and meta-analysis of cohort studies. J Affect Disord. 2022;302:332–51.

Lloyd-Richardson EE, Perrine N, Dierker L, Kelley ML. Characteristics and functions of non-suicidal self-injury in a community sample of adolescents. Psychol Med. 2007;37(8):1183–92.

Lockwood J, Townsend E, Daley D, Sayal K. Impulsivity as a predictor of self-harm onset and maintenance in young adolescents: a longitudinal prospective study. J Affect Disord. 2020a;274:583–92.

Lockwood J, Townsend E, Allen H, Daley D, Sayal K. What young people say about impulsivity in the short-term build up to self-harm: a qualitative study using card-sort tasks. PLoS One. 2020b;15(12):e0244319.

Lockwood J, Townsend E, Royes L, Daley D, Sayal K. What do young adolescents think about taking part in longitudinal self-harm research? Findings from a school-based study. Child Adolesc Psychiatry Ment Health. 2018;12:1–3.

Löffler A, Foell J, Bekrater-Bodmann R. Interoception and its interaction with self, other, and emotion processing: implications for the understanding of psychosocial deficits in borderline personality disorder. Curr Psychiatry Rep. 2018;20:1–9.

Löffler A, Kleindienst N, Neukel C, Bekrater-Bodmann R, Flor H. Pleasant touch perception in borderline personality disorder and its relationship with disturbed body representation. Borderline Personal Disord Emot Dysregul. 2022;9(1):3.

Lolas F, Gomez A, Suarez L. EPQ-R and suicide attempt: the relevance of psychoticism. Personal Individ Differ. 1991;12(9):899–902.

Lönnqvist J. Challenges for psychiatry in Finland-a personal view. Psychiatr Fenn. 2021;53:14–23.

Lu J, Ye Y, Lou J, Zhu H, Zhou X. Associations between unintentional injuries and deliberate self-harm behaviors of children and adolescents: a school-based cross-sectional survey. Gen Hosp Psychiatry. 2024;86:67–74.

Ludäscher P, Greffrath W, Schmahl C, Kleindienst N, Kraus A, Baumgärtner U, Magerl W, Treede RD, Bohus M. A cross-sectional investigation of discontinuation of self-injury and normalizing pain perception in patients with borderline personality disorder. Acta Psychiatr Scand. 2009;120(1):62–70.

Ludäscher P, Valerius G, Stiglmayr C, Mauchnik J, Lanius RA, Bohus M, Schmahl C. Pain sensitivity and neural processing during dissociative states in patients with borderline personality disorder with and without comorbid posttraumatic stress disorder: a pilot study. J Psychiatry Neurosci. 2010;35(3):177–84.
Lüdtke J, In-Albon T, Michel C, Schmid M. Predictors for DSM-5 nonsuicidal self-injury in female adolescent inpatients: the role of childhood maltreatment, alexithymia, and dissociation. Psychiatry Res. 2016;239:346–52.
Lutz NM, Chamberlain SR, Goodyer IM, Bhardwaj A, Sahakian BJ, Jones PB, Wilkinson PO. Behavioral measures of impulsivity and compulsivity in adolescents with nonsuicidal self-injury. CNS Spectr. 2022;27(5):604–12.
Lynam DR, Hoyle RH, Newman JP. The perils of partialling: cautionary tales from aggression and psychopathy. Assessment. 2006;13(3):328–41.
Lynam DR, Miller JD, Miller DJ, Bornovalova MA, Lejuez CW. Testing the relations between impulsivity-related traits, suicidality, and nonsuicidal self-injury: a test of the incremental validity of the UPPS model. Personal Disord Theory Res Treat. 2011;2(2):151.
Macintyre VG, Mansell W, Pratt D, Tai SJ. The psychological pathway to suicide attempts: a strategy of control without awareness. Front Psychol. 2021;12:588683.
MacLaren VV, Best LA. Nonsuicidal self-injury, potentially addictive behaviors, and the Five Factor Model in undergraduates. Personal Individ Differ. 2010;49(5):521–5.
Madge N, Hewitt A, Hawton K, Wilde EJ, Corcoran P, Fekete S, Heeringen KV, Leo DD, Ystgaard M. Deliberate self-harm within an international community sample of young people: comparative findings from the Child & Adolescent Self-harm in Europe (CASE) study. J Child Psychol Psychiatry. 2008;49(6):667–77.
Maddock GR, Carter GL, Murrell ER, Lewin TJ, Conrad AM. Distinguishing suicidal from nonsuicidal deliberate self-harm events in women with Borderline Personality Disorder. Aust NZ J Psychiatr. 2010;44(6):574–82.
Maes T, Dom G. Alcohol, other psychoactive substance use disorders, and suicide, 2021.
Magerl W, Burkart D, Fernandez A, Schmidt LG, Treede RD. Persistent antinociception through repeated self-injury in patients with borderline personality disorder. Pain. 2012;153(3):575–84.
Maniglio R. The role of child sexual abuse in the etiology of suicide and non-suicidal self-injury. Acta Psychiatr Scand. 2011;124(1):30–41.
Mann JJ. Neurobiology of suicidal behaviour. Nat Rev Neurosci. 2003;4(10):819–28.
Marco JH, Garcia-Alandete J, Pérez S, Guillen V, Jorquera M, Espallargas P, Botella C. Meaning in life and nonsuicidal self-injury: a follow-up study with participants with borderline personality disorder. Psychiatry Res. 2015;230(2):561–6.
Mars B, Heron J, Biddle L, Donovan JL, Holley R, Piper M, Potokar J, Wyllie C, Gunnell D. Exposure to, and searching for, information about suicide and self-harm on the Internet: Prevalence and predictors in a population based cohort of young adults. J Affect Disord. 2015;185:239–45.
Mars B, Burrows S, Hjelmeland H, Gunnell D. Suicidal behaviour across the African continent: a review of the literature. BMC Public Health. 2014;14:1–4.
Mars B, Heron J, Klonsky ED, Moran P, O'Connor RC, Tilling K, Wilkinson P, Gunnell D. Predictors of future suicide attempt among adolescents with suicidal thoughts or nonsuicidal self-harm: a population-based birth cohort study. Lancet Psychiatry. 2019;6(4):327–37.
Marshall SK, Tilton-Weaver LC, Stattin H. Nonsuicidal self-injury and depressive symptoms during middle adolescence: a longitudinal analysis. J Youth Adolesc. 2013;42:1234–42.
Martin J, Bureau JF, Yurkowski K, Lafontaine MF, Cloutier P. Heterogeneity of relational backgrounds is associated with variation in nonsuicidal self-injurious behavior. J Abnorm Child Psychol. 2016;44:511–22.
Martinez-Ales G, Hernandez-Calle D, Khauli N, Keyes KM. Why are suicide rates increasing in the United States? Towards a multilevel reimagination of suicide prevention. In: Behavioral neurobiology of suicide and self harm; 2020. p. 1–23.
Martorana G. Characteristics and associated factors of nonsuicidal self-injury among Italian young people: a survey through a thematic website. J Behav Addict. 2015;4(2):93–100.

Matel-Anderson DM, Bekhet AK, Garnier-Villarreal M. Mediating effects of positive thinking and social support on suicide resilience. West J Nurs Res. 2019;41(1):25–41.
Matera E, Margari M, Serra M, Petruzzelli MG, Gabellone A, Piarulli FM, Pugliese A, Tassiello AR, Croce F, Renna C, Margari A. Nonsuicidal self-injury: an observational study in a sample of adolescents and young adults. Brain Sci. 2021;11(8):974.
May AM, Klonsky ED. Assessing motivations for suicide attempts: development and psychometric properties of the inventory of motivations for suicide attempts. Suicide Life Threat Behav. 2013;43(5):532–46.
May AM, Klonsky ED. What distinguishes suicide attempters from suicide ideators? A meta-analysis of potential factors. Clin Psychol Sci Pract. 2016;23(1):5.
McAndrew S, Warne T. Hearing the voices of young people who self-harm: implications for service providers. Int J Ment Health Nurs. 2014;23(6):570–9.
McCann SJ. Emotional health and the Big Five personality factors at the American state level. J Happiness Stud. 2011;12:547–60.
McClelland H, Cleare S, O'Connor RC. Suicide risk in personality disorders: a systematic review. Curr Psychiatry Rep. 2023;25(9):405–17.
McCrae RR, Costa PT. Validation of the five-factor model of personality across instruments and observers. J Pers Soc Psychol. 1987;52(1):81.
McMain SF, Fitzpatrick S, Boritz T, Barnhart R, Links P, Streiner DL. Outcome trajectories and prognostic factors for suicide and self-harm behaviors in patients with borderline personality disorder following one year of outpatient psychotherapy. J Personal Disord. 2018;32(4):497–512.
McGirr A, Renaud J, Bureau A, Seguin M, Lesage A, Turecki G. Impulsive-aggressive behaviours and completed suicide across the life cycle: a predisposition for younger age of suicide. Psychol Med. 2008;38(3):407–17.
McGlashan TH. The Chestnut Lodge follow-up study: III. Long-term outcome of borderline personalities. Arch Gen Psychiatry. 1986;43(1):20–30.
McKenzie KC, Gross JJ. Nonsuicidal self-injury: an emotion regulation perspective. Psychopathology. 2014;47(4):207–19.
McManus S, Gunnell D. Trends in mental health, non-suicidal self-harm and suicide attempts in 16–24-year old students and non-students in England, 2000–2014. Soc Psychiatry Psychiatr Epidemiol. 2020;55(1):125–8.
Mendez I, Sintes A, Pascual JC, Puntí J, Lara A, Briones-Buixassa L, Nicolaou S, Schmidt C, Romero S, Fernández M, i Farrés CC. Borderline personality traits mediate the relationship between low perceived social support and nonsuicidal self-injury in a clinical sample of adolescents. J Affect Disord. 2022;302:204–13.
Meszaros G, Horvath LO, Balazs J. Self-injury and externalizing pathology: a systematic literature review. BMC Psychiatry. 2017;17:1–21.
Mettler J, Stern M, Lewis SP, Heath NL. Perceived vs. actual emotion reactivity and regulation in individuals with and without a history of NSSI. Front Psychol. 2021;12:612792.
Mettler J, Cho S, Stern M, Heath NL. Negative and positive emotional reactivity in women with and without a history of self-injury. Psychol Rep. 2023;29:00332941231180118.
Miller AB, Prinstein MJ. Adolescent suicide as a failure of acute stress-response systems. Annu Rev Clin Psychol. 2019;15(1):425–50.
Mirkovic B, Delvenne V, Robin M, Pham-Scottez A, Corcos M, Speranza M. Borderline personality disorder and adolescent suicide attempt: the mediating role of emotional dysregulation. BMC Psychiatry. 2021;21:1–0.
Misra N, Ghanekar A. Personality profiles of suicide ideators, attempters, completers and suicide note writers versus non-writers. In: Handbook of suicidal behaviour; 2017. p. 371–86.
Moberly NJ, Watkins ER. Ruminative self-focus, negative life events, and negative affect. Behav Res Ther. 2008;46(9):1034–9.
Møhl B. Assessment and treatment of nonsuicidal self-injury: a clinical perspective. Routledge; 2019.
Møhl B. Assessment and treatment of non-suicidal self-injury: a clinical perspective. Routledge; 2019 Jun 14.

Möller-Leimkühler AM. The gender gap in suicide and premature death or: why are men so vulnerable? Eur Arch Psychiatry Clin Neurosci. 2003;253:1–8.

Moran P, Coffey C, Romaniuk H, Olsson C, Borschmann R, Carlin JB, Patton GC. The natural history of self-harm from adolescence to young adulthood: a population-based cohort study. Lancet. 2012;379(9812):236–43.

Morgan S, Rickard E, Noone M, Boylan C, Carthy A, Crowley S, Butler J, Guerin S, Fitzpatrick C. Parents of young people with self-harm or suicidal behaviour who seek help–a psychosocial profile. Child Adolesc Psychiatry Ment Health. 2013;7:1–0.

Morgan ER, Rivara FP, Ta M, Grossman DC, Jones K, Rowhani-Rahbar A. Incarceration and subsequent risk of suicide: a statewide cohort study. Suicide Life Threat Behav. 2022;52(3):467–77.

Mortier P, Demyttenaere K, Auerbach RP, Green JG, Kessler RC, Kiekens G, Nock MK, Bruffaerts R. The impact of lifetime suicidality on academic performance in college freshmen. J Affect Disord. 2015;186:254–60.

Moscoso A, Speranza M, Delvenne V, Corcos M, Pham-Scottez A. Parental risk for suicide and attachment patterns among adolescents with borderline personality disorder. A clinical-based study. Front Psych. 2019;9:771.

Moselli M, Frattini C, Williams R, Ronningstam E. The study of motivation in the suicidal process: the motivational interview for suicidality. Front Psych. 2021a;11:598866.

Moselli M, Casini MP, Frattini C, Williams R. Suicidality and personality pathology in adolescence: a systematic, vol. 54; 2021b. p. 290.

Moutier CY. Innovative and timely approaches to suicide prevention in medical education. Acad Psychiatry. 2021a;45(3):252–6.

Moutier C. Suicide prevention in the COVID-19 era: transforming threat into opportunity. JAMA Psychiatry. 2021b;78(4):433–8.

Motz A. Self-harm as a sign of hope. Psychoanal Psychother. 2010;24(2):81–92.

Muehlenkamp JJ, Gutierrez PM, Osman A, Barrios FX. Validation of the Positive and Negative Suicide Ideation (PANSI) Inventory in a diverse sample of young adults. J Clin Psychol. 2005;61(4):431–45.

Muehlenkamp JJ, Walsh BW, McDade M. Preventing non-suicidal self-injury in adolescents: the signs of self-injury program. J Youth Adolesc. 2010;39:306–14.

Muehlenkamp JJ, Gutierrez PM. An investigation of differences between self-injurious behavior and suicide attempts in a sample of adolescents. Suicide Life Threat Behav. 2004;34(1):12–23.

Muehlenkamp JJ, Gutierrez PM. Risk for suicide attempts among adolescents who engage in nonsuicidal self-injury. Arch Suicide Res. 2007;11(1):69–82.

Muehlenkamp JJ, Ertelt TW, Miller AL, Claes L. Borderline personality symptoms differentiate non-suicidal and suicidal self-injury in ethnically diverse adolescent outpatients. J Child Psychol Psychiatry. 2011;52(2):148–55.

Muehlenkamp JJ, Claes L, Havertape L, Plener PL. International prevalence of adolescent nonsuicidal self-injury and deliberate self-harm. Child Adolesc Psychiatry Ment Health. 2012;6:1–9.

Muehlenkamp J, Brausch A, Quigley K, Whitlock J. Interpersonal features and functions of nonsuicidal self-injury. Suicide Life Threat Behav. 2013;43(1):67–80.

Muehlenkamp JJ, Brausch AM, Washburn JJ. How much is enough? Examining frequency criteria for NSSI disorder in adolescent inpatients. J Consult Clin Psychol. 2017;85(6):611.

Muehlenkamp JJ, Xhunga N, Brausch AM. Self-injury age of onset: a risk factor for NSSI severity and suicidal behavior. Arch Suicide Res. 2018;23:551.

Muehlenkamp JJ, Brausch AM, Littlefield A. Concurrent changes in nonsuicidal self-injury and suicide thoughts and behaviors. Psychol Med. 2023;53(11):4898–903.

Mullins-Sweatt SN, Lengel GJ, Grant DM. Non-suicidal self-injury: the contribution of general personality functioning. Personal Ment Health. 2013;7(1):56–68.

Nakar O, Brunner R, Schilling O, Chanen A, Fischer G, Parzer P, Carli V, Wasserman D, Sarchiapone M, Wasserman C, Hoven CW. Developmental trajectories of self-injurious behavior, suicidal behavior and substance misuse and their association with adolescent borderline personality pathology. J Affect Disord. 2016;197:231–8.

Neeleman J, Wessely S, Wadsworth M. Predictors of suicide, accidental death, and premature natural death in a general-population birth cohort. Lancet. 1998;351(9096):93–7.

Nicolai KA, Wielgus MD, Mezulis A. Identifying risk for self-harm: rumination and negative affectivity in the prospective prediction of nonsuicidal self-injury. Suicide Life Threat Behav. 2016;46(2):223–33.

Niedtfeld I, Schulze L, Kirsch P, Herpertz SC, Bohus M, Schmahl C. Affect regulation and pain in borderline personality disorder: a possible link to the understanding of self-injury. Biol Psychiatry. 2010;68(4):383–91.

Niu S, Yin X, Pan B, Chen H, Dai C, Tong C, Chen F, Feng X. Understanding comorbidity between nonsuicidal self-injury and depressive symptoms in a clinical sample of adolescents: a network analysis. Neuropsychiatr Dis Treat. 2024;Volume 20:1–7.

Nixon MK, Cloutier PF, Aggarwal S. Affect regulation and addictive aspects of repetitive self-injury in hospitalized adolescents. J Am Acad Child Adolesc Psychiatry. 2002;41(11):1333–41.

Nixon MK, Cloutier P, Jansson SM. Nonsuicidal self-harm in youth: a population-based survey. CMAJ. 2008;178(3):306–12.

Nock MK, Borges G, Bromet EJ, Cha CB, Kessler RC, Lee S. Suicide and suicidal behavior. Epidemiol Rev. 2008;30(1):133.

Nock MK, Green JG, Hwang I, McLaughlin KA, Sampson NA, Zaslavsky AM, Kessler RC. Prevalence, correlates, and treatment of lifetime suicidal behavior among adolescents: results from the National Comorbidity Survey Replication Adolescent Supplement. JAMA Psychiatry. 2013;70(3):300–10.

Nock MK. Why do people hurt themselves? New insights into the nature and functions of self-injury. Curr Dir Psychol Sci. 2009;18(2):78–83.

Nock MK. Future directions for the study of suicide and self-injury. J Clin Child Adolesc Psychol. 2012;41(2):255–9.

Nock MK. Self-injury. Annu Rev Clin Psychol. 2010;6(1):339–63.

Nock MK, Banaji MR. Prediction of suicide ideation and attempts among adolescents using a brief performance-based test. J Consult Clin Psychol. 2007;75(5):707.

Nock MK, Favazza AR. Nonsuicidal self-injury: definition and classification, 2009.

Nock MK, Kessler RC. Prevalence of and risk factors for suicide attempts versus suicide gestures: analysis of the National Comorbidity Survey. J Abnorm Psychol. 2006;115(3):616.

Nock MK, Joiner TE Jr, Gordon KH, Lloyd-Richardson E, Prinstein MJ. Nonsuicidal self-injury among adolescents: diagnostic correlates and relation to suicide attempts. Psychiatry Res. 2006;144(1):65–72.

Nock MK. Distinguishing suicide attempts from nonsuicidal self-harming behaviors. J Am Acad Child Adolesc Psychiatry. 2008;48(10):1039–40.

Nock MK, Hwang I, Sampson N, Kessler RC, Angermeyer M, Beautrais A, Borges G, Bromet E, Bruffaerts R, De Girolamo G, De Graaf R. Cross-national analysis of the associations among mental disorders and suicidal behavior: findings from the WHO World Mental Health Surveys. PLoS Med. 2009;6(8):e1000123.

Nock MK, Prinstein MJ. A functional approach to the assessment of self-mutilative behavior. J Consult Clin Psychol. 2004;72(5):885.

Nock MK, Millner AJ, Joiner TE, Gutierrez PM, Han G, Hwang I, King A, Naifeh JA, Sampson NA, Zaslavsky AM, Stein MB. Risk factors for the transition from suicide ideation to suicide attempt: results from the Army Study to Assess Risk and Resilience in Servicemembers (Army STARRS). J Abnorm Psychol. 2018;127(2):139.

Nolen-Hoeksema S. Emotion regulation and psychopathology: the role of gender. Annu Rev Clin Psychol. 2012;8(1):161–87.

Nolen-Hoeksema S, Morrow J. A prospective study of depression and posttraumatic stress symptoms after a natural disaster: the 1989 Loma Prieta earthquake. J Pers Soc Psychol. 1991;61(1):115.

Nordentoft M, Mortensen PB, Pedersen CB. Absolute risk of suicide after first hospital contact in mental disorder. Arch Gen Psychiatry. 2011;68(10):1058–64.

Norström T, Ramstedt M. The link between per capita alcohol consumption and alcohol-related harm in Sweden, 1987–2015. J Stud Alcohol Drugs. 2018;79(4):578–84.
Nurullah AS. Gender differences in distress: the mediating influence of life stressors and psychological resources. Asian Soc Sci. 2010;6(5):27.
Ochsner KN, Ray RR, Hughes B, McRae K, Cooper JC, Weber J, Gabrieli JD, Gross JJ. Bottom-up and top-down processes in emotion generation: common and distinct neural mechanisms. Psychol Sci. 2009;20(11):1322–31.
O'connor RC. Towards an integrated motivational–volitional model of suicidal behaviour. In: International handbook of suicide prevention: research, policy and practice; 2011. p. 181–98.
O'Connor RC, Kirtley OJ, Melson AJ. Future-oriented constructs and their role in suicidal ideation and enactment. In: A positive psychological approach to suicide: theory, research, and prevention; 2018. p. 17–36.
Oldham JM. Borderline personality disorder and suicidality. Am J Psychiatry. 2006;163(1):20–6.
Oquendo MA, Sullivan GM, Sudol K, Baca-Garcia E, Stanley BH, Sublette ME, Mann JJ. Toward a biosignature for suicide. Am J Psychiatry. 2014;171(12):1259–77.
Orcutt HK, Pickett SM, Pope EB. Experiential avoidance and forgiveness as mediators in the relation between traumatic interpersonal events and posttraumatic stress disorder symptoms. J Soc Clin Psychol. 2005;24(7):1003–29.
Ormel J, Oerlemans AM, Raven D, Laceulle OM, Hartman CA, Veenstra R, Verhulst FC, Vollebergh W, Rosmalen JG, Reijneveld SA, Oldehinkel AJ. Functional outcomes of child and adolescent mental disorders. Current disorder most important psychiatric history matters as well. Psychol Med. 2017;47(7):1271–82.
Oumaya M, Friedman S, Pham A, Abou Abdallah T, Guelfi JD, Rouillon F. Personnalité borderline, automutilations et suicide: revue de la littérature. L'Encéphale. 2008;34(5):452–8.
Pan L, Segreti A, Almeida J, Jollant F, Lawrence N, Brent D, Phillips M. Preserved hippocampal function during learning in the context of risk in adolescent suicide attempt. Psychiatry Res Neuroimaging. 2013;211(2):112–8.
Panagioti M, Gooding PA, Pratt D, Tarrier N. An empirical investigation of suicide schemas in individuals with Posttraumatic Stress Disorder. Psychiatry Res. 2015;227(2–3):302–8.
Paris J. Clinical features of borderline personality disorder. In: Handbook of personality disorders: theory, research, and treatment, vol. 2; 2018. p. 419.
Paris J. Suicidality in borderline personality disorder. Medicina. 2019;28;55(6):223.
Paris J, Zweig-Frank H, Kin NN, Schwartz G, Steiger H, Nair NP. Neurobiological correlates of diagnosis and underlying traits in patients with borderline personality disorder compared with normal controls. Psychiatry Res. 2004;121(3):239–52.
Pattison EM, Kahan J. The deliberate self-harm syndrome. Am J Psychiatry. 1983;140(7):867–72.
Paul E, Tsypes A, Eidlitz L, Ernhout C, Whitlock J. Frequency and functions of nonsuicidal self-injury: associations with suicidal thoughts and behaviors. Psychiatry Res. 2015;225(3):276–82.
Peckham AD, Jones P, Snorrason I, Wessman I, Beard C, Björgvinsson T. Age-related differences in borderline personality disorder symptom networks in a transdiagnostic sample. J Affect Disord. 2020;274:508–14.
Peh CX, Shahwan S, Fauziana R, Mahesh MV, Sambasivam R, Zhang Y, Ong SH, Chong SA, Subramaniam M. Emotion dysregulation as a mechanism linking child maltreatment exposure and self-harm behaviors in adolescents. Child Abuse Negl. 2017;67:383–90.
Pennel L, Quesada JL, Dematteis M. Neuroticism and anxious attachment as potential vulnerability factors of repeat suicide attempts. Psychiatry Res. 2018;264:46–53.
Perez-Rodriguez MM, Hazlett EA, Rich EL, Ripoll LH, Weiner DM, Spence N, Goodman M, Koenigsberg HW, Siever LJ, New AS. Striatal activity in borderline personality disorder with comorbid intermittent explosive disorder: sex differences. J Psychiatr Res. 2012;46(6):797–804.
Perez S, Lorca F, Marco JH. Dissociation, posttraumatic stress symptoms, emotional dysregulation, and invalidating environments as correlates of NSSI in borderline personality disorder patients. J Trauma Dissociation. 2020;21(5):520–35.
Perlman G, Gromatsky M, Salis KL, Klein DN, Kotov R. Personality correlates of self-injury in adolescent girls: disentangling the effects of lifetime psychopathology. J Abnorm Child Psychol. 2018;46(8):1677–85.

Peters EM, John A, Bowen R, Baetz M, Balbuena L. Neuroticism and suicide in a general population cohort: results from the UK Biobank Project. B J Psych open. 2018;4(2):62–8.

Phillips ML, Ladouceur CD, Drevets WC. A neural model of voluntary and automatic emotion regulation: implications for understanding the pathophysiology and neurodevelopment of bipolar disorder. Mol Psychiatry. 2008;13(9):833–57.

Pickles A, Aglan A, Collishaw S, Messer J, Rutter M, Maughan B. Predictors of suicidality across the life span: the Isle of Wight study. Psychol Med. 2010;40(9):1453–66.

Plener PL, Schumacher TS, Munz LM, Groschwitz RC. The longitudinal course of nonsuicidal self-injury and deliberate self-harm: a systematic review of the literature. Borderline Personal Disord Emot Dysregul. 2015;2:1–1.

Pompili M, Serafini G, Innamorati M, Dominici G, Ferracuti S, Kotzalidis GD, Serra G, Girardi P, Janiri L, Tatarelli R, Sher L. Suicidal behavior and alcohol abuse. Int J Environ Res Public Health. 2010;7(4):1392–431.

Pompili M. Can we expect a rise in suicide rates after the Covid-19 pandemic outbreak? Eur Neuropsychopharmacol. 2021;52:1.

Pompili M, Murri MB, Patti S, Innamorati M, Lester D, Girardi P, Amore M. The communication of suicidal intentions: a meta-analysis. Psychol Med. 2016;46(11):2239–53.

Pompili M, Girardi P, Ruberto A, Tatarelli R. Suicide in borderline personality disorder: a meta-analysis. Nord J Psychiatry. 2005;59(5):319–24.

Preece D, Kiekens G, Boyes M, Mortier P, Nock M, Kessler R, Bruffaerts R, Hasking P. Acquired capability for suicide among Belgian and Australian University students: psychometric properties of the German capability for suicide questionnaire and a test of the interpersonal theory of suicide. Suicide Life Threat Behav. 2021;51(3):403–15.

Putnam KM, Silk KR. Emotion dysregulation and the development of borderline personality disorder. Dev Psychopathol. 2005;17(4):899–925.

Rausch J, Flach E, Panizza A, Brunner R, Herpertz SC, Kaess M, Bertsch K. Associations between age and cortisol awakening response in patients with borderline personality disorder. J Neural Transm. 2021;128(9):1425–32.

Rappaport LM, Flint J, Kendler KS. Clarifying the role of neuroticism in suicidal ideation and suicide attempt among women with major depressive disorder. Psychol Med. 2017;47(13):2334–44.

Reichl C, Kaess M. Self-harm in the context of borderline personality disorder. Curr Opin Psychol. 2021;37:139–44.

Reinhardt M, Rice KG, Horváth Z. Nonsuicidal self-injury motivations in the light of self-harm severity indicators and psychopathology in a clinical adolescent sample. Front Psych. 2022;13:1046576.

Renaud J, Berlim MT, McGirr A, Tousignant M, Turecki G. Current psychiatric morbidity, aggression/impulsivity, and personality dimensions in child and adolescent suicide: a case-control study. J Affect Disord. 2008;105(1–3):221–8.

Ribeiro JD, Yen S, Joiner T, Siegler IC. Capability for suicide interacts with states of heightened arousal to predict death by suicide beyond the effects of depression and hopelessness. J Affect Disord. 2015;188:53–9.

Ribeiro JD, Franklin JC, Fox KR, Bentley KH, Kleiman EM, Chang BP, Nock MK. Self-injurious thoughts and behaviors as risk factors for future suicide ideation, attempts, and death: a meta-analysis of longitudinal studies. Psychol Med. 2016;46(2):225–36.

Ribeiro JD, Huang X, Fox KR, Franklin JC. Depression and hopelessness as risk factors for suicide ideation, attempts and death: meta-analysis of longitudinal studies. Br J Psychiatry. 2018;212(5):279–86.

Riley EN, Combs JL, Jordan CE, Smith GT. Negative urgency and lack of perseverance: identification of differential pathways of onset and maintenance risk in the longitudinal prediction of nonsuicidal self-injury. Behav Ther. 2015;46(4):439–48.

Roche SP, Rogers ML, Pridemore WA. A cross-national study of the population-level association between alcohol consumption and suicide rates. Drug Alcohol Depend. 2018;188:16–23.

Rockett IR, Ali B, Caine ED, Shepard DS, Banerjee A, Nolte KB, Connery HS, Larkin GL, Stack S, White FM, Jia H. Escalating costs of self-injury mortality in the 21st century United States: an interstate observational study. BMC Public Health. 2023;23(1):285.

Romero S, Colom F, Iosif AM, Cruz N, Pacchiaroti I, Sanchez-Moreno J, Vieta E. Relevance of family history of suicide in the long-term outcome of bipolar disorders. J Clin Psychiatry. 2007;68(10):1517–21.
Roemer L, Salters K, Raffa SD, Orsillo SM. Fear and avoidance of internal experiences in GAD: preliminary tests of a conceptual model. Cogn Ther Res. 2005;29:71–88.
Rosenthal MZ, Fang CM, Chapman AL. Ambulatory measurement of emotional dysfunction in borderline personality disorder. Curr Opin Psychol. 2015;3:75–9.
Rosenthal MZ, Cukrowicz KC, Cheavens JS, Lynch TR. Self-punishment as a regulation strategy in borderline personality disorder. J Personal Disord. 2006;20(3):232–46.
Rönnqvist I, Nilsson FK, Nordenskjöld A. Electroconvulsive therapy and the risk of suicide in hospitalized patients with major depressive disorder. JAMA Netw Open. 2021;4(7):e2116589.
Ross S, Heath NL, Toste JR. Non-suicidal self-injury and eating pathology in high school students. Am J Orthopsychiatry. 2009;79(1):83–92.
Roy A. Distal risk factors for suicidal behavior in alcoholics: replications and new findings. J Affect Disord. 2003;77(3):267–71.
Rubæk L, Møhl B. Direct and indirect self-injury. In: The Oxford handbook of nonsuicidal self-injury. Oxford University Press; 2023.
Rudd MD, Joiner TE, Rumzek H. Childhood diagnoses and later risk for multiple suicide attempts. Suicide Life Threat Behav. 2004;34(2):113–25.
Rudd MD, Joiner T, Rajab MH. Relationships among suicide ideators, attempters, and multiple attempters in a young-adult sample. J Abnorm Psychol. 1996;105(4):541.
Runeson B, Beskow J. Borderline personality disorder in young Swedish suicides. J Nerv Ment Dis. 1991;179(3):153–6.
Rüsch N, Lieb K, Göttler I, Hermann C, Schramm E, Richter H, Jacob GA, Corrigan PW, Bohus M. Shame and implicit self-concept in women with borderline personality disorder. Am J Psychiatry. 2007;164(3):500–8.
Russ MJ, Campbell SS, Kakuma T, Harrison K, Zanine E. EEG theta activity and pain insensitivity in self-injurious borderline patients. Psychiatry Res. 1999;89(3):201–14.
Rutter LA, Norton DJ, Brown TA. The impact of self-reported depression severity and age on facial emotion recognition in outpatients with anxiety and mood disorders. J Psychopathol Behav Assess. 2020;42(1):86–92.
Rutter LA, Norton DJ, Brown TA. Visual attention toward emotional stimuli: anxiety symptoms correspond to distinct gaze patterns. PLoS One. 2021;16(5):e0250176.
Sadeh N, Londahl-Shaller EA, Piatigorsky A, Fordwood S, Stuart BK, McNiel DE, Klonsky ED, Ozer EM, Yaeger AM. Functions of nonsuicidal self-injury in adolescents and young adults with Borderline Personality Disorder symptoms. Psychiatry Res. 2014;216(2):217–22.
Saffer BY, Glenn CR, David KE. Clarifying the relationship of parental bonding to suicide ideation and attempts. Suicide Life Threat Behav. 2015;45(4):518–28.
San Too L, Spittal MJ, Bugeja L, Reifels L, Butterworth P, Pirkis J. The association between mental disorders and suicide: a systematic review and meta-analysis of record linkage studies. J Affect Disord. 2019;259:302–13.
Santangelo PS, Koenig J, Funke V, Parzer P, Resch F, Ebner-Priemer UW, Kaess M. Ecological momentary assessment of affective and interpersonal instability in adolescent nonsuicidal self-injury. J Abnorm Child Psychol. 2017;45:1429–38.
Sapyta J, Goldston DB, Erkanli A, Daniel SS, Heilbron N, Mayfield A, Treadway SL. Evaluating the predictive validity of suicidal intent and medical lethality in youth. J Consult Clin Psychol. 2012;80(2):222.
Sarfati Y, Bouchaud B, Hardy-Baylé MC. Cathartic effect of suicide attempts not limited to depression: a short-term prospective study after deliberate self-poisoning. Crisis J Crisis Interve Suicide Prevent. 2003;24(2):73.
Sarchiapone M, Zeppegno P. Personality disorders and suicidality. In: Psychosis and personality disorders: unmet needs in early diagnosis and treatment. Cham: Springer International Publishing; 2022. p. 145–61.

Sareen J, Cox BJ, Afifi TO, De Graaf R, Asmundson GJ, Ten Have M, Stein MB. Anxiety disorders and risk for suicidal ideation and suicide attempts: a population-based longitudinal study of adults. Arch Gen Psychiatry. 2005;62(11):1249–57.

Schmahl CG, Vermetten E, Elzinga BM, Bremner JD. A positron emission tomography study of memories of childhood abuse in borderline personality disorder. Biol Psychiatry. 2004;55(7):759–65.

Scala JW, Levy KN, Johnson BN, Kivity Y, Ellison WD, Pincus AL, Wilson SJ, Newman MG. The role of negative affect and self-concept clarity in predicting self-injurious urges in borderline personality disorder using ecological momentary assessment. J Personal Disord. 2018;32(Supplement):36–57.

Selby EA. Understanding the relationship between emotional and behavioral dysregulation: a cascade of emotions, 2007.

Selby EA. A real-time evaluation of emotional cascades in borderline personality disorder (Doctoral dissertation, The Florida State University). 2011.

Selby EA, Joiner TE Jr. Cascades of emotion: the emergence of borderline personality disorder from emotional and behavioral dysregulation. Rev Gen Psychol. 2009;13(3):219–29.

Selby EA, Anestis MD, Joiner TE. Understanding the relationship between emotional and behavioral dysregulation: emotional cascades. Behav Res Ther. 2008;46(5):593–611.

Selby EA, Anestis MD, Bender TW, Joiner TE Jr. An exploration of the emotional cascade model in borderline personality disorder. J Abnorm Psychol. 2009;118(2):375.

Selby EA, Connell LD, Joiner TE. The pernicious blend of rumination and fearlessness in nonsuicidal self-injury. Cogn Ther Res. 2010;34:421–8.

Selby EA, Doyle P, Crosby RD, Wonderlich SA, Engel SG, Mitchell JD, Le Grange D. Momentary emotion surrounding bulimic behaviors in women with bulimia nervosa and borderline personality disorder. J Psychiatr Res. 2012;46(11):1492–500.

Selby EA, Franklin J, Carson-Wong A, Rizvi SL. Emotional cascades and self-injury: investigating instability of rumination and negative emotion. J Clin Psychol. 2013a;69(12):1213–27.

Selby EA, Ribeiro JD, Joiner TE Jr. What dreams may come: emotional cascades and nightmares in borderline personality disorder. Dreaming. 2013b;23(2):126.

Selby EA, Yen S, Spirito A. Time varying prediction of thoughts of death and suicidal ideation in adolescents: weekly ratings over 6-month follow-up. J Clin Child Adolesc Psychol. 2013c;42(4):481–95.

Selby EA, Kranzler A, Panza E. Development of emotional cascades in borderline personality disorder. In: Handbook of borderline personality disorder in children and adolescents. New York: Springer New York; 2014a. p. 159–76.

Selby EA, Joiner TE Jr, Ribeiro JD. Comprehensive theories of suicidal. In: The Oxford handbook of suicide and self-injury, vol. 8; 2014b. p. 286.

Selby EA, Nock MK, Kranzler A. How does self-injury feel? Examining automatic positive reinforcement in adolescent self-injurers with experience sampling. Psychiatry Res. 2014c;215(2):417–23.

Selby EA, Cornelius T, Fehling KB, Kranzler A, Panza EA, Lavender JM, Wonderlich SA, Crosby RD, Engel SG, Mitchell JE, Crow SJ. A perfect storm: examining the synergistic effects of negative and positive emotional instability on promoting weight loss activities in anorexia nervosa. Front Psychol. 2015a;6:1260.

Selby EA, Kranzler A, Fehling KB, Panza E. Nonsuicidal self-injury disorder: the path to diagnostic validity and final obstacles. Clin Psychol Rev. 2015b;38:79–91.

Selby EA, Gardner K. A latent profile analysis of suicidal and self-injurious behavior, other dysregulated behaviors, and borderline personality disorder symptoms. J Exp Psychopathol. 2015;6(4):356–68.

Selby EA, Kondratyuk S, Lindqvist J, Fehling K, Kranzler A. Temporal Bayesian Network modeling approach to evaluating the emotional cascade model of borderline personality disorder. Personal Disord Theory Res Treat. 2021;12(1):39.

Selby EA, Harnedy LE, Hiner M, Kim J. Developmental and momentary dynamics in the onset and maintenance of nonsuicidal self-injurious behavior and borderline personality disorder. Curr Psychiatry Rep. 2022;24(12):897–909.
Shaffer D, Jacobson C. Proposal to the DSM-V childhood disorder and mood disorder work groups to include nonsuicidal self-injury (NSSI) as a DSM-V disorder. American Psychiatric Association. 2009;2009:1–21.
Shafii M. Storm, stress, and suicide during adolescence. PsycCRITIQUES. 1985;30(7):568.
Shafti M, Taylor PJ, Forrester A, Pratt D. The co-occurrence of self-harm and aggression: a cognitive-emotional model of dual-harm. Front Psychol. 2021;12:586135.
Shah R, Zanarini MC. Comorbidity of borderline personality disorder: current status and future directions. Psychiatr Clin. 2018;41(4):583–93.
Sharp C, Vanwoerden S, Wall K. Adolescence as a sensitive period for the development of personality disorder. Psychiatr Clin. 2018;41(4):669–83.
Sharp C, Wall K. Personality pathology grows up: adolescence as a sensitive period. Curr Opin Psychol. 2018;21:111–6.
Shepherd-McMullen C, Mearns J, Stokes JE, Mechanic MB. Negative mood regulation expectancies moderate the relationship between psychological abuse and avoidant coping. J Interpers Violence. 2015;30(9):1553–66.
Shepard DS, Gurewich D, Lwin AK, Reed GA Jr, Silverman MM. Suicide and suicidal attempts in the United States: costs and policy implications. Suicide Life Threat Behav. 2016;46(3):352–62.
Sheppes G, Levin Z. Emotion regulation choice: selecting between cognitive regulation strategies to control emotion. Front Hum Neurosci. 2013;7:179.
Sheppes G, Scheibe S, Suri G, Gross JJ. Emotion-regulation choice. Psychol Sci. 2011;22(11):1391–6.
Silver J, Olino TM, Carlson GA, Dougherty LR, Klein DN. Utility of self-and parent-reported suicidal ideation in early childhood: prediction of suicidal ideation and psychopathology in adolescence. Suicide Life Threat Behav. 2023;53(1):89–99.
Silverman MM, Berman AL, Sanddal ND, O'carroll PW, Joiner TE Jr. Rebuilding the tower of Babel: a revised nomenclature for the study of suicide and suicidal behaviors. Part 2: suicide-related ideations, communications, and behaviors. Suicide Life Threat Behav. 2007a;37(3):264–77.
Silverman MM, Berman AL, Sanddal ND, O'carroll PW, Joiner TE Jr. Rebuilding the tower of Babel: a revised nomenclature for the study of suicide and suicidal behaviors. Part 1: background, rationale, and methodology. Suicide Life Threat Behav. 2007b;37(3):248–63.
Silvers JA, Hubbard AD, Chaudhury S, Biggs E, Shu J, Grunebaum MF, Fertuck E, Weber J, Kober H, Carson-Wong A, Brodsky BS. Suicide attempters with borderline personality disorder show differential orbitofrontal and parietal recruitment when reflecting on aversive memories. J Psychiatr Res. 2016;81:71–8.
Sitton MJ, Du Rocher ST, Byrne C. Psychosocial prediction of self-injurious behavior: a comparison of two populations. Prof Counsel. 2021;11(2):218–32.
Skegg K. Self-harm. Lancet. 2005;366(9495):1471–83.
Skodol AE, Gunderson JG, McGlashan TH, Dyck IR, Stout RL, Bender DS, Grilo CM, Shea MT, Zanarini MC, Morey LC, Sanislow CA. Functional impairment in patients with schizotypal, borderline, avoidant, or obsessive-compulsive personality disorder. Am J Psychiatry. 2002;159(2):276–83.
Slabbert A, Hasking P, Greene D, Boyes M. Measurement invariance of the distress tolerance scale among university students with and without a history of non-suicidal self-injury. PeerJ. 2021;9:e10915.
Slabbert A, Hasking P, Boyes M. Riding the emotional roller coaster: the role of distress tolerance in non-suicidal self-injury. Psychiatry Res. 2018;269:309–15.
Slabbert A, Hasking P, Notebaert L, Boyes M. Assessing distress tolerance using a modified version of the Emotional Image Tolerance task. J Exp Psychopathol. 2021;12(2):20438087211007597.
Slabbert A, Hasking P, Notebaert L, Boyes M. The role of distress tolerance in the relationship between affect and NSSI. Arch Suicide Res. 2022;26(2):761–75.

Slee N, Garnefski N, Spinhoven P, Arensman E. The influence of cognitive emotion regulation strategies and depression severity on deliberate self-harm. Suicide Life Threat Behav. 2008;38(3):274–86.

Sleuwaegen E, Houben M, Claes L, Berens A, Sabbe B. The relationship between nonsuicidal self-injury and alexithymia in borderline personality disorder:"Actions instead of words". Compr Psychiatry. 2017;77:80–8.

Smith T, Jalkanen JP, Anderson BA, Corbett JJ, Faber J, Hanayama S. 2014. General social surveys. 1972.

Smith AU, Reidy D. Bullying and suicide risk among sexual minority youth in the United States. Prev Med. 2021;153:106728.

Soloff P, White R, Diwadkar VA. Impulsivity, aggression and brain structure in high and low lethality suicide attempters with borderline personality disorder. Psychiatry Res Neuroimaging. 2014;222(3):131–9.

Somma A, Sharp C, Borroni S, Fossati A. Borderline personality disorder features, emotion dysregulation and non-suicidal self-injury: preliminary findings in a sample of community-dwelling Italian adolescents. Personal Ment Health. 2017;11(1):23–32.

Soto CJ, John OP. Traits in transition: the structure of parent-reported personality traits from early childhood to early adulthood. J Pers. 2014;82(3):182–99.

Soloff PH, Abraham K, Ramaseshan K, Burgess A, Diwadkar VA. Hyper-modulation of brain networks by the amygdala among women with Borderline Personality Disorder: network signatures of affective interference during cognitive processing. J Psychiatr Res. 2017;88:56–63.

Soloff PH. Emotional regulation and emotional processing. In: Handbook of personality disorders: theory, research, and treatment; 2018. p. 271–82.

Soloff PH, Chowdury A, Diwadkar VA. Affective interference in borderline personality disorder: the lethality of suicidal behavior predicts functional brain profiles. J Affect Disord. 2019;252:253–62.

Soloff PH, Lynch KG, Kelly TM, Malone KM, Mann JJ. Characteristics of suicide attempts of patients with major depressive episode and borderline personality disorder: a comparative study. Am J Psychiatry. 2000;157(4):601–8.

Spirito A, Esposito-Smythers C. Attempted and completed suicide in adolescence. Annu Rev Clin Psychol. 2006;2(1):237–66.

Spitzen TL, Tull MT, Baer MM, Dixon-Gordon KL, Chapman AL, Gratz KL. Predicting engagement in nonsuicidal self-injury (NSSI) over the course of 12 months: the roles of borderline personality disorder pathology and emotional consequences of NSSI. J Affect Disord. 2020;277:631–9.

Stänicke LI, Haavind H, Gullestad SE. How do young people understand their own self-harm? A meta-synthesis of adolescents' subjective experience of self-harm. Adolesc Res Rev. 2018;3(2):173–91.

Stanley IH, Hom MA, Boffa JW, Stage DR, Joiner TE. PTSD from a suicide attempt: an empirical investigation among suicide attempt survivors. J Clin Psychol. 2019;75(10):1879–95.

Stanley B, Brodsky BS, Gratch I. Dialectical behavior therapy. In: The American Psychiatric Association publishing textbook of personality disorders, vol. 31; 2021. p. 361.

Stead VE, Boylan K, Schmidt LA. Longitudinal associations between nonsuicidal self-injury and borderline personality disorder in adolescents: a literature review. Borderline Personal Disord Emot Dysregul. 2019;6:1–2.

Stepp SD, Whalen DJ, Scott LN, Zalewski M, Loeber R, Hipwell AE. Reciprocal effects of parenting and borderline personality disorder symptoms in adolescent girls. Dev Psychopathol. 2014;26(2):361–78.

Stone MH. A new look at borderline personality disorder and related disorders: hyper-reactivity in the limbic system and lower centers. Psychodynam Psychiatr. 2013;41(3):437–66.

Stone MH. Determining amenability to psychotherapy in patients with borderline disorders. Psychiatr Ann. 2004;34(6):437–45.

Stone MH. Borderline patients: 25 to 50 years later: with commentary on outcome factors. Psychodynam Psychiatr. 2017;45(2):259–96.
Stefa-Missagli S, Unterrainer HF, Giupponi G, Holasek SJ, Kapfhammer HP, Conca A, Sarlo M, Erbuto D, Rogante E, Moujaes-Droescher H, Davok K. Suicide and personality traits: a multicenter study of Austrian and Italian psychiatric patients and students. Suicide Life Threat Behav. 2020;50(1):220–32.
Sublette ME, Milak MS, Galfalvy HC, Oquendo MA, Malone KM, Mann JJ. Regional brain glucose uptake distinguishes suicide attempters from non-attempters in major depression. Arch Suicide Res. 2013;17(4):434–47.
Swannell SV, Martin GE, Page A, Hasking P, St John NJ. Prevalence of nonsuicidal self-injury in nonclinical samples: systematic review, meta-analysis and meta-regression. Suicide Life Threat Behav. 2014;44(3):273–303.
Tang H, Xiong T, Shi J, Chen Y, Liu X, Zhang S, Wang H, Lu Q, Yao Z. Global and reflective rumination are related to suicide attempts among patients experiencing major depressive episodes. BMC Psychiatry. 2021;21:1–9.
Tang J, Ma Y, Lewis SP, Chen R, Clifford A, Ammerman BA, Gazimbi MM, Byrne A, Wu Y, Lu X, Chang H. Association of internet addiction with nonsuicidal self-injury among adolescents in China. JAMA Netw Open. 2020;3(6):e206863.
Tangney JP, Dearing RL. Shame and guilt. Guilford Press; 2003.
Tatnell R, Hasking P, Lipp OV, Boyes M, Dawkins J. Emotional responding in NSSI: examinations of appraisals of positive and negative emotional stimuli, with and without acute stress. Cognit Emot. 2018;32(6):1304–16.
Taylor CD, Bee P, Haddock G. Does schema therapy change schemas and symptoms? A systematic review across mental health disorders. Psychol Psychother Theory Res Pract. 2017;90(3):456–79.
Taylor PJ, Jomar K, Dhingra K, Forrester R, Shahmalak U, Dickson JM. A meta-analysis of the prevalence of different functions of nonsuicidal self-injury. J Affect Disord. 2018;227:759–69.
Teismann T, Forkmann T, Michalak J, Brailovskaia J. Repetitive negative thinking about suicide: associations with lifetime suicide attempts. Clin Psychol Eur. 2021;3(3):e5579.
Teismann T, Forkmann T, Glaesmer H, Alpers GW, Brakemeier EL, Brockmeyer T, Christiansen H, Fehm L, Glombiewski J, Heider J, Hermann A. Prevalence of suicidal ideation in German psychotherapy outpatients: a large multicenter assessment. J Affect Disord. 2024;351:971–6.
Temes CM, Frankenburg FR, Fitzmaurice GM, Zanarini MC. Deaths by suicide and other causes among patients with borderline personality disorder and personality-disordered comparison subjects over 24 years of prospective follow-up. J Clin Psychiatry. 2019;80(1):4039.
Tonta KE, Hasking P, Boyes M, Howell J, McEvoy P, Kiekens G. Measurement invariance of three brief measures of rumination in young adults with and without a history of self-injury. Eur J Psychol Assess. 2020;18
Tonta KE, Boyes M, Howell J, McEvoy P, Johnson A, Hasking P. Modeling pathways to non-suicidal self-injury: the roles of perfectionism, negative affect, rumination, and attention control. J Clin Psychol. 2022;78(7):1463–77.
Tresno F, Ito Y, Mearns J. Self-injurious behavior and suicide attempts among Indonesian college students. Death Stud. 2012;36(7):627–39.
Trull TJ, Widiger TA, Lynam DR, Costa PT Jr. Borderline personality disorder from the perspective of general personality functioning. Focus. 2005;112(3):193–464.
Trull TJ, Tomko RL, Brown WC, Scheiderer EM. Borderline personality disorder in 3-D: dimensions, symptoms, and measurement challenge. Soc Personal Psychol Compass. 2010;4(11):1057–69.
Trull TJ, Solhan MB, Tragesser SL, Jahng S, Wood PK, Piasecki TM, Watson D. Affective instability: measuring a core feature of borderline personality disorder with ecological momentary assessment. J Abnorm Psychol. 2008;117(3):647.
Tschan T, Peter-Ruf C, Schmid M, In-Albon T. Temperament and character traits in female adolescents with nonsuicidal self-injury disorder with and without comorbid borderline personality disorder. Child Adolesc Psychiatry Ment Health. 2017;11:1–0.

Tschan T, Schmid M, In-Albon T. Parenting behavior in families of female adolescents with non-suicidal self-injury in comparison to a clinical and a nonclinical control group. Child Adolesc Psychiatry Ment Health. 2015;9:1–9.

Tsiachristas A, Geulayov G, Casey D, Ness J, Waters K, Clements C, Kapur N, McDaid D, Brand F, Hawton K. Incidence and general hospital costs of self-harm across England: estimates based on the multicentre study of self-harm. Epidemiol Psychiatr Sci. 2020;29:e108.

Tsoh JY, Delucchi KL, Hall SM, Lam JN. Smoking and depression in Chinese Americans. Am J Med Sci. 2003;326(4):187–91.

Tsoh J, Chiu HF, Duberstein PR, Chan SS, Chi I, Yip PS, Conwell Y. Attempted suicide in elderly Chinese persons: a multi-group, controlled study. Am J Geriatr Psychiatry. 2005;13(7):562–71.

Turecki G. Dissecting the suicide phenotype: the role of impulsive–aggressive behaviours: 2003 CCNP Young Investigator Award Paper. J Psychiatry Neurosci. 2005;30(6):398–408.

Turner BJ, Layden BK, Butler SM, Chapman AL. How often, or how many ways: clarifying the relationship between non-suicidal self-injury and suicidality. Arch Suicide Res. 2013;17(4):397–415.

Turner BJ, Kleiman EM, Nock MK. Psychopathology and risk of suicide, 2018.

Turner K, Sveticic J, Almeida-Crasto A, Gaee-Atefi T, Green V, Grice D, Kelly P, Krishnaiah R, Lindsay L, Mayahle B, Patist C. Implementing a systems approach to suicide prevention in a mental health service using the Zero Suicide Framework. Austr New Zealand J Psychiatr. 2021;55(3):241–53.

Turner BJ, Helps CE, Ames ME. Stop self-injuring, then what? Psychosocial risk associated with initiation and cessation of nonsuicidal self-injury from adolescence to early adulthood. J Psychopathol Clin Sci. 2022;131(1):45.

Turp M. The physicality of the self, 2003.

Tyrer P, Reed GM, Crawford MJ. Classification, assessment, prevalence, and effect of personality disorder. Lancet. 2015;385(9969):717–26.

Um M, Hershberger AR, Whitt ZT, Cyders MA. Recommendations for applying a multi-dimensional model of impulsive personality to diagnosis and treatment. Borderline Personal Disord Emot Dysregul. 2018;5:1–7.

Useda JD, Duberstein PR, Conner KR, Beckman A, Franus N, Tu X, Conwell Y. Personality differences in attempted suicide versus suicide in adults 50 years of age or older. J Consult Clin Psychol. 2007;75(1):126.

Vaartstra LD, Taone T, Mezulis A. Cognitive reactivity as a risk factor for nonsuicidal self-injury in young adults. J Am Coll Heal. 2023;12:1–7.

Valencia J, Sinambela FC. Nonsuicidal self-injury in those dealing with borderline personality disorder or separation from parents. KnE Soc Sci. 2020:50–64.

Valencia-Agudo F, Burcher GC, Ezpeleta L, Kramer T. Nonsuicidal self-injury in community adolescents: a systematic review of prospective predictors, mediators and moderators. J Adolesc. 2018;65:25–38. https://doi.org/10.18502/kss.v4i15.8190

van Dijk F, Schellekens A, van den Broek P, Kan C, Verkes RJ, Buitelaar J. Do cognitive measures of response inhibition differentiate between attention deficit/hyperactivity disorder and borderline personality disorder? Psychiatry Res. 2014;215(3):733–9.

Van den Broeck K, Claes L, Pieters G, Berens A, Raes F. Autobiographical memory specificity and nonsuicidal self-injury in borderline personality disorder. J Exp Psychopathol. 2015;6(4):398–410.

Van Heeringen K, Mann JJ. The neurobiology of suicide. Lancet Psychiatry. 2014;1(1):63–72.

Vansteenkiste M, Ryan RM. On psychological growth and vulnerability: basic psychological need satisfaction and need frustration as a unifying principle. J Psychother Integr. 2013;23(3):263.

Vartanian LR. When the body defines the self: self-concept clarity, internalization, and body image. J Soc Clin Psychol. 2009;28(1):94–126.

Vartanian LR, Pinkus RT, Smyth JM. Experiences of weight stigma in everyday life: implications for health motivation. Stigma Health. 2018;3(2):85.

Vega D, Sintes A, Fernández M, Puntí J, Soler J, Santamarina P, Soto À, Lara A, Méndez I, Martínez-Giménez R, Romero S. Review and update on nonsuicidal self-injury: who, how and why? Actas espanolas de psiquiatria. 2018;46(4):146–55.

Victor SE, Klonsky ED. Daily emotion in non-suicidal self-injury. J Clin Psychol. 2014a;70(4):364–75.
Victor SE, Klonsky ED. Correlates of suicide attempts among self-injurers: a meta-analysis. Clin Psychol Rev. 2014b;34(4):282–97.
Victor SE, Styer D, Washburn JJ. Characteristics of nonsuicidal self-injury associated with suicidal ideation: evidence from a clinical sample of youth. Child Adolesc Psychiatry Ment Health. 2015;9:1–8.
Vijayakumar L, Phillips M. Suicide prevention in low-and middle-income countries. In: The international handbook of suicide prevention; 2016. p. 505–23.
Voon D, Hasking P, Martin G. The roles of emotion regulation and ruminative thoughts in non-suicidal self-injury. Br J Clin Psychol. 2014;53(1):95–113.
Voracek M, Loibl LM, Kandrychyn S. Testing the Finno-Ugrian suicide hypothesis: replication and refinement with regional suicide data from Eastern Europe. Percept Mot Skills. 2007;104(3):985–94.
Wadman R, Vostanis P, Sayal K, Majumder P, Harroe C, Clarke D, Armstrong M, Townsend E. An interpretative phenomenological analysis of young people's self-harm in the context of interpersonal stressors and supports: parents, peers, and clinical services. Soc Sci Med. 2018;212:120–8.
Walsh BW, Rosen PM. Self-mutilation: theory, research, and treatment. The Guilford Press; 1988.
Wang YJ, Li X, Ng CH, Xu DW, Hu S, Yuan TF. Risk factors for nonsuicidal self-injury (NSSI) in adolescents: a meta-analysis. E Clin Med. 2022;1:46.
Watson D, Clark LA. Extraversion and its positive emotional core. In: Handbook of personality psychology. Academic Press; 1997. p. 767–93.
Watt-McMahon K, Mildred H, King R, Craigie G, Hyder S, Hall K. Understanding chronic suicidality in borderline personality disorder through comparison with depressive disorder: a systematic review. Clin Psychol. 2023;27(2):232–58.
Wedig MM, Frankenburg FR, Reich DB, Fitzmaurice G, Zanarini MC. Predictors of suicide threats in patients with borderline personality disorder over 16 years of prospective follow-up. Psychiatry Res. 2013;208(3):252–6.
Weierich MR, Nock MK. Posttraumatic stress symptoms mediate the relation between childhood sexual abuse and nonsuicidal self-injury. J Consult Clin Psychol. 2008;76(1):39.
Weintraub MJ, Van de Loo MM, Gitlin MJ, Miklowitz DJ. Self-harm, affective traits, and psychosocial functioning in adults with depressive and bipolar disorders. J Nerv Ment Dis. 2017;205(11):896–9.
Weis D, Rothenberg L, Moshe L, Brent DA, Hamdan S. The effect of sleep problems on suicidal risk among young adults in the presence of depressive symptoms and cognitive processes. Arch Suicide Res. 2015;19(3):321–34.
Westad YA, Hagen K, Jonsbu E, Solem S. Cessation of deliberate self-harm behavior in patients with borderline personality traits treated with outpatient dialectical behavior therapy. Front Psychol. 2021;12:578230.
Whitlock J, Muehlenkamp J, Purington A, Eckenrode J, Barreira P, Baral Abrams G, Marchell T, Kress V, Girard K, Chin C, Knox K. Nonsuicidal self-injury in a college population: general trends and sex differences. J Am Coll Heal. 2011;59(8):691–8.
Whitlock J, Eckenrode J, Silverman D. Self-injurious behaviors in a college population. Pediatrics. 2006;117(6):1939–48.
Whitlock J, Muehlenkamp J, Eckenrode J. Variation in nonsuicidal self-injury: identification and features of latent classes in a college population of emerging adults. J Clin Child Adolesc Psychol. 2008;37(4):725–35.
Whitlock J, Prussien K, Pietrusza C. Predictors of self-injury cessation and subsequent psychological growth: results of a probability sample survey of students in eight universities and colleges. Child Adolesc Psychiatry Ment Health. 2015;9:1–2.
Widiger TA, Costa PT Jr. Personality disorders and the five-factor model of personality: rationale for the. 3rd ed. American Psychological Association; 2013.

Wilcox HC, Arria AM, Caldeira KM, Vincent KB, Pinchevsky GM, O'Grady KE. Longitudinal predictors of past-year nonsuicidal self-injury and motives among college students. Psychol Med. 2012;42(4):717–26.

Wilson ML, Dunlavy AC, Viswanathan B, Bovet P. Suicidal expression among school-attending adolescents in a middle-income sub-Saharan country. Int J Environ Res Public Health. 2012;9(11):4122–34.

Wilkinson P. Nonsuicidal self-injury. Eur Child Adolesc Psychiatry. 2013;22:75–9.

Wilkinso4n P, Kelvin R, Roberts C, Dubicka B, Goodyer I. Clinical and psychosocial predictors of suicide attempts and nonsuicidal self-injury in the Adolescent Depression Antidepressants and Psychotherapy Trial (ADAPT). Am J Psychiatry. 2011;168(5):495–501.

Wilkinson PO, Qiu T, Jesmont C, Neufeld SA, Kaur SP, Jones PB, Goodyer IM. Age and gender effects on nonsuicidal self-injury, and their interplay with psychological distress. J Affect Disord. 2022;306:240–5.

Williams AE, Yelland C, Hollamby S, Wigley M, Aylward P. A new therapeutic group to help women with borderline personality disorder and their infants. J Psychiatr Pract. 2018;24(5):331–40.

Witt K, Boland A, Lamblin M, McGorry PD, Veness B, Cipriani A, Hawton K, Harvey S, Christensen H, Robinson J. Effectiveness of universal programmes for the prevention of suicidal ideation, behaviour and mental ill health in medical students: a systematic review and meta-analysis. BMJ Ment Health. 2019;22(2):84–90.

Wolff JC, Thompson E, Thomas SA, Nesi J, Bettis AH, Ransford B, Scopelliti K, Frazier EA, Liu RT. Emotion dysregulation and nonsuicidal self-injury: a systematic review and meta-analysis. Eur Psychiatry. 2019;59:25–36.

World Health Organization. WHO guidelines on mental health at work. World Health Organization; 2022.

World Health Organization. The WHO special initiative for mental health (2019–2023): universal health coverage for mental health. World Health Organization; 2019.

World Health Organization (WHO), 2014

Wyder M, De Leo D. Behind impulsive suicide attempts: indications from a community study. J Affect Disord. 2007;104(1–3):167–73.

Xie GD, Chang JJ, Yuan MY, Wang GF, He Y, Chen SS, Su PY. Childhood abuse and borderline personality disorder features in Chinese undergraduates: the role of self-esteem and resilience. BMC Psychiatry. 2021;21:1–9.

Xie X, Li Y, Liu J, Zhang L, Sun T, Zhang C, Liu Z, Liu J, Wen L, Gong X, Cai Z. The relationship between childhood maltreatment and non-suicidal self-injury in adolescents with depressive disorders. Psychiatry Res. 2024;331:115638.

Xiao Q, Song X, Huang L, Hou D, Huang X. Global prevalence and characteristics of nonsuicidal self-injury between 2010 and 2021 among a non-clinical sample of adolescents: a meta-analysis. Front Psych. 2022a;13:912441.

Xiao H, Double KS, Walker SA, Kunst H, MacCann C. Emotionally intelligent people use more high-engagement and less low-engagement processes to regulate others' emotions. J Intelligence. 2022b;10(4):76.

Xuan Z, Naimi TS, Kaplan MS, Bagge CL, Few LR, Maisto S, Saitz R, Freeman R. Alcohol policies and suicide: a review of the literature. Alcohol Clin Exp Res. 2016;40(10):2043–55.

Yakeley J, Burbridge-James W. Psychodynamic approaches to suicide and self-harm. B J Psych Adv. 2018;24(1):37–45.

Yates TM. Developmental pathways from child maltreatment to nonsuicidal self-injury, 2004.

Yen S, Johnson J, Costello E, Simpson EB. A 5-day dialectical behavior therapy partial hospital program for women with borderline personality disorder: predictors of outcome from a 3-month follow-up study. J Psychiatr Pract. 2009;15(3):173–82.

Yen S, Shea MT, Sanislow CA, Grilo CM, Skodol AE, Gunderson JG, McGlashan TH, Zanarini MC, Morey LC. Borderline personality disorder criteria associated with prospectively observed suicidal behavior. Am J Psychiatry. 2004;161(7):1296–8.

Yen S, Gagnon K, Spirito A. Borderline personality disorder in suicidal adolescents. Personal Ment Health. 2013;7(2):89–101.

Yen CF, Liu TL, Yang P, Hu HF. Risk and protective factors of suicidal ideation and attempt among adolescents with different types of school bullying involvement. Arch Suicide Res. 2015;19(4):435–52.

Yen S, Ranney ML, Krek M, Peters JR, Mereish E, Tezanos KM, Kahler CW, Solomon J, Beard C, Spirito A. Skills to enhance positivity in suicidal adolescents: results from a pilot randomized clinical trial. J Posit Psychol. 2020;15(3):348–61.

You J, Leung F, Lai CM, Fu K. The associations between nonsuicidal self-injury and borderline personality disorder features among Chinese adolescents. J Personal Disord. 2012;26(2): 226–37.

Ystgaard M, Hestetun I, Loeb M, Mehlum L. Is there a specific relationship between childhood sexual and physical abuse and repeated suicidal behavior? Child Abuse Negl. 2004;28(8): 863–75.

Zaki J. Cue integration: a common framework for social cognition and physical perception. Perspect Psychol Sci. 2013;8(3):296–312.

Zaki SM, Abd El-Kader NM, Fahmy HD, Abd El-Aziz AM, EL-Magd MH. Impulsivity, depression and aggression among psychiatric patients. J Biol Agric Healthc. 2013a;3(15)

Zaki LF, Coifman KG, Rafaeli E, Berenson KR, Downey G. Emotion differentiation as a protective factor against nonsuicidal self-injury in borderline personality disorder. Behav Ther. 2013b;44(3):529–40.

Zanarini MC. Childhood experiences associated with the development of borderline personality disorder. Psychiatr Clin N Am. 2000;23(1):89–101.

Zanarini MC, Frankenburg FR. The essential nature of borderline psychopathology. J Personal Disord. 2007;21(5):518–35.

Zanarini MC, Frankenburg FR, Reich DB, Fitzmaurice G, Weinberg I, Gunderson JG. The 10-year course of physically self-destructive acts reported by borderline patients and axis II comparison subjects. Acta Psychiatr Scand. 2008;117(3):177–84.

Zanarini MC, Horwood J, Wolke D, Waylen A, Fitzmaurice G, Grant BF. Prevalence of DSM-IV borderline personality disorder in two community samples: 6,330 English 11-year-olds and 34,653 American adults. J Personal Disord. 2011;25(5):607–19.

Zalta AK, Tirone V, Orlowska D, Blais RK, Lofgreen A, Klassen B, Held P, Stevens NR, Adkins E, Dent AL. Examining moderators of the relationship between social support and self-reported PTSD symptoms: a meta-analysis. Psychol Bull. 2021;147(1):33.

Zelkowitz RL, Cole DA. Measures of emotion reactivity and emotion regulation: convergent and discriminant validity. Personal Individ Differ. 2016;102:123–32.

Zettle RD, Hocker TR, Mick KA, Scofield BE, Petersen CL, Song H, Sudarijanto RP. Differential strategies in coping with pain as a function of level of experiential avoidance. Psychol Rec. 2005;55:511–24.

Zlotnick C, Mattia JI, Zimmerman M. Clinical correlates of self-mutilation in a sample of general psychiatric patients. J Nerv Ment Dis. 1999;187(5):296–301.

Chapter 13
Post-Traumatic Stress Disorder (PTSD)/ Complex Post-Traumatic Stress Disorder (C-PTSD) and Borderline Personality Disorder

Introduction

Borderline personality disorder (BPD) is a serious mental issue (Pascual et al. 2023; APA 2022; Bohus et al. 2021), contributing to substantial personal, social, and economic devastation (Van Asselt et al. 2007; Dixon-Gordon et al. 2013a). Individuals with BPD are characterized by disturbed interpersonal relationships, emotional instability, emotion dysregulation, heightened impulsivity especially under stress, destructive behaviors, suicidal ideation or attempts, deliberated self-injurious behaviors, and identity disturbance (American Psychiatric Association 2022; Jowett et al. 2020; Selby et al. 2022), cognitive impairment with a great tendency to focus on negative information (Kelly Grealy et al. 2022), and executive functions issues such as attention, learning, memory, planning, and visuospatial skills (Ruocco 2005). BPD is the most prevalent personality disorder, influencing 1.8–2.7% of the general population (Winsper et al. 2020; APA 2022; Bohus et al. 2021). According to several prevalence estimations of BPD, the lifetime prevalence is reported at 5.9% in the general population (Grant et al. 2008; Gross et al. 2002; Trull et al. 2010; Gunderson et al. 2018a, b; Stepp et al. 2016), with 10–20% of psychiatry outpatients and 15–50% of inpatients suffering from BPD (Lieb et al. 2004; Gunderson et al. 2018a, b; Stepp et al. 2016). In primary care settings, the prevalence rates of BPD in psychiatric outpatients and inpatients have been reported at 6%, 11–12%, and 22%, respectively (Zimmerman and Becker 2023; Ellison et al. 2018, 2020).

Exposure to trauma and traumatic life events is common across the world (Olff 2020; Kessler et al. 2017; Krause-Utz 2021). Approximately, 50–60% of people in the USA and nearly 70% of individuals all over the world (Kessler et al. 2017; Shalev et al. 2017) are prone to experience a traumatic, stressful event in their lifetime, such as physical or sexual assaults, natural disasters, accidents, man-made violence, war, or motor vehicle accidents (Olff 2020; Kessler et al. 2017; Feeney

M. Salavati, E. A. Selby, *Theories of Borderline Personality Disorder*,
https://doi.org/10.1007/978-3-031-75503-3_13

and Kenny 2022; Hébert and Amédée 2020; Gluck et al. 2021). In a large representative sample that included 68,894 adults from 24 countries, more than 70% of participants reported experiencing a traumatic event (Benjet et al. 2016; Kessler et al. 2017). However, authors have discussed the role of early childhood trauma in contributing to changes in child development that go far beyond the major symptoms of PTSD (Ford 2015a, b; Hébert and Amédée 2020). Exposure to traumatic life experiences has been revealed to be frequent in psychiatric populations, especially when involved in multiple exposures (Grubaugh et al. 2011; Gottlieb et al. 2018; Møller et al. 2020). The majority of individuals who experienced traumatic events do not develop significantly long-term psychopathology (Kessler et al. 2013; Lewis and Grenyer 2009), whereas only a considerable minority of them continue to experience a constellation of symptoms diagnosed as post-traumatic stress disorder (PTSD) (Feeney and Kenny 2022; Møller et al. 2020; Mauritz et al. 2013, 2021, 2022), and approximately 3.9–5.6% of traumatized individuals show PTSD symptoms (Koenen et al. 2017). PTSD, a well-known reaction to trauma (Powers et al. 2022a, b), which is characterized by re-experiencing the traumatic event in the form of nightmares, flashbacks, or vivid intrusive memories accompanied with fear and horror, avoidance of reminders of traumatic events, and persistent perceptions of increased threat such as hypervigilance (Møller et al. 2021), distorted negative beliefs and expectation, distorted cognitions revealed in self-criticize, and feelings of detachment or isolation from others (Karatzias et al. 2017; Simon et al. 2016; Friedman 2013). PTSD is characterized by traumatic re-experiencing, avoidance of traumatic reminders, and hypervigilance (WHO, ICD-11 2018; World Health Organization 2018). After being exposed to a traumatic event, the estimated risk for the development of PTSD is 5–10% (Kessler et al. 2017; Snoek et al. 2021), which can be higher depending on the nature of the traumatic event (Breslau et al. 1998; Snoek et al. 2021). Experiencing trauma can contribute to substantial distress, functional disturbances, and may lead to the development of trauma-related disorders (Gluck et al. 2021; George et al. 2016; Ressler et al. 2022). PTSD is a common disorder that causes a disabling condition among patients, and emerges after experiencing a sudden, catastrophic, or threatening event (Gratz and Tull 2012; Murray and El-Leithy 2022), contributing to the development of severe and persistent psychiatric symptoms (Gratz and Tull 2012). Among any psychiatric disorder, PTSD manifests the most serious and varied pattern of comorbidity (Brown et al. 2011; Brown and McNiff 2009; Galatzer-Levy et al. 2013), reporting 75% comorbidity with at least one other mental disorder (Kessler et al. 2017), especially depression, anxiety, and substance use disorder (Murray and El-Leithy 2022). Mood disorders have the most frequent comorbidity with BPD (Pascual et al. 2023), with an estimated one or more episodes of major depressive disorder (MDD) in 80% of individuals diagnosed with BPD in their lifetime, and 10–30% of MDD patients showed co-occurring BPD (Bohus et al. 2021; Trull et al. 2010; Gunderson et al. 2004; Jowett et al. 2020). The lifetime comorbidity of BPD and anxiety disorders is significantly high estimated at 84.8%, and it was shown that individuals with BPD are 14 times more likely to show anxiety symptoms and disorders, especially panic disorder with agoraphobia, GAD, and PTSD (Tomko et al. 2014; Shah and Zanarini 2018).

Frequent traumatic experiences are common in individuals suffering from BPD, and 20–75% of BPD patients report traumatic experiences during childhood (Yen et al. 2004; McGlashan et al. 2005). Although experiencing trauma is neither crucial nor sufficient to elucidate the psychopathology of BPD (Tragesser et al. 2007) and is not a prerequisite for assigning a diagnosis of BPD (Rosenstein et al. 2018), a substantial body of investigations has indicated high rates of traumatic life events that can directly lead to the development of BPD (Akiskal 1994; Masland et al. 2023; Rosenstein et al. 2018), and other psychiatric issues such as dissociation (Frewen et al. 2014; Reinders et al. 2023).

On the authority of nationally representative samples, it was demonstrated that one-fourth of individuals with PTSD met the criteria for BPD as well (Pagura et al. 2010), and more than 50% of individuals diagnosed with BPD met the criteria for lifetime PTSD (Scheiderer et al. 2015). Golier et al. (2003a) assessed the association between BPD and PTSD with regard to the role of trauma and its timing among a large, carefully characterized group of outpatients with one or more personality disorders. The results showed that high rates of early and lifetime trauma were obtained for all participants. Individuals with BPD indicated greater rates of childhood/adolescence physical abuse and were twice as likely to develop PTSD. In line with the path analysis of the association between BPD and PTSD, none of the different kinds of paths, including the direct paths, indirect paths through adulthood traumas, and paths sharing the antecedent of child abuse, were significant. The data showed that individuals with BPD were not more likely to be physically or sexually abused or to experience accidents, crimes, disasters, or other trauma in adulthood compared with participants diagnosed with other personality disorders. Participants with BPD were twice as likely to develop PTSD than individuals without BPD (Golier et al. 2003a, b).

BPD and Post-Traumatic Stress Disorder (PTSD)

The comorbidity of BPD and PTSD is notably well-documented (Harned et al. 2012, 2014), and is very common (Pascual et al. 2023), yet not well understood (Scheiderer et al. 2015, 2016). Numerous clinical and empirical studies have recognized the comorbidity of PTSD and BPD (e.g., Jowett et al. 2020; Cloitre et al. 2014; Brewin et al. 2017). As reported by studies, 24–68% of individuals with PTSD also met BPD criteria, and 25–39% of BPD cases also have PTSD symptoms (Pagura et al. 2010), with 10.42% total odds of lifetime BPD and PTSD (Carpenter et al. 2023a, b). The prevalence of PTSD among individuals who meet the BPD diagnostic threshold ranges from 34% to 46% (Slotema et al. 2018). Findings from treatment-seeking clinical samples have revealed rates of BPD among individuals with PTSD ranging from 10% to 76%, and rates of PTSD among people with BPD ranging from 25% to 58% (Pagura et al. 2010). The discrepant findings in this line of research present the existence of PTSD symptoms in some individuals with BPD (Gunderson and Sabo 2013; Sar et al. 2006) and suggest different rates of this comorbidity across studies due to the variety of diagnostic criteria, methods of sampling and assessment, and the management of extraneous variables such as demographics and other comorbidities (Scheiderer et al. 2015). Miller et al. (2012) clarified the association of BPD with symptoms to disorders of the internalizing and externalizing continuum among 214 trauma-exposed veterans with a high prevalence of PTSD. The findings of confirmatory analyses showed a three-factor model comprised of Externalizing, Fear, and Distress factors. Pursuant to the analyses, the location of BPD displayed significant cross-loadings for BPD on both Externalizing and Fear. Furthermore, structural equation models indicated that negative emotionality personality traits were significantly associated with all three comorbidity factors, in turn positive emotionality personality traits showed specific relations with Distress and Externalizing, particularly (Miller et al. 2012). In line with several investigations, nearly half of the patients diagnosed with PTSD also met the criteria for at least one personality disorder. In keeping with these studies, there is a substantial association between PTSD and BPD (Goldstein et al. 2021; Kolthof et al. 2022). For example, findings suggested that 25–30% of adult individuals with PTSD also are diagnosed with BPD, and 30–70% of adults with BPD meet the criteria for PTSD (Frías and Palma 2015). Depending on the type of studies, comorbidity of BPD and PTSD varies. Studies recruiting clinical samples presented rates of PTSD in BPD patients ranging from 25% to 58%, while rates of BPD among PTSD individuals ranging from 10% to 76% (Pagura et al. 2010). Epidemiological findings have revealed that 25–30% of individuals with PTSD also meet the criteria for BPD, 30%–70% of individuals with BPD show some criteria of PTSD during their lifetime (Frías and Palma 2015; Kolthof et al. 2022). Additionally, the prevalence rates of comorbid PTSD among BPD patients were reported to range from 30% to 50% (Pagura et al. 2010; Grant et al. 2008; McGlashan et al. 2000), while the comorbidity of BPD among PTSD cases ranged from 6.6% to 24% (Pagura et al. 2010; Pietrzak et al. 2011; Lezenweger et al. 2007). Ford and Courtois (2021) suggested that BPD and PTSD are associated with and overlap with other psychological conditions on a spectrum of post-traumatic syndromes that begin with childhood maltreatment and adverse childhood experiences, and then later develop into diagnoses with high rates of morbidity, including PTSD and BPD (Ford and Courtois 2021). Dell'Osso et al. (2019) identified the association between rumination, PTSD, and mood spectrum in BPD individuals with or without comorbid mood disorders among 50 BPD patients, divided into two groups: BPD (only) and BPD + Mood disorder. The findings revealed a significantly high level of PTSD, mood disorders, and rumination symptoms in both BPD groups. Moreover, rumination scores and PTSD symptoms were considerably associated with the presence of both BPD and BPD+MD. To summarize, these results supported the association between BPD and the PTSD spectrum, highlighting the role of rumination in BP pathology (Dell'Osso et al. 2019).

Through a literature review for the period between 1990 and 2013, Frías and Palma (2015) examined the major theoretical studies and research findings to describe the comorbidity of BPD and PTSD. The epidemiological results indicated a significantly higher prevalence of PTSD in subjects with BPD compared to the general population (Frías and Palma 2015), for instance, up to 58% of BPD individuals also met PTSD criteria (Zanarini et al. 2004). This association was elucidated based on two approaches: one disorder as a risk factor for the other, and the existence of third variables, with both approaches being considered complementary. In other words, it was hypothesized that childhood trauma may change the development of subcortical constructs, leading to increased vulnerability to elevated emotional dysregulation in interpersonal stressors (BPD), which contributes to increased likelihood of engaging in high-risk behaviors associated with traumatic memories in adulthood (PTSD). Difficulties in emotion regulation are a documented risk factor for the development and maintenance of PTSD (Coyne et al. 2023), and emotion dysregulation is a core feature of BPD as well (Aleva et al. 2023). The severity and complexity of difficulties in emotion regulation in individuals with BP pathology show substantial rates of co-occurring psychological disorders such as PTSD (Brown and Dahlin 2017). Experiencing violent events and exposure to violence may destroy the regulatory capacities of adolescents (Cummings et al. 2009), leading to issues in modulating severe emotional distress and arousal (Mennin et al. 2005). In line with Buckholdt et al. (2016), exposure to violence was associated with higher difficulties in emotion regulation, contributing to greater post-traumatic stress symptoms (PTSS) and BP pathology. Additionally, it was indicated that emotion dysregulation mediated the relations between exposure to violence and both PTSD and BP pathology (Buckholdt et al. 2016). A growing body of studies has shown a significant association between serious negative consequences and maladaptive behaviors related to the co-occurrence of BPD and PTSD (e.g., Miller and Resick 2007; Harned et al. 2018), comprising suicidal and other self-destructive behaviors (Connor et al. 2002; Harned et al. 2010; Brown and Dahlin 2017). Extant clinical studies (e.g., Harned et al. 2010) and community investigations (e.g., Pagura et al. 2010; Goldstein et al. 2011) have proposed that the comorbidity of BPD-PTSD reveals a variety of issues, such as general impairment, decreased levels of health-related quality of life, and heightened rate of usage of healthcare services (Scheiderer et al. 2016). In cases of comorbidity of BPD and PTSD, emotion regulation issues, suicidal ideation and behaviors, and self-injurious behaviors are noteworthy (Feeney and Kenny 2022). Approximately 79% of BPD individuals meet PTSD diagnostic criteria which can contribute to more functional impairments (Harned et al. 2013, 2018). Borderline personality disorder dispositions have been shown to play a significant role impacting severe PTSD symptoms and serious mental health matters such as NSSI (e.g., Deng et al. 2023), and greater functional disturbances and psychological distress (Boritz et al. 2016; Frías and Palma 2015).

According to the current literature, borderline and avoidant personality disorders (AVPD) particularly are the most common personality disorders among PTSD cases (Bollinger et al. 2000) and relevant to deliberate self-harm (Gratz and Tull 2012), especially because of the strong link between BPD and impaired tolerance of emotional distress and several distress regulation issues (Linehan 1993; Taylor et al. 2006; Chapman 2019; Gratz et al. 2010; Gratz and Tull 2012). In addition, in compliance with recent findings, BPD pathology moderates the relationship between deliberate self-harm and emotional responding (Gratz et al. 2010). Recent studies have indicated that individuals with substance use disorders display heightened rates of both BPD and PTSD in comparison to the general population (Brady et al. 2017), Gratz and Tull (2012) investigated the moderating roles of BPD and AVPD in the association between PTSD and deliberate self-harm (DSH) among 61 substance use disorder (SUD) inpatients. They hypothesized that substantial core impacts of PTSD, BPD, and AVPD diagnostic status on the frequency of DSH would be more elevated among SUD cases with vs. without these disorders. The findings demonstrated higher frequency of DSH among individuals with vs. without PTSD, provided significant evidence for the moderating role of AVPD in this association. Furthermore, increased levels of DSH were revealed among PTSD cases with AVPD. Surprisingly, they did not explore any findings to support an association between BPD and DSH frequency among their sample (Gratz and Tull 2012). Cunningham et al. (2019) expanded current investigations via examining PTSD, BPD, NSSI, and suicidal ideation in 728 male veterans of the US military to identify the role of NSSI and BPD features as risk factors for suicidal ideation in veterans suffering from PTSD. Results showed highly common rates of NSSI and BPD features among participants, and the potential importance of NSSI and BPD features in increasing suicidal risk among PTSD veterans (Cunningham et al. 2019). Harned et al. (2010) examined the influence of co-occurrence of PTSD on 94 female cases of BPD with suicide attempts in the preceding year (53 participants with a comorbid diagnosis of PTSD and 41 with no PTSD diagnosis). These two groups were compared in relation to the severity of BPD, the characteristics of trauma history, suicide and NSSI, comorbid axis I & II disorders, emotion regulation, psychosocial functioning, and history of using mental health treatment (medical and psychotherapy). The findings revealed differences in the lethality, intent, and triggering for deliberate self-harm, trauma history, emotion regulation, and axis I comorbidity among BPD individuals with and without PTSD. Consistent with the results, severe disturbances were found in individuals with both BPD and PTSD, suggesting some unique characteristics associated with the co-occurrence of BPD and PTSD (Harned et al. 2010).

As mentioned before, numerous findings have shown substantial overlap and a considerable rate of co-occurrence between BPD and PTSD (Eichelman 2010; Pagura et al. 2010; Sar et al. 2006). Dixon-Gordon et al. (2013a, b) examined the relation between borderline personality based on both subjective (e.g., self-report) and biological (e.g., cortisol) emotional reactivity. In addition, they identified the moderating role of PTSD symptoms in these associations. Moreover, the interactive influences of BPD and PTSD symptoms on emotional reactivity among 171 substance use disorder (SUD) participants with heightened rates of BPD and PTSD were examined. The results indicated a substantial impact of BPD pathology on subjective emotional reactivity, as well as a considerable interaction between BPD pathology and PTSD symptoms in the anticipation of cortisol reactivity including the association between BPD pathology and increased cortisol reactivity only in the group with low levels of PTSD symptoms. Corresponding findings were obtained when identifying the interaction between BPD pathology and the re-experiencing and avoidance/numbing symptoms of PTSD. Subsequently, it can be inferred from these findings that symptoms of PTSD likely play a moderating role in the BP-reactivity relation (Dixon-Gordon et al. 2013a, b).

Regarding mental health, a growing body of literature has documented the association between BPD and PTSD with adverse childhood experiences (Hoeboer et al. 2021, 2024; Bohus et al. 2019, 2020; Hailes et al. 2019; Messman-Moore and Bhuptani 2017; Kampling et al. 2022), child abuse (Sheridan and Carr 2020), and childhood trauma (Bozzatello et al. 2021). Numerous studies have demonstrated that "BPD+PTSD" comorbidity is reported to have a more frequent history of traumatic experiences in comparison to BPD alone, or to PTSD alone (Connor et al. 2002). Furthermore, among individuals with a comorbidity of BPD and PTSD compared to PTSD alone, trauma had more severe features, comprising earlier experience of sexual abuse and highly frequent physical and verbal abuse (Clarke et al. 2008). According to Ford and Courtois (2021), there are substantial associations and overlap between PTSD and BPD, which suggests that post-traumatic symptoms initiate with childhood maltreatment or other types of traumatic victimization, and then are exacerbated with high levels of additional trauma through adolescence and young adulthood. Experiencing trauma in childhood can have several impacts on PTSD during adulthood in various ways, including (1) childhood trauma can directly contribute to the development of PTSD in several ways: (1a) PTSD can be a pathologic consequence of experiencing childhood trauma that persist into adulthood and (1b) individuals may experience constant traumatic situations during childhood, but PTSD emerges in adulthood; (2) like other psychological disorders, childhood trauma can lead to an elevated risk of later PTSD development in adulthood, due to two different factors, consisting of (2a) highly frequent experiences of being exposed to traumatic events from early childhood over time, which contributes to an increasing risk of the development of PTSD in adulthood; (2a) childhood trauma can change the psychological processes and environmental elements during childhood leading to elevating the chance of developing later PTSD; and (2c) neurological and neuropsychological changes as well as hormonal alterations caused by being exposed to childhood trauma, may contribute to the development of later PTSD. Similarly, the impact of child sexual abuse in the development of the comorbidity of BPD and PTSD has been indicated (Ford and Courtois 2021). Most of the research has investigated BPD-PTSD comorbidity in clinical settings, yet few studies have assessed this comorbidity in the general population (Scheiderer et al. 2015). By using a large, nationally representative sample from Wave 2 of the *National Epidemiological Survey on Alcohol and Related Conditions* (NESARC, Grant et al. 2018), Pagura et al. (2010) examined differences in psychopathology, traumatic childhood experiences, and health-related quality of life (HRQOL) among individuals with BPD, PTSD, and the comorbidity of BPD-PTSD. The findings indicated poorer HRQOL, higher Axis I comorbidity, heightened rates of lifetime suicide attempt, and greater prevalence of repeated traumatic experiences in childhood among people with comorbid BPD-PTSD compared to individuals with either diagnosis alone. Furthermore, results showed significantly lower mental HRQOL scores in participants with comorbid BPD-PTSD in comparison with individuals with BPD-only or PTSD-only, and individuals with comorbid BPD-PTSD and

PTSD-only, indicated substantially lower physical HRQOL than those with BPD-only. Moreover, the severity of symptoms was greater in individuals with comorbid BPD-PTSD than participants with BPD-only or PTSD-only (Pagura et al. 2010). Through a face-to-face survey study, using data from Wave 2 of the National Epidemiological Survey on Alcohol and Related Conditions (NESAEC, Grant et al. 2018), Scheiderer et al. (2015) studied the relation between this comorbidity with reduction in health-related quality of life in 4104 BPD and PTSD participants, and also, the significance of child sexual abuse as a predictive factor for BPD and PTSD comorbidity in a general population sample. The results showed that lifetime comorbidity of BPD and PTSD was associated with more dysfunction than either individual disorder (BPD-only or PTSD-only), as well as the factors including gender, age, and child sexual abuse revealed significant influences on the prediction of the comorbidity of BPD and PTSD and the relevance decreased in health-related quality of life (Scheiderer et al. 2015). Through a cross-sectional study, Deng et al. (2023) examined the influence of BPD tendencies and subjective well-being on NSSI in 2160 Chinese secondary vocational students with PTSD. The findings indicated that sex, BPD tendencies, and subjective well-being were independent factors that anticipated NSSI in secondary vocational students with PTSD. Additionally, BPD tendencies showed a positive correlation with NSSI frequency. Family functioning indicated a significant positive correlation with subjective well-being, as well as a negative correlation with BPD tendencies (Deng et al. 2023).

BPD and Complex Post-Traumatic Stress Disorder (c-PTSD)

A growing attention has been paid over the last few decades to a construct called complex post-traumatic stress disorder (c-PTSD) (Shing Chiu et al. 2023; Nestgaard Rød and Schmidt 2021). This term was introduced by Judith Herman (1992) and Bessel van der Kolk et al. (2005) as a syndrome distinguished from PTSD, which occurs after experiencing extreme stress, comprising symptoms in addition to PTSD for the first time (Ford and Courtois 2021; Heim et al. 2022). In line with Ford and Courtois (2021), complex psychological trauma is characterized by (1) interpersonal experiences and events such as relational betrayal, (2) prolonged, pervasive, long-term, and sometimes current events, (3) directly being involved in attack, harm, abuse, neglect, and abandonment by irresponsible or neglectful caregivers, (4) happening at developmentally critical times in the victim's life, especially early childhood, and (5) having considerable devastating physical and psychological influences during the life span (Ford and Courtois 2014, 2021; Courtois and Ford 2012). The symptoms of c-PTSD have been displayed among people exposed to extremely traumatic situations, such as child abuse and domestic violence, which extend beyond the PTSD diagnosis (Herman 1992), comprising dissociation, emotion dysregulation, somatization, and changed core schemas including self-relationship and sustaining beliefs about both morality and spirituality (Ford and Courtois 2021). The 11th revision of the International Classification of Disease (ICD-11) includes distinguished alterations in the diagnostics of post-traumatic stress. Besides PTSD, a new sibling disorder, complex Post-Traumatic Stress Disorder (c-PTSD) has been included (WHO 2022; ICD-11 2018; Fung et al. 2022; Cloitre 2020), encompassing three clusters of symptoms, including re-experiencing, avoidance, and persistent, negative self-perception, and increased perception of ongoing threat (Gelezelyte et al. 2022; Ki Lam et al. 2023; Schiess-Jokanovic et al. 2021; Hébert and Amédée 2020; Böttche et al. 2018), which is associated with distinguished individual and social consequences (Ki Lam et al. 2023). In addition to all PTSD symptoms, the c-PTSD significant symptoms comprise dysregulated emotion processing such as self-soothing issues and stress tolerance difficulties, problematic interpersonal relationships such as avoidance of relationships and relational insecurity, alteration in consciousness and self-perception, and negative self-concept such as beliefs about oneself as a failure, changed perception of aggressor, interpersonal issues, and various alterations in the value system (Hyland et al. 2017; Fernández-Guerrero 2023; Krause-Utz 2021; Ford and Courtois 2014; Shing Chiu et al. 2023; Redican et al. 2022; Torres 2023), and clinically substantial levels of disturbances in self-organization (DSO) consisting of bodily integrity (WHO 2019; ICD-11 2018; Ford and Courtois 2014; Shing Chiu et al. 2023; Redican et al. 2022; Torres 2023; Schiess-Jokanovic et al. 2021; Ford et al. 2020). Evidence suggests that the prevalence of c-PTSD varies from 7.7% to 69.1% in different population, comprising the general population, non-treatment seeking trauma-exposed individuals, and clinical population (Saraiya et al. 2021; Morris et al. 2021; Hyland et al. 2020; Fernández-Fillol et al. 2021). In line with growing investigations, various factors have been revealed which can make individuals more vulnerable to c-PTSD, comprising repeated interpersonal trauma (Kazlauskas et al. 2020, 2024; Haselgruber et al. 2020; Daniunaite et al. 2021; Torres 2023), repeated cumulative trauma (Haselgruber et al. 2020; Cloitre et al. 2019; Darby et al. 2023), female gender (Haselgruber et al. 2020; Perkonigg et al. 2016), more comorbid psychopathology (Torres 2023), and different social factors (Daniunaite et al. 2021).

With an ever-growing number of studies, both PTSD and c-PTSD can be developed following exposure to a traumatic event or a series of aversive, traumatic events, contributing to significant dysfunctions (Gelezelyte et al. 2022; Rink and Lipinska 2020; Hyland et al. 2017; Harned et al. 2018). Furthermore, robust evidence has revealed the association between PTSD and c-PTSD with psychiatric disorders (Nestgaard Rød and Schmidt 2021; Coventry et al. 2020), such as schizophrenia, bipolar disorder, and personality disorder (Nestgaard Rød and Schmidt 2021; Bebbington and Freeman 2017), mood disorder (Fox et al. 2020; Fedorenko et al. 2023), alcohol use disorder (Fox et al. 2020), fear and anxiety disorders (Fedorenko et al. 2023; López-Castro et al. 2019; Jobson et al. 2022), behavioral disorders, and emotion dysregulation (Møller et al. 2020; López-Castro et al. 2019; Jobson et al. 2022; Weiss et al. 2020), substance misuse (Nguyen et al. 2022; Weiss et al. 2015; Contractor et al. 2019; Roberts 2023), and psychosis (Nestgaard Rød and Schmidt 2021; Panayi et al. 2022), suicidal behaviors, and self-injurious behaviors (Dixon-Gordon et al. 2014; Stanley et al. 2019; Raudales et al. 2021; Smith et al. 2024) risky sexual behaviors (Weiss et al. 2019), and emotionally unstable personality disorder (EUPD), characterized by emotional instability, interpersonal issues, impulsivity, and impaired self-concept (WHO 1992; Webb et al. 2022). In addition, the estimated prevalence rates were reported as 0.5% (Maercker et al. 2018) and 11.6% (Daniunaite et al. 2021) for c-PTSD, 1.5% (Maercker et al. 2018) and 10.4% (Daniunaite et al. 2021) for PTSD, and the rates of PTSD and c-PTSD were 1.5–3.4%, respectively (Redican et al. 2022).

However, although PTSD, c-PTSD, and BPD have not revealed completely shared symptoms, numerous studies have highlighted the overlaps between these disorders based on descriptive and empirical research (Saraiya et al. 2021; Ford 2019; Jowett et al. 2020; Hyland et al. 2021; Dell et al. 2024). The overlap between symptoms of BPD and those of c-PTSD is a subject of debate. Proposed questions include whether c-PTSD can be considered just as a re-packaging or only a duplication of BPD or whether it presents a logical foundation for boosting the accuracy of assessment, diagnosis, and various treatment options for people whose BPD symptoms and related disturbances are caused or worsened by complex traumatic stress reactions (Driessen et al. 2004; Ford and Courtois 2014). In other words, despite conceptual similarities in symptomatic presentations, it is not clear whether these are two distinct disorders (Lewis and Grenyer 2009) or not. Augmenting evidence endorses the discrimination validity of c-PTSD and BPD in accordance with categorical models of psychopathology. According to dimensional models of psychopathology, such as the Hierarchical Taxonomy of Psychopathology model (HiTOP model), it is possible to identify common vulnerabilities across apparently discrete disorders (Frost et al. 2020). Numerous clinical and experimental investigations have been conducted to explore the association between these two disorders among the general population as well as clinical samples. A constellation of analytic methods including factor analysis, latent class analysis, and network analysis has been utilized to identify these relationships. Although, some of these studies have shown a group who fulfill criteria for both BPD and c-PTSD, these two disorders are generally distinguishable at the symptomatic level (Karatzias et al. 2023). For instance, PTSD overlaps core symptoms including re-experience, avoidance, and blunting with c-PTSD and BPD (Dell et al. 2024). Furthermore, some symptoms consisting of sensitivity, worry, guilt, and detachment are shared between c-PTSD and BPD (Cloitre et al. 2014). Although BPD is associated with high rates of impulsivity and suicidal ideation and behaviors, self-injurious behaviors, these features may be present in c-PTSD as well (Cloitre et al. 2014; Karatzias et al. 2023). Furthermore, it has been found that experiencing early trauma in BPD individuals is related to fear of abandonment, while PTSD cases reported experiences of traumatic resurgences, as well as the tendency toward the development of BPD when the trauma happens in early life, while PTSD/c-PTSD tends to be developed in a more mature brain (Amad et al. 2016). Biskin and Paris (2012) proposed that emotion dysregulation is ego-dystonic, stressor-specific, and variable over time among individuals with c-PTSD, while in people with BPD, difficulties in emotion regulation and mood instability seem to be ego-syntonic and persistent over time (Biskin and Paris 2012). Karatzias et al. (2023) suggested that self-concept issues reflect an instability in the sense of self consisting of altered goals and beliefs, while a consistent and stable negative sense of self has been found among individuals with c-PTSD. Moreover, although feelings of low self-esteem are a common matter in both BPD and c-PTSD, a change in the view of self supports a BPD diagnosis (Karatzias et al. 2023). Frost et al. (2020) identified the distinct and common features of c-PTSD and BPD based on dimensional modeling methods. The latent structure of BPD and c-PTSD symptoms was elucidated by a bifactorial model, comprising one *general* factor such as vulnerability to all symptoms, and three *specific* factors like vulnerability to PTSD, BPD, and disturbances in self-organization. The findings indicated that c-PTSD symptoms were more differentiable from the general factor, while BPD symptoms were not easily distinguishable from the general factors. Moreover, the most typical feature of c-PTSD and BPD associated with the general factor included a negative self-concept in c-PTSD and an alternating self-concept in BPD. Most risk factors were related to the general factor, congruent with the explanation of dimensional models of psychopathology (Frost et al. 2020). Numerous descriptive and empirical studies have considered the differences between BPD and c-PTSD (e.g., Ford and Courtois 2021). In accordance with findings, BPD and c-PTSD manifest overlaps in the type of problems in emotion regulation, self-concept, and interpersonal relationships; however, significant distinctions have been obtained which reflect how these overlapped symptoms exhibit in either BPD or c-PTSD (Powers et al. 2022a, b; Brewin et al. 2019). Based on a latent class analysis, the following features were proposed by Cloitre et al. (2014) as a clear distinction between BPD and c-PTSD: (a) experiencing early traumatic events is not crucial to identify a BPD diagnosis, (b) fear of abandonment, frantic efforts to avoid abandonment, and distorted self-image are specific to BPD, (c) difficulties in interpersonal relationships are reported in both BPD and c-PTSD, albeit this issue is found to be associated with chaotic attachment in BPD and social avoidance in c-PTSD, and (d) distinguished differences in expression of emotional instability, increased reactivity, mismatched responses, anger, and irritability are reported in both BPD and c-PTSD, yet NSSH and suicidal behaviors are found specifically in BPD (Cloitre et al. 2014). In current conceptualizations, three core domains have been assumed as basic foundations of the complexity and heterogeneity of BPD symptoms comprising emotion dysregulation encompassing stress-related impulsivity (dysfunctional and destructive coping behaviors such as NSSI and suicidal attempts), impaired self-image, and interpersonal relationship disturbances (Bohus et al. 2021). Based on the findings of a study utilizing network analysis, c-PTSD represented associated symptoms, yet the BPD symptom network was found to be rather sparse with a fragile connection to c-PTSD symptoms (Knefel et al. 2016). Hyland et al. (2019) examined the phenomenological similarities and differences and discriminant validity of BPD and c-PTSD symptoms in 546 trauma-exposed participants from the United Kingdom. According to a three-factor model, findings identified multiple symptoms distinctive to related constructs, such as interpersonal relationship difficulties and suicidality, and shared symptoms with constructs such as affective dysregulation as well. In addition, the symptoms unique to the disturbances of self-organization factor consisted of emotional avoidance, interpersonal isolation and numbing, yet the symptoms unique to BPD included emotional and interpersonal reactivity, fears of abandonment, relationship ups-and-downs, and suicidal and self-injurious behaviors. Furthermore, it was revealed that exposure to several childhood interpersonal traumas was significantly associated with the PTSD, PBD, and disturbances in self-organization latent variables (Hyland et al. 2019).

It has been suggested that diagnostic symptoms associated with emotion dysregulation are endorsed across BPD and c-PTSD. And therefore, they are proposed to be common features in BPD and c-PTSD (Owczarek et al. 2023). Herman and van der Kolk (2020) proposed generally similar disturbances in both BPD and c-PTSD in five domains, including affect regulation, impulse control, reality testing, interpersonal relationships, and self-integration, from which some specific symptoms were identified as core similar domains for both BPD and PTSD that consisted of affect regulation, depression, severe anger, irritability, chronic emptiness, impulse control problems, reality testing issues, and self-integration (Lewis and Grenyer 2009). Related to the nosological status of BPD-PTSD comorbidity, results proposed that BPD and PTSD are independent clinical qualities, with a risk of fake comorbidity as similar clinical phenotypes like "complex PTSD," a clinical entity comprising a sub-group of PTSD-BPD participants (Frías and Palma 2015). To distinguish symptoms of PTSD, c-PTSD, and BPD, Powers et al. (2022a, b) used exploratory structural equation modeling to replicate previous findings on the association between these disorders among 470 trauma-exposed urban samples. The results showed that a three-factor ESEM model of c-PTSD and BPD symptoms best fit the data and endorsed the discriminatory validity between factors across trauma-related avoidance, aggressive behavior, and anxious attachment (Powers et al. 2022a, b). Through a latent class analysis, Saraiya et al. (2021) examined the social-emotional profiles of PTSD, c-PTSD, and BPD among 197 trauma-exposed participants, represented the symptoms of PTSD, c-PTSD, and BPD. They assigned four classes, including (1) high PTSD+c-PTSD+BPD class, displayed high level of all symptoms for the three diagnoses; (2) moderate PTSD+c-PTSD+BPD class, characterized by some symptoms across all three diagnoses, (3) a PTSD class, endorsed the *ICD-11* PTSD criteria, and (4) healthy class, by low symptoms for all three diagnoses. The findings revealed the highest levels of psychological distress, history of traumatic events, adverse childhood experiences, and PTSD symptoms in the high PTSD+c-PTSD+BPD class. In addition, shame was the only social emotion that revealed significant difference between the classes, which can be considered as a central emotion that distinguishes these manifestations following trauma exposure (Saraiya et al. 2021). Lawless and Tarren-Sweeney (2023) examined the alignment between mental health symptoms profiles obtained by cluster analysis and the nominal diagnosis of c-PTSD and BPD in a sample of 230 adolescents to identify the extent BPD and c-PTSD are parallel with complex symptomology presented in adolescents. The results indicated a low c-PTSD prevalence, displaying low concordance between PTSD and disturbances in self-organization case assignment. Moreover, the BPD and c-PTSD cases showed alignment with a higher complex and severe symptom profiles, including core symptoms and clinical signs of BPD. In addition, the BPD and c-PTSD participants were characterized by clinical-level inattention/over-activity and conduct difficulties (Lawless and Tarren-Sweeney 2023).

As mentioned earlier, individuals reporting a history of complex trauma, such as developmentally adverse interpersonal experiences, childhood maltreatment, prolonged domestic violence, and torture and exploitation, are prone to the development of not only PTSD but also other mental issues and psychiatric disorders encompassing personality disorders (Golier et al. 2003a, b; Westphal et al. 2013; Darby et al. 2023), especially BPD (Vermetten and Spiegel 2014; Zanarini et al. 2017). Substantially documented studies have proposed the association between c-PTSD and relational disturbances (fear of closeness or abandonment), affect dysregulation (over-regulation and under-regulation of affect), and changes in identity (positive or negative psycho-form or somatoform dissociation). Van Dijke et al. (2018) assessed the mediating role of affect dysregulation, relational impairment, and identity issues in the association between childhood trauma and c-PTSD independent of BPD symptoms, among 472 clinical adult sample. The findings indicated that the relation between childhood trauma and c-PTSD symptoms in adult was relatively mediated by under-regulation of emotion, negative psycho-form or somatoform dissociation, and fears of closeness and abandonment (Van Dijke et al. 2018). In spite of the similarities and overlaps between the symptoms of these two disorders, an index traumatic event and sequelae of exposure to traumatic stress is not inherent to diagnosis of BPD, which is crucial for c-PTSD diagnosis (Ford and Courtois 2014; Karatzias et al. 2023; de Aquino Ferreira et al. 2018), yet the majority of BPD individuals often report a history of severe childhood maltreatment and abuse with a great rate compared to other psychiatric disorders (Porter et al. 2020; Kleindienst et al. 2020). In other words, not all BPD individuals report a history of childhood maltreatment and trauma, and not all individuals who reported this history continue to the development of BP pathology (Lewis and Grenyer 2009). Prevalence findings have shown 81–91% of individuals suffering from BPD have a history of childhood trauma, whereas the remaining 9%–19% with BPD report no history of childhood trauma (Herman and van der Kolk 2020; Lewis and Grenyer 2009). Based on a latent class analysis (LCA), Cloitre et al. (2014) examined whether the symptoms of 280 female patients seeking treatment due to childhood maltreatment are consistent with diagnostic criteria for BPD, PTSD, and c-PTSD. The LCA showed four distinguished classifications of individuals, including (1) low symptom class (low endorsement of all symptoms); (2) a PTSD class (heightened symptoms of PTSD with low endorsements of symptoms of c-PTSD); (3) a c-PTSD class (increased symptoms of PTSD and self-organization symptoms, with the c-PTSD diagnosis showing low scores on the BPD symptoms); and (4) a BPD class (symptoms of BPD). The BPD class was clearly discrete in its endorsement of symptoms unique to BPD, although individuals diagnosed with BPD exhibited several symptoms of PTSD and c-PTSD. Also, the results indicated that four BPD symptoms were detected to considerably raise the odds of being in the BPD class in comparison to c-PTSD class: unstable sense of self, chaotic interpersonal relationship, frantic efforts to avoid abandonment, and impulsivity. The notable finding included a marked difference in the existence of suicidal and self-injurious behaviors in individuals in the BPD class compared to c-PTSD and PTSD classes. The only symptom of the BPD class which showed no difference from c-PTSD class was chronic feelings of emptiness, suggesting it does not discriminate between these two classes. Furthermore, although the issues in emotion regulation could not distinguish between BPD and c-PTSD, the severity and type of emotion dysregulation which manifested in symptoms such as suicidal attempts and self-harm behaviors have been found as characteristics of BPD, not c-PTSD. BPD is characterized by fears of abandonment, instability in the sense of self, unstable interpersonal relationships, impulsivity, and self-harm behaviors. Whereas, in PTSD and c-PTSD, little endorsement of items related to instability in self-representation and interpersonal relationships were reported (Cloitre et al. 2014).

In conclusion, as mentioned above, being exposed to traumatic life experiences has been documented to be common in psychiatric populations, especially experiencing multiple exposures. As shown, although most of the people exposed to traumatic events do not develop significantly long-term psychopathology, a substantial minority of them experienced complex symptoms diagnosed as PTSD/c-PTSD. The comorbidity of BPD and PTSD is considerably well-documented and common. In addition, several findings showed the existence of PTSD symptoms in some individuals with BPD. Furthermore, exposure to violence was related to severe difficulties in emotion regulation, leading to the development of post-traumatic stress symptoms (PTSS) and BP pathology. Additionally, emotion dysregulation mediated the relations between exposure to violence and both PTSS and BP pathology. Moreover, a remarkable association between negative consequences and maladaptive behaviors and the co-occurrence of BPD and PTSD were found, including suicidal and other self-destructive behaviors, reduced level of health-related quality of life, self-injurious behaviors, and more functional disturbances. Further, notable shared symptoms were reported between c-PTSD and BPD such as issues in self and problematic interpersonal relationships, which contributed to a challenging debate regarding whether c-PTSD and BPD have similar pathology or if they are discriminated with different diagnostic criteria.

References

Akiskal HS. The temperamental borders of affective disorders. Acta Psychiatr Scand. 1994;89:32–7.

Aleva A, Betts JK, Cotton SM, Laceulle OM, Hessels CJ, van Aken MA, Nicol K, Chanen AM. Personality disorders: theory, research, and treatment. Advance online publication; 2023.

Amad A, Ramoz N, Thomas P, Gorwood P. The age-dependent plasticity highlights the conceptual interface between borderline personality disorder and PTSD. Eur Arch Psychiatry Clin Neurosci. 2016;266:373–5.

American Psychiatric Association. Diagnostic and statistical manual of mental disorders. 5th ed, Text Revised (DSM-5-TR); 2022.

Bebbington P, Freeman D. Transdiagnostic extension of delusions: schizophrenia and beyond. Schizophr Bull. 2017;43(2):273–82.

Benjet C, Bromet E, Karam EG, Kessler RC, McLaughlin KA, Ruscio AM, Shahly V, Stein DJ, Petukhova M, Hill E, Alonso J. The epidemiology of traumatic event exposure worldwide: results from the World Mental Health Survey Consortium. Psychol Med. 2016;46(2):327–43.

Biskin RS, Paris J. Management of borderline personality disorder. CMAJ. 2012;184(17):1897–902.

Bohus M, Schmahl C, Fydrich T, Steil R, Müller-Engelmann M, Herzog J, Ludäscher P, Kleindienst N, Priebe K. A research programme to evaluate DBT-PTSD, a modular treatment approach for complex PTSD after childhood abuse. Borderline Personal Disord Emot Dysregul. 2019;6:1–6.

Bohus M, Kleindienst N, Hahn C, Müller-Engelmann M, Ludäscher P, Steil R, Fydrich T, Kuehner C, Resick PA, Stiglmayr C, Schmahl C. Dialectical behavior therapy for posttraumatic stress disorder (DBT-PTSD) compared with cognitive processing therapy (CPT) in complex presentations of PTSD in women survivors of childhood abuse: a randomized clinical trial. JAMA Psychiatry. 2020;77(12):1235–45.

Bohus M, Stoffers-Winterling J, Sharp C, Krause-Utz A, Schmahl C, Lieb K. Borderline personality disorder. Lancet. 2021;398(10310):1528–40.

Bollinger AR, Riggs DS, Blake DD, Ruzek JI. Prevalence of personality disorders among combat veterans with posttraumatic stress disorder. J Trauma Stress. 2000;13(2):255–70.

Boritz T, Barnhart R, McMain SF. The influence of posttraumatic stress disorder on treatment outcomes of patients with borderline personality disorder. J Personal Disord. 2016;30(3):395–407.

Böttche M, Ehring T, Krüger-Gottschalk A, Rau H, Schäfer I, Schellong J, Dyer A, Knaevelsrud C. Testing the ICD-11 proposal for complex PTSD in trauma-exposed adults: factor structure and symptom profiles. Eur J Psychotraumatol. 2018;9(1):1512264.

Bozzatello P, Rocca P, Baldassarri L, Bosia M, Bellino S. The role of trauma in early onset borderline personality disorder: a biopsychosocial perspective. Front Psych. 2021;12:721361.

Brady RE, Bujarski SJ, Feldner MT, Pyne JM. Examining the effects of alexithymia on the relation between posttraumatic stress disorder and over-reporting. Psychol Trauma Theory Res Pract Policy. 2017;9(1):80.

Breslau N, Kessler RC, Chilcoat HD, Schultz LR, Davis GC, Andreski P. Trauma and posttraumatic stress disorder in the community: the 1996 Detroit area survey of trauma. Arch Gen Psychiatry. 1998;55(7):626–32.

Brewin CR, Rumball F, Happé F. Neglected causes of post-traumatic stress disorder. BMJ. 2019;365:l2372.

Brewin CR, Cloitre M, Hyland P, Shevlin M, Maercker A, Bryant RA, Humayun A, Jones LM, Kagee A, Rousseau C, Somasundaram D. A review of current evidence regarding the ICD-11 proposals for diagnosing PTSD and complex PTSD. Clin Psychol Rev. 2017;58:1–5.

Brown MZ, Dahlin K. Dialectical behavior therapy for treating the effects of trauma, 2017.

Brown TA, McNiff J. Specificity of autonomic arousal to DSM-IV panic disorder and posttraumatic stress disorder. Behav Res Ther. 2009;47(6):487–93.

Brown TH, Mellman TA, Alfano CA, Weems CF. Sleep fears, sleep disturbance, and PTSD symptoms in minority youth exposed to Hurricane Katrina. J Trauma Stress. 2011;24(5):575–80.

Buckholdt KE, Kitzmann KM, Cohen R. Parent emotion coaching buffers the psychological effects of poor peer relations in the classroom. J Soc Pers Relat. 2016;33(1):23–41.

Carpenter RW, Hepp J, Trull TJ. Pain before, during, and after nonsuicidal self-injury: findings from a large web study. J Psychopathol Clin Sci. 2023a;132:984.

Carpenter RK, McAfee NW, Schumacher JA. Variations in trauma exposure, minority status, and considerations in course reduction in Mississippi University system. J Coll Stud Retent Res Theory Pract. 2023b;21:15210251231216345.

Chapman AL. Borderline personality disorder and emotion dysregulation. Dev Psychopathol. 2019;31(3):1143–56.

Chiu HT, Alberici A, Claxton J, Meiser-Stedman R. The prevalence, latent structure and psychosocial and cognitive correlates of complex post-traumatic stress disorder in an adolescent community sample. J Affect Disord. 2023;340:482–9.

Clarke SB, Rizvi SL, Resick PA. Borderline personality characteristics and treatment outcome in cognitivebehavioral treatments for PTSD in female rape victims. Behav Ther. 2008;39(1):72–8.

Cloitre M, Hyland P, Bisson JI, Brewin CR, Roberts NP, Karatzias T, Shevlin M. ICD-11 posttraumatic stress disorder and complex posttraumatic stress disorder in the United States: a population-based study. J Trauma Stress. 2019;32(6):833–42.

Cloitre M, Courtois CA, Ford JD, Green BL, Alexander P, Briere J, Van der Hart O. The ISTSS expert consensus treatment guidelines for complex PTSD in adults [Internet], 2012.

Cloitre M, Garvert DW, Weiss B, Carlson EB, Bryant RA. Distinguishing PTSD, complex PTSD, and borderline personality disorder: a latent class analysis. Eur J Psychotraumatol. 2014;5(1):25097.

Cloitre M. ICD-11 complex post-traumatic stress disorder: simplifying diagnosis in trauma populations. Br J Psychiatry. 2020;216(3):129–31.

Connor KM, Davidson JR, Hughes DC, Swartz MS, Blazer DG, George LK. The impact of borderline personality disorder on post-traumatic stress in the community: a study of health status, health utilization, and functioning. Compr Psychiatry. 2002;43(1):41–8.

Contractor AA, Weiss NH, Dixon-Gordon KL, Blumenthal H. Heterogeneity in the co-occurrence of substance use and posttraumatic stress disorder: a latent class analysis approach. J Dual Diagn. 2019;15(2):105–17.

Courtois CA, Ford JD. Treatment of complex trauma: A sequenced, relationship-based approach. Guilford Press; 2012.

Coventry PA, Meader N, Melton H, Temple M, Dale H, Wright K, Cloitre M, Karatzias T, Bisson J, Roberts NP, Brown JV. Psychological and pharmacological interventions for posttraumatic stress disorder and comorbid mental health problems following complex traumatic events: systematic review and component network meta-analysis. PLoS Med. 2020;17(8):e1003262.

Coyne SM, Warburton W, Swit C, Stockdale L, Dyer WJ. Who is most at risk for developing physical aggression after playing violent video games? An individual differences perspective from early adolescence to emerging adulthood. J Youth Adolesc. 2023;52(4):719–33.

Cummings EM, Goeke-Morey MC, Schermerhorn AC, Merrilees CE, Cairns E. Children and political violence from a social ecological perspective: implications from research on children and families in Northern Ireland. Clin Child Fam Psychol Rev. 2009;12:16–38.

Cunningham KC, Grossmann JL, Seay KB, Dennis PA, Clancy CP, Hertzberg MA, Berlin K, Ruffin RA, Dedert EA, Gratz KL, Calhoun PS. Nonsuicidal self-injury and borderline personality features as risk factors for suicidal ideation among male veterans with posttraumatic stress disorder. J Trauma Stress. 2019;32(1):141–7.

Daniunaite I, Cloitre M, Karatzias T, Shevlin M, Thoresen S, Zelviene P, Kazlauskas E. PTSD and complex PTSD in adolescence: discriminating factors in a population-based cross-sectional study. Eur J Psychotraumatol. 2021;12(1):1890937.

Darby RJ, Taylor EP, Cadavid MS. Phase-based psychological interventions for complex post-traumatic stress disorder: a systematic review. J Affect Disord Rep. 2023;20:100628.

de Aquino Ferreira LF, Pereira FH, Benevides AM, Melo MC. Borderline personality disorder and sexual abuse: a systematic review. Psychiatry Res. 2018;262:70–7.

Dell NA, Salas-Wright CP, Vaughn MG, Maldonado-Molina MM, Oh S, Bates M, Schwartz SJ. A machine learning approach using migration-related cultural stress to classify depression and post-traumatic stress disorder among hurricane survivors. J Affect Disord. 2024;347:77–84.

Dell'Osso L, Cremone IM, Carpita B, Dell'Oste V, Muti D, Massimetti G, Barlati S, Vita A, Fagiolini A, Carmassi C, Gesi C. Rumination, posttraumatic stress disorder, and mood symptoms in borderline personality disorder. Neuropsychiatr Dis Treat. 2019;13:1231–8.

Deng W, Yan S, Xu Y, Lu Z, Liu L, Zhou Y, Chen M. Effects of BPD tendencies and subjective well-being on NSSI in adolescents with PTSD. Front Psych. 2023;14:1152352.

Dixon-Gordon KL, Yiu A, Chapman AL. Borderline personality features and emotional reactivity: the mediating role of interpersonal vulnerabilities. J Behav Ther Exp Psychiatry. 2013a;44(2):271–8.

Dixon-Gordon KL, Gratz KL, Tull MT. Multimodal assessment of emotional reactivity in borderline personality pathology: the moderating role of posttraumatic stress disorder symptoms. Compr Psychiatry. 2013b;54(6):639–48.

Dixon-Gordon KL, Tull MT, Gratz KL. Self-injurious behaviors in posttraumatic stress disorder: an examination of potential moderators. J Affect Disord. 2014;166:359–67.

Driessen M, Beblo T, Mertens M, Piefke M, Rullkoetter N, Silva-Saavedra A, Reddemann L, Rau H, Markowitsch HJ, Wulff H, Lange W. Posttraumatic stress disorder and fMRI activation patterns of traumatic memory in patients with borderline personality disorder. Biol Psychiatry. 2004;55(6):603–11.

Eichelman B. Borderline personality disorder, PTSD, and suicide. Am J Psychiatry. 2010;167(10):1152–4.

Ellison WD, Rosenstein LK, Morgan TA, Zimmerman M. Community and clinical epidemiology of borderline personality disorder. Psychiatr Clin. 2018;41(4):561–73.

Ellison WD, Levy KN, Newman MG, Pincus AL, Wilson SJ, Molenaar P. Dynamics among borderline personality and anxiety features in psychotherapy outpatients: an exploration of nomothetic and idiographic patterns. Personal Disord Theory Res Treat. 2020;11(2):131.

Fedorenko EJ, Barnwell PV, Selby EA, Contrada RJ. Associations between the late positive potential and PTSD, anxiety, and depressive symptoms among trauma-exposed undergraduates. Biol Psychol. 2023;177:108499.

Feeney J, Kenny RA. Hair cortisol as a risk marker for increased depressive symptoms among older adults during the COVID-19 pandemic. Psychoneuroendocrinology. 2022;143:105847.

Fernández-Fillol C, Pitsiakou C, Perez-Garcia M, Teva I, Hidalgo-Ruzzante N. Complex PTSD in survivors of intimate partner violence: risk factors related to symptoms and diagnoses. Eur J Psychotraumatol. 2021;12(1):2003616.

Fernández-Guerrero MJ. Complex post-traumatic stress disorder and borderline personality disorder: the discussion goes on. Differential diagnosis proposal. Papeles del Psicólogo. 2023;44(3):172–9.

Ford JD. Commentary on the special section on complex PTSD: still going strong after all these years. J Trauma Stress. 2019;32(6):877–80.

Ford JD, Charak R, Modrowski CA, Kerig PK. PTSD and dissociation symptoms as mediators of the relationship between polyvictimization and psychosocial and behavioral problems among justice-involved adolescents. In: Polyvictimization. Routledge; 2020. p. 51–72.

Ford JD. Complex PTSD: research directions for nosology/assessment, treatment, and public health. Eur J Psychotraumatol. 2015a;6(1):27584.

Ford J. An affective cognitive neuroscience-based approach to PTSD psychotherapy: the TARGET model. J Cogn Psychother. 2015b;29(1):68–91.

Ford JD, Courtois CA. Complex PTSD, affect dysregulation, and borderline personality disorder. Borderline Personal Disord Emot Dysregul. 2014;1:1–7.

Ford JD, Courtois CA. Complex PTSD and borderline personality disorder. Borderline Personal Disord Emot Dysregul. 2021;8(1):16.

Fox R, Hyland P, Power JM, Coogan AN. Patterns of comorbidity associated with ICD-11 PTSD among older adults in the United States. Psychiatry Res. 2020;290:113171.

Frewen P, Kleindienst N, Lanius R, Schmahl C. Trauma-related altered states of consciousness in women with BPD with or without co-occurring PTSD. Eur J Psychotraumatol. 2014;5(1):24863.

Frías Á, Palma C. Comorbidity between post-traumatic stress disorder and borderline personality disorder: a review. Psychopathology. 2015;48(1):1–0.

Friedman MJ. Finalizing PTSD in DSM-5: getting here from there and where to go next. J Trauma Stress. 2013;26(5):548–56.

Frost R, Murphy J, Hyland P, Shevlin M, Ben-Ezra M, Hansen M, Armour C, McCarthy A, Cunningham T, McDonagh T. Revealing what is distinct by recognising what is common: distinguishing between complex PTSD and Borderline Personality Disorder symptoms using bifactor modelling. Eur J Psychotraumatol. 2020;11(1):1836864.

Fung HW, Chien WT, Lam SK, Ross CA. Investigating post-traumatic stress disorder (PTSD) and complex PTSD among people with self-reported depressive symptoms. Front Psych. 2022;13:953001.

Galatzer-Levy IR, Ankri Y, Freedman S, Israeli-Shalev Y, Roitman P, Gilad M, Shalev AY. Early PTSD symptom trajectories: persistence, recovery, and response to treatment: results from the Jerusalem Trauma Outreach and Prevention Study (J-TOPS). PLoS One. 2013;8(8):e70084.

Gelezelyte O, Roberts NP, Kvedaraite M, Bisson JI, Brewin CR, Cloitre M, Kairyte A, Karatzias T, Shevlin M, Kazlauskas E. Validation of the international trauma interview (ITI) for the clinical assessment of ICD-11 posttraumatic stress disorder (PTSD) and complex PTSD (CPTSD) in a Lithuanian sample. Eur J Psychotraumatol. 2022;13(1):2037905.

George LS, Park CL, Chaudoir SR. Examining the relationship between trauma centrality and posttraumatic stress disorder symptoms: a moderated mediation approach. Traumatology. 2016;22(2):85.

Gluck RL, Hartzell GE, Dixon HD, Michopoulos V, Powers A, Stevens JS, Fani N, Carter S, Schwartz AC, Jovanovic T, Ressler KJ. Trauma exposure and stress-related disorders in a large, urban, predominantly African-American, female sample. Arch Womens Ment Health. 2021;24:893–901.

Goldstein KE, Hazlett EA, Savage KR, Berlin HA, Hamilton HK, Zelmanova Y, Look AE, Koenigsberg HW, Mitsis EM, Tang CY, McNamara M. Dorso-and ventro-lateral prefrontal volume and spatial working memory in schizotypal personality disorder. Behav Brain Res. 2011;218(2):335–40.

Goldstein KE, Feinberg A, Corniquel MB, Szeszko JR, New AS, Haznedar MM, Goodman M, Chu KW, Tang CY, Hazlett EA. Anomalous amygdala habituation to unpleasant stimuli among unmedicated individuals with borderline personality disorder and a history of self-harming behavior. J Personal Disord. 2021;35(4):618–31.

Golier JA, Yehuda R, Bierer LM, Mitropoulou V, New AS, Schmeidler J, Silverman JM, Siever LJ. The relationship of borderline personality disorder to posttraumatic stress disorder and traumatic events. Am J Psychiatry. 2003a;160(11):2018–24.

Golier JA, Yehuda R, Lupien SJ, Harvey PD. Memory for trauma-related information in Holocaust survivors with PTSD. Psychiatry Res. 2003b;121(2):133–43.

Gottlieb JD, Poyato N, Valiente C, Perdigón A, Vázquez C. Trauma and posttraumatic stress disorder in Spanish public mental health system clients with severe psychiatric conditions: clinical and demographic correlates. Psychiatr Rehabil J. 2018;41(3):234.

Grant S, Colaiaco B, Motala A, Shanman R, Sorbero M, Hempel S. Acupuncture for the treatment of adults with posttraumatic stress disorder: a systematic review and meta-analysis. J Trauma Dissociation. 2018;19(1):39–58.

Grant BF, Chou SP, Goldstein RB, Huang B, Stinson FS, Saha TD, Smith SM, Dawson DA, Pulay AJ, Pickering RP, Ruan WJ. Prevalence, correlates, disability, and comorbidity of DSM-IV borderline personality disorder: results from the Wave 2 National Epidemiologic Survey on alcohol and related conditions. J Clin Psychiatry. 2008;69(4):533.

Gratz KL, Tull MT. Exploring the relationship between posttraumatic stress disorder and deliberate self-harm: the moderating roles of borderline and avoidant personality disorders. Psychiatry Res. 2012;199(1):19–23.

Gratz KL, Rosenthal MZ, Tull MT, Lejuez CW, Gunderson JG. An experimental investigation of emotional reactivity and delayed emotional recovery in borderline personality disorder: the role of shame. Compr Psychiatry. 2010;51(3):275–85.

Gros DF, Allan NP, Koscinski B, Keller S, Acierno R. Influence of comorbid social anxiety disorder in PTSD treatment outcomes for prolonged exposure in female military sexual trauma survivors with PTSD. J Clin Psychol. 2023;79(4):1039–50.

Gross R, Olfson M, Gameroff M, Shea S, Feder A, Fuentes M, Lantigua R, Weissman MM. Borderline personality disorder in primary care. Arch Intern Med. 2002;162(1):53–60.

Grubaugh AL, Zinzow HM, Paul L, Egede LE, Frueh BC. Trauma exposure and posttraumatic stress disorder in adults with severe mental illness: a critical review. Clin Psychol Rev. 2011;31(6):883–99.

Gunderson JG, Sabo AN. The phenomenological and conceptual interface between borderline personality disorder and PTSD. Person Person Disord. 2013;8:49–57.

Gunderson JG, Morey LC, Stout RL, Skodol AE, Shea MT, McGlashan TH, Zanarini MC, Grilo CM, Sanislow CA, Yen S, Daversa MT. Major depressive disorder and borderline personality disorder revisited: longitudinal interactions. J Clin Psychiatry. 2004;65(8):1049.

Gunderson JG, Herpertz SC, Skodol AE, Torgersen S, Zanarini MC. Borderline personality disorder. Nat Rev Dis Primers. 2018a;4(1):1–20.

Gunderson JG, Fruzzetti A, Unruh B, Choi-Kain L. Competing theories of borderline personality disorder. J Personal Disord. 2018b;32(2):148–67.

Hailes HP, Yu R, Danese A, Fazel S. Long-term outcomes of childhood sexual abuse: an umbrella review. Lancet Psychiatry. 2019;6(10):830–9.

Harned MS, Jackson SC, Comtois KA, Linehan MM. Dialectical behavior therapy as a precursor to PTSD treatment for suicidal and/or self-injuring women with borderline personality disorder. J Trauma Stress. 2010;23(4):421–9.

Harned MS, Korslund KE, Foa EB, Linehan MM. Treating PTSD in suicidal and self-injuring women with borderline personality disorder: development and preliminary evaluation of a dialectical behavior therapy prolonged exposure protocol. Behav Res Ther. 2012;50(6):381–6.

Harned MS, Tkachuck MA, Youngberg KA. Treatment preference among suicidal and self-injuring women with borderline personality disorder and PTSD. J Clin Psychol. 2013;69(7):749–61.

Harned MS, Korslund KE, Linehan MM. A pilot randomized controlled trial of dialectical behavior therapy with and without the dialectical behavior therapy prolonged exposure protocol for suicidal and self-injuring women with borderline personality disorder and PTSD. Behav Res Ther. 2014;55:7–17.

Harned MS, Wilks CR, Schmidt SC, Coyle TN. Improving functional outcomes in women with borderline personality disorder and PTSD by changing PTSD severity and post-traumatic cognitions. Behav Res Ther. 2018;103:53–61.

Haselgruber A, Sölva K, Lueger-Schuster B. Symptom structure of ICD-11 complex posttraumatic stress disorder (CPTSD) in trauma-exposed foster children: examining the international trauma questionnaire–child and adolescent version (ITQ-CA). Eur J Psychotraumatol. 2020;11(1):1818974.

Hébert M, Amédée LM. Latent class analysis of post-traumatic stress symptoms and complex PTSD in child victims of sexual abuse and their response to Trauma-Focused Cognitive Behavioural Therapy. Eur J Psychotraumatol. 2020;11(1):1807171.

Heim E, Karatzias T, Maercker A. Cultural concepts of distress and complex PTSD: future directions for research and treatment. Clin Psychol Rev. 2022;93:102143.

Herman JL. Complex PTSD: a syndrome in survivors of prolonged and repeated trauma. J Trauma Stress. 1992;5(3):377–91.

Herman JL, van der Kolk BA. Treating complex traumatic stress disorders in adults: scientific foundations and therapeutic models. Guilford Publications; 2020.

Ho GW, Karatzias T, Cloitre M, Chan AC, Bressington D, Chien WT, Hyland P, Shevlin M. Translation and validation of the Chinese ICD-11 international trauma questionnaire (ITQ) for the assessment of posttraumatic stress disorder (PTSD) and complex PTSD (CPTSD). Eur J Psychotraumatol. 2019;10(1):1608718.

Hoeboer CM, de Kleine RA, Oprel DA, Schoorl M, van der Does W, van Minnen A. Does complex PTSD predict or moderate treatment outcomes of three variants of exposure therapy. J Anxiety Disord. 2021;80:102388.

Hoeboer CM, Kullberg ML, Oprel DA, Schoorl M, van Minnen A, Antypa N, Mouthaan J, de Kleine RA, van der Does W. Impact of three variants of prolonged exposure therapy on comorbid diagnoses in patients with childhood abuse-related PTSD. Cogn Behav Ther. 2024;26:1–7.

Hruska B, Pacella ML, George RL, Delahanty DL. The association between daily PTSD symptom severity and alcohol-related outcomes in recent traumatic injury victims. Psychol Addict Behav. 2017;31(3):326.

Hyland P, Murphy J, Shevlin M, Vallières F, McElroy E, Elklit A, Christoffersen M, Cloitre M. Variation in post-traumatic response: the role of trauma type in predicting ICD-11 PTSD and CPTSD symptoms. Soc Psychiatry Psychiatr Epidemiol. 2017;52:727–36.

Hyland P, Karatzias T, Shevlin M, Cloitre M. Examining the discriminant validity of complex posttraumatic stress disorder and borderline personality disorder symptoms: results from a United Kingdom population sample. J Trauma Stress. 2019;32(6):855–63.

Hyland P, Shevlin M, Fyvie C, Cloitre M, Karatzias T. The relationship between ICD-11 PTSD, complex PTSD and dissociative experiences. J Trauma Dissociation. 2020;21(1):62–72.

Hyland P, Karatzias T, Shevlin M, McElroy E, Ben-Ezra M, Cloitre M, Brewin CR. Does requiring trauma exposure affect rates of ICD-11 PTSD and complex PTSD? Implications for DSM–5. Psychol Trauma Theory Res Pract Policy. 2021;13(2):133.

Jobson L, Willoughby C, Specker P, Wong J, Draganidis A, Lau W, Liddell B. Investigating the associations between cognitive appraisals, emotion regulation and symptoms of posttraumatic stress disorder among Asian American and European American trauma survivors. Sci Rep. 2022;12(1):18127.

Jowett S, Karatzias T, Shevlin M, Albert I. Differentiating symptom profiles of ICD-11 PTSD, complex PTSD, and borderline personality disorder: a latent class analysis in a multiply traumatized sample. Personal Disord Theory Res Treat. 2020;11(1):36.

Kampling H, Kruse J, Lampe A, Nolte T, Hettich N, Brähler E, Sachser C, Fegert JM, Gingelmaier S, Fonagy P, Krakau L. Epistemic trust and personality functioning mediate the association between adverse childhood experiences and posttraumatic stress disorder and complex posttraumatic stress disorder in adulthood. Front Psych. 2022;13:919191.

Karatzias T, Bohus M, Shevlin M, Hyland P, Bisson JI, Roberts N, Cloitre M. Distinguishing between ICD-11 complex post-traumatic stress disorder and borderline personality disorder: clinical guide and recommendations for future research. Br J Psychiatry. 2023;223(3):403–6.

Karatzias T, Shevlin M, Fyvie C, Hyland P, Efthymiadou E, Wilson D, Roberts N, Bisson JI, Brewin CR, Cloitre M. Evidence of distinct profiles of posttraumatic stress disorder (PTSD) and complex posttraumatic stress disorder (CPTSD) based on the new ICD-11 trauma questionnaire (ICD-TQ). J Affect Disord. 2017;207:181–7.

Kazlauskas E, Zelviene P, Daniunaite I, Hyland P, Kvedaraite M, Shevlin M, Cloitre M. The structure of ICD-11 PTSD and complex PTSD in adolescents exposed to potentially traumatic experiences. J Affect Disord. 2020;265:169–74.

Kazlauskas E, Kairyte A, Zelviene P. Complex posttraumatic stress disorder in adolescence: a two-year follow-up study. Clin Child Psychol Psychiatry. 2024;29(2):466–78.

Kelly Grealy M, Godfrey E, Brady F, Whyte O'Sullivan E, Carroll GA, Burke T. Borderline personality disorder traits and mentalising ability: the self-other social cognition paradox. Front Psych. 2022;13:1023348.

Kessler RC, Sonnega A, Bromet E, Hughes M, Nelson CB. Posttraumatic stress disorder in the National Comorbidity Survey. In: Fear and anxiety. Routledge; 2013. p. 22–34.

Kessler RC, Aguilar-Gaxiola S, Alonso J, Benjet C, Bromet EJ, Cardoso G, Degenhardt L, de Girolamo G, Dinolova RV, Ferry F, Florescu S. Trauma and PTSD in the WHO world mental health surveys. Eur J Psychotraumatol. 2017;8(sup5):1353383.

Kleindienst N, Löffler A, Herzig M, Bertsch K, Bekrater-Bodmann R. Evaluation of the own body in women with current and remitted borderline personality disorder: evidence for long-lasting effects of childhood sexual abuse. Eur J Psychotraumatol. 2020;11(1):1764707.

Knefel M, Tran US, Lueger-Schuster B. The association of posttraumatic stress disorder, complex posttraumatic stress disorder, and borderline personality disorder from a network analytical perspective. J Anxiety Disord. 2016;43:70–8.

Koenen KC, Ratanatharathorn A, Ng L, McLaughlin KA, Bromet EJ, Stein DJ, Karam EG, Ruscio AM, Benjet C, Scott K, Atwoli L. Posttraumatic stress disorder in the world mental health surveys. Psychol Med. 2017;47(13):2260–74.

Kolthof KA, Voorendonk EM, Van Minnen A, De Jongh A. Effects of intensive trauma-focused treatment of individuals with both post-traumatic stress disorder and borderline personality disorder. Eur J Psychotraumatol. 2022;13(2):2143076.

Krause-Utz A. Stimulating research on childhood adversities, borderline personality disorder, and complex post-traumatic stress disorder. Borderline Personal Disord Emot Dysregul. 2021;8(1):11.

Lam SK, Ng AS, Zhou CR, Hung SL, Fung HW. Persistence and psychological predictors of ICD-11 complex PTSD: a six-month longitudinal study in Hong Kong. J Loss Trauma. 2023;17:1–21.

Lawless J, Tarren-Sweeney M. Alignment of borderline personality disorder and complex post-traumatic stress disorder with complex developmental symptomatology. J Child Adolesc Trauma. 2023;16(2):433–46.

Lenzenweger MF, Lane MC, Loranger AW, Kessler RC. DSM-IV personality disorders in the National Comorbidity Survey Replication. Biol Psychiatry. 2007;62(6):553–64.

Lewis KL, Grenyer BF. Borderline personality or complex posttraumatic stress disorder? An update on the controversy. Harv Rev Psychiatry. 2009;17(5):322–8.

Linehan M. Cognitive-behavioral treatment of borderline personality disorder. Guilford Press; 1993.

Lieb K, Zanarini MC, Schmahl C, Linehan MM, Bohus M. Borderline personality disorder. Lancet. 2004;364(9432):453–61.

López-Castro T, Saraiya T, Zumberg-Smith K, Dambreville N. Association between shame and posttraumatic stress disorder: a meta-analysis. J Trauma Stress. 2019;32(4):484–95.

Maercker A, Hecker T, Augsburger M, Kliem S. ICD-11 prevalence rates of posttraumatic stress disorder and complex posttraumatic stress disorder in a German nationwide sample. J Nerv Ment Dis. 2018;206(4):270–6.

Masland SR, Victor SE, Peters JR, Fitzpatrick S, Dixon-Gordon KL, Bettis AH, Navarre KM, Rizvi SL. Destigmatizing borderline personality disorder: a call to action for psychological science. Perspect Psychol Sci. 2023;18(2):445–60.

Matthews SR, Elizabeth M, Roberts LN, Nixon RD. Client versus clinicians' standards of clinically meaningful change and the effects of treatment expectations on therapeutic outcomes in individuals with posttraumatic stress disorder. Behav Ther. 2022;53(3):560–70.

Matthews M, Webb TL, Sheppes G. Do people choose the same strategies to regulate other people's emotions as they choose to regulate their own? Emotion. 2022;22(8):1723.

Mauritz MW, Goossens PJ, Draijer N, Van Achterberg T. Prevalence of interpersonal trauma exposure and trauma-related disorders in severe mental illness. Eur J Psychotraumatol. 2013;4(1):19985.

Mauritz MW, van Gaal BG, Goossens PJ, Jongedijk RA, Vermeulen H. Treating patients with severe mental illness with narrative exposure therapy for comorbid post-traumatic stress disorder. B J Psych Open. 2021;7(1):e12.

Mauritz M, Goossens P, Jongedijk R, Vermeulen H, van Gaal B. Investigating the efficacy and experiences with narrative exposure therapy in severe mentally ill patients with comorbid post-traumatic stress disorder receiving flexible assertive community treatment: a mixed methods study. Front Psych. 2022;13:804491.

McGlashan TH, Grilo CM, Skodol AE, Gunderson JG, Shea MT, Morey LC, Zanarini MC, Stout RL. The collaborative longitudinal personality disorders study: baseline axis I/II and II/II diagnostic co-occurrence. Acta Psychiatr Scand. 2000;102(4):256–64.

McGlashan TH, Grilo CM, Sanislow CA, Ralevski E, Morey LC, Gunderson JG, Skodol AE, Shea MT, Zanarini MC, Bender D, Stout RL. Two-year prevalence and stability of individual DSM-IV criteria for schizotypal, borderline, avoidant, and obsessive-compulsive personality disorders: toward a hybrid model of axis II disorders. Am J Psychiatry. 2005;162(5):883–9.

Mennin DS, Heimberg RG, Turk CL, Fresco DM. Preliminary evidence for an emotion dysregulation model of generalized anxiety disorder. Behav Res Ther. 2005;43(10):1281–310.

Messman-Moore TL, Bhuptani PH. A review of the long-term impact of child maltreatment on posttraumatic stress disorder and its comorbidities: an emotion dysregulation perspective. Clin Psychol Sci Pract. 2017;24(2):154.

Miller MW, Resick PA. Internalizing and externalizing subtypes in female sexual assault survivors: implications for the understanding of complex PTSD. Behav Ther. 2007;38(1):58–71.

Miller MW, Wolf EJ, Reardon A, Greene A, Ofrat S, McInerney S. Personality and the latent structure of PTSD comorbidity. J Anxiety Disord. 2012;26(5):599–607.

Møller L, Augsburger M, Elklit A, Søgaard U, Simonsen E. Traumatic experiences, ICD-11 PTSD, ICD-11 complex PTSD, and the overlap with ICD-10 diagnoses. Acta Psychiatr Scand. 2020;141(5):421–31.

Møller L, Bach B, Augsburger M, Elklit A, Søgaard U, Simonsen E. Structure of ICD-11 complex PTSD and relationship with psychoform and somatoform dissociation. Eur J Trauma Dissoc. 2021;5(3):100233.

Morris D, Webb EL, Fox E, Holmes J, Reynolds K, Head M, Lunn A, Canterbury R, McAllister P, Dionelis K, Kamath S. Examining the prevalence of complex PTSD in an inpatient DBT service for females with a primary diagnosis of EUPD. Abuse Int Impact J. 2021;2(1):79–95.

Murray H, El-Leithy S. Working with complexity in PTSD: a cognitive therapy approach. Routledge; 2022.

Nestgaard Rød Å, Schmidt C. Complex PTSD: what is the clinical utility of the diagnosis. Eur J Psychotraumatol. 2021;12(1):2002028.

Nguyen J, Whiteside LK, Bulger EM, Veach L, Moloney K, Russo J, Nehra D, Wang J, Zatzick DF. Post-traumatic stress disorder (PTSD) symptoms and alcohol and drug use comorbidity at 25 US level I trauma centers. Trauma Surg Acute Care Open. 2022;7(1):e000913.

Olff M. To share or not to share–10 years of European Journal of Psychotraumatology. Eur J Psychotraumatol. 2020;11(1):1844955.

Owczarek M, Karatzias T, McElroy E, Hyland P, Cloitre M, Kratzer L, Knefel M, Grandison G, Ho GW, Morris D, Shevlin M. Borderline personality disorder (BPD) and complex posttraumatic stress disorder (CPTSD): a network analysis in a highly traumatized clinical sample. J Personal Disord. 2023;37(1):112–29.

Pagura J, Stein MB, Bolton JM, Cox BJ, Grant B, Sareen J. Comorbidity of borderline personality disorder and posttraumatic stress disorder in the US population. J Psychiatr Res. 2010;44(16):1190–8.

Panayi P, Berry K, Sellwood W, Campodonico C, Bentall RP, Varese F. The role and clinical correlates of complex post-traumatic stress disorder in people with psychosis. Front Psychol. 2022;13:791996.

Pascual JC, Arias L, Soler J. Pharmacological management of borderline personality disorder and common comorbidities. CNS Drugs. 2023;37(6):489–97.

Perkonigg A, Höfler M, Cloitre M, Wittchen HU, Trautmann S, Maercker A. Evidence for two different ICD-11 posttraumatic stress disorders in a community sample of adolescents and young adults. Eur Arch Psychiatry Clin Neurosci. 2016;266:317–28.

Pietrzak RH, Goldstein RB, Southwick SM, Grant BF. Personality disorders associated with full and partial posttraumatic stress disorder in the US population: results from Wave 2 of the National Epidemiologic Survey on alcohol and related conditions. J Psychiatr Res. 2011;45(5):678–86.

Porter C, Palmier-Claus J, Branitsky A, Mansell W, Warwick H, Varese F. Childhood adversity and borderline personality disorder: a meta-analysis. Acta Psychiatr Scand. 2020;141(1):6–20.

Powers A, Stevens JS, O-Banion D, Stenson AF, Kaslow N, Jovanovic T, Bradley B. Intergenerational transmission of risk for PTSD symptoms in African American children: the roles of maternal and child emotion dysregulation. Psychol Trauma Theory Res Pract Policy. 2022a;14(7):1099.

Powers A, Petri JM, Sleep C, Mekawi Y, Lathan EC, Shebuski K, Bradley B, Fani N. Distinguishing PTSD, complex PTSD, and borderline personality disorder using exploratory structural equation modeling in a trauma-exposed urban sample. J Anxiety Disord. 2022b;88:102558.

Raudales AM, Darosh AG, Contractor AA, Schatten HT, Dixon-Gordon KL, Weiss NH. Positive emotion dysregulation identifies trauma-exposed community individuals at risk for suicide and nonsuicidal self-injury. J Nerv Ment Dis. 2021;209(6):434–42.

Redican E, Cloitre M, Hyland P, McBride O, Karatzias T, Murphy J, Shevlin M. The latent structure of ICD-11 posttraumatic stress disorder (PTSD) and complex PTSD in a general population sample from USA: a factor mixture modelling approach. J Anxiety Disord. 2022;85:102497.

Reinders AA, Young AH, Veltman DJ. Biomarkers of dissociation. B J Psych Open. 2023;9(4):e119.

Regier DA, Kuhl EA, Kupfer DJ. The DSM-5: classification and criteria changes. World Psychiatry. 2013;12(2):92–8.

Ressler KJ, Berretta S, Bolshakov VY, Rosso IM, Meloni EG, Rauch SL, Carlezon WA Jr. Post-traumatic stress disorder: clinical and translational neuroscience from cells to circuits. Nat Rev Neurol. 2022;18(5):273–88.

Rink J, Lipinska G. Evidence of distinct profiles of ICD-11 post-traumatic stress disorder (PTSD) and complex PTSD in a South African sample. Eur J Psychotraumatol. 2020;11(1):1818965.

Roberts AL, Malspeis S, Kubzansky LD, Feldman CH, Chang SC, Koenen KC, Costenbader KH. Association of trauma and posttraumatic stress disorder with incident systemic lupus erythematosus in a longitudinal cohort of women. Arthritis Rheumatol. 2017;69(11):2162–9.

Roberts DG. Understanding autistic communities need for substance use information: developing a pragmatic resource (Doctoral dissertation, Manchester Metropolitan University), 2023.

Roberts AL, Koenen KC, Chen Q, Gilsanz P, Mason SM, Prescott J, Ratanatharathorn A, Rimm EB, Sumner JA, Winning A, De Vivo I. Posttraumatic stress disorder and accelerated aging: PTSD and leukocyte telomere length in a sample of civilian women. Depress Anxiety. 2017;34(5):391–400.

Rosenstein LK, Ellison WD, Walsh E, Chelminski I, Dalrymple K, Zimmerman M. The role of emotion regulation difficulties in the connection between childhood emotional abuse and borderline personality features. Personal Disord Theory Res Treat. 2018;9(6):590.

Ruocco AC. The neuropsychology of borderline personality disorder: a meta-analysis and review. Psychiatry Res. 2005;137(3):191–202.

Sar V, Akyuz G, Kugu N, Ozturk E, Ertem-Vehid H. Axis I dissociative disorder comorbidity in borderline personality disorder and reports of childhood trauma. J Clin Psychiatry. 2006;67(10):1583–90.

Saraiya TC, Fitzpatrick S, Zumberg-Smith K, López-Castro TE, Back SA, Hien D. Social–emotional profiles of PTSD, complex PTSD, and borderline personality disorder among racially and ethnically diverse young adults: a latent class analysis. J Trauma Stress. 2021;34(1):56–68.

Scheiderer EM, Wood PK, Trull TJ. The comorbidity of borderline personality disorder and post-traumatic stress disorder: revisiting the prevalence and associations in a general population sample. Borderline Personal Disord Emot Dysregul. 2015;2:1–6.

Scheiderer EM, Wang T, Tomko RL, Wood PK, Trull TJ. Negative affect instability among individuals with comorbid borderline personality disorder and posttraumatic stress disorder. Clin Psychol Sci. 2016;4(1):67–81.

Schiess-Jokanovic J, Knefel M, Kantor V, Weindl D, Schäfer I, Lueger-Schuster B. Complex post-traumatic stress disorder and post-migration living difficulties in traumatised refugees and asylum seekers: the role of language acquisition and barriers. Eur J Psychotraumatol. 2021;12(1):2001190.

Selby EA, Harnedy LE, Hiner M, Kim J. Developmental and momentary dynamics in the onset and maintenance of nonsuicidal self-injurious behavior and borderline personality disorder. Curr Psychiatry Rep. 2022;24(12):897–909.

Shalev A, Liberzon I, Marmar C. Post-traumatic stress disorder. N Engl J Med. 2017; 376(25):2459–69.

Shah R, Zanarini MC. Comorbidity of borderline personality disorder: current status and future directions. Psychiatr Clin. 2018;41(4):583–93.

Sheridan G, Carr A. Survivors' lived experiences of posttraumatic growth after institutional childhood abuse: an interpretative phenomenological analysis. Child Abuse Negl. 2020;103:104430.

Simon VA, Feiring C, Cleland CM. Early stigmatization, PTSD, and perceived negative reactions of others predict subsequent strategies for processing child sexual abuse. Psychol Violence. 2016;6(1):112.

Slotema CW, Blom JD, Niemantsverdriet MB, Sommer IE. Auditory verbal hallucinations in borderline personality disorder and the efficacy of antipsychotics: a systematic review. Front Psych. 2018;9:347.

Smith C, Ford C, Baldwin G, Jensen TK, Karatzias T, Birkeland MS, Meiser-Stedman R. Do psychological treatments for PTSD in children and young people reduce trauma-related appraisals? A systematic review and meta-analysis. Behav Res Ther. 2024;26:104621.

Snoek A, Nederstigt J, Ciharova M, Sijbrandij M, Lok A, Cuijpers P, Thomaes K. Impact of comorbid personality disorders on psychotherapy for post-traumatic stress disorder: systematic review and meta-analysis. Eur J Psychotraumatol. 2021;12(1):1929753.

Stanley IH, Hom MA, Boffa JW, Stage DR, Joiner TE. PTSD from a suicide attempt: An empirical investigation among suicide attempt survivors. J Clin Psychol. 2019;75(10):1879–95.

Stepp SD, Lazarus SA, Byrd AL. A systematic review of risk factors prospectively associated with borderline personality disorder: taking stock and moving forward. Personal Disord Theory Res Treat. 2016;7(4):316.

Taylor S, Asmundson GJ, Carleton RN. Simple versus complex PTSD: a cluster analytic investigation. J Anxiety Disord. 2006;20(4):459–72.

Tomko RL, Trull TJ, Wood PK, Sher KJ. Characteristics of borderline personality disorder in a community sample: comorbidity, treatment utilization, and general functioning. J Personal Disord. 2014;28(5):734–50.

Torres M. A Systematic Literature Review on the Impact of Sensation Seeking on Risk, Impulsivity, and PTSD (Doctoral dissertation, California Southern University). 2023.

Tragesser SL, Solhan M, Schwartz-Mette R, Trull TJ. The role of affective instability and impulsivity in predicting future BPD features. J Personal Disord. 2007;21(6):603–14.

Trull TJ, Tomko RL, Brown WC, Scheiderer EM. Borderline personality disorder in 3-D: dimensions, symptoms, and measurement challenges. Soc Personal Psychol Compass. 2010;4(11):1057–69.

Van Asselt AD, Dirksen CD, Arntz A, Severens JL. The cost of borderline personality disorder: societal cost of illness in BPD-patients. Eur Psychiatry. 2007;22(6):354–61.

Van der Kolk BA, Roth S, Pelcovitz D, Sunday S, Spinazzola J. Disorders of extreme stress: the empirical foundation of a complex adaptation to trauma. J Trauma Stress. 2005;18(5):389–99.

van Dijke A, Hopman JA, Ford JD. Affect dysregulation, psychoform dissociation, and adult relational fears mediate the relationship between childhood trauma and complex posttraumatic stress disorder independent of the symptoms of borderline personality disorder. Eur J Psychotraumatol. 2018;9(1):1400878.

Vermetten E, Spiegel D. Trauma and dissociation: implications for borderline personality disorder. Curr Psychiatry Rep. 2014;16:1–0.

Weiss NH, Nelson RJ, Contractor AA, Sullivan TP. Emotion dysregulation and posttraumatic stress disorder: a test of the incremental role of difficulties regulating positive emotions. Anxiet Stress Cop. 2019;32(4):443–56.

Webb EK, Bird CM, deRoon-Cassini TA, Weis CN, Huggins AA, Fitzgerald JM, Miskovich T, Bennett K, Krukowski J, Torres L, Larson CL. Racial discrimination and resting-state functional connectivity of salience network nodes in trauma-exposed Black adults in the United States. JAMA Netw Open. 2022;5(1):e2144759.

Weiss NH, Tull MT, Sullivan TP, Dixon-Gordon KL, Gratz KL. Posttraumatic stress disorder symptoms and risky behaviors among trauma-exposed inpatients with substance dependence: the influence of negative and positiveurgency. Drug Alcohol Depend. 2015;155:147–53.

Weiss NH, Contractor AA, Forkus SR, Goncharenko S, Raudales AM. Positive emotion dysregulation among community individuals: the role of trauma exposure and posttraumatic stress disorder. J Trauma Stress. 2020;33(5):741–9.

Westphal M, Olfson M, Bravova M, Gameroff MJ, Gross R, Wickramaratne P, Pilowsky DJ, Neugebauer R, Shea S, Lantigua R, Weissman M. Borderline personality disorder, exposure to interpersonal trauma, and psychiatric comorbidity in urban primary care patients. Psychiatry Interpers Biolog Processes. 2013;76(4):365–80.

Winsper C, Bilgin A, Thompson A, Marwaha S, Chanen AM, Singh SP, Wang A, Furtado V. The prevalence of personality disorders in the community: a global systematic review and meta-analysis. Br J Psychiatry. 2020;216(2):69–78.

World Health Organization. ICD-11 for mortality and morbidity statistics, 2018.

World Health Organization. The WHO special initiative for mental health (2019–2023): universal health coverage for mental health. World Health Organization; 2019.

World Health Organization. WHO guidelines on mental health at work. World Health Organization; 2022.

Yen S, Shea MT, Sanislow CA, Grilo CM, Skodol AE, Gunderson JG, McGlashan TH, Zanarini MC, Morey LC. Borderline personality disorder criteria associated with prospectively observed suicidal behavior. Am J Psychiatry. 2004;161(7):1296–8.

Zanarini MC, Temes CM, Magni LR, Fitzmaurice GM, Aguirre BA, Goodman M. Prevalence rates of borderline symptoms reported by adolescent inpatients with BPD, psychiatrically healthy adolescents and adult inpatients with BPD. Personal Ment Health. 2017;11(3):150–6.

Zimmerman M, Becker L. The hidden borderline patient: patients with borderline personality disorder who do not engage in recurrent suicidal or self-injurious behavior. Psychol Med. 2023;53(11):5177–84.

Chapter 14
Eating Disorders and Borderline Personality Disorder

Introduction

Borderline personality disorder (BPD) is presented as one of the most serious psychiatric disorders, featured by emotional lability, cognitive, behavioral instability, and disturbed interpersonal relationships (APA, DSM-5-TR 2022; Temes et al. 2019). Individuals with BPD often become involved in dysregulated eating behaviors, such as binge eating and purging (Selby et al. 2010a). A great body of investigations have demonstrated that eating disorders (EDs) and disordered-eating behavior are partially common among individuals with BPD (Khosravi 2020; Miller et al. 2022), and notable comorbidities has been reported at 14–53% based on various findings (Lee and Vaillancourt 2023; Zanarini et al. 2010; Martinussen et al. 2017; Miller et al. 2022).

Eating disorders encompass a broad group of mental disorders distinguished by disordered eating or weight control behaviors contributing to changed food assumption or absorption (Treasure et al. 2020). Updated DSM-5 descriptions define two main types of EDs featured by disturbed eating behaviors: infant and youth feeding disorders and eating disorders (Gordon et al. 2024). Feeding and eating disorders are typically characterized by a persistent impairment of eating or eating-related behavior that causes changes in the consumption or absorption of food, remarkably disturbing physical health or psychological functioning (APA, DSM-5-TR 2022). EDs comprise of anorexia nervosa (AN), bulimia nervosa (BN), and binge-eating disorder (BED), other specified feeding or eating disorders (OSFED), and un specified feeding or eating disorders (UFED) (APA, DSM-5-TR 2022; Gordon et al. 2024). EDs include disturbances in eating, weight, and body image, which are severe and serious mental disorder (Swanson et al. 2011; Rappaport et al. 2024). Our knowledge about the population distribution and community burden of EDs has improved markedly over the past two decades. Substantial evidence has documented that EDs and their linked behaviors have higher prevalence among individuals from

M. Salavati, E. A. Selby, *Theories of Borderline Personality Disorder*,
https://doi.org/10.1007/978-3-031-75503-3_14

lower-income groups and its distribution is under gender diversity and age as well (Pike and Dunne 2015; Calzo et al. 2017; Hazzard et al. 2020). According to investigations, the highest prevalence rates of EDs have been observed in children and adolescents, in spite of several reports of incidence among older adults (Ackard et al. 2013). Using a systematic rapid review methodology for peer-reviewed studies published between 2009 and 2021, the global lifetime prevalence of all types of EDs was shown to range from 0.74% to 2.2% in males, and from 2.58% to 8.4% in females. In addition, results suggested that EDs are more prevalent in youth and adolescents, especially females (Hay 2023). Based on international reports, eating and feeding disorders are among the psychiatric disorders with the highest mortality and suicidal rates (Miskovic-Wheatley et al. 2023; Chesney et al. 2021). More than 3.3 million morbidities, as well as several disabilities because of medical and psychiatric complications have been reported due to EDs each year around the world (van Hoeken and Hoek 2020). Moreover, studies have suggested that the number of adolescents seeking treatment for EDs is substantially increasing (e.g., Asch et al. 2021). Based on a national database in a sample including 8652 inpatients, Rappaport et al. (2024) indicated a gradual increase in hospitalizations for patients with EDs before the COVID pandemic, as well as a large rising rate during the pandemic with the mean age of 15.8 years ascribing 85.9% female. Based on the findings, anorexia nervosa was the most common eating disorder (57.5%), as well as an increasing rate of hospitalization for patients with avoidant-restrictive food intake disorder. In a sample of 15 inpatient and outpatient adolescents, a significant increase in EDs during the COVID-19 pandemic was found (Hartman-Munick et al. 2022). In addition, remarkable number of patients with EDs received the diagnosis of depression (585%), anxiety disorders (57.8%), and suicide ideations (21.9%). These findings can document that hospitalizations for EDs among American adolescents have an escalated rate, especially co-occurrence with suicidal thoughts (Rappaport et al. 2024). Based on a systematic review encompassing 6537 studies, the association between EDs and mental health issues including depression, anxiety, obsessive-compulsive disorder, and social anxiety were explored. Further three studies were concentrated on the relation between EDs and attention deficit/hyperactivity disorder (ADHD), two studies focused on EDs and suicidal-related outcomes, and seven studies investigated the relations between EDs and bipolar disorders, personality disorders, and NSSI. The results indicated that depression, social anxiety, and ADHD were the most prevalent mental health problems among individuals with EDs (Tan et al. 2023). The development of EDs stemmed from a crossroad of childhood and adulthood, a contributive association with the mental and the somatic, the individual and the social (Stankovska et al. 2023). EDs are chronic in nature and typically being in early stages of young adult life, before the ages of 20–30 (Raykos et al. 2018; Turner et al. 2024; Gale et al. 2016; Accurso and Waller 2021).

According to a body of investigations, comorbidity is common among patient with AN, BN, and BED (Keski-Rahkonen adn Mustelin 2016, estimated 80% of individuals suffering from other psychiatric disorders reported EDs over their life (Newton 2019). Remarkable co-occurrences with other psychiatric disorders have been found among a substantial number of individuals with eating disorders, such as anxiety disorders, obsessive-compulsive disorder. EDs come with comorbid mental issues, severe physical complications with a high risk of chronicity and mortality (Arcelus et al. 2011; Smink et al. 2012, 2016). For instance, studies have shown that the rates of anxiety disorders among individuals with EDs ranged from 25% to 75% (Swinbourne and Touyz 2007), while it was reported that 65% of individuals with EDs had at least one anxiety disorder (Deboer and Smits 2013). Symptoms of eating disorders, clinically and subclinical, can contribute to remarkable distress and disruptive functioning for individuals and their family, considerable interpersonal relationship issues, and elevated risk of medical morbidities, psychiatric morbidities, early mortality because of high rates of physical complications or the probability of suicidal behaviors (Demmler et al. 2020, 2023).

Anorexia nervosa (AN) is a severe psychiatric disorder that manifests in refusal to maintain normal weight, intentional caloric restriction, combined with constant behaviors interfering with weight gain (APA 2022). AN can be considered as a model of chronic human starvation (Khiyami et al. 2023) and AN impacts up to 2.2% of women (Keski-Rahkonen et al. 2007). A high mortality index has been reported for AN (Papadopoulos et al. 2009), with a very high suicide rate occurring in addition to high medical mortality (Selby et al. 2010a, b). Among eating disorders, AN is one of the most remarkable challenging conditions for clinicians and health policymakers around the world. The diagnostic criteria of AN are comprised of restriction of energy intake relative to requirements causing remarkable low body weight, intensely severe fear of gaining weight or becoming fat, constant behavior which interferes with weight gain, impaired experiences of one's body weight or shape and disturbed self-evaluation, having a distorted perception related to weight and shape, and no recognition of the severe negative consequences of current low body weight (APA, DSM-5-TR 2022; Gordon et al. 2024). Two subtypes of AN include restricting type, and binge-eating/purging type, in which individuals with anorexia nervosa apply a series of purging behaviors such as self-induced vomiting, misuse of laxatives, diuretics, or enemas, as well as regularly purging after the consumption of small amounts of food (APA, DSM-5-TR 2022; Gordon et al. 2024). The prevalence of AN has been estimated to be 1.4% in women and 0.2% in men (Galmiche et al. 2019), a 12-month prevalence ranges from 0% to 0.8% in women/0% to 0.01% in men; and a lifetime prevalence ranges from 0.9% to 1.42% in women/0.12% to 0.3% in men (APA, DSM-5-TR 2022). To elucidate the pathogenesis of AN, it is broadly acknowledged that biological factors lead to the development, course, and progression of AN (Barakat et al. 2023), such as changes in neuroendocrine functions, hypothalamic pituitary axis regulation, alterations in appetite regulating hormones (Schorr and Miller 2017), changed neural bases of reward processes (Berner et al. 2019), and various forms of dysregulated inflammatory status (Butler et al. 2024; Dalton et al. 2018; Nilsson et al. 2020; Leuti et al. 2021; Collu et al. 2020; Caso et al. 2020).

Bulimia nervosa (BN) is diagnosed as recurrent episodes of binge eating characterized by eating in a discrete period time, eating a much larger amount of food than what individuals eat regularly in a similar period of time, a sense of lack of control over eating during the episode, recurrent inappropriate compensatory behaviors to stop over-weight such as self-induced vomiting, misuse of laxatives, diuretics, fasting, and excessive exercise, and self-evaluation is unduly effected by based on body shape and weight. These symptoms last at least once a week for 3 months and should not coincide with episodes of AN (APA, DSM-5-TR 2022; Hessler et al. 2019; Goldschmidt et al. 2014). BN is manifested by recurrent episodes of heightened uncontrolled overeating that are followed by various types of compensatory behaviors, accompanied by extreme concerns about body weight and shape (Stankovska et al. 2023; World Health Organization, WHO 2019). However, individuals with BN retain normal weight; BN is a grave disorder with serious secondary symptoms, which has shown chronicity in nature and a tendency to co-occur with other psychiatric disorders (Hessler et al. 2019). The 12-month prevalence of BN ranges from 0.14% to 0.3% (0.22–0.5% in women; 0.05–0.1% in men), as well as the lifetime prevalence ranges from 0.28% to 1.0% (0.46–1.5% in women; 0.05–0.08% in men) in two adult community sample in the USA (APA, DSM-5-TR 2022).

Binge-eating disorder (BED) consists of episodes characterized by eating a larger than regular amount of food, in spite of not necessarily feeling physically hungry, in a discrete period of time and more than others would typically eat in a similar period of time, and a sense of lack of control over eating during the episode. Additionally, the episodes of binge eating are related with eating much more rapidly than normal, continuing eating until feeling uncomfortably full, eating alone due to feeling embarrassed, and feeing disgusted with oneself, depressed, or very guilty afterward, which occurs at least once a week for 3 months (APA, DSM-5-TR 2022). BED is one of the most common subtypes of feeding and eating disorders (American Psychiatric Association 2013), with a lifetime prevalence in general population about 2.03% in the USA (Cossrow et al. 2016). In contrast to BN, inappropriate compensatory behaviors have not occurred in individuals with BED (APA 2022). In line with recent findings, some certain metacognitive beliefs related to food and eating have been found in individuals with BED contributing to the maintenance of BED symptoms, encompassing: (a) negative beliefs (ideas of having no control over eating); (b) positive beliefs (thoughts about mood is improved by eating); and permissive beliefs (thought that a person should let himself to binge eating) (Burton et al. 2018).

There are several other forms of eating disorders and exploratory eating disorder diagnoses that are not discussed here due to a lower co-occurrence with BPD (e.g., avoidant/restrictive food intake disorder; ARFID; purging disorder), and likewise we do not cover information on non-psychiatric eating-related health concerns here (e.g., obesity, poor nutrition, diminished access to healthy food options). Although these issues are not discussed further, it is important to be aware that other EDs and eating-related health problems can increase the complexity of issues when presenting as comorbid with BPD.

Comorbidity and Common Symptoms Between BPD and Eating Disorders

Among psychiatric disorders, BPD and eating disorders are comparatively common, even in various populations with different gender and age (Khosravi 2020). According to experimental and clinical studies, the majority of individuals with an have shown comorbidity with personality disorders, specifically BPD (Martinussen et al. 2017; Miller et al. 2022; Voderholzer et al. 2021; Robinson et al. 2014). The comorbidity of EDs with BPD is common and highlights potential shared risk factors, phenotypes, and behavioral traits encompassing attachment issues, adverse childhood experience, NSSI, interpersonal relationship difficulties, and comorbid maladaptive mood and dysregulated behaviors (McDonald 2019). BPD symptoms such as impulsivity, affective instability, outbursts of anger, and suicidal behaviors are frequently studied in the context of EDs (Amianto et al. 2012; Claes et al. 2015; Newton 2019). The rates of EDs in individuals with BPD were reported to be 21.7% for AN and 24.1% for BN comorbidity (Zanarini et al. 2010), and based on a meta-analysis, the prevalence of personality disorders in patients with EDs was such that 28% of BN had BPD, provided 25% of AN binge-eating/purging subtype and 10.8% of AN restrictive subtype had BPD (Sansone et al. 2004). Bulimia nervosa and anorexia nervosa symptoms have shown significant correlation with BPD symptomology (Miller et al. 2022); however, the focus of investigations studying ED-BPD comorbidity has been concentrated on BN rather than AN (Miller et al. 2022). According to a meta-analysis assessing the prevalence of personality disorders among individuals with EDs, it was revealed that the most common comorbid personality disorder in EDs is BPD: 28.4% for BPD+BN; 25.5% for BPD+AN-binge-eating/purging subtype; and 11.7% for BPD+BED (Sansone et al. 2005). Based on meta-analyses studies, it has been estimated that one-quarter to one-third of individuals with BN meet criteria for BPD (Martinussen et al. 2017; Sansone et al. 2005). Considering a global prevalence of BN, around 1 million individuals would be assumed to meet both BN and BPD (BN+BPD) criteria (Reas et al. 2013). A systematic review and series of meta-analysis was performed to examine: (1) which of the nine BPD symptoms are specifically increased among individuals with EDs versus individuals without EDs, (2) whether a specific symptom of EDs have escalated levels of particular BPD symptoms, and (3) which one of the BPD symptoms remain unstudied/understudied in association with eating disorders. Across 122 studies, 9 separate meta-analyses for each 9 BPD symptoms were done to compare levels of symptoms among individuals with BPD and healthy controls. The findings showed emotional instability was found as the most elevated BPD symptom, while anger was shown as the least elevated, among individuals with BPD compared to controls. Based on comparisons of effect size across ED subtypes, AN binge-eating/purging subtype indicated the largest number of BPD symptoms, provided effect size for AN restrictive subtype were not remarkably larger than those other EDs for any BPD symptom. Based on the result, it was found that identity disturbances and interpersonal relationship issues were the least studied BPD symptoms (Miller et al. 2022).

Due to high rates of comorbidity between BN and BPD (Pearson et al. 2023; Selby et al. 2012; Cassin 2005), it has been suggested that there is potentially interacting etiologies which may contribute to the exacerbation of the likelihood of BN or BPD in the presence of each of them (Sansone et al. 2005), shared impulsivity (Zapolski et al. 2010), affective instability (Santangelo et al. 2014; Kockler et al. 2017), and difficulties in emotion regulation (Selby et al. 2012). It has been suggested that BPD symptoms may lead to EDs onset, presentation, and treatment course (Miller et al. 2022). For instance, longitudinal investigations have demonstrated that interpersonal issues (Shanmugam et al. 2014) and identity disturbances in adolescents (Verschueren et al. 2024) predict elevation in ED symptoms over time (Miller et al. 2022). On the other hand, in spite of several reports documented highly prevalent comorbidities of BPD and EDs, few studies have been done to elucidate whether this noteworthy comorbidity can be considered as an indicator of relatively causal associations (Sansone et al. 2011). Through applying data from a community-based cohort study and maintaining a developmental and psychosocial framework, Lee and Vaillancourt (2023) investigated the course of eating disorder and BPD features, shared trajectories and patterns of co-occurrence, temporal precedence, unique and common probabilities of childhood risk factors, and burden of likely clinical cases ascribable to each risk factors in a sample of 544 adolescents aged 14–18 years. The results indicated that 5% of adolescents followed a high symptom trajectory of eating issues, while this amount was 21% for BPD features. Based on findings, nearly a quarter of symptomatic adolescents had a report of co-occurring EDs and BPD features, as well as greater levels of EDs were more significant indicator of high levels of BPD features. Furthermore, non-modifiable factors were the most significant predictors belonging to a high trajectory group (girls and LGBTQ + youth). Moreover, bullying perpetration and clinical hyperactivity were specifically reported just for BPD features, while bullying victimization led to temporarily the largest population attributable fractions to eating disorder and BPD feature (Lee and Vaillancourt 2023). Based on a network analysis, the associations between certain groupings of BPD and ED symptoms, and other transdiagnostic variables encompassing insecure attachment, rejection sensitivity, emotion dysregulation, a theory of mind, and emotion recognition were explored among 753 adults (109 of them had a lifetime ED diagnosis). The findings indicated that the comorbidity between BPD and ED symptoms was merely relatively conceptualized via transdiagnostic variables. The centrality indices from network analysis revealed the emotion dysregulation and abandonment were core components in the network. While the theory of mind and emotion recognition showed weak connections with the other transdiagnostic variables (De Paoli et al. 2020). Miller et al. (2022) clarified the association between BN and AN symptoms and BPD symptomatology to answer two questions: (1) whether the nine BPD diagnostic criteria differentially associate with BN and AN, and (2) whether a compound measure of BPD symptoms differentially correlate with symptoms of BN versus AN. The results demonstrated greater AN and BN symptoms among individuals who experienced unstable interpersonal relationships, emotional instability, emptiness, identity disturbances, inappropriate anger, dissociation/paranoia, and suicidal behaviors. Further, avoidance abandonment was neither associated with BN nor AN (Miller et al. 2022). There are complicated associations between BPD symptoms and EDs, and it is assumed that BPD symptoms can be considered as a predisposing or severity factor of EDs (Pope Jr and Hudson 1989; Sansone and Sansone 2007). Wildes et al. (2011) found that individuals with AN with an "uncontrolled" personality profile, such as impulsivity, emotion dysregulation, and self-inflicted injurious behaviors, showed poorer outcomes at discharge and greater rates of readmission to treatment (Wildes et al. 2011). Furthermore, common psychopathology features contribute to a more complex clinical picture and more challenging issues within therapeutic interventions (Zeeck et al. 2007; Chen et al. 2009). Miller et al. (2022) proposed that certain symptoms of BPD have a considerable role in the comorbidity between BPD and EDs compared to others (Miller et al. 2022). Emotional instability, impulsivity, and anger indicated a remarkably greater association with BN in comparison to AN, while identity disturbance showed a stronger correlation with AN than with BN (Miller et al. 2022).

Anger and aggression are two core psychopathologic traits among individuals with EDs (Fassino et al. 2001), which have significant association with ED subtypes (Fassino et al. 2001), the severity levels of ED symptoms (Abbate-Daga et al. 2005), comorbidities with other psychiatric disorders (Fassino et al. 2003), biochemical dysfunction (Coccaro et al. 2010), disturbed endocrinologic functions (Costes et al. 2006), and impaired treatment outcome (Fassino et al. 2003). Miotto et al. (2008) found significantly higher levels of anger among individuals with BN compared to AN and healthy controls (Miotto et al. 2008). Krug et al. (2008) found that ED symptoms and specific personality traits were positively correlated with various forms of anger expression and higher rates of self-harm behaviors (Krug et al. 2008).

Emotion dysregulation has been documented as a core pathology in BPD contributing to severe clinical manifestations of BPD symptoms (Linehan 1993; Daros and Williams 2019; Chapman 2019; Chapman et al. 2020), as well as it is frequently reported in clinical populations (Prefit et al. 2019). Emotion regulation refers to attempts to impact which emotion one has, when one has them, and how one experiences or expresses these emotions (Gross 1998, 2024, 2015, 2013). Emotion dysregulation comprises (1) a lack of awareness/understanding of emotions; (2) difficulty with behavioral control in the context of emotions; (3) issues in using appropriate strategies to alter the duration and/or level of emotional responses to involve in goal-directed behavior; and (4) an unwillingness to experience emotions in the context of continuing significant/meaningful activities (Gratz and Roemer 2004). Further, emotion regulation difficulties have consistently been reported to be increased in individuals with all ED subtypes in comparison to controls (Lavender et al. 2015; Horvath et al. 2024; Ruscitti et al. 2016). Kockler et al. (2017) identified seven dysregulated sequences in BPD in comparison to healthy controls, and they compared these emotion sequences among individuals with BPD to patients with PTSD and BN. In line with findings, individuals with BPD more often switch between feelings of anxiety and sadness, and higher experiences of anxiety prior to experiencing anger compared to healthy controls. Further, none revealed greater frequencies compared to the PTSD group and the BN group, despite more frequent switching from anger to disgust among patients with BN (Kockler et al. 2017).

In line with emotion regulation models of dysregulated behaviors, binge eating, and vomiting occurring following elevated levels of negative emotions, contributing to formation behaviors to decline the levels of negative emotions (Selby et al. 2008). Substantial body of studies have documented that individuals with AN or BN revealed higher levels of impairment in their ability to regulate emotions, such as managing emotions in achieving goals while experiencing negative emotions, impulsive reaction to distress, and applying functional coping strategies in comparison to individuals with binge-eating disorder (Ruscitti et al. 2016; Svaldi et al. 2012a; Gratz and Roemer 2004; Brockmeyer et al. 2014). Ruscitti et al. (2016) investigated whether individuals with EDs indicate similar emotion dysregulation as patients without EDs, as well as whether patients with ED not-otherwise specified (EDNOS) show similar difficulties in emotion regulation in comparison to patients without eating disorders. The results revealed that individuals with EDs showed greater difficulties in emotion regulation in most domains of emotion regulation and that those with BED and EDNOS indicated the most remarkable differences in emotion regulation in comparison to patients without eating disorders. Further, no significant differences were found in terms of specific difficulties in emotion regulation among individuals with ED subtypes (Ruscitti et al. 2016). Difficulties in emotions are the major shared features in BPD and EDs, including issues in recognizing emotions named *alexithymia*, and emotional dysregulation (Khosravi 2020; Miller et al. 2022). Based on explanations about the disease mechanisms, EDs have joint characteristics of emotion dysregulation disorders such as BPD (Kolar et al. 2016). Emotion regulation issues observed in EDs encompass greater levels of emotion intensity, lower acceptance of emotions, less emotional awareness and clarity, and high level of using maladaptive emotion regulation strategies (Lavender et al. 2015). Like BPD, individuals with higher emotional instability may be engaged in more maladaptive eating-related behaviors, including binge and purging to regulate intensely negative emotions and rapid mood fluctuations (Miller et al. 2022; Telch et al. 2000). According to theoretical conceptualizations, applying various emotion regulation strategies encompassing rumination, suppression, and avoidance by individuals with BPD and EDs may contribute to highlighting the significant role of emotion regulation as a transdiagnostic structure in the development of BPD and EDs (Sloan et al. 2017). Based on a cross-sectional study, Khosravi (2020) studied the prevalence and psychopathology of feeding or eating disorders (FEDs) among 220 individuals with BPD (38 with BPD; 72 with BPD+FEDs; and 110 healthy controls. The findings indicated a 65.4% (n = 72) prevalence of FEDs, with the greatest and lowest prevalence rates for other specified FEDs (51.3%) and BN (6.9%), respectively. The results revealed the mediating role of anxiety and depression in the association between alexithymia and eating-disordered behaviors (Khosravi 2020).

A great body of empirical investigation and clinical observations have documented individuals with BN report co-occurrence of BPD (BPD+BN), which have shown to cause more severe effects on the outcome of treatment (e.g., Hessler et al.

2019). Several studies have documented that difficulties in emotion regulation play a major role in the development and maintenance of both BN and BPD symptomatology (Selby et al. 2012; Svaldi et al. 2012a, b; Pearson et al. 2023). BPD and BN are disorders that become engaged in emotion dysregulation, especially for negative emotion, impulsive behaviors beyond eating and vomiting as well (Selby et al. 2012). Experimental classification investigations proposed that individuals with BN with higher scores on emotion dysregulation traits, an "interpersonal-emotional" personality cluster, tend to display the highest frequency of daily binge eating and purging (Wonderlich et al. 2007). However, most individuals with BN display emotional dysregulation and impulsive behaviors (over binge eating and vomiting), even with no diagnosis of BPD simultaneously (Crosby et al. 2009; Myers and Derakshan 2015). Selby et al. (2012) investigated emotional responding surrounding binge eating and vomiting among 133 women with BN and no BPD diagnosis (BN) in comparison to women with BN and diagnostic levels of BPD (BN+BPD). They hypothesized that among BN+BPD group compared to BN alone would indicate greater daily variability in levels of negative and positive emotion which contribute largely on days when bulimic events occurred, elevated trajectories of negative emotion and positive emotion preceding binge/vomit behaviors, and escalated trajectories of negative or positive emotions following binge/vomit behaviors. The results demonstrated no significant elevated emotional variability among individuals with BPD in comparison to those without. For both groups, negative emotional variability was increased on bulimic event days, proposing that emotional variability may have led to binge eating and/or vomiting. Additionally, negative emotion prior to a binge was increased for the BN+BPD group compared to BN-BPD, while there were no significant group differences in increases in positive emotion were as a function of time leading up to binge episodes (Selby et al. 2012). Among 133 participants with BN from EMA data, Pearson et al. (2017) examined the associations between four identified BPD-like traits (including emotional lability, insecure attachment, identity issues, and cognitive dysregulation) and subsequent state factors, consisting of frequency of stressful events, perception of stressful events, emotional reactivity to stressful events. Three types of stressful events were studied: interpersonal, work/environment, and general daily hassles. Findings indicated that individuals' differences in BPD traits anticipated the state experience of triggers of bulimic behaviors in women with BN. The results showed that women with BN and higher scores on BPD traits reported more experience of a higher frequency of stressful events, tendency to perceive stressful events as stressful, and those with higher score in insecure attachment were more likely to react to interpersonal stressful events with higher negative emotion (Pearson et al. 2017). Santangelo et al. (2014) investigated the specificity of affective instability in individuals with BPD compared to clinical and healthy controls, among 43 female patients with BPD, 28 female healthy controls, and female clinical controls including PTSD ($n = 28$) and BN ($n = 20$). The findings indicated heightened affective instability for emotional valence and distress in comparison to healthy controls. Patients with PTSD or BN displayed a similar elevated instability of emotional valence and distress compared to the BPD group; however, there was no evidence supporting that affective instability was specific to individuals with BPD (Santangelo et al. 2014).

Few studies have been done to examine individuals with AN and BPD (Voderholzer et al. 2021; Selby et al. 2010a, b). A considerable tendency toward being involved in more compulsive behaviors such as hoarding food have been reported among individuals with AN; however, those with purging and binge-eating disorder (BED) subtypes tend to manifest heightened levels of behavioral dysregulation (Tozzi et al. 2006). Selby et al. (2010a, b) proposed that one of the most significant problems which should be noted regarding exploring BPD and dysregulated behaviors among individuals with BPD is the co-occurring AN and BPD that may contribute to synergistic effects, provided that both disorders escalate issues with behavioral dysregulation more so than either disorder alone (Selby et al. 2010b). To refine behavioral dysregulation in BPD, Selby et al. (2010a, b) investigated the association between dysregulated behaviors in BPD and a variety of potentially dysregulated behaviors among a large sample consisting of 718 females diagnosed with AN, among them, 41 participants were diagnosed with BPD. Findings supported a relation between BPD and alcohol misuse, hitting someone/breaking things, provoking fights/arguments, self-injurious behaviors, overdosing, street drug use, binge-eating, impulsive spending, shop lifting/stealing, and risky sexual behaviors. Differences were found in anticipating behavioral dysregulation applying dichotomous BPD diagnoses and a continuous measure of BPD (Selby et al. 2010b). Selby et al. (2015) explored the association between positive emotional instability and weight loss activities among 118 women with AN to investigate the synergic effects of positive and negative emotional instability on enhancing weight loss activities. The findings revealed higher levels of positive and negative emotional instability, and an interaction between the two which showed an association with highly frequent weight-loss activities, beyond AN subtype and mean levels of emotional instability (Selby et al. 2015).

Insufficient strategies of emotion regulation seem to be crucial in understanding the development and maintenance of binge-eating disorder (BED) (Walenda et al. 2021). Research findings have shown that the inability to regulate emotions adaptively may be considered as core factors for the development and sustaining BED (Svaldi et al. 2012a, b; Brockmeyer et al. 2014). The emotion regulation model provided by Polivy (1993) considers the function of binges in mitigating negative emotion, contributing to secondary reinforcement for maladaptive coping mechanisms which becomes learned and automated (Cardi et al. 2015). Binge eating is suggested as an impulsive behavior in individuals with BPD (Sebastian et al. 2013). Walenda et al. (2021) examined a broader range emotion regulation strategy (including acceptance, refocusing on planning, positive refocusing, positive reappraisal, putting into perspective, self-blame, rumination, and catastrophizing). In addition, they assessed the associations between those strategies and binge-eating-related beliefs (comprising negative, positive, and permissive), and clinical variables (EDs symptoms, both anxiety, depression, and alexithymia) among 35 individuals with BED and 41 female health control group. The results showed a significantly higher level of difficulties in emotion regulation, such as non-acceptance of emotional responses, lack of emotional clarity, difficulties involving goal-directed behavior, impulse control issues, and restricted access to emotion regulation strategies in comparison to healthy controls. Further, individuals were remarkably more likely to apply maladaptive strategies, including rumination and self-blame; and less likely to use adaptive strategies comprising positive refocusing and putting into perspective, as well. Among participants in a clinical group, different issues in emotion regulation happened which were positively correlated with greater level of alexithymia, anxiety, and depressive symptomatology. Positive associations were found in self-blame and catastrophizing and anxiety symptoms, with a significant relation between catastrophizing and the severity of EDs psychopathology (Walenda et al. 2021). Mahmoud Shaker et al. (2022) studied the frequency of binge-eating behavior in 70 patients with BPD, and its associations with impulsivity and emotion dysregulation. Findings showed medium emotional regulation propensity among individuals with BPD, mainly moderate in impulsivity in BPD, and significant relations between BE behavior and fear of abandonment, and clarity of feeling compared to non-binge group (Shaker et al. 2022).

Depression, anxiety, and *alexithymia* are suggested as shared psychopathology in BPD and EDs, as well as eating-related behaviors considered as common comorbidity between these two disorders (Khosravi 2020). Higher levels of anxiety, depression, and more extreme general psychopathology and life-threatening behaviors, higher levels of suffering from emotional dysregulation, and more problems in decreasing ED symptoms compared to individuals with EDs alone have been demonstrated (Chen et al. 2009; Ben-Porath et al. 2009). It has been shown that in individuals with BPD, emptiness is associated with lower levels of daily positive affect and higher levels of depressive mood (Hampton et al. 2021). The severity of depressive symptoms and higher level of anhedonia have been reported to remarkably anticipate ED symptom severity (Dingemans et al. 2020; Dolan et al. 2022). Further, individuals with BPD often experience pervasively undesirable and chronic shame and guilt over their behaviors (Cameron et al. 2021), characterized by negative, inadequate, or flawed self-perceptions (Jovev and Jackson 2004). In addition, both shame and guilt as disturbing emotional states are related to EDs (Carden et al. 2020). Individuals with borderline pathology often experience a limited form of guilt while more clear feeling of shame. Rather, individuals diagnosed with EDs manifest shame and guilt as self-conscious and moral emotions evoked in response to self-evaluation (Doyle et al. 2022).

In addition to these findings, the Five Factor model perspective has demonstrated higher levels of neuroticism, lower agreeableness, and low conscientiousness that are the characteristics of ED, especially BN, and simultaneously are substantially associated with BPD, impulsiveness, binge, and purging (Farstad et al. 2016; Claes et al. 2006; Tan et al. 2023). A meta-analysis of the prevalence indicated that all ED diagnoses are featured by increased perfectionism, neuroticism, and avoidance motivation, elevated sensitivity to social rewards, and lower levels of extraversion and self-directedness compared to controls. In addition, higher levels of impulsiveness in individuals with BN than AN were found. The findings revealed that BPD and paranoid PD were more common in individuals with AN binge-eating/purging,

BN, and ED not otherwise specified (Farstad et al. 2016). In line with cluster analyses of personality traits, three groups of individuals with EDs were suggested: under-controlled/deregulated; over-controlled; and resilient. Under-controlled patients with significantly high level of impulsivity and low levels of control reported greater BPD symptoms, binge eating, and purging in comparison to the other two profile groups (Wildes and Marcus 2013). Jackson (2021) compared personality styles (over-controlled, under-controlled, and resilience with four groups of individuals with EDs including AN restricting, BN, AN—being eating/purging, and atypical AN. Based on their findings, restricting and atypical AN showed the highest level of over-control, BPD indicated the greatest level of under-control, and BN and community samples were in between. Additionally, no significant differences were reported between the ED group and community sample. Moreover, the mental capacity to understand oneself and others in terms of mental states, mentalizing, has been suggested to be impaired in both BPD and eating disorders. Sacchetti et al. (2019) studied systematically mentalizing disturbances in 53 individuals with EDs and investigated whether impairments in mentalizing were associated with BPD features compared to BN. The results indicated that the scores of mentalizing were lower among patients with EDs compared to healthy controls, which were partially accounted for by BPD features, and partially by bulimic symptoms (Sacchetti et al. 2019).

Numerous studies have documented notable associations between EDs and impulsivity (Schag et al. 2015, 2019), and impulsivity has been proposed as a transdiagnostic feature of individuals with EDs (Mallorquí-Bagué et al. 2020). Impulsivity in BPD is manifested when patients experience unpleasant and undesirable emotions (Faraji and Özarabacı 2022; Klonsky 2008), while eating disorders are based on impulsive behaviors (Sneed 2012). Faraji and Oğur (2023) examined the association between BP traits, eating attitudes, guilt, and shame among 213 female and 18 male university students. The findings demonstrated positive correlations between shame and BP traits, emotion indecision, self-image, sense of emptiness, and intense anger. Further, significant positive correlation was reported between bulimia and preoccupation with eating and BP traits impulsivity (Faraji and Oğur 2023). Pellegrini et al. (2022) identified the clinical and psychometric characteristics of patients with EDs and disordered eating, with emphasis on impulsivity, among two groups of BPD inpatients based on the presence/non-presence of disordered-eating behaviors. The findings showed patients with BPD+disordered eating reported more lifetime suicide attempts and hospitalization, greater levels of impulsivity, especially attentional impulsivity, and higher depressive symptoms. Further, a significant correlation was found between attentional impulsivity and all of EDs subtypes, except the restriction type (Pellegrini et al. 2022).

Following on prior discussion, BPD is a severe chronic psychiatric disorder characterized by recurrent suicide attempt(s) and/or nonsuicidal self-injury (NSSI), with at least three-quarters of individuals with BPD attempting suicide and 10% dying by suicide (Lieb et al. 2004; Tan et al. 2023). EDs are proposed as a substantial risk factor for suicide, with a considerable association between suicide risk and EDs (Pisetsky et al. 2017; Thornton et al. 2016). Suicide is one of the most notable factors and leading causes of death in individuals with EDs, in particular among individuals with BN (Kostro et al. 2014; Bodell et al. 2014; Goldstein and Gvion 2019). In addition, empirical evidence and clinical observation have demonstrated a strong association between AN and NSSI (Oudijn et al. 2022). Self-destructive eating-disordered behavior and other types of NSSI appear during the course of AN which may contribute to considering them as a symptom of AN, similar to BPD symptom (Oudijn et al. 2022). To elucidate the association between suicidal thoughts and suicidal attempts in EDs, motivational and volition model as well as contributing factors may be useful. This model encompasses the stages of pre-motivation, motivation, and volition of suicidal behavior. The first stage, pre-motivation, integrates diathesis and stress factors, and the second stage elucidates the development of suicidal thoughts by factors including thwarted belongingness, perceived burdensomeness, lack of social support, and decreased resilience, and coping mechanisms. Consequently, suicidal behaviors and attempts are associated with elements such as being exposed to suicide, impulsivity, physical pain sensitivity, and fearlessness of death (O'Connor and Kirtley 2018). Several documented findings have indicated that the association between EDs pathology and factors leading to formation of suicidal ideation and suicidal behaviors, such as thwarted belongingness, perceived burdensomeness (Kwan et al. 2017), feeling of being a burden to others due to body dissatisfaction (Forrest et al. 2016), increased pain tolerance and fearlessness about death because of starvation and purging behaviors as types of self-harm behaviors (Joiner Jr et al. 2005; Crow et al. 2014). Using a retrospective chart review covering a 25-year period among 382 inpatients aged 9–18 years, Arnold et al. (2023) examined the rates of suicidal thoughts and behaviors in children and adolescents with AN and BN. The findings indicated about half of youth inpatients with AN (binge-eating type) and BN reported lifetime suicidal thoughts, and also, one-tenth of patients with AN (binge-eating type) had a history of attempting suicide (Arnold et al. 2023). In line with some studies, higher rates of suicidal attempts and NSSI have been found in more than half of BN samples (Svirko and Hawton 2007; Franko and Keel 2006; Franko et al. 2018), and also, higher rates of suicidal behaviors have been suggested in the anorexia nervosa binge-eating/purging subtypes as in BN (Nagata et al. 2000). Importantly, co-occurring presentation of BPD and EDs is correlated with greater levels of distress, psychological impairments, suicidal behaviors, and nonsuicidal self-injury compared to only one disorder (Ben-Porath et al. 2009). Claes et al. (2015) compared NSSI in female patients with ED (n = 98; NSSI+BPD) and without BPD (n = 45; NSSI-only). The results demonstrated that EDs patients with NSSI+BPD were different from those with NSSI-only associated with the frequency of suicidal thoughts and ideation, alcohol/drug/medication abuse, internalizing/externalizing psychopathology, interpersonal relationship difficulties, and coping strategies. In addition, ED patients with NSSI+BPD group indicated higher levels of impairments in each of the mentioned domains (Claes et al. 2018). Based on several investigations, it has been found that the co-occurrence of BPD and EDs is associated with a greater risk of repeated suicidal attempts; the co-occurring of BPD and AN is related to an escalated risk of repeated nonsuicidal self-harm, and BPD with co-occurring BED is associated with a greater rate of other psychiatric disorders other than EDs (Chen et al. 2009). Few studies have compared suicidal behaviors and NSSI between BPD groups with and without EDs (Chen et al. 2009). Chen et al. (2009) investigated the degree of association between EDs and the recurrence and severity of suicide attempts, NSSI, rates of comorbidities of mental disorders, and psychosocial functioning among 135 treatment-seeking females with BPD. The findings showed a significant association between BN and higher risk of recurrent suicide attempts, while current AN was related to increased risk of recurrent NSSI. Additionally, individuals with BPD and comorbid AN or BN were associated with a higher number of non-Ed current psychiatric disorders (Chen et al. 2009). Claes et al. (2015) indicated that individuals with EDs reported higher rates of NSSI and impulsivity compared to healthy controls, importantly the scores of BN were higher than those with AN (Claes et al. 2015). In reviewing 36 cross-sectional and 2 longitudinal studies, Goldstein and Gvion (2019) proposed that EDs with purging behavior, impulsivity, and certain interpersonal characteristics were associated with higher risk of suicidal behaviors (Goldstein and Gvion 2019).

The construct of *rejection sensitivity*, an elevated tendency toward misinterpretation of ambiguous social cues as being rejecting in nature (Downey and Feldman 1996), has been experimentally and theoretically linked with BPD (Lakatos 2012), and is suggested as a shared deficit in BPD and EDs (De Paoli et al. 2020). Rejection sensitivity is a tendency to worry about rejection or to expect being rejected in most situations (Selby et al. 2010a, b). Studies have indicated that rejection sensitivity is a related construct to abandonment avoidance, and it is a mediator in the association between BPD and EDs symptoms in a clinical outpatient sample (Al-Salom and Boylan 2019). High levels of rejection sensitivity cause a misinterpretation of interpersonal conversation (Al-Salom and Boylan 2019). Rejection sensitivity may induce emotion dysregulation and can be specifically associated with dysregulated sensitivity behaviors in BPD, and it is found as a factor that contributed to emotion dysregulation in both BPD and dysregulated eating behaviors. Finally, Selby et al. (2010a, b) examined the roles of rejection sensitivity and emotion dysregulation in the association between BPD and dysregulated eating behaviors among 94 college students (26 participants met BPD criteria). The findings indicated that BPD symptoms anticipated high levels of rejection sensitivity, which contribute to elevated levels of difficulties in emotion dysregulation and subsequent dysregulated eating behaviors. Additionally, an indirect considerable impact for rejection sensitivity on dysregulated behaviors, through emotion dysregulation, was explored (Selby et al. 2010a, b).

Thus, the connections between EDs and BPD involve many fundamental underlying vulnerabilities, and cases of comorbidity should be treated with a high degree of care and evaluation of the interplay between the two symptom sets. Furthermore, treatments that target emotion dysregulation—such as dialectical behavior therapy—may be particularly ideal for working with such complex comorbidity cases.

References

Abbate-Daga G, Pierò A, Gramaglia C, Fassino S. Factors related to severity of vomiting behaviors in bulimia nervosa. Psychiatry Res. 2005;134(1):75–84.

Accurso EC, Waller G. Concordance between youth and caregiver report of eating disorder psychopathology: development and psychometric properties of the eating disorder-15 for parents/caregivers (ED-15-P). Int J Eat Disord. 2021;54(7):1302–6.

Ackard DM, Richter S, Frisch MJ, Mangham D, Cronemeyer CL. Eating disorder treatment among women forty and older: increases in prevalence over time and comparisons to young adult patients. J Psychosom Res. 2013;74(2):175–8.

Al-Salom P, Boylan K. Borderline personality disorder and disordered eating behaviour: the mediating role of rejection sensitivity. J Can Acad Child Adolesc Psychiatry. 2019;28(2):72.

American Psychiatric Association DS. Diagnostic and statistical manual of mental disorders: DSM-5. Washington, DC: American Psychiatric Association; 2013.

American Psychiatric Association. Diagnostic and statistical manual of mental disorders. 5th ed, Text Revised (DSM-5-TR); 2022.

Amianto F, Siccardi S, Abbate-Daga G, Marech L, Barosio M, Fassino S. Does anger mediate between personality and eating symptoms in bulimia nervosa? Psychiatry Res. 2012;200(2–3):502–12.

Arcelus J, Mitchell AJ, Wales J, Nielsen S. Mortality rates in patients with anorexia nervosa and other eating disorders: a meta-analysis of 36 studies. Arch Gen Psychiatry. 2011;68(7):724–31.

Arnold S, Correll CU, Jaite C. Frequency and correlates of lifetime suicidal ideation and suicide attempts among consecutively hospitalized youth with anorexia nervosa and bulimia nervosa: results from a retrospective chart review. Borderline Personal Disord Emot Dysregul. 2023;10(1):10.

Asch DA, Buresh J, Allison KC, Islam N, Sheils NE, Doshi JA, Werner RM. Trends in US patients receiving care for eating disorders and other common behavioral health conditions before and during the COVID-19 pandemic. JAMA Netw Open. 2021;4(11):e2134913.

Barakat S, McLean SA, Bryant E, Le A, Marks P, Touyz S, Maguire S. Risk factors for eating disorders: findings from a rapid review. J Eat Disord. 2023;11(1):8.

Ben-Porath DD, Wisniewski L, Warren M. Differential treatment response for eating disordered patients with and without a comorbid borderline personality diagnosis using a dialectical behavior therapy (DBT)-informed approach. Eat Disord. 2009;17(3):225–41.

Berner LA, Wang Z, Stefan M, Lee S, Huo Z, Cyr M, Marsh R. Subcortical shape abnormalities in bulimia nervosa. Biol Psych Cogn Neurosci Neuroimag. 2019;4(12):1070–9.

Bodell L, Forney KJ, Keel P, Gutierrez P, Joiner TE. Consequences of making weight: a review of eating disorder symptoms and diagnoses in the United States military. Clin Psychol Sci Pract. 2014;21(4):398–409.

Brockmeyer T, Skunde M, Wu M, Bresslein E, Rudofsky G, Herzog W, Friederich HC. Difficulties in emotion regulation across the spectrum of eating disorders. Compr Psychiatry. 2014;55(3):565–71.

Burton AL, Mitchison D, Hay P, Donnelly B, Thornton C, Russell J, Swinbourne J, Basten C, Goldstein M, Touyz S, Abbott MJ. Beliefs about binge eating: psychometric properties of the eating beliefs questionnaire (EBQ-18) in eating disorder, obese, and community samples. Nutrients. 2018;10(9):1306.

Butler RM, Crumby EK, Christian C, Brosof LC, Vanzhula IA, Levinson CA. Facing eating disorder fears: an open trial adapting prolonged exposure to the treatment of eating disorders. Behav Ther. 2024;55(2):347–60.

Calzo JP, Blashill AJ, Brown TA, Argenal RL. Eating disorders and disordered weight and shape control behaviors in sexual minority populations. Curr Psychiatry Rep. 2017;19:1–0.

Cameron AY, Benz M, Reed KP. The role of guilt and shame in psychosocial functioning in a sample of women with borderline personality disorder. J Nerv Ment Dis. 2021;209(1):13–6.

Carden LJ, Saini P, Seddon C, Watkins M, Taylor PJ. Shame and the psychosis continuum: a systematic review of the literature. Psychol Psychother Theory Res Pract. 2020;93(1):160–86.
Cardi V, Corfield F, Leppanen J, Rhind C, Deriziotis S, Hadjimichalis A, Hibbs R, Micali N, Treasure J. Emotional processing, recognition, empathy and evoked facial expression in eating disorders: an experimental study to map deficits in social cognition. PLoS One. 2015;10(8):e0133827.
Caso JR, Graell M, Navalón A, MacDowell KS, Gutiérrez S, Soto M, Leza JC, Carrasco JL, Marsá MD. Dysfunction of inflammatory pathways in adolescent female patients with anorexia nervosa. Prog Neuro-Psychopharmacol Biol Psychiatry. 2020;96:109727.
Cassin SE. Adapted motivational interviewing for women with binge eating disorder (Doctoral dissertation, University of Calgary), 2005.
Chapman AL. Borderline personality disorder and emotion dysregulation. Dev Psychopathol. 2019;31(3):1143–56.
Chapman HC, Visser KF, Mittal VA, Gibb BE, Coles ME, Strauss GP. Emotion regulation across the psychosis continuum. Dev Psychopathol. 2020;32(1):219–27.
Chen EY, Brown MZ, Harned MS, Linehan MM. A comparison of borderline personality disorder with and without eating disorders. Psychiatry Res. 2009;170(1):86–90.
Chesney TR, Coburn N, Mahar AL, Davis LE, Zuk V, Zhao H, Hsu AT, Wright F, Haas B, Hallet J, Menjak I. Allcause and cancer-specific death of older adults following surgery for cancer. JAMA Surg. 2021;156(7):e211425.
Claes L, Nederkoorn C, Vandereycken W, Guerrieri R, Vertommen H. Impulsiveness and lack of inhibitory control in eating disorders. Eat Behav. 2006;7(3):196–203.
Claes L, Luyckx K, Bijttebier P, Turner B, Ghandi A, Smets J, Norre J, Van Assche L, Verheyen E, Goris Y, Hoksbergen I. Non-suicidal self-injury in patients with eating disorder: associations with identity formation above and beyond anxiety and depression. Eur Eat Disord Rev. 2015;23(2):119–25.
Claes L, Turner B, Dierckx E, Luyckx K, Verschueren M, Schoevaerts K. Different clinical presentations in eating disorder patients with nonsuicidal self-injury based on the co-occurrence of borderline personality disorder. Psychologica Belgica. 2018;58(1):243.
Coccaro EF, Lee R, Kavoussi RJ. Aggression, suicidality, and intermittent explosive disorder: serotonergic correlates in personality disorder and healthy control subjects. Neuropsychopharmacology. 2010;35(2):435–44.
Collu R, Post JM, Scherma M, Giunti E, Fratta W, Lutz B, Fadda P, Bindila L. Altered brain levels of arachidonic acid-derived inflammatory eicosanoids in a rodent model of anorexia nervosa. Biochim Biophys Acta Molecular and Cell Biology of Lipids. 2020;1865(4):158578.
Cossrow N, Pawaskar M, Witt EA, Ming EE, Victor TW, Herman BK, Wadden TA, Erder MH. Estimating the prevalence of binge eating disorder in a community sample from the United States: comparing DSM-IV-TR and DSM-5 criteria. J Clin Psychiatry. 2016;77(8):15456.
Costes S, Broca C, Bertrand G, Lajoix AD, Bataille D, Bockaert J, Dalle S. ERK1/2 control phosphorylation and protein level of cAMP-responsive element–binding protein: a key role in glucose-mediated pancreatic β-cell survival. Diabetes. 2006;55(8):2220–30.
Crosby RD, Wonderlich SA, Engel SG, Simonich H, Smyth J, Mitchell JE. Daily mood patterns and bulimic behaviors in the natural environment. Behav Res Ther. 2009;47(3):181–8.
Crow SJ, Swanson SA, Le Grange D, Feig EH, Merikangas KR. Suicidal behavior in adolescents and adults with bulimia nervosa. Compr Psychiatry. 2014;55(7):1534–9.
Dalton B, Bartholdy S, Robinson L, Solmi M, Ibrahim MA, Breen G, Schmidt U, Himmerich H. A meta-analysis of cytokine concentrations in eating disorders. J Psychiatr Res. 2018;103(103):252–64.
Daros AR, Williams GE. A meta-analysis and systematic review of emotion-regulation strategies in borderline personality disorder. Harv Rev Psychiatry. 2019;27(4):217–32.
De Paoli T, Fuller-Tyszkiewicz M, Huang C, Krug I. A network analysis of borderline personality disorder symptoms and disordered eating. J Clin Psychol. 2020;76(4):787–800.
DeBoer LB, Smits JA. Anxiety and disordered eating. Cogn Ther Res. 2013;37:887–9.

Demmler JC, Brophy ST, Marchant A, John A, Tan JO. Shining the light on eating disorders, incidence, prognosis and profiling of patients in primary and secondary care: national data linkage study. Br J Psychiatry. 2020;216(2):105–12.

Demmler KM, Beal T, Ghadirian MZ, Neufeld LM. Characteristics of global data on adolescent's dietary intake: a systematic scoping review. Curr Dev Nutr. 2023;1:102054.

Dingemans AE, van Son GE, Vanhaelen CB, van Furth EF. Depressive symptoms rather than executive functioning predict group cognitive behavioural therapy outcome in binge eating disorder. Eur Eat Disord Rev. 2020;28(6):620–32.

Dolan SC, Reilly EE, Brown TA, Shott ME, Frank GK. Anticipatory and consummatory pleasure in eating disorders. J Eat Disord. 2022;10(1):161.

Downey G, Feldman SI. Implications of rejection sensitivity for intimate relationships. J Pers Soc Psychol. 1996;70(6):1327.

Doyle JN, Watt MC, Cohen JN, Couture ME, Smith MM. Relations between anxiety sensitivity and attachment in outpatients with borderline personality disorder. J Personal Disord. 2022;36(5):606–22.

Faraji H, Oğur S. Examining the relationship between borderline personality traits and eating attitudes, and guilt and shame, 2023.

Faraji H, Özarabacı T. The relationships between borderline personality traits, offence-related feelings of shame and guilt and attitudes towards violence. Üsküdar Üniversitesi Sosyal Bilimler Dergisi. 2022;15:291–308.

Farstad SM, McGeown LM, von Ranson KM. Eating disorders and personality, 2004–2016: a systematic review and meta-analysis. Clin Psychol Rev. 2016;46:91–105.

Fassino S, Daga GA, Piero A, Leombruni P, Rovera GG. Anger and personality in eating disorders. J Psychosom Res. 2001;51(6):757–64.

Fassino S, Leombruni P, Pierò A, Abbate-Daga G, Rovera GG. Mood, eating attitudes, and anger in obese women with and without binge eating disorder. J Psychosom Res. 2003;54(6):559–66.

Ford BQ, Gross JJ. Emotion regulation: why beliefs matter. Can Psychol. 2018;59(1):1.

Forrest LN, Bodell LP, Witte TK, Goodwin N, Bartlett ML, Siegfried N, Eddy KT, Thomas JJ, Franko DL, Smith AR. Associations between eating disorder symptoms and suicidal ideation through thwarted belongingness and perceived burdensomeness among eating disorder patients. J Affect Disord. 2016;195:127–35.

Franko DL, Keel PK. Suicidality in eating disorders: occurrence, correlates, and clinical implications. Clin Psychol Rev. 2006;26(6):769–82.

Franko DL, Tabri N, Keshaviah A, Murray HB, Herzog DB, Thomas JJ, Coniglio K, Keel PK, Eddy KT. Predictors of long-term recovery in anorexia nervosa and bulimia nervosa: data from a 22-year longitudinal study. J Psychiatr Res. 2018;96:183–8.

Gale L, Channon S, Larner M, James D. Experiences of using pro-eating disorder websites: a qualitative study with service users in NHS eating disorder services. Eat Weight Disord. 2016;21:427–34.

Galmiche M, Déchelotte P, Lambert G, Tavolacci MP. Prevalence of eating disorders over the 2000–2018 period: a systematic literature review. Am J Clin Nutr. 2019;109(5):1402–13.

Goldschmidt AB, Wonderlich SA, Crosby RD, Engel SG, Lavender JM, Peterson CB, Crow SJ, Cao L, Mitchell JE. Ecological momentary assessment of stressful events and negative affect in bulimia nervosa. J Consult Clin Psychol. 2014;82(1):30.

Goldstein A, Gvion Y. Socio-demographic and psychological risk factors for suicidal behavior among individuals with anorexia and bulimia nervosa: a systematic review. J Affect Disord. 2019;245:1149–67.

Gordon AR, Beccia AL, Egan N, Lipson SK. Intersecting gender identity and racial/ethnic inequities in eating disorder risk factors, symptoms, and diagnosis among US college students: an intersectional multilevel analysis of individual heterogeneity and discriminatory accuracy. Int J Eat Disord. 2024;57(1):146–61.

Gratz KL, Roemer L. Multidimensional assessment of emotion regulation and dysregulation: development, factor structure, and initial validation of the difficulties in emotion regulation scale. J Psychopathol Behav Assess. 2004;26:41–54.

Gross F, Ford B. Handbook of emotion regulation. 3rd ed. Guilford Press; 2024.
Gross JJ. The extended process model of emotion regulation: elaborations, applications, and future directions. Psychol Inq. 2015;26(1):130–7.
Gross JJ. Emotion regulation: taking stock and moving forward. Emotion. 2013;13(3):359.
Gross JJ. The emerging field of emotion regulation: an integrative review. Rev Gen Psychol. 1998;2(3):271–99.
Hartman-Munick SM, Lin JA, Milliren CE, Braverman PK, Fisher MM, Jary JM, Lemly DC, Ornstein RM, Roche A, Rome ES, Rosen EL. 12. The impact of the COVID-19 pandemic on adolescent/young adult eating disorder patient visits: data from the National Eating Disorder Quality Improvement Collaborative. J Adolesc Health. 2022;70(4):S7.
Hampton-Anderson JN, Craighead LW. Psychosociocultural contributors to maladaptive eating behaviors in African American youth: recommendations and future directions. Am J Lifestyle Med. 2021;15(6):621–33.
Hampton C, Reeping D, Ozkan DS. Positionality statements in engineering education research: A look at the hand that guides the methodological tools. Stud Eng Educ. 2021;1(2):126–41.
Hay P. Disentangling eating disorder diagnostic schemes. Commentary on Walsh et al. "a systematic review comparing atypical anorexia nervosa and anorexia nervosa". Int J Eat Disord. 2023;56(4):841–3.
Hazzard VM, Loth KA, Hooper L, Becker CB. Food insecurity and eating disorders: a review of emerging evidence. Curr Psychiatry Rep. 2020;22:1–9.
Hessler JB, Heuser J, Schlegl S, Bauman T, Greetfeld M, Voderholzer U. Impact of comorbid borderline personality disorder on inpatient treatment for bulimia nervosa: analysis of routine data. Borderline Personal Disord Emot Dysregul. 2019;6:1–9.
Horvath SA, Keel PK, Forney KJ. Examining negative urgency as a predictor of eating disorder maintenance in purging syndromes. J Clin Psychol. 2024;80:1607.
Jackson AM. Body image, eating behavior, and dietary intake in adults. Washington State University; 2021.
Joiner TE Jr, Brown JS, Wingate LR. The psychology and neurobiology of suicidal behavior. Annu Rev Psychol. 2005;56:287–314.
Jovev M, Jackson HJ. Early maladaptive schemas in personality disordered individuals. J Personal Disord. 2004;18(5):467–78.
Keski-Rahkonen A, Mustelin L. Epidemiology of eating disorders in Europe: prevalence, incidence, comorbidity, course, consequences, and risk factors. Curr Opin Psychiatry. 2016;29(6):340–5.
Keski-Rahkonen A, Hoek HW, Susser ES, Linna MS, Sihvola E, Raevuori A, Bulik CM, Kaprio J, Rissanen A. Epidemiology and course of anorexia nervosa in the community. Am J Psychiatry. 2007;164(8):1259–65.
Khiyami A, Mehrotra N, Venugopal S, Mahmud H, Zenonos GA, Gardner PA, Fazeli PK. IGF-1 is positively associated with BMI in patients with acromegaly. Pituitary. 2023;26(2):221–6.
Khosravi M. Eating disorders among patients with borderline personality disorder: understanding the prevalence and psychopathology. J Eat Disord. 2020;8(1):38.
Klonsky ED. What is emptiness? Clarifying the 7th criterion for borderline personality disorder. J Personal Disord. 2008;22(4):418–26.
Kockler TD, Tschacher W, Santangelo PS, Limberger MF, Ebner-Priemer UW. Specificity of emotion sequences in borderline personality disorder compared to posttraumatic stress disorder, bulimia nervosa, and healthy controls: an e-diary study. Borderline Personal Disord Emot Dysregul. 2017;4:1–8.
Kolar DR, Hammerle F, Jenetzky E, Huss M, Bürger A. Aversive tension in female adolescents with Anorexia Nervosa: a controlled ecological momentary assessment using smartphones. BMC Psychiatry. 2016;16:1–1.
Kostro K, Lerman JB, Attia E. The current status of suicide and self-injury in eating disorders: a narrative review. J Eat Disord. 2014;2:1–9.

Krug I, Treasure J, Anderluh M, Bellodi L, Cellini E, Collier D, Di Bernardo M, Granero R, Karwautz A, Nacmias B, Penelo E. Associations of individual and family eating patterns during childhood and early adolescence: a multicentre European study of associated eating disorder factors. Br J Nutr. 2008;101(6):909–18.

Kwan MY, Gordon KH, Minnich AM, Carter DL, Troop-Gordon W. Peer victimization and eating disorder symptoms in college students. J Soc Clin Psychol. 2017;36(5):419–36.

Lakatos SC. Would exposure therapy be effective for reducing rejection sensitivity in borderline personality disorder? Grad Stud J Psychol. 2012;14:61–72.

Lavender JM, Wonderlich SA, Engel SG, Gordon KH, Kaye WH, Mitchell JE. Dimensions of emotion dysregulation in anorexia nervosa and bulimia nervosa: a conceptual review of the empirical literature. Clin Psychol Rev. 2015;40:111–22.

Lee KS, Vaillancourt T. Trajectories, comorbidity, and risk factors for adolescent disordered eating and borderline personality disorder features. Dev Psychopathol. 2023;17:1–2.

Leuti A, Fava M, Pellegrini N, Maccarrone M. Role of specialized pro-resolving mediators in neuropathic pain. Front Pharmacol. 2021;12:717993.

Lieb K, Zanarini MC, Schmahl C, Linehan MM, Bohus M. Borderline personality disorder. Lancet. 2004;364(9432):453–61.

Linehan M. Cognitive-behavioral treatment of borderline personality disorder. Guilford Press; 1993.

Mallorquí-Bagué N, Testa G, Lozano-Madrid M, Vintró-Alcaraz C, Sánchez I, Riesco N, Granero R, Perales JC, Navas JF, Megías-Robles A, Martínez-Zalacaín I. Emotional and non-emotional facets of impulsivity in eating disorders: from anorexia nervosa to bulimic spectrum disorders. Eur Eat Disord Rev. 2020;28(4):410–22.

Martinussen M, Friborg O, Schmierer P, Kaiser S, Øvergård KT, Neunhoeffer AL, Martinsen EW, Rosenvinge JH. The comorbidity of personality disorders in eating disorders: a meta-analysis. Eat Weight Disord Stud Anorexia, Bulimia Obes. 2017;22:201–9.

Marcos YQ, Sebastián MQ, Aubalat LP, Ausina JB, Treasure J. Peer and family influence in eating disorders: a meta-analysis. Eur Psychiatry. 2013;28(4):199–206.

McDonald S. Understanding the genetics and epigenetics of bulimia nervosa/bulimia spectrum disorder and comorbid borderline personality disorder (BN/BSD-BPD): a systematic review. Eat Weight Disord. 2019;24:799–814.

Miller AE, Trolio V, Halicki-Asakawa A, Racine SE. Eating disorders and the nine symptoms of borderline personality disorder: a systematic review and series of meta-analyses. Int J Eat Disord. 2022;55(8):993–1011.

Miotto P, Pollini B, Restaneo A, Favaretto G, Preti A. Aggressiveness, anger, and hostility in eating disorders. Compr Psychiatry. 2008;49(4):364–73.

Miskovic-Wheatley J, Bryant E, Ong SH, Vatter S, Le A, Touyz S, Maguire S. Eating disorder outcomes: findings from a rapid review of over a decade of research. J Eat Disord. 2023;11(1):85.

Myers LB, Derakshan N. The relationship between two types of impaired emotion processing: repressive coping and alexithymia. Front Psychol. 2015;6:138065.

Nagata T, Kawarada Y, Kiriike N, Iketani T. Multi-impulsivity of Japanese patients with eating disorders: primary and secondary impulsivity. Psychiatry Res. 2000;94(3):239–50.

Newton JR. Borderline personality disorder and eating disorders: a trans-diagnostic approach to unravelling diagnostic complexity. Australas Psychiatry. 2019;27(6):556–8.

Nilsson D, Lejonclou A, Holmqvist R. Psychoform and somatoform dissociation among individuals with eating disorders. Nord J Psychiatry. 2020;74(1):1–8.

O'Connor RC, Kirtley OJ. The integrated motivational–volitional model of suicidal behaviour. Philos Trans R Soc Biol Sci. 2018;373(1754):20170268.

Oudijn M, Linders J, Mocking R, Lok A, van Elburg A, Denys DJ. Psychopathological and neurobiological overlap between anorexia nervosa and self-injurious behavior: a narrative review and conceptual hypotheses. Front Psych. 2022;13:756238.

Papadopoulos FC, Ekbom A, Brandt L, Ekselius L. Excess mortality, causes of death and prognostic factors in anorexia nervosa. Br J Psychiatry. 2009;194(1):10–7.

Pearson CM, Lavender JM, Cao L, Wonderlich SA, Crosby RD, Engel SG, Mitchell JE, Peterson CB, Crow SJ. Associations of borderline personality disorder traits with stressful events and emotional reactivity in women with bulimia nervosa. J Abnorm Psychol. 2017;126(5):531.
Pearson JK, Davies PT, Sturge-Apple ML. The moderating role of adrenocortical reactivity in the associations between interparental conflict, emotional reactivity, and school adjustment. Dev Psychopathol. 2023;35(4):1878–90.
Pellegrini D, Grennan L, Bhatnagar N, McVey G, Couturier J. Virtual prevention of eating disorders in children, adolescents, and emerging adults: a scoping review. J Eat Disord. 2022;10(1):94.
Pike KM, Dunne PE. The rise of eating disorders in Asia: a review. J Eat Disord. 2015;3:1–4.
Pisetsky EM, Haynos AF, Lavender JM, Crow SJ, Peterson CB. Associations between emotion regulation difficulties, eating disorder symptoms, nonsuicidal self-injury, and suicide attempts in a heterogeneous eating disorder sample. Compr Psychiatry. 2017;73:143–50.
Polivy J. Etiology of binge eating: psychological mechanisms, 1993.
Pope HG Jr, Hudson JI. Are eating disorders associated with borderline personality disorder? A critical review. Int J Eat Disord. 1989;8(1):1–9.
Prefit AB, Candea DM, Szentagotai-Tătar A. Emotion regulation across eating pathology: a meta-analysis. Appetite. 2019;143(143):104438.
Rappaport DI, O'Connor M, Reedy C, Vo M. Clinical characteristics of US adolescents hospitalized for eating disorders 2010–2022. Hosp Pediatr. 2024;14(1):52–8.
Raykos BC, Erceg-Hurn DM, McEvoy PM, Fursland A, Waller G. Severe and enduring anorexia nervosa? Illness severity and duration are unrelated to outcomes from cognitive behaviour therapy. J Consult Clin Psychol. 2018;86(8):702.
Reas DL, Rø Ø, Karterud S, Hummelen B, Pedersen G. Eating disorders in a large clinical sample of men and women with personality disorders. Int J Eat Disord. 2013;46(8):801–9.
Ruscitti C, Rufino K, Goodwin N, Wagner R. Difficulties in emotion regulation in patients with eating disorders. Borderline Personal Disord Emot Dysregul. 2016;3:1–7.
Robinson P, Barrett B, Bateman A, Hakeem A, Hellier J, Lemonsky F, Rutterford C, Schmidt U, Fonagy P. Study protocol for a randomized controlled trial of mentalization based therapy against specialist supportive clinical management in patients with both eating disorders and symptoms of borderline personality disorder. BMC Psychiatry. 2014;14:1–0.
Sacchetti S, Robinson P, Bogaardt A, Clare A, Ouellet-Courtois C, Luyten P, Bateman A, Fonagy P. Reduced mentalizing in patients with bulimia nervosa and features of borderline personality disorder: a case-control study. BMC Psychiatry. 2019;19:1–2.
Sansone RA, Levitt JL, Sansone LA. An overview of psychotherapy strategies for the management of selfharm behavior. In: Self-harm behavior and eating disorders; 2005. p. 139–52.
Sansone RA, Sansone LA. Childhood trauma, borderline personality, and eating disorders: a developmental cascade. Eat Disord. 2007;15(4):333–46.
Sansone RA, Levitt JL, Sansone LA. The prevalence of personality disorders among those with eating disorders. Eat Disord. 2004;13(1):7–21.
Sansone RA, Chu JW, Wiederman MW, Lam C. Eating disorder symptoms and borderline personality symptomatology. Eat Weight Disord. 2011;16:e81–5.
Sansone RA, Sansone LA, Levitt JL. Borderline personality disorder: self-harm and eating disorders. In: Self-harm behavior and eating disorders. Routledge; 2005. p. 79–92.
Santangelo P, Reinhard I, Mussgay L, Steil R, Sawitzki G, Klein C, Trull TJ, Bohus M, Ebner-Priemer UW. Specificity of affective instability in patients with borderline personality disorder compared to posttraumatic stress disorder, bulimia nervosa, and healthy controls. J Abnorm Psychol. 2014;123(1):258.
Schag K, Leehr EJ, Martus P, Bethge W, Becker S, Zipfel S, Giel KE. Impulsivity-focused group intervention to reduce binge eating episodes in patients with binge eating disorder: study protocol of the randomised controlled IMPULS trial. BMJ Open. 2015;5(12):e009445.
Schag K, Rennhak SK, Leehr EJ, Skoda EM, Becker S, Bethge W, Martus P, Zipfel S, Giel KE. IMPULS: impulsivity-focused group intervention to reduce binge eating episodes in

patients with binge eating disorder–a randomised controlled trial. Psychother Psychosom. 2019;88(3):141–53.
Schorr M, Miller KK. The endocrine manifestations of anorexia nervosa: mechanisms and management. Nat Rev Endocrinol. 2017;13(3):174–86.
Sebastian A, Jacob G, Lieb K, Tüscher O. Impulsivity in borderline personality disorder: a matter of disturbed impulse control or a facet of emotional dysregulation? Curr Psychiatry Rep. 2013;15:1–8.
Selby EA, Braithwaite SR, Joiner TE Jr, Fincham FD. Features of borderline personality disorder, perceived childhood emotional invalidation, and dysfunction within current romantic relationships. J Fam Psychol. 2008;22(6):885.
Selby EA, Ward AC, Joiner TE Jr. Dysregulated eating behaviors in borderline personality disorder: are rejection sensitivity and emotion dysregulation linking mechanisms? Int J Eat Disord. 2010a;43(7):667–70.
Selby EA, Bulik CM, Thornton L, Brandt HA, Crawford S, Fichter MM, Halmi KA, Jacoby GE, Johnson CL, Jones I, Kaplan AS. Refining behavioral dysregulation in borderline personality disorder using a sample of women with anorexia nervosa. Personal Disord Theory Res Treat. 2010b;1(4):250.
Selby EA, Doyle P, Crosby RD, Wonderlich SA, Engel SG, Mitchell JD, Le Grange D. Momentary emotion surrounding bulimic behaviors in women with bulimia nervosa and borderline personality disorder. J Psychiatr Res. 2012;46(11):1492–500.
Selby EA, Cornelius T, Fehling KB, Kranzler A, Panza EA, Lavender JM, Wonderlich SA, Crosby RD, Engel SG, Mitchell JE, Crow SJ. A perfect storm: examining the synergistic effects of negative and positive emotional instability on promoting weight loss activities in anorexia nervosa. Front Psychol. 2015;6:1260.
Shaker NM, Azzam LA, Zahran RM, Hashem RE. Frequency of binge eating behavior in patients with borderline personality disorder and its relation to emotional regulation and impulsivity. Eat Weight Disord Stud Anorexia Bulimia Obes. 2022;27(7):2497–506.
Shanmugam V, Jowett S, Meyer C. Interpersonal difficulties as a risk factor for athletes' eating psychopathology. Scand J Med Sci Sports. 2014;24(2):469–76.
Sloan E, Hall K, Moulding R, Bryce S, Mildred H, Staiger PK. Emotion regulation as a transdiagnostic treatment construct across anxiety, depression, substance, eating and borderline personality disorders: a systematic review. Clin Psychol Rev. 2017;57:141–63.
Smink FR, Van Hoeken D, Hoek HW. Epidemiology of eating disorders: incidence, prevalence and mortality rates. Curr Psychiatry Rep. 2012;14(4):406–14.
Smink FR, van Hoeken D, Donker GA, Susser ES, Oldehinkel AJ, Hoek HW. Three decades of eating disorders in Dutch primary care: decreasing incidence of bulimia nervosa but not of anorexia nervosa. Psychol Med. 2016;46(6):1189–96.
Sneed MM. Blogging in the fatosphere: a qualitative study of perceptions of personal risks and benefits for women who blog about weight, weight loss, and dieting issues (Doctoral dissertation, East Tennessee State University), 2012.
Stankovska G, Memedi I, Nuhii N. Relationship between bulimia nervosa and psychological problems in period of adolescence: perfectionism, self-esteem, and beyond. In: Eating disorders. Cham: Springer International Publishing; 2023. p. 723–45.
Svaldi J, Philipsen A, Matthies S. Risky decision-making in borderline personality disorder. Psychiatry Res. 2012a;197(1–2):112–8.
Svaldi J, Griepenstroh J, Tuschen-Caffier B, Ehring T. Emotion regulation deficits in eating disorders: a marker of eating pathology or general psychopathology? Psychiatry Res. 2012b;197(1–2):103–11.
Svirko E, Hawton K. Self-injurious behavior and eating disorders: the extent and nature of the association. Suicide Life Threat Behav. 2007;37(4):409–21.
Swanson SA, Crow SJ, Le Grange D, Swendsen J, Merikangas KR. Prevalence and correlates of eating disorders in adolescents: results from the national comorbidity survey replication adolescent supplement. Arch Gen Psychiatry. 2011;68(7):714–23.

Swinbourne JM, Touyz SW. The co-morbidity of eating disorders and anxiety disorders: a review. Eur Eat Disord Rev Prof J Eat Disord Assoc. 2007;15(4):253–74.
Tan EJ, Raut T, Le LK, Hay P, Ananthapavan J, Lee YY, Mihalopoulos C. The association between eating disorders and mental health: an umbrella review. J Eat Disord. 2023;11(1):51.
Telch MJ, Valentiner DP, Ilai D, Petruzzi D, Hehmsoth M. The facilitative effects of heart-rate feedback in the emotional processing of claustrophobic fear. Behav Res Ther. 2000;38(4):373–87.
Temes CM, Frankenburg FR, Fitzmaurice GM, Zanarini MC. Deaths by suicide and other causes among patients with borderline personality disorder and personality-disordered comparison subjects over 24 years of prospective follow-up. J Clin Psychiatry. 2019;80(1):4039.
Thornton LM, Welch E, Munn-Chernoff MA, Lichtenstein P, Bulik CM. Anorexia nervosa, major depression, and suicide attempts: shared genetic factors. Suicide Life Threat Behav. 2016;46(5):525–34.
Tozzi F, Thornton LM, Mitchell J, Fichter MM, Klump KL, Lilenfeld LR, Reba L, Strober M, Kaye WH, Bulik CM, Price Foundation Collaborative Group. Features associated with laxative abuse in individuals with eating disorders. Psychosom Med. 2006;68(3):470–7.
Treasure J, Willmott D, Ambwani S, Cardi V, Clark Bryan D, Rowlands K, Schmidt U. Cognitive interpersonal model for anorexia nervosa revisited: the perpetuating factors that contribute to the development of the severe and enduring illness. J Clin Med. 2020;9(3):630.
Turner BJ, McKnight B, Helps CE, Yeo SN, Barbic S. Peer support for borderline personality disorder: a critical review of its feasibility, acceptability, and alignment with concepts of recovery. In: Personality disorders: theory, research, and treatment; 2024.
van Hoeken D, Hoek HW. Review of the burden of eating disorders: mortality, disability, costs, quality of life, and family burden. Curr Opin Psychiatry. 2020;33(6):521–7.
Verschueren M, Claes L, Palmeroni N, Raemen L, Moons P, Bruckers L, Molenberghs G, Dierckx E, Schoevaerts K, Luyckx K. Identity functioning in patients with an eating disorder: developmental trajectories throughout treatment. Nutrients. 2024;16(5):591.
Voderholzer U, Favreau M, Schlegl S, Hessler-Kaufmann JB. Impact of comorbid borderline personality disorder on the outcome of inpatient treatment for anorexia nervosa: a retrospective chart review. Borderline Personal Disord Emot Dysregul. 2021;8:1–2.
Walenda A, Kostecka B, Santangelo PS, Kucharska K. Examining emotion regulation in binge-eating disorder. Borderline Personal Disord Emot Dysregul. 2021;8:1–0.
Wildes JE, Marcus MD. Alternative methods of classifying eating disorders: models incorporating comorbid psychopathology and associated features. Clin Psychol Rev. 2013;33(3):383–94.
Wildes JE, Marcus MD, Crosby RD, Ringham RM, Dapelo MM, Gaskill JA, Forbush KT. The clinical utility of personality subtypes in patients with anorexia nervosa. J Consult Clin Psychol. 2011;79(5):665.
World Health Organization. The WHO special initiative for mental health (2019–2023): universal health coverage for mental health. World Health Organization; 2019.
Wonderlich SA, Rosenfeldt S, Crosby RD, Mitchell JE, Engel SG, Smyth J, Miltenberger R. The effects of childhood trauma on daily mood lability and comorbid psychopathology in bulimia nervosa. J Trauma Stress. 2007;20(1):77–87.
Zanarini MC, Reichman CA, Frankenburg FR, Reich DB, Fitzmaurice G. The course of eating disorders in patients with borderline personality disorder: a 10-year follow-up study. Int J Eat Disord. 2010;43(3):226–32.
Zapolski TC, Settles RE, Cyders MA, Smith GT. Borderline personality disorder, bulimia nervosa, antisocial personality disorder, ADHD, substance use: common threads, common treatment needs, and the nature of impulsivity. Independ Pract (Lutterworth, England). 2010;30(1):20.
Zeeck A, Birindelli E, Sandholz A, Joos A, Herzog T, Hartmann A. Symptom severity and treatment course of bulimic patients with and without a borderline personality disorder. Eur Eat Disord Rev Prof J Eat Disord Assoc. 2007;15(6):430–8.

Chapter 15
Attention-Deficit/Hyperactivity Disorder (ADHD) and Borderline Personality Disorder

Introduction

Borderline personality disorder (BPD) is characterized by instability in interpersonal relationship, emotional states, self-image, substantial impulsivity, and self-destructive behavioral embark (DSM-5-TR; American Psychiatric Association 2022). BPD is a complicated mental state with a high probability of comorbidity and co-occurring psychological issues and psychiatric disorders (Shen et al. 2017; Zanarini et al. 2004; Grant et al. 2008). Notably, the symptoms of BPD can potentially coincide with or be complicated by co-occurring attentional or hyperactivity symptoms, especially in youth cases.

Attention-deficit/hyperactivity disorder (ADHD) is a common and chronic neurological and heritable neurodevelopmental disorder (Zoromski et al. 2015; Evans et al. 2018; Jacobsson et al. 2021; Pelham et al. 2017; Williams 2023; Langevin et al. 2023), with a persistent pattern of inattention and/or hyperactivity/impulsivity, and restlessness which contribute to impairment in functioning or development (DSM-5-TR; 2022; Yadav 2021; Perroud et al. 2016). ADHD is featured by an early onset which is persistent in adult, with several notable impairments in social and academic functioning (Evans et al. 2018; Currie and Stabile 2006; Faraone et al. 2006). Individuals with a diagnosis of ADHD have manifested higher levels of depressive symptoms, difficulties in marriage functioning and several issues in interpersonal relationships across life span contributed to functional impairments (Pan et al. 2024; Goodman 2007). ADHD is featured based on three clusters of symptoms comprising inattention (impaired attention control), hyperactivity (motor restlessness), and impulsivity (Weiner et al. 2019; Perroud et al. 2016). *Inattention* is frequently displayed behaviorally in ADHD as straying from tasks, failing to follow through on instructions or completing work or chores, several issues in maintaining concentration, and being disorganized which cannot be attributed to defiance

M. Salavati, E. A. Selby, *Theories of Borderline Personality Disorder*,
https://doi.org/10.1007/978-3-031-75503-3_15

or lack of comprehension (DSM-5-TR; 2022). *Hyperactivity* is defined as inappropriate excessive motor activity, or excessive fidgeting, tapping, or talkativeness. In addition, the manifestation of hyperactivity in adults includes extreme restlessness or exhausting others with their activity (DSM-5-TR; 2022). *Impulsivity* is recognized by hasty behaviors that happen in the moment with no forethought, which may contribute to the potential of the person (DSM-5-TR; 2022). Briefly, impulsivity is defined as "acting without reflecting the consequences" (Ditrich et al. 2021). Impulsive behaviors may show a desire for immediate reward and reinforcements or the lack of ability to delay gratification, which are manifested as social intrusiveness and/or making crucial decisions without any consideration of long-term consequences. Additionally, yet inattention, hyperactivity, and impulsivity are proposed as core symptoms of ADHD (Posner et al. 2014), *emotional lability,* featured by low frustration tolerance, irritability, and mood lability, is a common characteristic contributing to the experience of high distress in people and their families (APA 2013; Moukhtarian et al. 2018, 2020, 2021). *Emotion dysregulation* or emotional impulsivity has been reported as common associated features in children and adults with ADHD (DSM-5-TR 2022). In ADHD, emotion regulation is featured by issues in temper control, irritability, frequent outbursts of negative emotions, emotional over-reactivity, considerably decreased in ability to manage certain life stresses, feelings of being overwhelmed and hassled, mood lability, rapid and unpredictable mood switching from normal mood to depression, or mild excitement (Reimherr et al. 2005; Moukhtarian et al. 2018, 2020, 2021). Emotion dysregulation as a clinical feature in ADHD can predict a persistent course of ADHD symptoms in adulthood (Biederman et al. 2012). The rates of diagnosed ADHD have escalated over the last decades, both in children (Thomas et al. 2015a, b; Kazda et al. 2023; Xu et al. 2018) and adults (Song et al. 2021). Based on one systematic meta-review, the risk factors of ADHD encompass a wide range of biological (Ronald et al. 2021), maternal (Li et al. 2020; Ai et al. 2021; Guo et al. 2020; Rowland and Wilson 2021; Schwartz et al. 2021; Min et al. 2021), environmental (Asarnow et al. 2021; Caye et al. 2020), social (Russell et al. 2016), and nutritional factors (Del-Ponte et al. 2019; Farsad-Naeimi et al. 2020). Etiological approaches propose both (1) within-child correlates; and (2) risk factors that lead to the disorder including gene and environmental influences (Nigg 2017).

According to the DSM-5-TR (2022), population surveys indicate that ADHD occurs worldwide in approximately 7.2% in children and adolescents; while based on cross-national prevalence, it ranges from 0.1% to 10.2% of children and adolescent, and 2.5% in adults (DSM-5-TR 2022). Based on epidemiological findings, ADHD has revealed an estimated adult prevalence of 2–3% (Kenter et al. 2021). Depending on meta-analytical rates, the prevalence rates of ADHD ranged from 2% to 7.1–7.2% (Sayal et al. 2018; Langevin et al. 2023; Thomas et al. 2015a, b), and 2.5–5% in adults (Song et al. 2021; Bálint et al. 2009; Willcutt 2012; Young et al. 2020).

ADHD has been indicated to be notably associated with a wide range of mental disorders, encompassing anxiety and mood disorders, reading disorders, learning and language disorders, conduct disorder, oppositional and antisocial personalities, disruptive mood dysregulation disorder, autism spectrum disorder, developmental coordination disorder, self-injurious behaviors, substance use disorder (Porter et al. 2020; Williams 2023; Young and Cocallis 2019; Mayes and Zickgraf 2019), and borderline personality disorder (Philipsen et al. 2008). Furthermore, ADHD in adult populations is markedly correlated with comorbid mental disorders, such as autism spectrum disorder, anxiety and mood disorders, obsessive compulsive disorder, substance use disorders, eating disorders, bipolar disorder, personality disorders and impulse control disorders, which contributes to making recognition, diagnosis, and management more complicated (Katzman et al. 2017; Sobanski 2006; Kessler et al. 2006). A growing body of epidemiological investigations have shown that among 80% of adults with ADHD, at least one coexisting psychiatric disorder has been reported, such as mood and anxiety disorders, substance use disorders, and personality disorders (Torgersen et al. 2006; Sobanski et al. 2007). According to experimental investigation, more that 80% of children and adults with ADHD have displayed at least one other psychiatric disorder (Barkley et al. 2010), including 40–60% for oppositional defiant disorder (ODD); 25% for an anxiety disorder; 20–25% for conduct disorder; 10% for a tic disorder, and 5% for an emotional disorder (Altszuler 2019).

ADHD is well recognized among pediatric professionals as a common childhood disorder, which in most cases has childhood onset (Katzman et al. 2017; APA 2022; Langevin et al. 2023) followed by a wide spectrum of social-academic functioning impairments (Katzman et al. 2017), the concentration has been shifted to identifying and treatment of ADHD in adults (Katzman et al. 2017). There is now a growing body of evidence to cite that ADHD symptoms persist into adulthood (O'malley et al. 2016; Moukhtarian et al. 2018, 2020, 2021; Cheung et al. 2016; Mahadevan et al. 2019), and it is considered a lifelong disorder for most individuals (APA 2013; Evans et al. 2019). According to a meta-analysis of longitudinal studies published in 2005, it was indicated that more than one-third of children with ADHD continued to fulfill diagnostic criteria into their 20 s, approximately 65% continuing to experience disturbing symptoms (Faraone et al. 2006). According to the DSM, childhood onset of ADHD is a requirement which applied widely for diagnosing ADHD in adult (Porter et al. 2020). In comparison with ADHD in childhood, the epidemiological studies of adult ADHD have been relatively neglected, due to the lack of documented valid diagnostic criteria (Porter et al. 2020). Based on investigations, ADHD influences nearly 4.4–5.2% of adults between 18 and 44 years of age (Ginsberg et al. 2014; Goodman 2009; Fayyad et al. 2007), as well as the prevalence in older adults have ranges between 2.8% and 3.5% (Mahadevan et al. 2019). According to a large population-based research, Das et al. (2014) reported a prevalence of 2.2% in older adults (68–74 years) in comparison with 6.2% in middle-aged adults (48–52 years) (Das et al. 2014). Moreover, despite current clinical controversy, a great body of evidence proposes that ADHD remains under-recognized and under-treated in adult patients (Katzman et al. 2016); however, substantial improvements have been achieved in the clinical and functional outcomes of adult ADHD including significant components of psychosocial functioning such as social relationships, workplace performance and parenting skills (Biederman et al. 2009; Katzman et al. 2017). Moreover, it has been indicated that ADHD in adults is highly associated with poorer health, lower educational achievements, and increased rates of unemployment (Ebejer et al. 2012).

Adult ADHD is characterized by inattentiveness (the most prevalent symptom which has been estimated to occur in 90% of cases), impulsivity, hyperactivity (the least prevalent), and restlessness (Young et al. 2020; Wilson et al. 2011; Sobanski et al. 2008; Rasmussen and Levander 2009), and is identified by the DSM to match into three various subtypes including hyperactive, or impulsive, inattentive, and restlessness (Singh and Singh 2015). Emotion dysregulation has been identified as a significant symptom and core feature of ADHD in adults (Surman et al. 2011; Surman and Goodman 2017; Corbisiero et al. 2013; Barkley et al. 2010). Furthermore, difficulties with motivation, emotional recognition, excessive mind wandering, and behavioral self-regulation have been reported (Mahadevan et al. 2019). Earlier studies have revealed that adults with ADHD demonstrate more pessimistic, introverted, rebellious, and aggressive symptoms (May and Bos 2000), display greater levels of mental distress, dissatisfaction, lower capacity to be organized and self-disciplined, as well as lower levels of sociability, altruism, and sympathy to others (Miller et al. 2008; Richter et al. 2007). Additionally, adult ADHD is proposed as a part of the externalizing spectrum which contributes to the shared homotypic comorbidity and heterotypic continuity across the lifespan. Studies have shown a lag in brain maturation specifically in the areas of the brain associated with executive functioning, including prefrontal and cingulate cortices which may contribute to the preference for immediate small rewards combined with impairment in reward processing (Mahadevan et al. 2019). In line with experimental and clinical investigations, the manifestations of ADHD alter from childhood to adulthood, embodying decreased hyperactivity (Biederman et al. 2000), an increase in self-destructive and dangerous behaviors associated with inattention and impulsivity, risky sexual behaviors and substance use, and severe impairments in academic functioning (Kent et al. 2011; Evans et al. 2019).

Shared Overlapping Symptoms of ADHD and BPD

The association between ADHD and BPD has received considerable attention due to the similar clinical features in these disorders (Distel et al. 2011). Recently, remarkable shared overlapped symptoms and considerable co-occurring have been reported in clinical manifestations between ADHD and BPD (Fossati et al. 2002; Matthies and Philipsen 2014; Philipsen et al. 2008), which have contributed to an increase in research activities in this field (Matthies and Philipsen 2014; Kouppis et al. 2022; Weiner et al. 2019). Both BPD and ADHD have indicated high prevalence, for instance, about 5% for ADHD (Polanczyk et al. 2007) and about 1–2% for BPD (Lieb et al. 2004). In line with a body of scientific literature, remarkably prevalent co-occurring ADHD and BPD have been reported (e.g., Richter et al. 2007; Ferrer et al. 2010; Weiner et al. 2019). Moreover, ADHD and BPD have shared common behavioral and neuropsychological disturbances, which may elucidate the putative developmental associations between these two disorders (Stepp et al. 2013). Across several current studies, an estimated 38% of patients with BPD have also reported co-occurrence with ADHD, as well as more than 60% of BPD individuals meet criteria for ADHD during childhood (van Dijk et al. 2014; Ferrer et al. 2010; O'malley et al. 2016). In a large national study of 34,000 adults in the USA, the lifetime comorbidity of ADHD and BPD was reported to be 33.7% (Bernardi et al. 2012). In both BPD and ADHD, phenotypic manifestations are at times inharmonious, with only some overlap between them at a dimensional level. In line with a dimensional perspective, it has been demonstrated that the co-occurrence between ADHD and BPD can be elucidated based on two communal dimensions, including impulsivity and emotion dysregulation (Weiner et al. 2019). In clinical settings, it has been found that patients who initially meet BPD diagnostic criteria developed a clinical picture suggesting ADHD comorbidity (Ferrer et al. 2010; Matthies and Philipsen 2014). Substantial experimental and clinical studies have demonstrated a notable association between ADHD diagnoses in childhood and later the development of personality disorders in adulthood (Mahadevan et al. 2019; Stepp et al. 2013). Females with ADHD and BPD have shown more shared clinical features than when ADHD presents in males (Philipsen et al. 2009; Van Dijke 2012), and a noteworthy association has been found between retrospectively assessed ADHD symptoms and current BPD features only in female samples (Fossati et al. 2015). Korsgaard et al. (2016) found adolescent girls with ADHD reported more personality disorders features than boys, especially antisocial and borderline personality pathology (Korsgaard et al. 2016, 2022). There is also substantial co-occurrence of adult ADHD with BPD, which is considered as one of the most common overlaps, with 40% of individuals diagnosed with BPD likely to have a diagnosis of ADHD (Cumyn et al. 2009; Ferrer et al. 2010). Higher ADHD scores were found among children aged 5–17 years with BPD symptomatology in comparison to children with other types of personality disorders features (Coolidge et al. 2000). Considering gender differences, Black et al. (2007) showed that adult male and female prisoners with BPD indicated ADHD symptoms 3.4 times more than prisoners with no BPD pathology, and Rösler et al. (2009) reported that female prisoners with ADHD had BPD features 52 times more than female prisoners without ADHD. Numerous investigations have demonstrated the frequent co-occurrence of ADHD and BPD as life-long comorbidities (Stepp et al. 2013; Davids and Gastpar 2005; Storebø and Simonsen 2014), resulting in severe health-related matters regarding psychopathology, quality of life, and psychosocial functioning (Matthies and Philipsen 2014). Additionally, a growing body of investigations have reported the shared common symptoms between ADHD and BPD (e.g., Stepp et al. 2013; Barkley 2011; Kouppis et al. 2022; Weiner et al. 2019), encompassing impulsivity, poor self-regulation, impaired executive function, anger control deficits, disturbed inhibitory control, and aggression (Dowson et al. 2004; Philipsen 2006; Connor et al. 2010; Harty et al. 2009; Jensen et al. 2007; Leichsenring et al. 2013). Akça et al. (2020) compared 550 adolescent inpatients with ADHD, BPD, and ADHD+BPD to determine the severity of co-occurring disorders. The results demonstrated that the severity of nearly all comorbid disorders, aggression, self-harm, suicidal thoughts, and substance use were significantly higher in the ADHD+BPD group (Akça et al. 2020).

Retrospective findings have highlighted that childhood ADHD can be considered as a potential precursor of BPD in adulthood (Fossati et al. 2002; Philipsen et al. 2008). In a national prospective longitudinal study of twins in Sweden, Tiger et al. (2022) demonstrated an association between childhood ADHD symptoms which were assessed at age 9–12 and adult BPD was identified by impulsivity in contrast to inattention and hyperactivity (Tiger et al. 2022). Philipsen et al. (2008) reported that 59.5% of BPD subjects showed related indicators of likely childhood ADHD diagnosis. According to their findings, in a sample of 118, female BPDs indicated 41.5% prevalence rate of childhood ADHD (Philipsen et al. 2008). According to parent-report and child-report, the severity of hyperactivity, impulsivity, and inattention at ages 14–15 can anticipate BPD at ages 16–18 (Beeney et al. 2021). In a prospective study in twins, Belsky et al. (2012) found an association between maternal-rated and teacher-rated symptoms of impulsivity at age 5 and BPD at age 12 (Belsky et al. 2012). Based on retrospective research, Fischer et al. (2005) found a relation between ADHD and BPD, and reported that children with ADHD aged 4–12 years showed higher rates of BPD as young adults, mean age at follow-up age of 20–21 years, in comparison to community controls (Fischer et al. 2005). Distel et al. (2011) investigated the genetic and environmental contributions to the relation between borderline personality traits (BPT) and ADHD symptoms among 7233 twins and siblings aged 18–90 years. The heritability of BPT and ADHD symptoms was estimated at 45% and 36%, and the genetic and environmental correlations between BPT and ADHD symptoms were reported to be 0.71 and 0.51, respectively (Distel et al. 2011).

Some findings have suggested relations between presentations or types of ADHD and BPD. For instance, Cumyn et al. (2009) found a greater prevalence rate of comorbid BPD in the combined type of ADHD (24%), and for inattentive presentation of ADHD 10% (Cumyn et al. 2009). O'Grady and Hinshaw (2023) examined whether hyperactivity/impulsivity, internalizing/externalizing behaviors, and adversity/trauma can predict young adult BPD in a sample of females with ($n = 140$) and without ($n = 88$) childhood ADHD diagnosis. The results indicated both childhood hyperactivity/impulsivity and childhood adverse experiences/trauma anticipated might be considered as predictors of young adult BPD dimensional features. In addition, internalizing/externalizing symptoms were remarkably anticipated as young adult BPD dimensional features (O'Grady and Hinshaw 2023).

Following recent investigations, the associations between ADHD and borderline personality feature (BPF) have been documented (Fossati et al. 2015), and higher rate of the links between BPF and aggression have been revealed in females (Mancke et al. 2015). The manifestations of aggression in individuals with BPD appear in self-destructive behavior (i.e., as self-injury and suicidal behaviors) or externally directed aggression and impulsivity (Látalová and Praško 2010; Ross and Babcock 2009). Impulsive behaviors also have been reported among individuals with ADHD, varying from low frustration tolerance to recurrent temper tantrums (Connor et al. 2010). BPD may be a pertinent risk factor for aggression among girls with ADHD, specifically ADHD females with issues involving emotion regulation, hostile cognitions, and interpersonal problems with peers (McQuade et al. 2014), contributing to an increased probability of BPF manifestations. Emotional impulsivity and interpersonal sensitivity features of BPF may lead to higher aggressive relationships among girls with ADHD (Babinski et al. 2021). Bertsch et al. (2019) proposed that a diminished level of ability to control one's impulses in BPD is biologically related to deficits in prefrontal emotional processing, which makes the individual more prone to outbursts of anger and aggressive behaviors in comparison to an ADHD case (Bertsch et al. 2019). Moreover, emotional dysregulation, hostility, and social impairments have been reported as difficulties in oppositional defiant disorder (ODD), and also, it has been suggested that (ODD) may contribute to the development of BPF (Burke and Austin 2010), and also a heightened rate of aggression in BPF (Babinski and McQuade 2019). In addition, studies suggest that both childhood ADHD and ODD symptoms may lead to an increased risk for BPF in adolescence (Stepp 2012). Babinski and McQuade (2019) studied the role of BPF as a mediator of the correlation between ADHD and ODD symptoms and aggression in girls. The results indicated a significant correlation between ADHD, ODD, and BPF which were associated with aggression. Based on parents' and youth reports, BPF completely mediated the relation between all ODD symptom severity and relational and physical aggression. Additionally, a significant link between BPF and girls' manifestations of ADHD/ODD symptoms may exist, as it was indicated that hyperactivity/impulsivity and oppositional behavior were uniquely related to BPF among girls. Furthermore, the findings showed a remarkable association between ADHD and ODD severity and both physical and relational aggression in girls (Babinski et al. 2021). In spite of the notable influence of stress on anger and aggression in BPD and ADHD, few studies have investigated these impacts. Cackowski et al. (2017) investigated the various aspects of anger and aggression among 29 female BPD and 28 ADHD patients and 30 healthy controls. The results revealed significantly higher trait aggression and hostility, more tendency to show provoked anger among individuals with BPD while ADHD patients reported greater levels of anger under stress in comparison with controls, which approved the influence of stress on anger in BPD, yet no aggressive behavior were reported (Cackowski et al. 2017).

Impulsivity is reported as a main symptom of both ADHD and BPD (Ditrich et al. 2021; Fossati et al. 2002; Ferrer et al. 2010; Sebastian et al. 2014; Barkley 2011; Weiner et al. 2019; APA 2022). Based on a growing body of studies, elevated levels of impulsivity and aggression have been revealed in individuals with BPD and also ADHD (Krause-Utz et al. 2013; Grant et al. 2008; Philipsen et al. 2008; Dowson and Blackwell 2010; New et al. 2009; Perez-Rodriguez et al. 2012; O'Grady and Hinshaw 2023). Impulsive behaviors are defined as behaviors with undesirable consequences because these behaviors are not based on sufficient thought-out, and inappropriately they occur in an untimely fashion (Moeller et al. 2001; Evenden 1999). Impulsivity is defined as self-harming behaviors which can occur under conditions of negative emotional distress (Sebastian et al. 2014). According to descriptive definitions applied in the DSM-criteria, the types of impulsivities in ADHD and BPD are not necessarily the same. Based on DSM-5-TR (2022), impulsivity is required to fulfill the diagnosis of BPD at least in two areas of potentially self-destructive behaviors such as excessive sex, substance use, binge eating, and self-injurious behaviors (APA 2022). In BPD, impulsivity is a core symptom and central element of neurobehavioral models of diseases (Lieb et al. 2004; Glenn and Klonsky 2010), and is defined as impulsive self-harm (Fossati et al. 2002). In BPD patients, impulsive behaviors are self-destructive comprising impulsive sexual behaviors, spending, binge eating, or reckless driving (MacDonald and Sadek 2023). In ADHD, impulsivity in ADHD typically refers to impatience when waiting, talking over people, interfering in the work of others, and interrupting others from what they are doing (Fossati et al. 2002; Glenn and Klonsky 2010; MacDonald and Sadek 2023). A core issue of impulsivity in ADHD stems from difficulties in inhibition responses which is elucidated from a neuropsychological viewpoint (Barkley 2011) and is revealed by slower reactions to stop signals in stop-signal tasks (Alderson et al. 2013). MacDonald and Sadek (2023) proposed that in ADHD, both cognitive impulsivity and motor impulsivity are the main manifestations of impulsivity, while in BPD behavioral impulsivity are driven by intense emotional states and may be less provoked by cognitive and motor impulsivity (MacDonald and Sadek 2023). Additionally, it was shown that symptoms of BPD are associated with response inhibition, even after controlling for ADHD (Nigg et al. 2005), and it is also correlated with more intense emotional states (Jacob et al. 2010). Studies have indicated that individuals with ADHD and comorbid ADHD and BPD showed higher scores in impulsivity measurements and worse functioning in inhibitory tasks in comparison to BPD patients (Lampe et al. 2007; Ferrer et al. 2010; Speranza et al. 2011). Lampe et al. (2007) showed no difference in behavioral aspects of impulsivity comprising angry temperament and non-planning impulsiveness among patients with ADHD and BPD (Lampe et al. 2007). Studies have reported higher impulsivity scores and more ADHD diagnoses in BPD, as well as a significant correlation between ADHD symptoms and impulsivity (Kulacaoglu et al. 2017). In line with a neuropsychological laboratory study in adults with ADHD ($n = 40$) and adults with ADHD+BPD ($n = 20$), findings have shown higher rates of impulsivity and attention difficulties in ADHD+BPD compared with ADHD group, while there were no differences in self-rating impulsivity and response inhibition in ADHD and ADHD+BPD groups (O'malley et al. 2016). Krause-Utz et al. (2016) examined the role of stress in the association between ADHD and BPD in a sample comprising adult women with BPD ($n = 30$), adult women with ADHD ($n = 28$), and control group. The results revealed higher rates of impulsivity in ADHD compared with BPD and control group. No differences in impulsivity and action cancelation have been found among ADHD and BPD after increasing stress, but higher levels of impulsivity in BPD were shown in comparison with control through elevating stress (Krause-Utz et al. 2016).

Emotion dysregulation has been documented as a core mechanism of borderline pathology which is described directly in two of the DSM-5-TR criteria for the diagnosis of BPD (APA DSM-5-TR 2022; Glenn and Klonsky 2010; Moukhtarian et al. 2021). Furthermore, it is proposed as a significant symptom of ADHD, which has been estimated to be 34–70% of adults with ADHD reported emotion regulation issues (Rüfenacht et al. 2019; Faraone et al. 2019; Hirsch et al. 2019; Glenn and Klonsky 2010). Additionally, according to several investigations, emotion dysregulation is considered as a shared feature of ADHD and BPD (Stepp et al. 2013; Moukhtarian et al. 2021; Faraone et al. 2019; Skirrow et al. 2014). According to studies using ecological momentary assessment, it has been found that patients with BPD experience longer duration of unpleasant tension accompanying slower return to their baseline emotional state (Rüfenacht et al. 2019). It has been revealed that emotion dysregulation in ADHD is similar to what has been found in BPD patients, comprising escalated levels of instability and intensity of negative emotions and a slow return to affective baseline when activated (Skirrow et al. 2014; Weiner et al. 2019; Matthies and Philipsen 2014). However, difficulties in emotional management and regulation in BPD individuals with ADHD, few studies have investigated directly this issue in comorbid BPD+ADHD (Perroud et al. 2017; Cackowski et al. 2017; Cavelti et al. 2024). Emotion dysregulation has been reported to be a valuable transdiagnostic clinical pattern in ADHD and BPD, and it is able to distinguish between ADHD and BPD (Moukhtarian et al. 2021). Despite similarities of emotion dysregulation between BPD and ADHD, there are some considerable differences between these two disorders (Weiner et al. 2019; Cackowski et al. 2017). For example, the severity of self-destructive behaviors and emotion dysregulation seems to be worse in patients with BPD (Philipsen et al. 2009), causing higher rate of mortality due to unnatural accidents such as suicide among BPD cases (Dalsgaard et al. 2015; Rydkjaer et al. 2020; Björkenstam et al. 2018). In a cohort study of 15,847 female patients with BPD, it has been found that a subsequent clinical diagnosis of ADHD did not show any impact on the overall risk of mortality (Kouppis et al. 2022). By applying experience sampling method (ESM) and multilevel modeling, Moukhtarian et al. (2021) studied differences in emotional dynamics in daily life in ADHD and BPD. They investigated the dynamics of positive and negative emotions and found the occurrence and influence on intensity of negative emotions of self-reported aversive events, including *bad social* events (other individuals or social situations), and *bad functional* events (practical and everyday life tasks). The momentary changes in various reports of emotional symptoms were assessed in 98 adult females with ADHD only, BPD only, comorbid ADHD+BPD, and controls. The findings revealed that no differences in scores of the dynamics of emotional dysregulation have been found in patients with ADHD and those with BPD. In addition, the BPD and comorbid BPD+ADHD groups manifested remarkable differences in comparison to controls, with lesser positive and more negative intensity of emotions, as well as more instability of negative emotions. Based on obtained results, no significant differences have been found in the intensity of positive emotions between ADHD group and controls; however, increased intensity of specific negative emotions (irritability), and heightened instability of negative emotions (sadness, irritability, anger) in comparison to controls have been shown. According to findings, it was concluded that the intensity and instability of positive emotions do not have the ability to differentiate the patient with ADHD and controls. Additionally, it was indicated that individuals with BPD showed higher intensity of sadness and lesser intensity of happiness in comparison with individuals with ADHD. Additionally, results may have been due to emotional dysregulation with the findings showing a high incidence of *bad social* events in comparison to controls, and also a greater incidence of *bad functional* events have been reported in ADHD group when in comparison with controls. It was demonstrated that both bad *social* and *bad functional* events indicated a substantial influence on the intensity of negative emotions (Moukhtarian et al. 2021). Rüfenacht et al. (2019) assessed and compared emotional reactivity, cognitive emotional regulation strategies, and empathy among participants' suffering of ADHD individuals with those of patients with BPD, or comorbid ADHD and BPD (279 ADHD; 70 BPD; 60 BPD+ADHD). Also, the association between ADHD symptoms and emotion dysregulation severity was evaluated (Rüfenacht et al. 2019). The results indicated notably better emotion regulation, highly efficient emotion regulation strategies, lower emotional reactivity, better applying the adaptive cognitive strategies, and lesser use of non-adaptive strategies in ADHD patients in comparison to BPD and BPD+ADHD. Additionally, similar to BPD, poor cognitive emotion regulation strategies including rumination, self-blame, blaming others, and catastrophizing have significant role in emotion dysregulation among ADHD. Furthermore, less emotional sensitivity, and less persistence of the emotion was found in ADHD compared to BPD and BPD+ADHD patients. In sum, the findings showed similar inefficient cognitive emotional regulation skills contributing to emotion dysregulation in ADHD and BPD, in spite of greater use of adaptive cognitive emotional strategies and lower level of emotion dysregulation in ADHD in comparison to individuals with BPD (Rüfenacht et al. 2019).

Adult ADHD and BPD also exhibit shared warning signs and risk factors, supporting assumptions about the dimensional nature of the emergence of these disorders, rather than being categorical entities. Shared warning signs consist of impulsivity and anger considered as trait-like dimensions of BPD as well as some of the core mediators of ADHD symptoms in childhood and BPD diagnosis in adulthood (Carlotta et al. 2013). Although the symptoms of emotional dysregulation such as impulsivity and irritability are characteristically observed in both BPD and ADHD (Ditrich et al. 2021; Weiner et al. 2019; Moukhtarian et al. 2018; Matthies and Philipsen 2014), the nature of the association between ADHD and BPD requires specific recognition (Asherson et al. 2014). Adult ADHD and BPD manifest several shared clinical features such as emotional dysregulation and impulsivity (Philipsen et al. 2009), as well as impairments in executive functioning (Mcclure et al. 2016; Ruocco 2005; Unoka and Richman 2016). Moreover, issues in motivation, difficulties in emotional recognition, excessive mind wandering, and problems in behavioral self-regulation have been detected as overlapped symptoms in ADHD and BPD (Mahadevan et al. 2019). Higher level of trait-impulsivity has been reported in ADHD and ADHD +BPD in comparison to BPD alone, whereas trait-emotion dysregulation is reported higher in BPD and ADHD+BPD than ADHD alone, which may propose that impulsivity and emotion dysregulation in BPD are highly intrinsically related (Petrovic and Castellanos 2016; Sebastian et al. 2014).

Several explanatory models have suggested the associations between emotion-regulation related temperament/personality traits and disruptive behaviors (Matthies and Philipsen 2014). Martel et al. (2009) suggested that high negative and positive emotionality may be associated with disruptive behavior disorders generally, deficient control processes may have association with ADHD and low agreeableness specifically, and lower level of agreeableness may be specifically related to oppositional-defiant and conduct issues (Martel et al. 2009). In line with heritability investigations, ADHD and BPD share several temperament traits, especially novelty seeking and harm avoidance (Anckarsäter et al. 2007). Temperament (harm avoidance, novelty-seeking, and reward dependence) and dimensions of characterological traits (self-directedness, cooperativeness, and self-transcendence) (Cloninger 1994) are assumed to have a marked role in the developmental trajectories contributing to ADHD and BPD. The highest scores of novelty-seeking and harm avoidance were reported among patients with ADHD and BPD (Matthies and Philipsen 2014). Novelty seeking is associated with impulsiveness, which is highly related to male BPD (Fossati et al. 2001; Barnow et al. 2009), while harm avoidance has been indicated to be higher in female BPD (Barnow et al. 2009). Lower scores of self-directedness and cooperativeness were indicated in individuals with BPD (Matthies and Philipsen 2014). Additionally, studies have shown higher than average levels of novelty-seeking temperament strongly linked to ADHD than BPD, while harm avoidance was shown to be more linked to BPD (Van Dijke 2012). In line with similar findings, it has been concluded that the concept of ADHD should not be misclassified as personality disorder due to the higher scores of temperament/character traits in patients with ADHD, in contrast to lower scores of self-directedness and cooperativeness in BPD patients (Van Dijke 2012; Matthies and Philipsen 2014).

Interpersonal issues are also reported in both BPD and ADHD (Prada et al. 2014) which are associated with diminished quality of life and decreased self-esteem in both disorders (Euler et al. 2019; IsHak et al. 2013; O'Malley et al. 2016). Di Lonardo Burr et al. (2022) posited that although interpersonal deficits are one of the core features in BPD, when seen in ADHD, should be considered as an indirect influence rather than a core symptom (Di Lonardo Burr et al. 2022). This is likely due to effects of other factors that can contribute to interpersonal difficulties in ADHD, such as tardiness and error-prone behaviors in workplace environments (Harpin 2005). Based on DSM classification, interpersonal issues in BPD is one of the core symptoms of BPD diagnosis that are manifested by unstable, intense, and chaotic relationships with a shift between idealization and devaluation, accompanied by highly interpersonal sensitivity and severe efforts to avoid being abandoned (APA 2022; Euler et al. 2019). While interpersonal difficulties in ADHD have been proposed as being sequential to the three major symptoms: inattention, hyperactivity, and impulsivity, in addition to deficits in social cognition, which can be elucidated by the context of frontostriatal dysfunction (Uekermann et al. 2010). Sebastian et al. (2014) reported patients with BPD represented prefrontal dysfunctions across impulse control elements rather than orbitofrontal, dorsomedial, and dorsolateral regions, while individuals with ADHD exhibited impaired activity specifically in ventrolateral and media prefrontal regions. They concluded that a dissociation of impulse control is associated with frontal dysfunctions in BPD and ADHD patients (Sebastian et al. 2014). Adult with ADHD may represent disorganized or novelty-seeking behaviors, yet identity disturbances are specific to BPD that are displayed by chaotic behaviors and hyper-investment in interpersonal relationships and goals with no coherence over time (Wilkinson et al. 2011). Additionally, underlying feelings of stress and instability lead to self-destructive behaviors and provoke unstable relationships, insufficient sense of self, and dissociative or paranoid symptoms in BP which have not been observed in ADHD (Matthies and Philipsen 2014).

The most documented theory contributing to a comprehensive understanding of BPD proposes that BPD develops in the context of interaction between temperamental characteristics, especially impulsivity and emotion dysregulation, and an invalidating childhood environment featured by lack of tolerance toward any expression of private emotional experiences, being exposed to several adverse environments contributing to disability to learn how to effectively regulate emotional states, and also, being vacillated between emotional inhibition and extreme emotional instability (Linehan 1993). Despite interrelation between BPD, ADHD symptoms, and traumatic experiences, these associations remain the subject of debate (Matthies and Philipsen 2014). In line with several studies, it has been proposed that difficulties in child–parent interactions may contribute to ADHD symptoms in children which can lead to traumatic interactions and increased possibility of being under emotional abuse and neglect in these children (Johnston et al. 2012).

A great body of investigations has demonstrated that adverse and traumatic experiences are highly prevalent in personality disorders generally, and in ADHD patients as well (Björkenstam et al. 2017). Exposure to trauma including interpersonal abuse, neglect, conflict, or loss of home during childhood are associated with identity disturbances, which have been shown as much as 13 times more likely in BPD (Porter et al. 2020). In a cross-sectional study, Prada et al. (2014) investigated the possible role of childhood trauma in the association between ADHD and BPD in a clinical sample (n-415). The findings revealed that adult BPD patients displayed a greater number of childhood traumas compared with adult ADHD (Prada et al. 2014). Issues in emotion regulation have been revealed to be core mediators in the associations between childhood trauma and BPD (van Dijke et al. 2010). Philipsen et al. (2008) documented a significant association between the retrospective diagnosis of childhood ADHD in BPD females and a history of emotional abuse in childhood (Philipsen et al. 2008). Through a cross-sectional study, Ferrer et al. (2017) compared maltreatment history among adults suffering from BPD, ADHD, and BPD+ADHD to disentangle the relations between ADHD and child sexual abuse (CSA). The results showed that women with BPD and ADHD indicated higher scores of CSA in comparison with women without BPD and without ADHD. In addition, emotional abuse, physical abuse, and sexual abuse anticipated BPD+ADHD diagnosis (Ferrer et al. 2017). In a cross-sectional study based on a non-clinical sample, Dalbudak et al. (2015) demonstrated a significant association between depressive symptoms, emotional and physical abuse, and severity of ADHD symptoms with severity of borderline personality features. In addition, the results showed that these variables may have mediating role in the relationship between childhood ADHD and adult BPD (Dalbudak et al. 2015).

Thus, there are many common underlying vulnerabilities between ADHD and BPD, in addition to somewhat unclearly defined diagnostic criteria that can make it difficult to distinguish between the diagnoses in differential diagnosis scenarios (e.g., impulsivity). Given that ADHD is primarily treated with psychotropic medication whereas BPD is most effectively treated with psychotherapy, careful assessment of potentially comorbid cases is necessary, and in cases of true comorbidity a hybrid medication and psychotherapy approach may be most effective (e.g., Asheron et al. 2014).

References

Ai Y, Zhao J, Shi J, Zhu TT. Antibiotic exposure and childhood attention-deficit/hyperactivity disorder: systematic review and meta-analysis. Psychopharmacology. 2021;238:3055–62.

Akça ÖF, Wall K, Sharp C. Borderline personality disorder and attention deficit/hyperactivity disorder in adolescence: overlap and differences in a clinical setting. Bord Personal Disord Emot Dysregul. 2020;7:1–9.

Alderson RM, Kasper LJ, Hudec KL, Patros CH. Attention-deficit/hyperactivity disorder (ADHD) and working memory in adults: a meta-analytic review. Neuropsychology. 2013;27(3):287.

Altszuler A. The effect of methylphenidate on associative learning among youth with attention-deficit/hyperactivity disorder (Doctoral dissertation, Florida International University); 2019.

American Psychiatric Association DS. Diagnostic and statistical manual of mental disorders: DSM-5. Washington, DC: American psychiatric association; 2013.

American Psychiatric Association. Diagnostic and statistical manual of mental disorders. 5th ed. Text Revised (DSM-5-TR); 2022.

Anckarsäter H, Piechnik S, Tullberg M, Ziegelitz D, Sörman M, Bjellvi J, Karlsson E, Fernandez NV, Wikkelso C, Forsman A. Persistent regional frontotemporal hypoactivity in violent offenders at follow-up. Psychiatry Res Neuroimaging. 2007;156(1):87–90.

Asarnow RF, Newman N, Weiss RE, Su E. Association of attention-deficit/hyperactivity disorder diagnoses with pediatric traumatic brain injury: a meta-analysis. JAMA Pediatr. 2021;175(10):1009–16.

Asheron P, Young AH, Eich-Hochli D, et al. Differential diagnosis, comorbidity, and treatment of attention-deficit/hyperactivity disorder in relation to bipolar or borderline personality disorder in adults. Curr Med Res Opin. 2014;30(8):1657–72.

Asherson P, Manor I, Huss M. Attention-deficit/hyperactivity disorder in adults: update on clinical presentation and care. Neuropsychiatry. 2014;4(1):109.

Babinski DE, McQuade JD. Borderline personality features mediate the association between ADHD, ODD, and relational and physical aggression in girls. J Atten Disord. 2019;23(8):838–48.

Babinski DE, McQuade JD, Waschbusch DA. A latent profile analysis of borderline personality features and externalizing problems in youth. J Clin Psychol. 2021;77(3):732–44.

Bálint S, Czobor P, Komlósi S, Meszaros A, Simon V, Bitter I. Attention deficit hyperactivity disorder (ADHD): gender-and age-related differences in neurocognition. Psychol Med. 2009;39(8):1337–45.

Barkley RA. Is executive functioning deficient in ADHD? It depends on your definitions and your measures. ADHD Rep. 2011;19(4):1–9.

Barkley RA, Murphy KR, Fischer M. ADHD in adults: what the science says. Guilford press; 2010.

Barnow S, Stopsack M, Grabe HJ, Meinke C, Spitzer C, Kronmüller K, Sieswerda S. Interpersonal evaluation bias in borderline personality disorder. Behav Res Ther. 2009;47(5):359–65.

Beeney JE, Forbes EE, Hipwell AE, Nance M, Mattia A, Lawless JM, Banihashemi L, Stepp SD. Determining the key childhood and adolescent risk factors for future BPD symptoms using regularized regression: comparison to depression and conduct disorder. J Child Psychol Psychiatry. 2021;62(2):223–31.

Belsky DW, Caspi A, Arseneault L, Bleidorn W, Fonagy P, Goodman M, Houts R, Moffitt TE. Etiological features of borderline personality related characteristics in a birth cohort of 12-year-old children. Dev Psychopathol. 2012;24(1):251–65.

Bernardi S, Faraone SV, Cortese S, Kerridge BT, Pallanti S, Wang S, Blanco C. The lifetime impact of attention deficit hyperactivity disorder: results from the National Epidemiologic Survey on Alcohol and Related Conditions (NESARC). Psychol Med. 2012;42(4):875–87.

Bertsch K, Krauch M, Roelofs K, Cackowski S, Herpertz SC, Volman I. Out of control? Acting out anger is associated with deficient prefrontal emotional action control in male patients with borderline personality disorder. Neuropharmacology. 2019;156:107463.

Biederman J, Mick E, Faraone SV. Age-dependent decline of symptoms of attention deficit hyperactivity disorder: impact of remission definition and symptom type. Am J Psychiatry. 2000;157(5):816–8.

Biederman J, Monuteaux MC, Spencer T, Wilens TE, Faraone SV. Do stimulants protect against psychiatric disorders in youth with ADHD? A 10-year follow-up study. Pediatrics. 2009;124(1):71–8.

Biederman J, Petty CR, Woodworth KY, Lomedico A, Hyder LL, Faraone SV. Adult outcome of attention-deficit/hyperactivity disorder: a controlled 16-year follow-up study. J Clin Psychiatry. 2012;73(7):577.

Björkenstam E, Ekselius L, Burström B, Kosidou K, Björkenstam C. Association between childhood adversity and a diagnosis of personality disorder in young adulthood: a cohort study of 107,287 individuals in Stockholm County. Eur J Epidemiol. 2017;32:721–31.

Björkenstam E, Björkenstam C, Jablonska B, Kosidou K. Cumulative exposure to childhood adversity, and treated attention deficit/hyperactivity disorder: a cohort study of 543 650 adolescents and young adults in Sweden. Psychol Med. 2018;48(3):498–507.

Black DW, Gunter T, Allen J, Blum N, Arndt S, Wenman G, Sieleni B. Borderline personality disorder in male and female offenders newly committed to prison. Compr Psychiatry. 2007;48(5):400–5.

Burke A, Austin TL. The problem of identifying and diagnosing adult attention deficit hyperactive disorder (AADHD): results and implications of a South African study. J Psychol Afr. 2010;20(2):265–73.

Cackowski S, Krause-Utz A, Van Eijk J, Klohr K, Daffner S, Sobanski E, Ende G. Anger and aggression in borderline personality disorder and attention deficit hyperactivity disorder–does stress matter? Bord Personal Disord Emot Dysregul. 2017;4:1–3.

Carlotta D, Borroni S, Maffei C, Fossati A. On the relationship between retrospective childhood ADHD symptoms and adult BPD features: the mediating role of action-oriented personality traits. Compr Psychiatry. 2013;54(7):943–52.

Cavelti M, Blaha Y, Lerch S, Hertel C, Berger T, Reichl C, Koenig J, Kaess M. The evaluation of a stepped care approach for early intervention of borderline personality disorder. Bord Personal Disord Emot Dysregul. 2024;11:12.

Caye A, Petresco S, de Barros AJ, Bressan RA, Gadelha A, Goncalves H, Manfro AG, Matijasevich A, Menezes AM, Miguel EC, Munhoz TN. Relative age and attention-deficit/hyperactivity disorder: data from three epidemiological cohorts and a meta-analysis. J Am Acad Child Adolesc Psychiatry. 2020;59(8):990–7.

Cheung CH, Rijsdijk F, McLoughlin G, Brandeis D, Banaschewski T, Asherson P, Kuntsi J. Cognitive and neurophysiological markers of ADHD persistence and remission. Br J Psychiatry. 2016;208(6):548–55.

Cloninger CR. Temperament and personality. Curr Opin Neurobiol. 1994;4(2):266–73.

Connor DF, Chartier KG, Preen EC, Kaplan RF. Impulsive aggression in attention-deficit/hyperactivity disorder: symptom severity, co-morbidity, and attention-deficit/hyperactivity disorder subtype. J Child Adolesc Psychopharmacol. 2010;20(2):119–26.

Coolidge FL, Segal DL, Stewart SE, Ellett JA. Neuropsychological dysfunction in children with borderline personality disorder features: a preliminary investigation. J Res Pers. 2000;34(4):554–61.

Corbisiero S, Stieglitz RD, Retz W, Rösler M. Is emotional dysregulation part of the psychopathology of ADHD in adults? Atten Defic Hyperact Disord. 2013;5:83–92.

Cumyn L, French L, Hechtman L. Comorbidity in adults with attention-deficit hyperactivity disorder. Can J Psychiatry. 2009;54(10):673–83.

Currie J, Stabile M. Child mental health and human capital accumulation: the case of ADHD. J Health Econ. 2006;25(6):1094–118.

Dalbudak E, Evren C, Aldemir S, Taymur I, Evren B, Topcu M. The impact of sensation seeking on the relationship between attention deficit/hyperactivity symptoms and severity of internet addiction risk. Psychiatry Res. 2015;228(1):156–61.

Dalsgaard S, Østergaard SD, Leckman JF, Mortensen PB, Pedersen MG. Mortality in children, adolescents, and adults with attention deficit hyperactivity disorder: a nationwide cohort study. Lancet. 2015;385(9983):2190–6.

Das D, Cherbuin N, Easteal S, Anstey KJ. Attention deficit/hyperactivity disorder symptoms and cognitive abilities in the late-life cohort of the PATH through life study. PLoS One. 2014;9(1):e86552.

Davids E, Gastpar M. Attention deficit hyperactivity disorder and borderline personality disorder. Prog Neuro-Psychopharmacol Biol Psychiatry. 2005;29(6):865–77.

Del-Ponte B, Quinte GC, Cruz S, Grellert M, Santos IS. Dietary patterns and attention deficit/hyperactivity disorder (ADHD): a systematic review and meta-analysis. J Affect Disord. 2019;252:160–73.

Di Lonardo Burr SM, LeFevre JA, Arnold LE, Epstein JN, Hinshaw SP, Molina BS, Hechtman L, Hoza B, Jensen PS, Vitiello B, Pelham WE Jr. Paths to postsecondary education enrollment among adolescents with and without childhood attention-deficit/hyperactivity disorder (ADHD): a longitudinal analysis of symptom and academic trajectories. Child Dev. 2022;93(5):e563–80.

Distel MA, Carlier A, Middeldorp CM, Derom CA, Lubke GH, Boomsma DI. Borderline personality traits and adult attention-deficit hyperactivity disorder symptoms: a genetic analysis of comorbidity. Am J Med Genet B Neuropsychiatr Genet. 2011;156(7):817–25.

Ditrich I, Philipsen A, Matthies S. Borderline personality disorder (BPD) and attention deficit hyperactivity disorder (ADHD) revisited–a review-update on common grounds and subtle distinctions. Bord Personal Disord Emot Dysregul. 2021;8:1–2.

Dowson JH, Blackwell AD. Impulsive aggression in adults with attention-deficit/hyperactivity disorder. Acta Psychiatr Scand. 2010;121(2):103–10.

Dowson JH, McLean A, Bazanis E, Toone B, Young S, Robbins TW, Sahakian B. The specificity of clinical characteristics in adults with attention-deficit/hyperactivity disorder: a comparison with patients with borderline personality disorder. Eur Psychiatry. 2004;19(2):72–8.

Ebejer JL, Medland SE, van der Werf J, Gondro C, Henders AK, Lynskey M, Martin NG, Duffy DL. Attention deficit hyperactivity disorder in Australian adults: prevalence, persistence, conduct problems and disadvantage. PLoS One. 2012;7(10):e47404.

Euler S, Stalujanis E, Allenbach G, Kolly S, De Roten Y, Despland JN, Kramer U. Dialectical behavior therapy skills training affects defense mechanisms in borderline personality disorder: an integrative approach of mechanisms in psychotherapy. Psychother Res. 2019;29(8):1074–85.

Evans S, Ling M, Hill B, Rinehart N, Austin D, Sciberras E. Systematic review of meditation-based interventions for children with ADHD. Eur Child Adolesc Psychiatry. 2018;27:9–27.

Evans BC, Felton JW, Lagacey MA, Manasse SM, Lejuez CW, Juarascio AS. Impulsivity and affect reactivity prospectively predict disordered eating attitudes in adolescents: a 6-year longitudinal study. Eur Child Adolesc Psychiatry. 2019;28:1193–202.

Evenden JL. Varieties of impulsivity. Psychopharmacology. 1999;146(4):348–61.
Faraone SV, Rostain AL, Blader J, Busch B, Childress AC, Connor DF, Newcorn JH. Practitioner review: emotional dysregulation in attention-deficit/hyperactivity disorder–implications for clinical recognition and intervention. J Child Psychol Psychiatry. 2019;60(2):133–50.
Faraone SV, Biederman J, Spencer T, Mick E, Murray K, Petty C, Adamson JJ, Monuteaux MC. Diagnosing adult attention deficit hyperactivity disorder: are late onset and subthreshold diagnoses valid? Am J Psychiatry. 2006;163(10):1720–9.
Farsad-Naeimi A, Asjodi F, Omidian M, Askari M, Nouri M, Pizarro AB, Daneshzad E. Sugar consumption, sugar sweetened beverages and attention deficit hyperactivity disorder: a systematic review and meta-analysis. Complement Ther Med. 2020;53:102512.
Fayyad J, De Graaf R, Kessler R, Alonso J, Angermeyer M, Demyttenaere K, De Girolamo G, Haro JM, Karam EG, Lara C, Lepine JP. Cross-national prevalence and correlates of adult attention-deficit hyperactivity disorder. Br J Psychiatry. 2007;190(5):402–9.
Ferrer M, Andión Ó, Matalí J, Valero S, Navarro JA, Ramos-Quiroga JA, Torrubia R, Casas M. Comorbid attention-deficit/hyperactivity disorder in borderline patients defines an impulsive subtype of borderline personality disorder. J Personal Disord. 2010;24(6):812–22.
Ferrer M, Andión Ó, Calvo N, Ramos-Quiroga JA, Prat M, Corrales M, Casas M. Differences in the association between childhood trauma history and borderline personality disorder or attention deficit/hyperactivity disorder diagnoses in adulthood. Eur Arch Psychiatry Clin Neurosci. 2017;267:541–9.
Fischer M, Barkley RA, Smallish L, Fletcher K. Executive functioning in hyperactive children as young adults: attention, inhibition, response perseveration, and the impact of comorbidity. Dev Neuropsychol. 2005;27(1):107–33.
Fossati A, Gratz KL, Borroni S, Maffei C, Somma A, Carlotta D. The relationship between childhood history of ADHD symptoms and DSM-IV borderline personality disorder features among personality disordered outpatients: the moderating role of gender and the mediating roles of emotion dysregulation and impulsivity. Compr Psychiatry. 2015;56:121–7.
Fossati A, Di Ceglie A, Acquarini E, Barratt ES. Psychometric properties of an Italian version of the Barratt Impulsiveness Scale-11 (BIS-11) in nonclinical subjects. J Clin Psychol. 2001;57(6):815–28.
Fossati A, Novella L, Donati D, Donini M, Maffei C. History of childhood attention deficit/hyperactivity disorder symptoms and borderline personality disorder: a controlled study. Compr Psychiatry. 2002;43(5):369–77.
Ginsberg Y, Beusterien KM, Amos K, Jousselin C, Asherson P. The unmet needs of all adults with ADHD are not the same: a focus on Europe. Expert Rev Neurother. 2014;14(7):799–812.
Glenn CR, Klonsky ED. A multimethod analysis of impulsivity in nonsuicidal self-injury. Personal Disord Theory Res Treat. 2010;1(1):67.
Goodman DW. The consequences of attention-deficit/hyperactivity disorder in adults. J Psychiatr Pract. 2007;13(5):318–27.
Goodman DW. ADHD in adults: update for clinicians on diagnosis and assessment. Prim Psychiatry. 2009;16(11):38.
Grant BF, Chou SP, Goldstein RB, Huang B, Stinson FS, Saha TD, Smith SM, Dawson DA, Pulay AJ, Pickering RP, Ruan WJ. Prevalence, correlates, disability, and comorbidity of DSM-IV borderline personality disorder: results from the Wave 2 National Epidemiologic Survey on Alcohol and Related Conditions. J Clin Psychiatry. 2008;69(4):533.
Guo D, Ju R, Zhou Q, Mao J, Tao H, Jing H, Zhu C, Dai J. Association of maternal diabetes with attention deficit/hyperactivity disorder (ADHD) in offspring: a meta-analysis and review. Diabetes Res Clin Pract. 2020;165:108269.
Harpin VA. The effect of ADHD on the life of an individual, their family, and community from preschool to adult life. Arch Dis Child. 2005;90(suppl 1):i2–7.
Harty SC, Miller CJ, Newcorn JH, Halperin JM. Adolescents with childhood ADHD and comorbid disruptive behavior disorders: aggression, anger, and hostility. Child Psychiatry Hum Dev. 2009;40:85–97.

Hirsch O, Chavanon ML, Christiansen H. Emotional dysregulation subgroups in patients with adult attention-deficit/hyperactivity disorder (ADHD): a cluster analytic approach. Sci Rep. 2019;9(1):5639.

IsHak WW, Elbau I, Ismail A, Delaloye S, Ha K, Bolotaulo NI, Nashawati R, Cassmassi B, Wang C. Quality of life in borderline personality disorder. Harv Rev Psychiatry. 2013;21(3):138–50.

Jacob GA, Gutz L, Bader K, Lieb K, Tüscher O, Stahl C. Impulsivity in borderline personality disorder: impairment in self-report measures, but not behavioral inhibition. Psychopathology. 2010;43(3):180–8.

Jacobsson P, Hopwood CJ, Söderpalm B, Nilsson T. Adult ADHD and emerging models of maladaptive personality: a meta-analytic review. BMC Psychiatry. 2021;21:1–6.

Jensen PS, Arnold LE, Swanson JM, Vitiello B, Abikoff HB, Greenhill LL, Hechtman L, Hinshaw SP, Pelham WE, Wells KC, Conners CK. 3-year follow-up of the NIMH MTA study. J Am Acad Child Adolesc Psychiatry. 2007;46(8):989–1002.

Johnston C, Mash EJ, Miller N, Ninowski JE. Parenting in adults with attention-deficit/hyperactivity disorder (ADHD). Clin Psychol Rev. 2012;32(4):215–28.

Katzman MA, Bilkey T, Chokka PR, Fallu A, Klassen LJ. Re: is adult attention-deficit hyperactivity disorder being overdiagnosed? Can J Psychiatry. 2016;61(1):60–1.

Katzman MA, Bilkey TS, Chokka PR, Fallu A, Klassen LJ. Adult ADHD and comorbid disorders: clinical implications of a dimensional approach. BMC Psychiatry. 2017;17:1–5.

Kazda L, McGeechan K, Bell K, Thomas R, Barratt A. Increased diagnosis of attention-deficit hyperactivity disorder despite stable hyperactive/inattentive behaviours: evidence from two birth cohorts of Australian children. J Child Psychol Psychiatry. 2023;64(8):1140–8.

Kent KM, Pelham WE Jr, Molina BS, Sibley MH, Waschbusch DA, Yu J, Gnagy EM, Biswas A, Babinski DE, Karch KM. The academic experience of male high school students with ADHD. J Abnorm Child Psychol. 2011;39(3):451–62.

Kenter RM, Lundervold AJ, Nordgreen T. A self-guided internet-delivered intervention for adults with ADHD: a protocol for a randomized controlled trial. Internet Interv. 2021;26:100485.

Kessler RC, Adler L, Barkley R, Biederman J, Conners CK, Demler O, Faraone SV, Greenhill LL, Howes MJ, Secnik K, Spencer T. The prevalence and correlates of adult ADHD in the United States: results from the National Comorbidity Survey Replication. Am J Psychiatry. 2006;163(4):716–23.

Korsgaard HO, Ulberg R, Hummelen B, Midgley N, Thorén A, Dahl HS. Personality disorders as a possible moderator of the effects of relational interventions in short-term psychoanalytic psychotherapy with depressed adolescents. Int J Environ Res Public Health. 2022;19(17):10952.

Korsgaard HO, Torgersen S, Wentzel-Larsen T, Ulberg R. Personality disorders and Axis I comorbidity in adolescent outpatients with ADHD. BMC Psychiatry. 2016;16:1.

Kouppis E, Gerdin B, Björkenstam C, Björkenstam E, Ekselius L. Effect of comorbid ADHD on mortality in women with borderline personality disorder. Bord Personal Disord Emot Dysregul. 2022;9(1):25.

Krause-Utz A, Cackowski S, Daffner S, Sobanski E, Plichta MM, Bohus M, Ende G, Schmahl C. Delay discounting and response disinhibition under acute experimental stress in women with borderline personality disorder and adult attention deficit hyperactivity disorder. Psychol Med. 2016;46(15):3137–49.

Krause-Utz A, Sobanski E, Alm B, Valerius G, Kleindienst N, Bohus M, Schmahl C. Impulsivity in relation to stress in patients with borderline personality disorder with and without co-occurring attention-deficit/hyperactivity disorder: an exploratory study. J Nerv Ment Dis. 2013;201(2):116–23.

Kulacaoglu F, Solmaz M, Ardic FC, Akin E, Kose S. The relationship between childhood traumas, dissociation, and impulsivity in patients with borderline personality disorder comorbid with ADHD. Psychiatry Clin Psychopharmacol. 2017;27(4):393–402.

Lampe K, Konrad K, Kroener S, Fast K, Kunert HJ, Herpertz SC. Neuropsychological and behavioural disinhibition in adult ADHD compared to borderline personality disorder. Psychol Med. 2007;37(12):1717–29.

Langevin R, Marshall C, Wallace A, Gagné ME, Kingsland E, Temcheff C. Disentangling the associations between attention deficit hyperactivity disorder and child sexual abuse: a systematic review. Trauma Violence Abuse. 2023;24(2):369–89.
Látalová K, Praško J. Aggression in borderline personality disorder. Psychiatry Q. 2010;81:239–51.
Leichsenring F, Leibing E, Kruse J, New AS, Leweke F. Borderline personality disorder. Focus. 2013;11(2):249–60.
Li L, Lagerberg T, Chang Z, Cortese S, Rosenqvist MA, Almqvist C, D'Onofrio BM, Hegvik TA, Hartman C, Chen Q, Larsson H. Maternal pre-pregnancy overweight/obesity and the risk of attention-deficit/hyperactivity disorder in offspring: a systematic review, meta-analysis and quasi-experimental family-based study. Int J Epidemiol. 2020;49(3):857–75.
Linehan MM. Dialectical behavior therapy for treatment of borderline personality disorder: implications for the treatment of substance abuse. NIDA Res Monogr. 1993;137:201.
Lieb K, Zanarini MC, Schmahl C, Linehan MM, Bohus M. Borderline personality disorder. Lancet. 2004;364(9432):453–61.
MacDonald L, Sadek J. Management strategies for borderline personality disorder and bipolar disorder comorbidities in adults with ADHD: a narrative review. Brain Sci. 2023;13(11):1517.
Mahadevan J, Kandasamy A, Benegal V. Situating adult attention-deficit/hyperactivity disorder in the externalizing spectrum: etiological, diagnostic, and treatment considerations. Indian J Psychiatry. 2019;61(1):3–12.
Mancke F, Bertsch K, Herpertz SC. Gender differences in aggression of borderline personality disorder. Bord Personal Disord Emot Dysregul. 2015;2:1–2.
Martel MM, Nigg JT, Von Eye A. How do trait dimensions map onto ADHD symptom domains? J Abnorm Child Psychol. 2009;37(3):337–48.
Matthies SD, Philipsen A. Common ground in attention deficit hyperactivity disorder (ADHD) and borderline personality disorder (BPD)–review of recent findings. Bord Personal Disord Emot Dysregul. 2014;1:1–3.
May B, Bos J. Personality characteristics of ADHD adults assessed with the Millon clinical multiaxial inventory-II: evidence of four distinct subtypes. J Pers Assess. 2000;75(2):237–48.
Mayes SD, Zickgraf H. Atypical eating behaviors in children and adolescents with autism, ADHD, other disorders, and typical development. Res Autism Spectr Disord. 2019;64:76–83.
Mcclure G, Hawes DJ, Dadds MR. Borderline personality disorder and neuropsychological measures of executive function: a systematic review. Personal Ment Health. 2016;10(1):43–57.
McQuade JD, Vaughn AJ, Hoza B, Murray-Close D, Molina BS, Arnold LE, Hechtman L. Perceived social acceptance and peer status differentially predict adjustment in youth with and without ADHD. J Atten Disord. 2014;18(1):31–43.
Miller CJ, Miller SR, Newcorn JH, Halperin JM. Personality characteristics associated with persistent ADHD in late adolescence. J Abnorm Child Psychol. 2008;36:165–73.
Min X, Li C, Yan Y. Parental age and the risk of ADHD in offspring: a systematic review and meta-analysis. Int J Environ Res Public Health. 2021;18(9):4939.
Moeller FG, Barratt ES, Dougherty DM, Schmitz JM, Swann AC. Psychiatric aspects of impulsivity. Am J Psychiatry. 2001;158(11):1783–93.
Moukhtarian TR, Mintah RS, Moran P, Asherson P. Emotion dysregulation in attention-deficit/hyperactivity disorder and borderline personality disorder. Bord Personal Disord Emot Dysregul. 2018;5:1.
Moukhtarian TR, Reinhard I, Morillas-Romero A, Ryckaert C, Mowlem F, Bozhilova N, Moran P, Ebner-Priemer U, Asherson P. Wandering minds in attention-deficit/hyperactivity disorder and borderline personality disorder. Eur Neuropsychopharmacol. 2020;38:98–109.
Moukhtarian TR, Reinhard I, Moran P, Ryckaert C, Skirrow C, Ebner-Priemer U, Asherson P. Comparable emotional dynamics in women with ADHD and borderline personality disorder. Bord Personal Disord Emot Dysregul. 2021;8:1.
New AS, Hazlett EA, Newmark RE, Zhang J, Triebwasser J, Meyerson D, Lazarus S, Trisdorfer R, Goldstein KE, Goodman M, Koenigsberg HW. Laboratory induced aggression: a positron emission tomography study of aggressive individuals with borderline personality disorder. Biol Psychiatry. 2009;66(12):1107–14.

Nigg JT, Silk KR, Stavro GI, Miller TO. Disinhibition and borderline personality disorder. Dev Psychopathol. 2005;17(4):1129–49.

Nigg JT. Getting ahead of ADHD: what next-generation science says about treatments that work? In: And how you can make them work for your child. Guilford Publications; 2017.

O'Grady SM, Hinshaw SP. Developmental predictors of young adult borderline personality disorder: a prospective, longitudinal study of females with and without childhood ADHD. BMC Psychiatry. 2023;23(1):106.

O'malley GK, McHugh L, Mac Giollabhui N, Bramham J. Characterizing adult attention-deficit/hyperactivity-disorder and comorbid borderline personality disorder: ADHD symptoms, psychopathology, cognitive functioning and psychosocial factors. Eur Psychiatry. 2016;31:29–36.

Pan G, Han Y, Wang TC, Chen ZY, Wang XQ, Sun HB, Liu YH, Wang Q, Lin WH, Li JM, Zhou SZ. Attention deficit hyperactivity disorder in children with epilepsy: a multicenter cross-sectional analysis in China. World J Pediatr. 2024:1–9. https://doi.org/10.1007/s12519-024-00813-2.

Pelham WE, Smith BH, Evans SW, Bukstein O, Gnagy EM, Greiner AR, Sibley MH. The effectiveness of short-and long-acting stimulant medications for adolescents with ADHD in a naturalistic secondary school setting. J Atten Disord. 2017;21(1):40–5.

Perez-Rodriguez MM, Hazlett EA, Rich EL, Ripoll LH, Weiner DM, Spence N, Goodman M, Koenigsberg HW, Siever LJ, New AS. Striatal activity in borderline personality disorder with comorbid intermittent explosive disorder: sex differences. J Psychiatr Res. 2012;46(6):797–804.

Perroud N, Badoud D, Weibel S, Nicastro R, Hasler R, Küng AL, Luyten P, Fonagy P, Dayer A, Aubry JM, Prada P. Mentalization in adults with attention deficit hyperactivity disorder: comparison with controls and patients with borderline personality disorder. Psychiatry Res. 2017;256:334–41.

Perroud N, Hasler R, Golay N, Zimmermann J, Prada P, Nicastro R, Aubry JM, Ardu S, Herrmann FR, Giannakopoulos P, Baud P. Personality profiles in adults with attention deficit hyperactivity disorder (ADHD). BMC Psychiatry. 2016;16:1–9.

Petrovic P, Castellanos FX. Top-down dysregulation—from ADHD to emotional instability. Front Behav Neurosci. 2016;10:70.

Philipsen A. Differential diagnosis and comorbidity of attention-deficit/hyperactivity disorder (ADHD) and borderline personality disorder (BPD) in adults. Eur Arch Psychiatry Clin Neurosci. 2006;256:i42–6.

Philipsen A, Limberger MF, Lieb K, Feige B, Kleindienst N, Ebner-Priemer U, Barth J, Schmahl C, Bohus M. Attention-deficit hyperactivity disorder as a potentially aggravating factor in borderline personality disorder. Br J Psychiatry. 2008;192(2):118–23.

Philipsen A, Feige B, Hesslinger B, Scheel C, Ebert D, Matthies S, Limberger MF, Kleindienst N, Bohus M, Lieb K. Borderline typical symptoms in adult patients with attention deficit/hyperactivity disorder. Atten Defic Hyperact Disord. 2009;1:11–8.

Polanczyk G, De Lima MS, Horta BL, Biederman J, Rohde LA. The worldwide prevalence of ADHD: a systematic review and metaregression analysis. Am J Psychiatry. 2007;164(6):942–8.

Porter C, Palmier-Claus J, Branitsky A, Mansell W, Warwick H, Varese F. Childhood adversity and borderline personality disorder: a meta-analysis. Acta Psychiatr Scand. 2020;141(1):6–20.

Posner J, Park C, Wang Z. Connecting the dots: a review of resting connectivity MRI studies in attention-deficit/hyperactivity disorder. Neuropsychol Rev. 2014;24:3–15.

Prada P, Hasler R, Baud P, Bednarz G, Ardu S, Krejci I, Nicastro R, Aubry JM, Perroud N. Distinguishing borderline personality disorder from adult attention deficit/hyperactivity disorder: a clinical and dimensional perspective. Psychiatry Res. 2014;217(1–2):107–14.

Rasmussen K, Levander S. Untreated ADHD in adults: are there sex differences in symptoms, comorbidity, and impairment? J Atten Disord. 2009;12(4):353–60.

Reimherr FW, Marchant BK, Strong RE, Hedges DW, Adler L, Spencer TJ, West SA, Soni P. Emotional dysregulation in adult ADHD and response to atomoxetine. Biol Psychiatry. 2005;58(2):125–31.

Richter MM, Ehlis AC, Jacob CP, Fallgatter AJ. Cortical excitability in adult patients with attention-deficit/hyperactivity disorder (ADHD). Neurosci Lett. 2007;419(2):137–41.

Ronald A, de Bode N, Polderman TJ. Systematic review: how the attention-deficit/hyperactivity disorder polygenic risk score adds to our understanding of ADHD and associated traits. J Am Acad Child Adolesc Psychiatry. 2021;60(10):1234–77.

Rösler M, Retz W, Yaqoobi K, Burg E, Retz-Junginger P. Attention deficit/hyperactivity disorder in female offenders: prevalence, psychiatric comorbidity and psychosocial implications. Eur Arch Psychiatry Clin Neurosci. 2009;259:98–105.

Ross JM, Babcock JC. Proactive and reactive violence among intimate partner violent men diagnosed with antisocial and borderline personality disorder. J Fam Violence. 2009;24:607–17.

Rowland J, Wilson CA. The association between gestational diabetes and ASD and ADHD: a systematic review and meta-analysis. Sci Rep. 2021;11(1):5136.

Ruocco AC. The neuropsychology of borderline personality disorder: a meta-analysis and review. Psychiatry Res. 2005;137(3):191–202.

Rüfenacht E, Euler S, Prada P, Nicastro R, Dieben K, Hasler R, Pham E, Perroud N, Weibel S. Emotion dysregulation in adults suffering from attention deficit hyperactivity disorder (ADHD), a comparison with borderline personality disorder (BPD). Bord Personal Disord Emot Dysregul. 2019;6:1.

Russell AE, Ford T, Williams R, Russell G. The association between socioeconomic disadvantage and attention deficit/hyperactivity disorder (ADHD): a systematic review. Child Psychiatry Hum Dev. 2016;47:440–58.

Rydkjaer J, Jepsen JR, Pagsberg AK, Fagerlund B, Glenthoej BY, Oranje B. Do young adolescents with first-episode psychosis or ADHD show sensorimotor gating deficits? Psychol Med. 2020;50(4):607–15.

Sayal K, Prasad V, Daley D, Ford T, Coghill D. ADHD in children and young people: prevalence, care pathways, and service provision. Lancet Psychiatry. 2018;5(2):175–86.

Schwartz AN, Reyes LM, Meschke LL, Kintziger KW. Prenatal opioid exposure and ADHD childhood symptoms: a meta-analysis. Children. 2021;8(2):106.

Sebastian A, Jung P, Krause-Utz A, Lieb K, Schmahl C, Tüscher O. Frontal dysfunctions of impulse control–a systematic review in borderline personality disorder and attention-deficit/hyperactivity disorder. Front Hum Neurosci. 2014;8:698.

Shen CC, Hu LY, Hu YH. Comorbidity study of borderline personality disorder: applying association rule mining to the Taiwan national health insurance research database. BMC Med Inform Decis Mak. 2017;17:1.

Singh S, Singh S. The effectiveness of mindfulness therapy on self-esteem of adolescents with attention deficit hyperactivity disorder (ADHD). Indian J Health Well Being. 2015;6(3):267–72.

Skirrow C, Ebner-Priemer U, Reinhard I, Malliaris Y, Kuntsi J, Asherson P. Everyday emotional experience of adults with attention deficit hyperactivity disorder: evidence for reactive and endogenous emotional lability. Psychol Med. 2014;44(16):3571–83.

Sobanski E, Brüggemann D, Alm B, Kern S, Philipsen A, Schmalzried H, Heßlinger B, Waschkowski H, Rietschel M. Subtype differences in adults with attention-deficit/hyperactivity disorder (ADHD) with regard to ADHDsymptoms, psychiatric comorbidity and psychosocial adjustment. Eur Psychiatry. 2008;23(2):142–9.

Sobanski E, Brüggemann D, Alm B, Kern S, Deschner M, Schubert T, Philipsen A, Rietschel M. Psychiatric comorbidity and functional impairment in a clinically referred sample of adults with attention-deficit/hyperactivity disorder (ADHD). Eur Arch Psychiatry Clin Neurosci. 2007;257:371–7.

Sobanski E. Psychiatric comorbidity in adults with attention-deficit/hyperactivity disorder (ADHD). Eur Arch Psychiatry Clin Neurosci. 2006;256:i26–31.

Song P, Zha M, Yang Q, Zhang Y, Li X, Rudan I. The prevalence of adult attention-deficit hyperactivity disorder: a global systematic review and meta-analysis. J Glob Health. 2021;11:04009.

Speranza M, Revah-Levy A, Cortese S, Falissard B, Pham-Scottez A, Corcos M. ADHD in adolescents with borderline personality disorder. BMC Psychiatry. 2011;11:1–9.

Stepp SD. Development of borderline personality disorder in adolescence and young adulthood: introduction to the special section. J Abnorm Child Psychol. 2012;40:1–5.
Stepp SD, Olino TM, Klein DN, Seeley JR, Lewinsohn PM. Unique influences of adolescent antecedents on adult borderline personality disorder features. Personal Disord Theory Res Treat. 2013;4(3):223.
Storebø OJ, Simonsen E. Is ADHD an early stage in the development of borderline personality disorder? Nord J Psychiatry. 2014;68(5):289–95.
Surman CB, Goodman DW. Is ADHD a valid diagnosis in older adults? Atten Defic Hyperact Disord. 2017;9:161–8.
Surman CB, Biederman J, Spencer T, Yorks D, Miller CA, Petty CR, Faraone SV. Deficient emotional self-regulation and adult attention deficit hyperactivity disorder: a family risk analysis. Am J Psychiatry. 2011;168(6):617–23.
Thomas R, Sanders S, Doust J, Beller E, Glasziou P. Prevalence of attention-deficit/hyperactivity disorder: a systematic review and meta-analysis. Pediatrics. 2015a;135(4):e994–1001.
Thomas SR, O'Brien KA, Clarke TL, Liu Y, Chronis-Tuscano A. Maternal depression history moderates parenting responses to compliant and noncompliant behaviors of children with ADHD. J Abnorm Child Psychol. 2015b;43:1257–69.
Tiger A, Ohlis A, Bjureberg J, Lundström S, Lichtenstein P, Larsson H, Hellner C, Kuja-Halkola R, Jayaram-Lindström N. Childhood symptoms of attention-deficit/hyperactivity disorder and borderline personality disorder. Acta Psychiatr Scand. 2022;146(4):370–80.
Torgersen T, Gjervan B, Rasmussen K. ADHD in adults: a study of clinical characteristics, impairment and comorbidity. Nord J Psychiatry. 2006;60(1):38–43.
Uekermann J, Kraemer M, Abdel-Hamid M, Schimmelmann BG, Hebebrand J, Daum I, Wiltfang J, Kis B. Social cognition in attention-deficit hyperactivity disorder (ADHD). Neurosci Biobehav Rev. 2010;34(5):734–43.
Unoka Z, Richman MJ. Neuropsychological deficits in BPD patients and the moderator effects of co-occurring mental disorders: a meta-analysis. Clin Psychol Rev. 2016;44:1–2.
van Dijk F, Schellekens A, van den Broek P, Kan C, Verkes RJ, Buitelaar J. Do cognitive measures of response inhibition differentiate between attention deficit/hyperactivity disorder and borderline personality disorder? Psychiatry Res. 2014;215(3):733–9.
van Dijke A, Ford JD, van der Hart O, van Son M, van der Heijden P, Bühring M. Affect dysregulation in borderline personality disorder and somatoform disorder: differentiating under-and over-regulation. J Personal Disord. 2010;24(3):296–311.
Van Dijke A. Dysfunctional affect regulation in borderline personality disorder and in somatoform disorder. Eur J Psychotraumatol. 2012;3(1):19566.
Weiner L, Perroud N, Weibel S. Attention deficit hyperactivity disorder and borderline personality disorder in adults: a review of their links and risks. Neuropsychiatr Dis Treat. 2019;8:3115–29.
Wilson VB, Mitchell SH, Musser ED, Schmitt CF, Nigg JT. Delay discounting of reward in ADHD: application in young children. J Child Psychol Psychiatry. 2011;52(3):256–64.
Wilkinson P, Kelvin R, Roberts C, Dubicka B, Goodyer I. Clinical and psychosocial predictors of suicide attempts and nonsuicidal self-injury in the Adolescent Depression Antidepressants and Psychotherapy Trial (ADAPT). Am J Psychiatry. 2011;168(5):495–501.
Willcutt EG. The prevalence of DSM-IV attention-deficit/hyperactivity disorder: a meta-analytic review. Neurotherapeutics. 2012;9(3):490–9.
Williams DM. Improved academic achievement and self-efficacy through the participation in extracurricular activities of university students previously diagnosed with ADHD: a hermeneutic phenomenological study. Liberty University; 2023.
Xu G, Strathearn L, Liu B, Yang B, Bao W. Twenty-year trends in diagnosed attention-deficit/hyperactivity disorder among US children and adolescents, 1997–2016. JAMA Netw Open. 2018;1(4):e181471.
Yadav P. Pharmacological treatment of ADHD. In: New developments in diagnosing, assessing, and treating ADHD. IGI Global; 2021. p. 132–45.
Young S, Cocallis KM. Attention Deficit Hyperactivity Disorder (ADHD) in the prison system. Curr Psychiatry Rep. 2019;21:1–9.

Young S, Adamo N, Ásgeirsdóttir BB, Branney P, Beckett M, Colley W, Cubbin S, Deeley Q, Farrag E, Gudjonsson G, Hill P. Females with ADHD: an expert consensus statement taking a lifespan approach providing guidance for the identification and treatment of attention-deficit/hyperactivity disorder in girls and women. BMC Psychiatry. 2020;20:1–27.
Zanarini MC, Frankenburg FR, Hennen J, Reich DB, Silk KR. Axis I comorbidity in patients with borderline personality disorder: 6-year follow-up and prediction of time to remission. Am J Psychiatry. 2004;161(11):2108–14.
Zoromski AK, Owens JS, Evans SW, Brady CE. Identifying ADHD symptoms most associated with impairment in early childhood, middle childhood, and adolescence using teacher report. J Abnorm Child Psychol. 2015;43:1243–55.

Chapter 16
Other Psychiatric Comorbidities and Borderline Personality Disorder

Introduction

As mentioned across previous chapters, borderline personality disorder (BPD) has been demonstrated to have highly frequent comorbidity with psychiatric disorders and other personality disorders (e.g., Bornovalova et al. 2018). According to the DSM-5-TR (APA 2022), the most common comorbid disorders comprise depressive and bipolar disorders, substance use disorders, anxiety disorders, eating disorders, PTSD, and attention deficit/hyperactivity disorder (ADHD); also, BPD highly co-occurs with other personality disorders (APA 2022; Kessler et al. 2006; Martel 2009; Martel et al. 2014; Reimherr et al. 2015; Matthies and Philipsen 2014).

Several models have been provided with various explanations to elucidate the personality-psychopathology associations, most notably the predisposition, pathoplasty, and common cause models (Bornovalova et al. 2018; Durbin and Hicks 2014). According to the predisposition model, it proposes that BPD traits heighten the risk for the onset of a new disorder. The pathoplasty model suggests that BPD traits influence the course of disorders, and greater severity and/or chronicity of a disorder may be a contribution of higher BPD traits. Additionally, the common cause model suggests that there is a third variable, such as emotion regulation difficulties, which can provide an explanation for the comorbidity between BPD traits and other psychiatric disorders. Although these models are able to explain independently BPD-psychopathology correlations, it should be considered that they can elucidate these associations simultaneously (Bornovalova et al. 2018; Durbin and Hicks 2014).

M. Salavati, E. A. Selby, *Theories of Borderline Personality Disorder*,
https://doi.org/10.1007/978-3-031-75503-3_16

The Comorbidity of BPD and Bipolar I and II Disorders

Mood disorders are common and debilitating mental health issues with remarkable social costs (DeRubeis and Strunk 2017). These mood disorders encompass experiencing abnormal negative or positive moods, although the characteristics of these disorders are not restricted to aspects of mood (Strunk and Sasso 2017). Paris and Black (2015) described the differences between the concept of mood and the construct of personality. Mood is partially a straightforward concept with a variety of high, low, or unstable states, while the concept of personality is a complicated construct that encompasses traits that influence emotion, cognitions, and behavior, with a continuum of normal variations to abnormal states. In addition, depressed or manic mood can be recognized by clinicians, whereas personality is scaled by self-report systems and associated theoretical models, such as the five-factor model (Widiger and Costa 2012) and can be diagnosed via categorical classification, such as the DSM-5 (APA 2013, 2022). Further, mood disorders are treated with medications, whereas personality disorders are treated by psychotherapy (Paris and Black 2015).

Bipolar I disorder is characterized by a clinical course of recurring mood episodes including manic, depressive, and hypomanic, which is necessarily diagnosed by the occurrence of at least one manic episode (APA 2022). According to the DSM-5-TR (APA 2022), bipolar I disorder diagnostic criteria include a distinct period during which there is an abnormally, persistently elevated, expansive, or irritable mood accompanied by persistently heightened activity or energy lasting at least 1 week; inflated self-esteem or grandiosity, diminished levels of need for sleep; talkativeness; flight of ideas and sense of thought racing; distractibility; elevated goal-directed activities; engaging in high risk behaviors; and substantial impairment in social/occupational functioning. On the other hand, the mentioned features are the diagnostic criteria of bipolar II disorder, but the episode is not severe enough to cause significant disturbances in social and occupational functioning or to necessitate hospitalization (APA 2022).

Bipolar disorder and BPD are presented as the most frequent psychiatric disorders (Sanches 2019). In line with studies, it has been indicated that BD encompasses elements of depressive disorder (including dysphoric mood, anhedonia, psychomotor disorder), elements of mania (comprising a remarkable unusual increase in energy in various forms, disturbed judgement with disinhibition, and an unusual elevated or irritable mood), and subjective experiences related to elements consisting of emotional emptiness, irrational guilt, suicidal ideation, grandiose thoughts, elevated or depressed mood, and heightened creativity or disturbed cognitive functioning (Hosokawa et al. 2009; Parker and Fletcher 2009). Based on evidence, a markedly high prevalence of BPD has been found in bipolar disorders (e.g., Palmer et al. 2021; Zimmerman and Morgan 2013). Numerous reviews of literature have demonstrated that 20% of patients with BD have comorbid BPD, and almost 20% of individuals with BPD have BD (Fornaro et al. 2016; Frias et al. 2016). There is a substantial co-occurrence of personality disorders and bipolar disorders, and a high prevalence of various types of personality disorders among patients with BD has been reported, ranging from 30% to 40% (Schiavone et al. 2004; Garno et al. 2005; Antoniadis et al. 2012). The prevalence of BD and BPD has been reported as 21.6% and 18.5%, respectively (Fornaro et al. 2016). According to numerous findings, a remarkably high prevalence of bipolar disorder in individuals with BPD has been found in several studies (e.g., McGlashan et al. 2000; Fornaro et al. 2016; Patel et al. 2019; Tickle 2022; McDermid et al. 2015). One study reported that the prevalence of bipolar disorder was 14.1% in individuals with BPD. The results showed an approximately 15% prevalence of BD-BPD comorbidity (Zimmerman and Morgan 2013). The association between BPD and BD has been a subject of debate for several past decades (Stone 1981; Siever and Gunderson 1979; Boyce and Wood 2011). Although some findings have shown a greater prevalence of BPD in Bipolar II disorder (BIID) compared to BD-I, merely two studies, which compared the prevalence of BPD in these two, have shown no significant difference (Vieta et al. 2000; Zimmerman and Mattia 1999a, b). Based on a national cross-sectional study including 679 outpatients with personality disorders, Sjåstad et al. (2012) identified whether the prevalence of affective disorders is greater among individuals with BPD in comparison to other personality disorders. The findings indicated that individuals with BPD notably suffered from unipolar rather than bipolar disorders. Lower levels of depression and dysthymia were exhibited in BPD compared to other personality disorders. Odds ratios demonstrated a 34% lower risk for unipolar depression, 70% lower risk for dysthymia, and 66% greater risk for bipolar disorder in individuals with BPD in comparison to other personality disorders (Sjåstad et al. 2012).

Both bipolar disorder and BPD are proposed as remarkably severe psychiatric disorders, which have a substantial influence on daily functioning and quality of life, and are manifested by a chronic and recurrent illness course (Riemann et al. 2017). A substantial growing body of studies that directly compared patients with BPD and BD has indicated that individuals with both disorders vary in clinical features (Mneimne et al. 2018; Richard-Lepouriel et al. 2019), frequency of suicide attempts (Bayes et al. 2019, 2022; Perroud et al. 2016), neurobiological substrates (Bøen et al. 2019; Rossi et al. 2013), maladaptive schemas (Nilsson et al. 2010), temperament (Eich et al. 2014), history of child abuse, and neglect (Bayes et al. 2019, 2022; Mazer et al. 2019; Richard-Lepouriel et al. 2019). Through a review literature on the clinical influence of one disorder on the other, Frias et al. (2016) proposed that among patients with BD+BPD, they reported more mood episodes, an earlier age of onset of BD, higher suicidality, a higher level of hostility, and a greater prevalence of substance use (Frias et al. 2016). Zimmerman et al. (2021) assumed that patients with BPD/BD would present considerably higher rates of psychosocial morbidity compared to patients with only BPD or BD. They compared psychiatric outpatients with BPD and BD to patients with BPD without BD and patients with BPD/BD. The findings indicated that compared to patients with BD, the patients with BD and BPD revealed more comorbid disorders, psychopathology in their first-degree relatives, childhood trauma, suicidality, hospitalizations, time unemployed, and a likelihood of receiving disability payments. BPD+BD was related to more posttraumatic stress disorder in the patients as well as their family, greater rates of BD and substance use disorders in their relatives, a higher rate of childhood trauma, unemployment, disability, suicidality, suicide attempts, and hospitalizations (Zimmerman et al. 2021). According to a systematic review of cross-diagnostic studies, it was demonstrated that depressive symptoms have an earlier onset in BPD compared to BD, patients with BD manifested more mixed or manic symptoms. Additionally, it was found that individuals with BPD indicated more negative attitudes toward others and themselves, higher rates of difficulties in interpersonal relationships, and more maladaptive regulation strategies in affective instability with separate pathways. It was suggested that impulsivity is a trait in BPD instead of a state in BD. Moreover, BPD and BD showed a high overlap in depressive and anxious symptoms, dysphoria, different abnormal temperamental traits, suicidal ideation, and childhood trauma. Among both BPD and BD, shared deficits in neuropsychological and neuroimaging findings were reported (Masso Rodriguez et al. 2021).

BPD and BD comprise overlapped phenomenology which frequently contributes to diagnostic confusion (Palmer et al. 2021; Paris 2004; Baryshnikov et al. 2015; Durdurak et al. 2022). Both BPD (Berk et al. 2007) and BD (Leboyer and Kupfer 2010; MacNeil and Walhout 2011; Berk et al. 2007) are frequently over-diagnosed or misdiagnosed (Ghaemi and Sabokrouh 2015; Akiskal et al. 2005; Paris 2007; Ruggero et al. 2010), contributing to potentially adverse risks of physical and psychological consequences, as well as inappropriate medication and psychotherapeutic interventions and health status issues (Bassett 2012; Leboyer and Kupfer 2010; MacNeil and Walhout 2011; Berk et al. 2007). Ruggero et al. (2010) identified the extent to which certain characteristics of BPD may contribute to an increased risk of being misdiagnosed with BD. The results indicated that individuals with BPD faced remarkably greater odds of having been misdiagnosed, with nearly 40% of them reporting a previous misdiagnosis in comparison to merely 10% of patients with other disorders (Ruggero et al. 2010). Several investigations have been done to explore whether BPD and BD are two distinct disorders or if they are similar disorders across a continuum, contributing to suggesting a "bipolar-borderline continuum" (Renaud et al. 2012; Sanches 2019). For instance, Paris (2007) comprehensively examined the hypothesis to identify BPD as a bipolar spectrum disorder and argued that, based on their conclusion, BPD remains distinct from BD cross-sectionally and over time (Paris 2007). Albeit, BPD and BD have shared clinical features, and also, frequent co-occurance, their inter-relationship is controversial. Especifically, one of the most common diagnostic dilemma occurs in the differentiation of BPD from BD I & II, and a number of researchers have debated whether these disorders are independent or interdependent conditions. (Bayes et al. 2019, 2022; Riemann et al. 2017). Also, distinguishing BPD from BD is challenging and difficult (Bayes et al. 2016; Ghaemi and Barroilhet 2014; Sanches 2019). A remarkable body of investigations has demonstrated numerous indicative variables distinguishing BPD and BP, encompassing age of onset (Kernberg and Yeomans 2013), depressive (Kernberg and Yeomans 2013; Renaud et al. 2012) and elevated mood states (Ruggero et al. 2010; Renaud et al. 2012; Parker 2011), family history (Bassett 2012; Distel et al. 2008), illness course (Paris and Zweig-Frank 2001), self-identity

(Bassett 2012; Renaud et al. 2012), relationships quality (Gunderson et al. 2011), and mood state contextual nuances (Renaud et al. 2012; Parker 2011). To recognize characteristics distinguishing BD from BPD and to clarify variables to differentiate these two disorders, Bayes et al. (2016) found that predictors of BPD status differed according to diagnostic decisions, yet with the most consistent items being childhood sexual abuse, childhood depersonalization, personality variables associated with relationships issues and sensitivity to criticism, and the absence of any BP family history (Bayes et al. 2016). Barroilhet et al. (2013) proposed that the overlap of BPD and BD symptomatology is significantly fake, and they argued that the "core" characteristics of mood instability and impulsivity are not central to both disorders. In line with their argument, BP is presented as a disorder of psychomotor activation, while BPD criteria of abandonment, identity diffusion, recurrent suicidal or self-inflicted injurious behaviors, and dissociative symptoms differentiate BPD from BD (Barroilhet et al. 2013). To identify whether BPD and BIID can be distinguished from each other and from MDD, Wilson et al. (2012) compared depression severity, impulsiveness, and hostility in mood disorder among four groups: MDD with BPD, MDD with no personality disorders, BIID with BPD, and BIID with no personality disorders. The results indicated that individuals with BPD exhibited greater levels of impulsiveness and hostility, independent of other personality disorders. BIID patients demonstrated higher attentional impulsiveness compared to MDD patients, independent of BPD status, while individuals with BPD showed more non-planning impulsiveness compared to patients without BPD. No differences in depression severity were found; however, individuals with BPD reported more severe depression. The BPD group showed a higher score in cognitive factor and anxiety factor (Wilson et al. 2012). A great body of literature has emphasized the significant similarities and comorbidity of BPD and BD (Bassett 2012). Baryshnikov et al. (2015) studied the correlations of BD and BPD self-reported questionnaires to explore overlapping and non-overlapping symptoms of both of these disorders. Based on their findings, it was shown that affective instability, impulsivity, irritability, flight of thoughts, and distractibility appear to overlap (Baryshnikov et al. 2015). According to a latent class analysis of BPD and BD symptoms in 34,653 individuals with BPD, mania and depression, two separate syndromes (BPD and BD) were found (de la Rosa et al. 2017). In another investigation, the association between borderline personality features (BPF) and prospective illness course in 375 BD patients (including BID, BIID, BD Unspecified Bipolar and related disorders) was studied, and, also, the influence of current mood state on self-reported BPF profiles was recognized. The findings indicated that more BPF at baseline was related to greater episode frequency during subsequent follow-up. Additionally, affective instability, impulsivity, and self-mutilation/suicidality revealed an association with full-duration and brief episode frequency (Riemann et al. 2017). Clinical differentiation of bipolar disorder from BPD has been debated as a dilemmatic diagnostic subject (Paris 2007, 2018; Coulston et al. 2012; Bassett 2012) and can be challenging (Paris 2004; Paris and Zweig-Frank 2001). Shared specific symptom domains, including impulsivity, mood fluctuation, and emotional instability have been reported in both bipolar disorder and BPD. This symptomatological and phenomenological overlap contributes to a longstanding and unresolved debate about whether these two disorders can be considered as a continuum or should be viewed as separate diagnoses (Kernberg and Yeomans 2013; Zimmerman and Morgan 2013; Akiskal et al. 2005). Both BPD and BD can manifest with changed mood states, deliberated self-injurious behaviors and suicidality, impulsivity, sexually disinhibited behaviors, excessive spending, and alcohol and substance misuse (Ghaemi and Barroilhet 2014). Additionally, other researchers have highlighted the importance of the nature of emotion and affect, based on their different time course and quality in BPD compared to BD. For instance, studies indicated a slower time course of affective alteration in BD, whereas BPD affect is characterized by rapidly chaotic changes over time, whether in minutes, hours, or days (Renaud et al. 2012), switching between euthymia and anger (Bassett 2012), and is most of the time triggered by environmental and interpersonal factors (Renaud et al. 2012). It is suggested that a family history of MDD may contribute to the reinforcement of the diagnosis of BD (Souery et al. 2012; Zimmerman and Galione 2010), and also, the life trajectories of disabling BD symptoms are more prolonged than those with BPD (Paris 2004, 2007). Yen et al. (2015) identified the longitudinal influence of BPD on the course and outcome of BD among 271 pediatric patients and parents. The results showed that the number of BPD symptoms was substantially associated with a poor clinical course of BD, above and beyond BD features. Emotional dysregulation was indicated as the strongest association with poor course at the factor level; the individual symptoms were significantly associated with poor course and dissociation/stress-related paranoid ideation, impulsivity, and affective instability (Yen et al. 2015).

According to a literature review, it was revealed that BPD and BD are partially different in the sense of self, disturbed interpersonal relationships, family history of bipolar disorders, the benefits of medications, the level of cognitive deficits, the form of emotional dysregulation and mood shifting, the incidence of suicidality and suicide attempts, the form of psychotic episodes, a history of childhood sexual abuse, the loss of brain substance, changes in cortical activity, glucocorticoid receptor sensitivity, and mitochondrial dysfunction. Moreover, they found similarities in non-specific characteristics of emotional dysregulation, the incidence of atypical depressive features, self-injurious behaviors, and transporter polymorphisms, possible genetic linkages, overall decreases in limbic modulation, diminishment in the size of hippocampi and amygdala, and the incidence of sleep disruption (Bassett 2012). Additionally, Bayes et al. (2016) investigated the clinical differentiation of BIID from BPD and found key distinguishing elements comprising family history, onset pattern, clinical course, phenomenological profile of depressive and elevated mood states, and symptoms of emotional dysregulation (Bayes et al. 2016). To measure BPD pathology in comparison with BDs, Smith et al. (2008) investigated the issues of differentiation between BPD and 87 young participants with MDD, BD, and bipolar spectrum disorder. The findings showed that both BD and MDD groups indicated remarkably greater median levels of borderline features compared to the MDD group (Smith et al. 2008).

In line with clinical and empirical findings, it has been indicated that comorbidity of BPD-BD results in a more severe course of bipolar disorder, comprising episode frequency, emotional instability, self-injurious behaviors, and suicidality (Riemann et al. 2017). While, in spite of substantial rates of co-occurrence, longitudinal studies have revealed that BD comorbidity has no influence on BPD course, general functioning, and response to treatment (Frias et al. 2016). According to a meta-review of systematic reviews among 249 prospective studies, it was proposed that a family history of psychopathology, affective instability, attention deficit hyperactivity disorder, anxiety disorders, depression, sleep disturbances, substance abuse, psychotic symptoms, suicidality, childhood adversity, and temperament were reported as predisposing symptoms across both BPD and BD (Durdurak et al. 2022).

Several key aspects of the relevant clinical manifestations have been proposed. One of the most remarkable shared constructs between BPD and BD includes *emotional instability* which are featured by mood changes, temporal instability, high intensity, and delayed recovery from dysphoria (Koenigsberg 2010; Paris 2007; Benazzi 2007; Henry et al. 2001). In line with a substantial body of studies, BPD has constructs that overlap with BD in affective instability and impulsivity (Renaud et al. 2012). Emotional instability in BD is often misdiagnosed with personality disorders, especially BPD (Mesbah and Abolmaali 2021). However, while emotional instability is a common characteristic between BPD and BD, the patterns of it are different in these two disorders (Henry et al. 2001). In line with evidence, affective instability in individuals with BPD has a unique phenotype and differs from classical hypomania (Koenigsberg 2010; Paris and Black 2015). For instance, the switch from euthymia to depression or elevated mood is related to BD, while the switch from anger to euthymia is associated with BPD (Reich et al. 2012; Vannucci et al. 2022). In line with cross-sectional assessment, periods of affective instability among individuals with BPD are similar to hypomania (Kernberg and Yeomans 2013), contributing to a false diagnosis of BDs (Ruggero et al. 2010), while inter-episode residual symptoms in patients with BD, such as chronic dysphoria, can compromise diagnosis (Paykel et al. 2006). Based on clinical observations, rapid cycling of mood states has been suggested as a common component of both borderline and bipolar conditions (Bassett 2012). The fluctuating mood symptoms reported in both BPD and BD have contributed to the development of the assumption of an "ultra-rapid cycling" subtype of BD, which has led to the BP spectrum (MacKinnon 2015). Ecological momentary assessments (EMAs) studies have indicated that individuals with BPD in remission display highly overall negative emotion (Gruber et al. 2013; Havermans et al. 2010), and also greater fluctuations in both negative and positive emotionality in comparison to healthy controls (Knowles and Tarrier 2009). Although, certain features of BPD, including micro-psychosis symptoms and interpersonal issues, have not been clearly elucidated as associated with mood fluctuations, contributing to challenging a BP condition (Paris and Black 2015). Affective instability is suggested as a core manifestation of BPD, which happens in the episodes of BD (Koenigsberg 2010), although the underlying mechanisms for affective instability in BIID are more autonomous and internally driven, compared with BPD which is reactive to interpersonal stressors (Renaud et al. 2012). Studies have shown that individuals with BPD reveal greater levels of emotional reactivity in comparison with healthy controls (Aas et al. 2016), as well as stronger feelings of anger and frustration during euthymic states in individuals with BPD (Dutra et al. 2014; Johnson and Carver 2016). The severity of affective instability in bipolar II disorder is not as severe as BPD, also, mood shifts are from euthymia to depression or elation in bipolar II disorder, while it is from euthymia to anxiety or anger in BPD (Reich et al. 2012; Benazzi 2007; Henry et al. 2001; Bayes et al. 2019, 2022). In an investigation comparing BIID with BPD, it was concluded that maladaptive emotional regulation strategies, such as catastrophizing and rumination, were more severe in BPD compared to the BD group (Bayes et al. 2016). Studies have shown that individuals with BPD displayed a greater number of maladaptive emotion regulation strategies in comparison with BD patients, including deficient non-acceptance of emotional responses, limited access to emotion regulation strategies, lack of clarity of emotional awareness, issues in controlling impulsive behavior and tendency to self-blame, catastrophizing, and blame others (Bayes et al. 2016; Fletcher et al. 2015, 2019).

Experiencing *depressed mood* reported in BPD patients are manifested by emptiness, shame, and pain, while depressive states are characterized by diminished self-esteem and self-criticism in BD (Bayes et al. 2016; Meares et al. 2011). The occurrence of mood episodes in BD is spontaneous, while symptoms of BPD are reactive and usually are triggered by interpersonal relationships stimulus such as abandonment, rejection, or frustration (Kernberg and Yeomans 2013; Renaud et al. 2012; Paris 2007). Depressive mood is manifested as melancholic symptoms in BIID (Parker et al. 2013) and agitation (Benazzi 2006), while BPD is featured by non-melancholic depressive episodes reactive to interpersonal events (Russell et al. 2007). In line with studies, most of the BPD symptoms are reactive to interpersonal events such as perceived rejection and abandonment (Kernberg and Yeomans 2013), yet patients with BIID experience more spontaneous mood episodes compared to BPD (Renaud et al. 2012). Further, atypical manifestations of depression, such as hypersomnia and hyperphagia, are reported to be common to both BIID and BPD (Benazzi 1999; Perugi et al. 2011). It was found that typical depressive symptoms such as reduced self-esteem and self-criticism were connected to BIID, while BPD depressive features are more represented by emptiness and painful incoherence (Meares et al. 2011). Palmer et al. (2021) examined the diagnostic accuracy of the Mood Disorder Questionnaire (MDQ) and McLean Screening Instrument for BPD (MSI) in 757 inpatients, as well as, determined whether that individual screening items can differentiate bipolar disorder from BPD. The results indicated that both screening instruments showed remarkable specificity rather than sensitivity. MDQ individual items (elevated mood, grandiosity, increased energy, pressured speech, diminished need for sleep, hyperactivity) were remarkable predictors of bipolar disorder diagnosis and non-predictors of BPD diagnosis. MSI sub-items, including self-injurious behaviors and suicidal attempts could predict BPD in the absence of bipolar disorder, and also, distrust and irritability predicted BPD (Palmer et al. 2021). *Feelings of anger and irritability* have been presented as prominent symptoms of BD occurring during hypomania, depressive, and mixed mood states (Mesbah and Abolmaali 2021). The feeling of anger encompasses various constructs, including trait and state anger (Deffenbacher 2003). Trait anger is presented by the construct inclined to experience anger linked to the slightest provocation, while state anger is characterized by a high level of anger, which is defined as the temporary psychological emotional feeling that occurs in a specific time and situation, and varies from mild irritation to intense rage. State anger causes severe expression of anger, comprising anger attacks and aggression (Williams et al. 2017). According to the literature, anger is suggested as a part of difficulties in emotion regulation, and also, it is assumed that patients who suffer from the disorders report experiences of intense and more frequently fluctuating negative and positive emotions (Mesbah and Abolmaali 2021). A great body of studies have shown cross-sectional associations between bipolarity and anger (e.g., Ballester et al. 2022; Perlis et al. 2004; Akiskal and Benazzi 2006). Through a prospective study that comprised a sample of 255 BD, 85 non-BPD psychopathology, and 84 healthy controls (HC), individuals with BPD showed higher levels of anger and feelings of aggression in comparison with HC and psychiatric group across a 4-year follow-up (Ballester et al. 2014). Through a cross-sectional analysis, Mesbah and Abolmaali (2021) explored whether patients who converted to BD indicated greater feelings of anger, irritability, and borderline and antisocial personality traits in comparison with individuals with a history of unipolar depression who did not convert. The findings revealed the bipolar conversion group reported significantly greater levels of trait anger and aggression reactivity, and higher prevalence of "anger trait," "antisocial traits," and "borderline traits" in comparison to current and remitted depressive patients, as well. Additionally, based on prospective analyses, it was found that aggression reactivity can anticipate incident hypomania (Mesbah and Abolmaali 2021).

Impulsivity is another common construct between BPD and BD (Palmer et al. 2021), and also, as ambiguous association has been posited between impulsivity and BD and BPD (Durdurak et al. 2022). Impulsivity is characterized as a tendency for engaging in rapidly unpleasant behaviors and acting on urges without considering the aversive consequences (Critchfield et al. 2004; Oquendo and Mann 2000). Impulsivity is suggested as common phenotype of bipolar disorders and BPD (Paris 2007); however, they have various manifestations and clinical representations (Bayes et al. 2016). BPD has been represented as a core diagnostic criterion of BPD, which is suggested as a maladaptive strategy for managing intensely negative emotions via distraction or mitigate the aversive negative emotions (Lawrence et al. 2010), whereas impulsivity has been represented as a core diagnostic criterion of BPD (Swann et al. 2002, 2020). One research has shown a trait impulsivity of 41% in BIID, especially with hypomanic as against depressive BIID mood states (Benazzi 2007), considered to be on a spectrum with inter-episode trait impulsivity (Fergus et al. 2003; Swann et al. 2008; Peluso et al. 2007; Lawrence et al. 2010). A marked body of studies has directly investigated the similarities and differences of BIID and BPD (e.g., Henry et al. 2001; Patten and Paris 2008; Wilson et al. 2012). Evidence has shown higher levels of impulsiveness in individuals with BPD compared to BIID (Henry et al. 2001; Wilson et al. 2007; Bøen et al. 2012), as well as remarkably higher rates of impulsivity in patients with both disorders: BPD+BIID (Palmer et al. 2021). Wilson et al. (2007) indicated that patients with BIID have a notable tendency toward the *attentional impulsiveness* related to cognitive impairments (encompassing disturbed concentration, distractibility, and racing thoughts), as opposed to *motor and non-planning impulsiveness,* which is featured by issues in planning actions and thinking about consequences observed in individuals with BPD (Wilson et al. 2012). It has been demonstrated that impulsivity is higher during hypomanic episode in patients with BIID, whereas in individuals with BPD, impulsivity is not necessarily associated with mood states and is more likely to be represented as non-planning impulsiveness (Bayes et al. 2019, 2022). *Deliberate self-harm* happens in both BPD and BD, especially BIID during mixed states (Joyce et al. 2010), with a greater rate in BPD compared to BD (83% vs 49%) (Bayes et al. 2016; Bassett 2012). Self-injurious behaviors have been reported in mixed states of bipolar disorders and BPD (Joyce et al. 2010). Among 100 young individuals with early-onsetof BD, it has been pointed out that early onset of BD was related to the greatest risk of self-harm and suicide attempts (Moor et al. 2012). In order to differentiate NSSI in BPD and BD, the presence of other diagnostic criteria, including emotion dysregulation and cyclicity of symptoms and signs should be assessed. Further, evaluating the time course of the cyclicity can be useful: the presence of discrete, prolonged periods of emotional symptomatology (Bassett 2012). Studies have proposed that cluster B personality disorders are significantly associated with suicide attempts in patients with BID (e.g., Bezerra et al. 2017). Suicidality has been proposed to be a common core feature in both BPD and BIID (Rihmer and Döme 2016; Rihmer and Benazzi 2010; Zanarini et al. 2014), albeit the rates of suicidal attempts are substantially higher in BPD compared to BIID (60% vs 30%) (Bayes et al. 2016).

According to empirical and clinical literature, significant differences in *thinking styles* have been recognized in patients with BPD and BD, with implications for their emotional health and relationship quality (Bassett et al. 2012), such as substantial deficiencies in mindfulness (attention, awareness, and acceptance of the moment), interpersonal effectiveness, emotion regulation issues, and impulsivity in individuals with BPD (Wupperman et al. 2009). Based on findings, patients with BD display a greater level of maladaptive schemas and affective temperaments compared to controls, while a higher level of cyclothymic temperament and diminished self-control have been exhibited in individuals with BPD (Nilsson et al. 2010). *Psychotic symptoms* can occur in both BPD and BD with various patterns. Based on clinical observations, psychotic episodes show longer duration yet rarely last beyond several months. Transient experiences of dissociation and paranoid symptoms that are reactive to stressors have been reported in individuals with BPD (Adams and Sanders 2011; Barnow et al. 2010; Glaser et al. 2010; Goodwin 2007). Among individuals with BPD, transient psychotic features are more common especially under stressful conditions, whereas, psychotic features have not been identified in BIID (Bayes et al. 2019, 2022).

According to a body of literature, history of childhood abuse has been proposed as etiological factors of BD (Aas et al. 2016) and BPD (Cattane et al. 2017). Both BPD and BD have been shown to have strong association with remarkable incidence of *childhood trauma* (Bayes et al. 2016; Perroud et al. 2016; Saunders et al.

2015; Mazer et al. 2019; Bøen et al. 2015), and it has been reported to be 50% in BD and 60–80% in BPD (Álvarez-Tomás et al. 2019; Conus 2010; Fowke et al. 2012); however, there are notable differences in the form of childhood trauma or vulnerability to such trauma between these two disorders (Bassett 2012). Several studies have indicated the role of early life trauma in the etiology of both BPD and BD (Watson et al. 2006; Holmes 2003). A history of childhood maltreatment, including physical, emotional, and sexual abuse has been reported in both BIID and BPD patients. However, lower likelihood of childhood traumatic experiences has been reported among patients with BIID, whereas a greater likelihood of traumatic history with a female predominance in clinical settings has been found in individuals with BPD (Bayes et al. 2019, 2022). Mazer et al. (2019) proposed that emotional abuse, emotional neglect, and physical neglect in BPD can differentiate BPD from BD (Mazer et al. 2019). Fletcher et al. (2014) indicated that maladaptive strategies and maladaptive emotion regulation were associated with parental style in BPD and BIID, especially among individuals with BPD. It has been proposed that dysfunctional maternal relationships describe BPD, while dysfunctional paternal relationships contribute to emotional regulation issues in BPD and BD. Moreover, maternal abuse is related to intensified self-blame, whereas maternal over-control was linked to an increased tendency to catastrophize and blame others in BPD. Paternal abuse was associated with a diminished use of acceptance strategies in BPD, and parental over-control was negatively correlated with the use of positive refocusing and decreased levels of impulsive control behavior in BIID. Further, paternal relationships are identified by indifference in both BPD and BD, although a higher tendency for blaming others was found in BPD, and a greater tendency to rumination was reported in BIID (Fletcher et al. 2015, 2019).

The Comorbidity of BPD and Depressive Disorder

According to the DSM-5-TR, major depressive disorder (MDD) is recognized by the presence of at least one major episode occurring in the absence of a history of manic or hypomanic episodes. The core features of MDD include depressed mood, notably reduced interest or pleasure, weight loss or weight gain, insomnia or hypersomnia, psychomotor retardation or agitation, diminished ability to think or concentrate, or indecisiveness, recurrent thoughts of death, recurrent suicidal ideation, and suicidal attempts, which should be presented during the same 2-week period which a marked decrease in functioning (APA 2022). The world's population experiencing an episode of MDD has been estimated at 4.4–5.0% in any given 12-month period (WHO 2018; Ferrari et al. 2013), despite remarkable variation by country and region (Kessler et al. 2022). MDD and BPD are frequently co-occurring (Beatson and Rao 2012). According to other studies and clinical investigations, the lifetime prevalence of MDD in the course of BPD has been reported at 83% in one large study (Zanarini et al. 2000). The association between MDD and BPD is a subject of numerous debates and is the focus of numerous biological, phenomenological, and longitudinal investigations. The most prominent question is whether BPD is a distinct disorder from MDD, and also, why there is a great comorbidity between BPD and MDD (Goodman et al. 2015).

In MDD, severe levels of negative emotion are presented as a main diagnostic symptom. Depressed individuals specifically experience intense levels of inert negative emotion with large and slow switches in affect (Nelson et al. 2020). Although individuals with BPD experience unstable emotional states with rapid sudden alterations in affect (Ebner-Priemer et al. 2007). In line with a comprehensive meta-analysis, it was shown that depressed individuals retrospectively employed maladaptive regulation strategies (including rumination and suppression) remarkably most of the time and adaptive strategies (comprising cognitive reappraisal and acceptance) less often compared to healthy group (Visted et al. 2018). Meanwhile, based on findings, individuals with BPD retrospectively use expressive suppression and rumination more frequently and cognitive reappraisal and acceptance less often in comparison to healthy controls (Daros and Williams 2019). Zetsche et al. (2024) studied different emotion regulation strategies and their influence on subsequent emotions in the daily life of MDD and BPD patients and healthy controls. Based on findings, both MDD and BPS groups utilized rumination and suppression more frequently and acceptance less often compared to healthy control. Depressed participants reported higher rumination more often compared to individuals with BPD. Expressive suppression and rumination indicated negative impacts on subsequent emotions in participants in all groups. Substantially, both MDD and BPD groups were capable of benefitting from adaptive strategies (Zetsche et al. 2024). It has been demonstrated that BPD influences the severity and prognosis of an MDD diagnosis (Yoshimatsu and Palmer 2014), BPD may contribute to more severe and chronic course of MDD, and individuals with both disorders display a greater suicide risk (Sarhan et al. 2022; Söderholm et al. 2020). Through a cohort study, Söderholm et al. (2024) examined whether there are differences in suicide attempts and suicidal ideation among patients with MDD, BPD, and MDD+BPD, and also whether BPD and depression severity contribute to increased risks for suicide attempts and suicidal ideation and self-harm. The obtained findings indicated that the risk of suicide attempts among individuals with BPD was greater than for non-BPD individuals. Additionally, BPD severity was associated with a risk of suicide attempts and clinically significant suicide ideation. During follow-up, mean depression severity and alterations in depression symptoms showed an association with suicide ideation risk regardless of diagnosis (Söderholm et al. 2024). Chen et al. (2023) explored the association between BP features, emotional regulation, and NSSI in 1192 depressed adolescents. The obtained results showed that the majority of depressed adolescents had indicated NSSI in the past year, and a negative correlation between NSSI and BP features were exhibited, yet a positive correlation between NSSI and emotion regulation capacity was found, which was positively associated with the expression suppression dimension. Moreover, the occurrence of NSSI was positively related to BP features generally. Also, based on findings, emotional regulation was indicated as having a mediating role between BP traits and NSSI among adolescents with depression (Chen et al. 2023).

The Comorbidity of BPD and Anxiety Disorders

In line with a growing body of literature, anxiety disorders are greatly prevalent in individuals with BPD, with comorbidity rates of up to 90% (Harned and Valenstein 2013; Zanarini et al. 1998a, b; Zimmerman and Mattia 1999a, b). BPD is associated with remarkable rates of comorbidity with other psychiatric disorders, such as mood disorders, anxiety disorders, and psychotic disorders with a 4.2–4.8% lifetime prevalence (Zimmerman and Mattia 1999a, b; Harned et al. 2011, 2018, 2022). It was estimated that with approximately 75–90% of individuals with BPD exhibit at least one lifetime anxiety disorder (Linehan et al. 2006; Grant et al. 2008), it was shown that anxiety disorders significantly contribute to a negative prognostic in BPD (Zanarini et al. 2004). Studies have identified heightened clinical severity and diminished psychosocial functioning in patients with anxiety disorder co-occurring with personality disorders (Skodol et al. 1995; Ozkan and Altindag 2005). In BPD inpatients, it has been reported that 88% meet criteria for a lifetime anxiety disorder, comprising PTSD (56%), panic disorder (48%), social anxiety disorder (46%), specific phobia (32%), OCD (16%), generalized anxiety disorder (14%), and agoraphobia (12%) (Harned and Valenstein 2013; Zanarini et al. 1998a, b; Zimmerman and Mattia 1999a, b; McGlashan et al. 2000; Grant et al. 2008). In a 6-year follow-up of 284 Norwegian outpatients, it was indicated that BPD anticipated any anxiety disorder at follow-up (Alnaes and Torgersen 1990). Further, the findings have proposed that the presence of a personality disorder leads to the impairments of anxiety disorder outcome (Ansell et al. 2015). According to evidence-based treatment for BPD and anxiety disorders studies, it has been demonstrated that brief anxiety disorder treatments can be implemented effectively among individuals with BPD at a mild level of disorder (Feeney 2002; Clarke and Currie 2009). However, among individuals with BPD at a moderate level of disorder, intensive and longer therapeutic interventions are needed (Steil et al. 2011; Bohus and Kröger 2011; Bohus et al. 2021; Cloitre et al. 2014). Additionally, in individuals with severe levels of disorder (e.g., serious suicidal and non-suicidal behaviors), an integrated treatment for BPD and anxiety disorders has been suggested (Harned et al. 2012).

The Comorbidity of BPD and OCD

Obsessive-compulsive disorder (OCD) is a commonly occurring psychiatric disorder, and as a remarkably disabling condition that contributes to key decreases in quality of life (Tolin and Springer 2018). Based on the DSM-5-TR, OCD is recognized by the "presence of obsessions, and compulsion, or both. Obsessions are defined by recurrent and persistent thoughts, urges, or images that are experienced as intrusive and unwanted, and that cause marked anxiety or distress" (APA 2022, p. 314). Individuals who suffer from obsessions attempt to ignore or suppress these thoughts and urges, or neutralize them by performing a compulsion. Moreover, based on the DSM-5-TR, compulsion is defined by "repetitive behaviors or mental acts that the individual feels driven to perform in response to an obsession or according to rules that must be applied rigidly" (APA 2022, p. 314). The purpose of these behaviors or mental acts, which are not connected to reality, is preventing or diminishing anxiety or distress, and preventing unwanted and dread events or situations (APA 2022).

OCD most often co-occurs with several psychiatric disorders (Hofmeijer-Sevink et al. 2013; Subramaniam et al. 2012; Dams et al. 2020; Sharma et al. 2021). The comorbidity between personality disorders and OCD is reported commonly (Pinto and Cowan 2023; Thamby and Khanna 2019). The prevalence of BPD among OCD patients has been estimated at approximately 5% (Denys et al. 2004). In cross-sectional research, Melca et al. (2015) investigated the prevalence and correlates of BPD, OCPD, and schizotypal PD among 110 OCD patients. The results demonstrated that OCD patients with BPD exhibited greater comorbidity of mood, anxiety, and eating disorders; compulsions comprising interpersonal domains; a more remarkable association with impulsive-compulsive disorders such as skin picking disorders; a higher rate of mental compulsions; and motor impulsivity. To summarize, based on empirical findings, OCD patients with a personality disorder tend to be more severe; to display higher comorbidity rates; and to exhibit elevated severity of maladaptive impulsive and/or compulsive traits (Melca et al. 2015). Based on the findings of three case reports comprising of patients with BPD and OCD, Hayashi (1996) proposed that identifiable characteristics of OCD symptoms that overlap with BPD encompass pervasiveness, poor insight, and resistance, and obsessive control evident in personal relationships. It was concluded that comorbidity is not a simple association, and the symptomatology of the comorbid patients originates from OCD pathology connected to the personality disorders rather than from independent BPD pathology (Hayashi 1996).

The Comorbidity of BPD and Substance Use and Alcohol Use Disorders

Substance use disorders (SUDSs) encompass patterns of recurrent substance use contributing to considerable issues and difficulties, including *disturbed control* (taking more substance than intended, attempting unsuccessfully to stop using, spending a remarkable amount of time obtaining and using the substance, and craving, or strong desire for substance use), *social impairment* (failing to fulfill responsibilities and obligations at school, work, or home, continuing substance use in spite of numerous problems, giving up other activities because of substance use), and *risky use* (using substances in dangerous situations such as driving, continuing substance use in spite of serious physical or psychological consequences), *exhibiting symptoms of tolerance or withdrawal* (US Department of Health and Human Services 2014). Several investigations have demonstrated the comorbidity between personality disorders and SUDs (Penzenstadler et al. 2019; Korsgaard et al. 2016), especially among individuals with BPD (13%) (Langås et al. 2012), which ranges from 10% to 14.8% in the normal population and from 34.8% to 73.0% among individuals treated for SUDs (Parmar and Kaloiya 2018). Korsgaard et al. (2016) investigated the association between personality disorders and SUDs among 153 adolescents referred to a mental health outpatient center. The findings indicate a greatly significant association between the number of personality symptoms and having one or more SUDs (Korsgaard et al. 2016, 2022). According to a systematic review, approximately 38–57% of individuals with BPD also have an SUD diagnosis (Trull et al. 2005, 2008, 2010), and 5–32% of individuals with SUDs have met the criteria of BPD (Brooner et al. 2002). Individuals with BPD often use dependence-producing substances to mitigate intensely negative emotions, or to replace negative emotions with a pleasant state and feel intoxicated. Further, using addictive substances may be triggered by socio-environmental factors such as peer pressure (McMain et al. 2009, 2012; Kienast et al. 2014).

According to the literature, increased prevalence rates of BPD and SUDs comorbidity have been found, for instance, a rate of nearly 57% in alcohol-related disorders (Kienast et al. 2014). The comorbidity between BPD and substance-related disorders has been reported to be approximately 78% (Tomko et al. 2015). In a sample of 147 patients, Barth (2015) found the most common comorbidities in BPD with SUDs: tobacco dependence (54%), alcohol dependence (47%), and drug dependence (22%). One study indicated that the prevalence of BPD in people seeking bupropion treatment for opioid addiction was over 40% (Sansone and Sansone 2013), and almost 50% of individuals with BPD reported a history of prescription drug abuse (Sansone and Sansone 2009). Based on a large survey study, it was found that 50.7% of individuals with BPD also met a diagnosis of an SUD over the previous 12 months. In addition, it was shown that among individuals with a lifetime diagnosis of SUDs, 9.5% reported to also having a lifetime diagnosis of BPD (Grant et al. 2008). A longitudinal study revealed that 62% of individuals with BPD met the criteria for SUDs at the beginning stage of study, and beyond 90% of patients with BPD comorbid with SUDs experienced remission of the SUDs by the time of the study's 10-year follow-up. The author found that the rate of recurrence was 40% for alcohol and 35% for drugs. The rate of new onset of SUDs was reported as 21% for drugs and 23% for alcohol (Zanarini et al. 2011). Individuals with BPD reported greater rates of new SUDs onsets even when their BPD symptoms had recovered (Walter et al. 2023).

Across several empirical studies, it has been demonstrated that the levels of impulsivity, suicidality, and self-injurious behaviors related to BPD can be intensified by the use of alcohol or drugs (Bosch et al. 2001; Van Den Bosch et al. 2003). Moreover, the presence of BPD symptoms may lead to the severity of SUDs symptomatology (Morgenstern et al. 1997), and the course of SUDs treatment can be more complicated because of BPD pathology (Center for Substance Abuse Treatment 2005). The behaviors of patients with the comorbidity of BPD and SUDs are characterized by higher levels of impulsivity compared with patients with only one of the two disorders. Based on clinical manifestations, a tendency toward short-term rewards and diminished capability to work towards mid-term and long-term rewards has been revealed (Wilson et al. 2006; Coffey et al. 2011). According to contemporary theories, emotion regulation and impulsivity are two prominent features in both BPD and SUDs (Littlefield et al. 2021; Conrod and Nikolaou 2016; Crowell et al. 2009; Gunderson et al. 2018). Moreover, it has been suggested that the co-occurrence of BPD and SUDs may reflect shared etiological processes of disturbed impulse control and emotion regulation difficulties (Littlefield et al. 2021). Some investigations suggested a shared genetic impact and genetic correlations for BPD and SUDs (e.g., Bornovalova et al. 2013), such as between BP traits and nicotine and cannabis use (Distel et al. 2012), between BP traits and alcohol, nicotine, and alcohol dependence (Few et al. 2016), between BPD symptoms and alcohol and cannabis use and alcohol and cannabis use disorders (Long et al. 2020; Gillespie et al. 2021). Few et al. (2016) indicated that the genetic correlation between BPD and SUDs can be associated with common personality traits like neuroticism and affective instability (Few et al. 2016).

To sum up, BPD has been indicated to have high frequent comorbidity with other psychiatric disorders and other personality disorders, which contribute to more therapeutically complicated conditions leading to a poor prognosis. As mentioned, bipolar disorder and BPD have the most frequent co-occurrence with each other, encompassing depressive disorder, mania, components of emotional emptiness, irrational guilt, suicidal ideation, grandiose thoughts, elevated or depressed mood, and heightened creativity or disturbed cognitive functioning. Furthermore, two significant shared constructs have been found between BD and BPD, including emotion dysregulation and impulsivity. In addition, highly substantial comorbidity has been reported in MDD or anxiety disorders and BPD, and overlapped symptomatology that contributes to complicated conditions for therapeutic clinical interventions. Moreover, a remarkable co-occurrence has been found among OCD and BPD, contributing to more severe conditions in OCD patients, including poor insight and resistance, and obsessive control evident in personal relationships. Additionally, since individuals with BPD often use dependence-producing substances to avoid experiencing intense emotions, or to substitute negative emotions with a pleasant emotion, highly frequent comorbidities have been found in BPD and SUDs and alcohol-related disorders.

References

Aas M, Henry C, Andreassen OA, Bellivier F, Melle I, Etain B. The role of childhood trauma in bipolar disorders. Int J Bipolar Disord. 2016;4:1.

Adams B, Sanders T. Experiences of psychosis in borderline personality disorder: a qualitative analysis. J Ment Health. 2011;20(4):381–91.

Akiskal HS, Benazzi F. The DSM-IV and ICD-10 categories of recurrent [major] depressive and bipolar II disorders: evidence that they lie on a dimensional spectrum. J Affect Disord. 2006;92(1):45–54.

Akiskal KK, Savino M, Akiskal HS. Temperament profiles in physicians, lawyers, managers, industrialists, architects, journalists, and artists: a study in psychiatric outpatients. J Affect Disord. 2005;85(1–2):201–6.

Alnaes R, Torgersen S. MCMI personality disorders among patients with major depression with and without anxiety disorders. J Personal Disord. 1990;4(2):141–9.

Álvarez-Tomás I, Ruiz J, Guilera G, Bados A. Long-term clinical and functional course of borderline personality disorder: a meta-analysis of prospective studies. Eur Psychiatry. 2019;56(1):75–83.

American Psychiatric Association. Diagnostic and statistical manual of mental disorders. 5th ed. Text Revised (DSM-5-TR); 2022.

Ansell EB, Wright AG, Markowitz JC, Sanislow CA, Hopwood CJ, Zanarini MC, Yen S, Pinto A, McGlashan TH, Grilo CM. Personality disorder risk factors for suicide attempts over 10 years of follow-up. Personal Disord Theory Res Treat. 2015;6(2):161.

Antoniadis D, Samakouri M, Livaditis M. The association of bipolar spectrum disorders and borderline personality disorder. Psychiatry Q. 2012;83:449–65.

American Psychiatric Association DS. Diagnostic and statistical manual of mental disorders: DSM-5. Washington, DC: American Psychiatric Association; 2013.

Ballester J, Goldstein B, Goldstein TR, Yu H, Axelson D, Monk K, Hickey MB, Diler RS, Sakolsky DJ, Sparks G, Iyengar S. Prospective longitudinal course of aggression among adults with bipolar disorder. Bipolar Disord. 2014;16(3):262–9.

Ballester L, Alayo I, Vilagut G, Mortier P, Almenara J, Cebria AI, Echeburua E, Gabilondo A, Gili M, Lagares C, Piqueras JA. Predictive models for first-onset and persistence of depression and anxiety among university students. J Affect Disord. 2022;308:432–41.

Barnow S, Arens EA, Sieswerda S, Dinu-Biringer R, Spitzer C, Lang S. Borderline personality disorder and psychosis: a review. Curr Psychiatry Rep. 2010;12:186–95.

Barroilhet S, Vöhringer PA, Ghaemi SN. Borderline versus bipolar: differences matter. Acta Psychiatr Scand. 2013;128(5):385.

Barth FD. Alexithymia, affect regulation, and binge drinking in college students. J Coll Stud Psychother. 2015;29(2):132–46.

Baryshnikov I, Aaltonen K, Koivisto M, Näätänen P, Karpov B, Melartin T, Heikkinen M, Ketokivi M, Joffe G, Isometsä E. Differences and overlap in self-reported symptoms of bipolar disorder and borderline personality disorder. Eur Psychiatry. 2015;30(8):914–9.

Bassett D. Borderline personality disorder and bipolar affective disorder. Spectra or spectre? A review. Aust N Z J Psychiatry. 2012;46(4):327–39.

Bassett DS, Nelson BG, Mueller BA, Camchong J, Lim KO. Altered resting state complexity in schizophrenia. NeuroImage. 2012;59(3):2196–207.

Bayes A, Parker G, McClure G. Emotional dysregulation in those with bipolar disorder, borderline personality disorder and their comorbid expression. J Affect Disord. 2016;204:103–11.

Bayes A, Parker G, Paris J. Differential diagnosis of bipolar II disorder and borderline personality disorder. Curr Psychiatry Rep. 2019;21:1–1.

Bayes A, Spoelma M, Parker G. Comorbid bipolar disorder and borderline personality disorder: diagnosis using machine learning. J Psychiatr Res. 2022;152:1–6.

Beatson JA, Rao S. Depression and borderline personality disorder. Med J Aust. 2012;197(11):620–1.

Benazzi F. Impulsivity in bipolar-II disorder: trait, state, or both? Eur Psychiatry. 2007;22(7):472–8.

Benazzi F. Prevalence of bipolar II disorder in atypical depression. Eur Arch Psychiatry Clin Neurosci. 1999;249:62–5.

Benazzi F. Borderline personality–bipolar spectrum relationship. Prog Neuro-Psychopharmacol Biol Psychiatry. 2006;30(1):68–74.

Berk MS, Jeglic E, Brown GK, Henriques GR, Beck AT. Characteristics of recent suicide attempters with and without borderline personality disorder. Arch Suicide Res. 2007;11(1):91–104.

Bezerra S, Galvao-de-Almeida A, Studart P, Martins DF, Caribé AC, Schwingel PA, Miranda-Scippa Â. Suicide attempts in bipolar I patients: impact of comorbid personality disorders. Braz J Psychiatry. 2017;39:133–9.

Bøen E, Hummelen B, Elvsåshagen T, Boye B, Andersson S, Karterud S, Malt UF. Different impulsivity profiles in borderline personality disorder and bipolar II disorder. J Affect Disord. 2015;170:104–11.

Bøen E, Hjørnevik T, Hummelen B, Elvsåshagen T, Moberget T, Holtedahl JE, Babovic A, Hol PK, Karterud S, Malt UF. Patterns of altered regional brain glucose metabolism in borderline personality disorder and bipolar II disorder. Acta Psychiatr Scand. 2019;139(3):256–68.

Bøen H, Dalgard OS, Johansen R, Nord E. A randomized controlled trial of a senior Centre group programme for increasing social support and preventing depression in elderly people living at home in Norway. BMC Geriatr. 2012;12:1–1.

Bohus M, Kröger C. Psychopathology and psychotherapy of borderline personality disorder: state of the art. Nervenarzt. 2011;82:16–24.

Bohus M, Stoffers-Winterling J, Sharp C, Krause-Utz A, Schmahl C, Lieb K. Borderline personality disorder. Lancet. 2021;398(10310):1528–40.

Bornovalova MA, Hicks BM, Iacono WG, McGue M. Longitudinal twin study of borderline personality disorder traits and substance use in adolescence: developmental change, reciprocal effects, and genetic and environmental influences. Personal Disord Theory Res Treat. 2013;4(1):23.

Bornovalova MA, Verhulst B, Webber T, McGue M, Iacono WG, Hicks BM. Genetic and environmental influences on the codevelopment among borderline personality disorder traits, major depression symptoms, and substance use disorder symptoms from adolescence to young adulthood. Dev Psychopathol. 2018;30(1):49–65.

Bosch LM, Verheul R, Brink WV. Substance abuse in borderline personality disorder: clinical and etiological correlates. J Personal Disord. 2001;15(5):416–24.

Boyce CJ, Wood AM. Personality prior to disability determines adaptation: agreeable individuals recover lost life satisfaction faster and more completely. Psychol Sci. 2011;22(11):1397–402.

Brooner RK, Schmidt CW Jr, Herbst JH. Personality trait characteristics of opioid abusers with and without comorbid personality disorders. In: Personality disorders and the five-factor model of personality; 2002. https://doi.org/10.1037/10423-015.

Cattane N, Rossi R, Lanfredi M, Cattaneo A. Borderline personality disorder and childhood trauma: exploring the affected biological systems and mechanisms. BMC Psychiatry. 2017;17:1–4.

Center for Substance Abuse Treatment (US). Medication-assisted treatment for opioid addiction in opioid treatment programs. 2005.

Chen P, Feng Y, Li XH, Li JX, Wang YY, Zheng WY, Su Z, Cheung T, Ungvari GS, Ng CH, Sha S. Systematic reviews and meta-analyses on major depressive disorder: a bibliometric perspective. Front Psych. 2023;14:1136125.

Clarke DM, Currie KC. Depression, anxiety and their relationship with chronic diseases: a review of the epidemiology, risk and treatment evidence. Med J Aust. 2009;190:S54–60.

Cloitre M, Garvert DW, Weiss B, Carlson EB, Bryant RA. Distinguishing PTSD, complex PTSD, and borderline personality disorder: a latent class analysis. Eur J Psychotraumatol. 2014;5(1):25097.

Coffey SF, Schumacher JA, Baschnagel JS, Hawk LW, Holloman G. Impulsivity and risk-taking in borderline personality disorder with and without substance use disorders. Personal Disord Theory Res Treat. 2011;2(2):128.

Conrod JP, Nikolaou K. Annual research review: on the developmental neuropsychology of substance use disorders. J Child Psychol Psychiatry. 2016;57(3):371–94.

Conus P. Part 4. Diagnosing bipolar disorder. Focus issue. Cutting edge psychiatry in practice: the management of bipolar spectrum disorder: 168; 2010.

Coulston CM, Tanious M, Mulder RT, Porter RJ, Malhi GS. Bordering on bipolar: the overlap between borderline personality and bipolarity. Aust N Z J Psychiatry. 2012;46(6):506–21.

Critchfield KL, Levy KN, Clarkin JF. The relationship between impulsivity, aggression, and impulsive-aggression in borderline personality disorder: an empirical analysis of self-report measures. J Personal Disord. 2004;18(6):555–70.

Crowell SE, Beauchaine TP, Linehan MM. A biosocial developmental model of borderline personality: elaborating and extending Linehan's theory. Psychol Bull. 2009;135(3):495.

Dams GM, Calamari JE, Rector NA, Riemann BC. Identification of belief-based subtypes in obsessive-compulsive disorder using latent profile analysis. J Obsessive Compuls Relat Disord. 2020;26:100555.

Daros AR, Williams GE. A meta-analysis and systematic review of emotion-regulation strategies in borderline personality disorder. Harv Rev Psychiatry. 2019;27(4):217–32.

de la Rosa I, Oquendo MA, García G, Stanley B, González-Pinto A, Liu SM, Blanco C. Determining if borderline personality disorder and bipolar disorder are alternative expressions of the same disorder: results from the National Epidemiologic Survey on Alcohol and Related Conditions. J Clin Psychiatry. 2017;78(8):1939.

Deffenbacher JL. Anger disorders. Med Psychiatry. 2003;22:89–112.

Denys D, Zohar J, Westenberg HG. The role of dopamine in obsessive-compulsive disorder: preclinical and clinical evidence. J Clin Psychiatry. 2004;65(Suppl 14):11–7.

DeRubeis RJ, Strunk DR, editors. The Oxford handbook of mood disorders. Oxford University Press; 2017.

Distel MA, Trull TJ, Derom CA, Thiery EW, Grimmer MA, Martin NG, Willemsen G, Boomsma DI. Heritability of borderline personality disorder features is similar across three countries. Psychol Med. 2008;38(9):1219–29.

Distel MA, Trull TJ, de Moor MM, Vink JM, Geels LM, van Beek JH, Bartels M, Willemsen G, Thiery E, Derom CA, Neale MC. Borderline personality traits and substance use: genetic factors underlie the association with smoking and ever use of cannabis, but not with high alcohol consumption. J Personal Disord. 2012;26(6):867–79.

Durbin CE, Hicks BM. Personality and psychopathology: a stagnant field in need of development. Eur J Personal. 2014;28(4):362–86.

Durdurak BB, Altaweel N, Upthegrove R, Marwaha S. Understanding the development of bipolar disorder and borderline personality disorder in young people: a meta-review of systematic reviews. Psychol Med. 2022;52(16):3769–82.

Dutra SJ, West TV, Impett EA, Oveis C, Kogan A, Keltner D, Gruber J. Rose-colored glasses gone too far? Mania symptoms predict biased emotion experience and perception in couples. Motiv Emot. 2014;38:157–65.

Ebner-Priemer UW, Kuo J, Kleindienst N, Welch SS, Reisch T, Reinhard I, Lieb K, Linehan MM, Bohus M. State affective instability in borderline personality disorder assessed by ambulatory monitoring. Psychol Med. 2007;37(7):961–70.

Eich D, Gamma A, Malti T, Wehrli MV, Liebrenz M, Seifritz E, Modestin J. Temperamental differences between bipolar disorder, borderline personality disorder, and attention deficit/hyperactivity disorder: some implications for their diagnostic validity. J Affect Disord. 2014;169:101–4.

Feeney JA. Attachment-related dynamics: what can we learn from self-reports of avoidance and anxiety? Attach Hum Dev. 2002;4(2):193–200.

Fergus EL, Miller RB, Luckenbaugh DA, Leverich GS, Findling RL, Speer AM, Post RM. Is there progression from irritability/dyscontrol to major depressive and manic symptoms? A retrospective community survey of parents of bipolar children. J Affect Disord. 2003;77(1):71–8.

Ferrari AJ, Charlson FJ, Norman RE, Patten SB, Freedman G, Murray CJ, Vos T, Whiteford HA. Burden of depressive disorders by country, sex, age, and year: findings from the global burden of disease study 2010. PLoS Med. 2013;10(11):e1001547.

Few LR, Miller JD, Grant JD, Maples J, Trull TJ, Nelson EC, Oltmanns TF, Martin NG, Lynskey MT, Agrawal A. Trait-based assessment of borderline personality disorder using the NEO five-factor inventory: phenotypic and genetic support. Psychol Assess. 2016;28(1):39.

Fletcher K, Yang Y, Johnson SL, Berk M, Perich T, Cotton S, Jones S, Lapsley S, Michalak E, Murray G. Buffering against maladaptive perfectionism in bipolar disorder: the role of self-compassion. J Affect Disord. 2019;250:132–9.

Fletcher I, Taylor K, Lobban F. Exploring the links between the phenomenology of creativity and bipolar disorder. J Affect Disord. 2015;174:658–64.

Fletcher K, Parker G, Bayes A, Paterson A, McClure G. Emotion regulation strategies in bipolar II disorder and borderline personality disorder: differences and relationships with perceived parental style. J Affect Disord. 2014;157:52–9.
Fornaro M, Orsolini L, Marini S, De Berardis D, Perna G, Valchera A, Ganança L, Solmi M, Veronese N, Stubbs B. The prevalence and predictors of bipolar and borderline personality disorders comorbidity: systematic review and meta-analysis. J Affect Disord. 2016;195:105–18.
Fowke A, Ross S, Ashcroft K. Childhood maltreatment and internalized shame in adults with a diagnosis of bipolar disorder. Clin Psychol Psychother. 2012;19(5):450–7.
Frias A, Palma C, Farriols N, Gonzalez L, Horta A. Anxious adult attachment may mediate the relationship between childhood emotional abuse and borderline personality disorder. Personal Ment Health. 2016;10(4):274–84.
Garno JL, Goldberg JF, Ramirez PM, Ritzler BA. Bipolar disorder with comorbid cluster B personality disorder features: impact on suicidality. J Clin Psychiatry. 2005;66(3):339–45.
Ghaemi SN, Barroilhet S. Bipolar illness versus borderline personality: red skies versus red apples. In: Borderline personality and mood disorders: comorbidity and controversy. New York: Springer; 2014. p. 97–115.
Ghaemi F, Sabokrouh F. The relationship between personality traits and metacognitive listening strategies among Iranian EFL learners, ELT. Int J Engl Lang Teach. 2015;5(2)
Gillespie D, Hatchard J, Squires H, Gilmore A, Brennan A. Conceptualising changes to tobacco and alcohol policy as affecting a single interlinked system. BMC Public Health. 2021;21:1–2.
Glaser JP, Van Os J, Thewissen V, Myin-Germeys I. Psychotic reactivity in borderline personality disorder. Acta Psychiatr Scand. 2010;121(2):125–34.
Goodman JH, Prager J, Goldstein R, Freeman M. Perinatal dyadic psychotherapy for postpartum depression: a randomized controlled pilot trial. Arch Womens Ment Health. 2015;18:493–506.
Goodwin KA. Dissociative effects of true and false recall as a function of different encoding strategies. Memory. 2007;15(1):93–103.
Grant BF, Chou SP, Goldstein RB, Huang B, Stinson FS, Saha TD, Smith SM, Dawson DA, Pulay AJ, Pickering RP, Ruan WJ. Prevalence, correlates, disability, and comorbidity of DSM-IV borderline personality disorder: results from the wave 2 National Epidemiologic Survey on Alcohol and Related Conditions. J Clin Psychiatry. 2008;69(4):533.
Gruber J, Kogan A, Mennin D, Murray G. Real-world emotion? An experience-sampling approach to emotion experience and regulation in bipolar I disorder. J Abnorm Psychol. 2013;122(4):971.
Gunderson JG, Stout RL, McGlashan TH, Shea MT, Morey LC, Grilo CM, Zanarini MC, Yen S, Markowitz JC, Sanislow C, Ansell E. Ten-year course of borderline personality disorder: psychopathology and function from the collaborative longitudinal personality disorders study. Arch Gen Psychiatry. 2011;68(8):827–37.
Gunderson JG, Herpertz SC, Skodol AE, Torgersen S, Zanarini MC. Borderline personality disorder. Nat Rev Dis Primers. 2018;4(1):1–20.
Harned MS, Valenstein HR. Treatment of borderline personality disorder and co-occurring anxiety disorders. F1000Prime Rep. 2013;5:5.
Harned MS, Dimeff LA, Woodcock EA, Skutch JM. Overcoming barriers to disseminating exposure therapies for anxiety disorders: a pilot randomized controlled trial of training methods. J Anxiety Disord. 2011;25(2):155–63.
Harned MS, Korslund KE, Foa EB, Linehan MM. Treating PTSD in suicidal and self-injuring women with borderline personality disorder: development and preliminary evaluation of a dialectical behavior therapy prolonged exposure protocol. Behav Res Ther. 2012;50(6):381–6.
Harned MS, Wilks CR, Schmidt SC, Coyle TN. Improving functional outcomes in women with borderline personality disorder and PTSD by changing PTSD severity and post-traumatic cognitions. Behav Res Ther. 2018;103:53–61.
Harned MS, Garcia NM, Coyle TN. Exposure therapy when patients present with comorbid borderline personality disorder. In: Clinical guide to exposure therapy: beyond phobias. Cham: Springer International Publishing; 2022. p. 125–41.
Havermans R, Nicolson NA, Berkhof J, deVries MW. Mood reactivity to daily events in patients with remitted bipolar disorder. Psychiatry Res. 2010;179(1):47–52.

Hayashi N. The wish to be held: female patients with borderline personality disorder. Psychiatry Clin Neurosci. 1996;50(5):267–70.

Henry C, Mitropoulou V, New AS, Koenigsberg HW, Silverman J, Siever LJ. Affective instability and impulsivity in borderline personality and bipolar II disorders: similarities and differences. J Psychiatr Res. 2001;35(6):307–12.

Hofmeijer-Sevink MK, van Oppen P, van Megen HJ, Batelaan NM, Cath DC, van der Wee NJ, van den Hout MA, van Balkom AJ. Clinical relevance of comorbidity in obsessive compulsive disorder: The Netherlands OCD Association study. J Affect Disord. 2013;150(3):847–54.

Holmes J. Borderline personality disorder and the search for meaning: an attachment perspective. Aust N Z J Psychiatry. 2003;37(5):524–31.

Hosokawa T, Momose T, Kasai K. Brain glucose metabolism difference between bipolar and unipolar mood disorders in depressed and euthymic states. Prog Neuro-Psychopharmacol Biol Psychiatry. 2009;33(2):243–50.

Johnson SL, Carver CS. Emotion-relevant impulsivity predicts sustained anger and aggression after remission in bipolar I disorder. J Affect Disord. 2016;189:169–75.

Joyce PR, Light KJ, Rowe SL, Cloninger CR, Kennedy MA. Self-mutilation and suicide attempts: relationships to bipolar disorder, borderline personality disorder, temperament and character. Aust N Z J Psychiatry. 2010;44(3):250–7.

Kernberg OF, Yeomans FE. Borderline personality disorder, bipolar disorder, depression, attention deficit/hyperactivity disorder, and narcissistic personality disorder: practical differential diagnosis. Bull Menn Clin. 2013;77(1):1–22.

Kessler RC, Akiskal HS, Angst J, Guyer M, Hirschfeld RM, Merikangas KR, Stang PE. Validity of the assessment of bipolar spectrum disorders in the WHO CIDI 3.0. J Affect Disord. 2006;96(3):259–69.

Kessler RC, Ruhm CJ, Puac-Polanco V, Hwang IH, Lee S, Petukhova MV, Sampson NA, Ziobrowski HN, Zaslavsky AM, Zubizarreta JR. Estimated prevalence of and factors associated with clinically significant anxiety and depression among US adults during the first year of the COVID-19 pandemic. JAMA Netw Open. 2022;5(6):e2217223.

Kienast T, Stoffers J, Bermpohl F, Lieb K. Borderline personality disorder and comorbid addiction: epidemiology and treatment. Dtsch Arztebl Int. 2014;111(16):280.

Knowles RE, Tarrier N. Evaluation of the effect of prospective patient diaries on emotional Well-being in intensive care unit survivors: a randomized controlled trial. Crit Care Med. 2009;37(1):184–91.

Koenigsberg HW. Affective instability: toward an integration of neuroscience and psychological perspectives. J Personal Disord. 2010;24(1):60–82.

Korsgaard HO, Torgersen S, Wentzel-Larsen T, Ulberg R. Personality disorders and axis I comorbidity in adolescent outpatients with ADHD. BMC Psychiatry. 2016;16:1.

Korsgaard HO, Ulberg R, Hummelen B, Midgley N, Thorén A, Dahl HS. Personality disorders as a possible moderator of the effects of relational interventions in short-term psychoanalytic psychotherapy with depressed adolescents. Int J Environ Res Public Health. 2022;19(17):10952.

Langås AM, Malt UF, Opjordsmoen S. In-depth study of personality disorders in first-admission patients with substance use disorders. BMC Psychiatry. 2012;12:1.

Lawrence KA, Allen JS, Chanen AM. Impulsivity in borderline personality disorder: reward-based decision-making and its relationship to emotional distress. J Personal Disord. 2010;24(6):785–99.

Leboyer M, Kupfer DJ. Bipolar disorder: new perspectives in health care and prevention. J Clin Psychiatry. 2010;71(12):1971.

Linehan MM, Comtois KA, Murray AM, Brown MZ, Gallop RJ, Heard HL, Korslund KE, Tutek DA, Reynolds SK, Lindenboim N. Two-year randomized controlled trial and follow-up of dialectical behavior therapy vs therapy by experts for suicidal behaviors and borderline personality disorder. Arch Gen Psychiatry. 2006;63(7):757–66.

Littlefield AK, Lane SP, Gette JA, Watts AL, Sher KJ. The "big everything": integrating and investigating dimensional models of psychopathology, personality, personality pathology, and cognitive functioning. Personal Disord Theory Res Treat. 2021;12(2):103.

Long MT, Massaro JM, Hoffmann U, Benjamin EJ, Naimi TS. Alcohol use is associated with hepatic steatosis among persons with presumed nonalcoholic fatty liver disease. Clin Gastroenterol Hepatol. 2020;18(8):1831–41.

MacKinnon DF. Depressive disorders: major depressive disorder and persistent depressive disorder. Psychiatry. 2015;23:902–65.

MacNeil LT, Walhout AJ. Gene regulatory networks and the role of robustness and stochasticity in the control of gene expression. Genome Res. 2011;21(5):645–57.

Martel MM. Conscientiousness as a mediator of the association between masculinized finger-length ratios and attention-deficit/hyperactivity disorder (ADHD). J Child Psychol Psychiatry. 2009;50(7):790–8.

Martel MM, Gremillion ML, Tackett JL. Personality traits elucidate sex differences in attention-deficit/hyperactivity disorder comorbidity during early childhood. J Psychopathol Behav Assess. 2014;36:237–45.

Masso Rodriguez A, Hogg B, Gardoki-Souto I, Valiente-Gómez A, Trabsa A, Mosquera D, García-Estela A, Colom F, Perez V, Padberg F, Moreno-Alcazar A. Clinical features, neuropsychology and neuroimaging in bipolar and borderline personality disorder: a systematic review of cross-diagnostic studies. Front Psych. 2021;12:681876.

Matthies SD, Philipsen A. Common ground in attention deficit hyperactivity disorder (ADHD) and borderline personality disorder (BPD)–review of recent findings. Bord Personal Disord Emot Dysregul. 2014;1:1–3.

Mazer AK, Cleare AJ, Young AH, Juruena MF. Bipolar affective disorder and borderline personality disorder: differentiation based on the history of early life stress and psychoneuroendocrine measures. Behav Brain Res. 2019;357:48–56.

McDermid J, Sareen J, El-Gabalawy R, Pagura J, Spiwak R, Enns MW. Co-morbidity of bipolar disorder and borderline personality disorder: findings from the National Epidemiologic Survey on Alcohol and Related Conditions. Compr Psychiatry. 2015;58:18–28.

McGlashan TH, Grilo CM, Skodol AE, Gunderson JG, Shea MT, Morey LC, Zanarini MC, Stout RL. The collaborative longitudinal personality disorders study: baseline axis I/II and II/II diagnostic co-occurrence. Acta Psychiatr Scand. 2000;102(4):256–64.

McMain SF, Links PS, Gnam WH, Guimond T, Cardish RJ, Korman L, Streiner DL. A randomized trial of dialectical behavior therapy versus general psychiatric management for borderline personality disorder. Am J Psychiatry. 2009;166(12):1365–74.

McMain SF, Guimond T, Streiner DL, Cardish RJ, Links PS. Dialectical behavior therapy compared with general psychiatric management for borderline personality disorder: clinical outcomes and functioning over a 2-year follow-up. Am J Psychiatry. 2012;169(6):650–61.

Meares R, Gerull F, Stevenson J, Korner A. Is self-disturbance the core of borderline personality disorder? An outcome study of borderline personality factors. Aust N Z J Psychiatry. 2011;45(3):214–22.

Melca IA, Yücel M, Mendlowicz MV, de Oliveira-Souza R, Fontenelle LF. The correlates of obsessive–compulsive, schizotypal, and borderline personality disorders in obsessive–compulsive disorder. J Anxiety Disord. 2015;33:15–24.

Mesbah Z, Abolmaali AK. Living experience of female adolescents with irrational beliefs in a narrative analysis study. J Excell Couns Psychother. 2021;10(38):21–35.

Mneimne M, Fleeson W, Arnold EM, Furr RM. Differentiating the everyday emotion dynamics of borderline personality disorder from major depressive disorder and bipolar disorder. Personal Disord Theory Res Treat. 2018;9(2):192.

Morgenstern J, Langenbucher J, Labouvie E, Miller KJ. The comorbidity of alcoholism and personality disorders in a clinical population: prevalence rates and relation to alcohol typology variables. J Abnorm Psychol. 1997;106(1):74.

Moor S, Crowe M, Luty S, Carter J, Joyce PR. Effects of comorbidity and early age of onset in young people with bipolar disorder on self harming behaviour and suicide attempts. J Affect Disord. 2012;136(3):1212–5.

Nelson J, Klumparendt A, Doebler P, Ehring T. Everyday emotional dynamics in major depression. Emotion. 2020;20(2):179.

Nilsson AK, Jørgensen CR, Straarup KN, Licht RW. Severity of affective temperament and maladaptive self-schemas differentiate borderline patients, bipolar patients, and controls. Compr Psychiatry. 2010;51(5):486–91.

Oquendo MA, Mann JJ. The biology of impulsivity and suicidality. Psychiatr Clin N Am. 2000;23(1):11–25.

Ozkan M, Altindag A. Comorbid personality disorders in subjects with panic disorder: do personality disorders increase clinical severity? Compr Psychiatry. 2005;46(1):20–6.

Palmer BA, Pahwa M, Geske JR, Kung S, Nassan M, Schak KM, Alarcon RD, Frye MA, Singh B. Self-report screening instruments differentiate bipolar disorder and borderline personality disorder. Brain Behav. 2021;11(7):e02201.

Paris J. Borderline or bipolar? Distinguishing borderline personality disorder from bipolar spectrum disorders. Harv Rev Psychiatry. 2004;12(3):140–5.

Paris J. The nature of borderline personality disorder: multiple dimensions, multiple symptoms, but one category. J Personal Disord. 2007;21(5):457–73.

Paris J. Clinical features of borderline personality disorder. In: Handbook of personality disorders: theory, research, and treatment, vol. 2. New York: The Guilford Press; 2018. p. 419.

Paris J, Black DW. Borderline personality disorder and bipolar disorder: what is the difference and why does it matter? J Nerv Ment Dis. 2015;203(1):3–7.

Paris J, Zweig-Frank H. A 27-year follow-up of patients with borderline personality disorder. Compr Psychiatry. 2001;42(6):482–7.

Parker G. Clinical differentiation of bipolar II disorder from personality-based "emotional dysregulation" conditions. J Affect Disord. 2011;133(1–2):16–21.

Parker GB, Fletcher K. Is bipolar II depression phenotypically distinctive? Acta Psychiatr Scand. 2009;120(6):446–55.

Parker G, McCraw S, Hadzi-Pavlovic D, Fletcher K. Costs of the principal mood disorders: a study of comparative direct and indirect costs incurred by those with bipolar I, bipolar II and unipolar disorders. J Affect Disord. 2013;149(1–3):46–55.

Parmar A, Kaloiya G. Comorbidity of personality disorder among substance use disorder patients: a narrative review. Indian J Psychol Med. 2018;40(6):517–27.

Patten SB, Paris J. The bipolar spectrum—a bridge too far? Can J Psychiatry. 2008;53(11):762–8.

Patel RS, Manikkara G, Chopra A. Bipolar disorder and comorbid borderline personality disorder: patient characteristics and outcomes in US hospitals. Medicina. 2019;55(1):13.

Paykel ES, Abbott R, Morriss R, Hayhurst H, Scott J. Sub-syndromal and syndromal symptoms in the longitudinal course of bipolar disorder. Br J Psychiatry. 2006;189(2):118–23.

Peluso MA, Hatch JP, Glahn DC, Monkul ES, Sanches M, Najt P, Bowden CL, Barratt ES, Soares JC. Trait impulsivity in patients with mood disorders. J Affect Disord. 2007;100(1–3):227–31.

Penzenstadler L, Soares C, Anci E, Molodynski A, Khazaal Y. Effect of assertive community treatment for patients with substance use disorder: a systematic review. Eur Addict Res. 2019;25(2):56–67.

Perlis RH, Miyahara S, Marangell LB, Wisniewski SR, Ostacher M, DelBello MP, Bowden CL, Sachs GS, Nierenberg AA, Investigators S-B. Long-term implications of early onset in bipolar disorder: data from the first 1000 participants in the systematic treatment enhancement program for bipolar disorder (STEP-BD). Biol Psychiatry. 2004;55(9):875–81.

Perroud N, Zewdie S, Stenz L, Adouan W, Bavamian S, Prada P, Nicastro R, Hasler R, Nallet A, Piguet C, Paoloni-Giacobino A. Methylation of serotonin receptor 3A in ADHD, borderline personality, and bipolar disorders: link with severity of the disorders and childhood maltreatment. Depress Anxiety. 2016;33(1):45–55.

Perugi G, Fornaro M, Akiskal HS. Are atypical depression, borderline personality disorder and bipolar II disorder overlapping manifestations of a common cyclothymic diathesis? World Psychiatry. 2011;10(1):45.

Pinto A, Cowan E. Personality features of obsessive-compulsive and related disorders. In: The Oxford handbook of obsessive-compulsive and related disorders. New York: Oxford University Press; 2023. p. 214.

Reich DB, Zanarini MC, Fitzmaurice G. Affective lability in bipolar disorder and borderline personality disorder. Compr Psychiatry. 2012;53(3):230–7.

Reimherr FW, Marchant BK, Gift TE, Steans TA, Wender PH. Types of adult attention-deficit hyperactivity disorder (ADHD): baseline characteristics, initial response, and long-term response to treatment with methylphenidate. Atten Defic Hyperact Disord. 2015;7:115–28.

Renaud S, Corbalan F, Beaulieu S. Differential diagnosis of bipolar affective disorder type II and borderline personality disorder: analysis of the affective dimension. Compr Psychiatry. 2012;53(7):952–61.

Richard-Lepouriel H, Kung AL, Hasler R, Bellivier F, Prada P, Gard S, Ardu S, Kahn JP, Dayer A, Henry C, Aubry JM. Impulsivity and its association with childhood trauma experiences across bipolar disorder, attention deficit hyperactivity disorder and borderline personality disorder. J Affect Disord. 2019;244:33–41.

Riemann G, Weisscher N, Post RM, Altshuler L, McElroy S, Frye MA, Keck PE, Leverich GS, Suppes T, Grunze H, Nolen WA. The relationship between self-reported borderline personality features and prospective illness course in bipolar disorder. Int J Bipolar Disord. 2017;5:1–7.

Rihmer Z, Benazzi F. Impact on suicidality of the borderline personality traits impulsivity and affective instability. Ann Clin Psychiatry. 2010;22(2):121–8.

Rihmer Z, Döme P. Major mood disorders and suicidal behavior. In: The international handbook of suicide prevention. Chichester: Wiley, Blackwell; 2016. p. 74–92.

Rossi R, Pievani M, Lorenzi M, Boccardi M, Beneduce R, Bignotti S, Borsci G, Cotelli M, Giannakopoulos P, Magni LR, Rillosi L. Structural brain features of borderline personality and bipolar disorders. Psychiatry Res Neuroimaging. 2013;213(2):83–91.

Ruggero CJ, Carlson GA, Kotov R, Bromet EJ. Ten-year diagnostic consistency of bipolar disorder in a first-admission sample. Bipolar Disord. 2010;12(1):21–31.

Russell JJ, Moskowitz DS, Zuroff DC, Sookman D, Paris J. Stability and variability of affective experience and interpersonal behavior in borderline personality disorder. J Abnorm Psychol. 2007;116(3):578.

Sanches M. The limits between bipolar disorder and borderline personality disorder: a review of the evidence. Diseases. 2019;7(3):49.

Sansone RA, Sansone LA. Borderline personality and criminality. Psychiatry (Edgmont). 2009;6(10):16.

Sansone RA, Sansone LA. Responses of mental health clinicians to patients with borderline personality disorder. Innov Clin Neurosci. 2013;10(5–6):39.

Sarhan AL, Modallal S, Mahamid FA, Berte DZ. Depression symptoms and associated factors among thalassemia patients in the Palestinian territories: a cross-sectional study. Middle East Curr Psychiatr. 2022;29:1–8.

Saunders KE, Bilderbeck AC, Price J, Goodwin GM. Distinguishing bipolar disorder from borderline personality disorder: a study of current clinical practice. Eur Psychiatry. 2015;30(8):965–74.

Schiavone P, Dorz S, Conforti D, Scarso C, Borgherini G. Comorbidity of DSM–IV personality disorders in unipolar and bipolar affective disorders: a comparative study. Psychol Rep. 2004;95(1):121–8.

Sharma E, Sharma LP, Balachander S, Lin B, Manohar H, Khanna P, Lu C, Garg K, Thomas TL, Au AC, Selles RR. Comorbidities in obsessive-compulsive disorder across the lifespan: a systematic review and meta-analysis. Front Psych. 2021;12:703701.

Siever LJ, Gunderson JG. Genetic determinants of borderline conditions. Schizophr Bull. 1979;5(1):59–86.

Sjåstad HN, Gråwe RW, Egeland J. Affective disorders among patients with borderline personality disorder. PLoS One. 2012;7(12):e50930.

Skodol AE, Oldham JM, Hyler SE, Stein DJ, Hollander E, Gallaher PE, Lopez AE. Patterns of anxiety and personality disorder comorbidity. J Psychiatr Res. 1995;29(5):361–74.

Smith DJ, Kyle S, Forty L, Cooper C, Walters J, Russell E, Caesar S, Farmer A, McGuffin P, Jones I, Jones L. Differences in depressive symptom profile between males and females. J Affect Disord. 2008;108(3):279–84.

Söderholm JJ, Socada JL, Rosenström T, Ekelund J, Isometsä ET. Borderline personality disorder with depression confers significant risk of suicidal behavior in mood disorder patients—a comparative study. Front Psych. 2020;11:290.

Söderholm JJ, Socada JL, Ekelund J, Isometsä E. How changes in depression severity and borderline personality disorder intensity are linked–a cohort study of depressed patients with and without borderline personality disorder. Bord Personal Disord Emot Dysregul. 2024;11(1):3.

Souery D, Zaninotto L, Calati R, Linotte S, Mendlewicz J, Sentissi O, Serretti A. Depression across mood disorders: review and analysis in a clinical sample. Compr Psychiatry. 2012;53(1):24–38.

Steil R, Dyer A, Priebe K, Kleindienst N, Bohus M. Dialectical behavior therapy for posttraumatic stress disorder related to childhood sexual abuse: a pilot study of an intensive residential treatment program. J Trauma Stress. 2011;24(1):102–6.

Stone MH. Borderline syndromes: a consideration of subtypes and an overview, directions for research. Psychiatr Clin. 1981;4(1):3–24.

Strunk DR, Sasso K. Phenomenology and course of mood disorders. In: The Oxford handbook of mood disorders; 2017. p. 37–48.

Subramaniam M, Abdin E, Vaingankar JA, Chong SA. Obsessive–compulsive disorder: prevalence, correlates, help-seeking and quality of life in a multiracial Asian population. Soc Psychiatry Psychiatr Epidemiol. 2012;47:2035–43.

Swann SW, William B. Encyclopedia of personality and individual differences; 2020. p. 5337–42.

Swann AC, Bjork JM, Moeller FG, Dougherty DM. Two models of impulsivity: relationship to personality traits and psychopathology. Biol Psychiatry. 2002;51(12):988–94.

Swann AC, Steinberg JL, Lijffijt M, Moeller FG. Impulsivity: differential relationship to depression and mania in bipolar disorder. J Affect Disord. 2008;106(3):241–8.

Thamby A, Khanna S. The role of personality disorders in obsessive-compulsive disorder. Indian J Psychiatry. 2019;61(Suppl 1):S114–8.

Tickle EV. Borderline personality disorder among individuals with bipolar disorder: prevalence, correlates, and experiences of the comorbid diagnosis (Doctoral dissertation, University of Worcester); 2022.

Tolin DF, Springer KS. Obsessive-compulsive and related disorders. Oxford: Oxford University Press; 2018.

Tomko RL, Lane SP, Pronove LM, Treloar HR, Brown WC, Solhan MB, Wood PK, Trull TJ. Undifferentiated negative affect and impulsivity in borderline personality and depressive disorders: a momentary perspective. J Abnorm Psychol. 2015;124(3):740.

Trull TJ, Widiger TA, Lynam DR, Costa PT Jr. Borderline personality disorder from the perspective of general personality functioning. Focus. 2005;112(3):193–464.

Trull TJ, Solhan MB, Tragesser SL, Jahng S, Wood PK, Piasecki TM, Watson D. Affective instability: measuring a core feature of borderline personality disorder with ecological momentary assessment. J Abnorm Psychol. 2008;117(3):647.

Trull TJ, Tomko RL, Brown WC, Scheiderer EM. Borderline personality disorder in 3-D: dimensions, symptoms, and measurement challenges. Soc Personal Psychol Compass. 2010;4(11):1057–69.

US Department of Health and Human Services. SAMHSA's concept of trauma and guidance for a trauma-informed approach. 2014.

Van Den Bosch LM, Verheul R, Langeland W, Van Den Brink W. Trauma, dissociation, and posttraumatic stress disorder in female borderline patients with and without substance abuse problems. Aust N Z J Psychiatry. 2003;37(5):549–55.

Vannucci C, Bonsall MB, Di Simplicio M, Cairns A, Holmes EA, Burnett HS. Positive moods are all alike? Differential affect amplification effects of 'elated'versus 'calm'mental imagery in young adults reporting hypomanic-like experiences. Transl Psychiatry. 2022;12(1):453.

Vieta E, Colom F, Martínez-Arán A, Benabarre A, Reinares M, Gastó C. Bipolar II disorder and comorbidity. Compr Psychiatry. 2000;41(5):339–43.
Visted E, Vøllestad J, Nielsen MB, Schanche E. Emotion regulation in current and remitted depression: a systematic review and meta-analysis. Front Psychol. 2018;9:322567.
Watson S, Chilton R, Fairchild H, Whewell P. Association between childhood trauma and dissociation among patients with borderline personality disorder. Aust N Z J Psychiatry. 2006;40(5):478–81.
Walter ZC, Carlyle M, Kerswell N, Mefodeva V, Nixon RD, Cobham VE, Hides L. Study protocol: implementing and evaluating a trauma-informed model of care in residential youth treatment for substance use disorders. Front Psych. 2023;14:1169794.
Widiger TA, Costa PT. Integrating normal and abnormal personality structure: the five-factor model. J Pers. 2012;80(6):1471–506.
Wilson ST, Stanley B, Brent DA, Oquendo MA, Huang YY, Haghighi F, Hodgkinson CA, Mann JJ. Interaction between tryptophan hydroxylase I polymorphisms and childhood abuse is associated with increased risk for borderline personality disorder in adulthood. Psychiatr Genet. 2012;22(1):15–24.
Wilson ST, Fertuck EA, Kwitel A, Stanley MC, Stanley B. Impulsivity, suicidality and alcohol use disorders in adolescents and young adults with borderline personality disorder. Int J Adolesc Med Health. 2006;18(1):189–96.
Wilson ST, Stanley B, Oquendo MA, Goldberg P, Zalsman G, Mann JJ. Comparing impulsiveness, hostility, and depression in borderline personality disorder and bipolar II disorder. J Clin Psychiatry. 2007;68(10):1533–9.
Williams R, Holliday R, Clem M, Anderson E, Morris EE, Surís A. Borderline personality disorder and military sexual trauma: analysis of previous traumatization and current psychiatric presentation. J Interpers Violence. 2017;32(15):2223–36.
World Health Organization. WHO report on surveillance of antibiotic consumption: 2016–2018 early implementation. 2018.
Wupperman P, Neumann CS, Whitman JB, Axelrod SR. The role of mindfulness in borderline personality disorder features. J Nerv Ment Dis. 2009;197(10):766–71.
Yen S, Frazier E, Hower H, Weinstock LM, Topor DR, Hunt J, Goldstein TR, Goldstein BI, Gill MK, Ryan ND, Strober M. Borderline personality disorder in transition age youth with bipolar disorder. Acta Psychiatr Scand. 2015;132(4):270–80.
Yoshimatsu K, Palmer B. Depression in patients with borderline personality disorder. Harv Rev Psychiatry. 2014;22(5):266–73.
Zanarini MC. Childhood experiences associated with the development of borderline personality disorder. Psychiatr Clin N Am. 2000;23(1):89–101.
Zanarini MC, Frankenburg FR, Reich DB, Wedig MM, Conkey LC, Fitzmaurice GM. Prediction of time-toattainment of recovery for borderline patients followed prospectively for 16 years. Acta Psychiatr Scand. 2014;130(3):205–13.
Zanarini MC, Frankenburg FR, DeLuca CJ, Hennen J, Khera GS, Gunderson JG. The pain of being borderline: dysphoric states specific to borderline personality disorder. Harv Rev Psychiatry. 1998a;6(4):201–7.
Zanarini MC, Frankenburg FR, Dubo ED, Sickel AE, Trikha A, Levin A, Reynolds V. Axis I comorbidity of borderline personality disorder. Am J Psychiatry. 1998b;155(12):1733–9.
Zanarini MC, Frankenburg FR, Hennen J, Reich DB, Silk KR. Axis I comorbidity in patients with borderline personality disorder: 6-year follow-up and prediction of time to remission. Am J Psychiatry. 2004;161(11):2108–14.
Zanarini MC, Laudate CS, Frankenburg FR, Reich DB, Fitzmaurice G. Predictors of self-mutilation in patients with borderline personality disorder: a 10-year follow-up study. J Psychiatr Res. 2011;45(6):823–8.
Zetsche U, Neumann P, Bürkner PC, Renneberg B, Koster EH, Hoorelbeke K. Computerized cognitive control training to reduce rumination in major depression: a randomized controlled trial. Behav Res Ther. 2024;177:104521.

Zimmerman M, Galione J. Psychiatrists† and nonpsychiatrist physicians† reported use of the DSM-IV criteria for major depressive disorder. J Clin Psychiatry. 2010;71(3):15975.
Zimmerman M, Mattia JI. Axis I diagnostic comorbidity and borderline personality disorder. Compr Psychiatry. 1999a;40(4):245–52.
Zimmerman M, Mattia JI. Psychiatric diagnosis in clinical practice: is comorbidity being missed? Compr Psychiatry. 1999b;40(3):182–91.
Zimmerman M, Morgan TA. The relationship between borderline personality disorder and bipolar disorder. Dialogues Clin Neurosci. 2013;15(2):155–69.
Zimmerman M, Balling C, Chelminski I, Dalrymple K. Patients with borderline personality disorder and bipolar disorder: a descriptive and comparative study. Psychol Med. 2021;51(9):1479–90.

Index

A

Abandonment, 13–15, 23–25, 38, 45, 47, 48, 62, 156, 165, 208, 212, 213, 215, 226, 234, 276, 299, 300, 310, 358, 360–364, 382, 383, 387, 390, 425, 428
Acceptance and change, 135
Acceptance and commitment therapy (ACT), 247–259
Adverse childhood experiences (ACEs), 47, 48, 57, 58, 63–66, 68–70, 72, 75, 76, 208, 211, 215, 277, 354, 357, 362, 381
Affect, 7, 14, 17, 19, 38, 43, 46, 66, 70, 76, 96, 101, 104, 108, 127–130, 151, 166, 173, 180, 226, 227, 290, 307, 310, 317, 362, 363, 426, 432
Affective instability, 1, 2, 14–17, 64, 73, 95, 101, 104, 109, 148, 152, 155, 304, 305, 381, 382, 385, 386, 424–428, 436
Aggression, 2, 7, 14, 16, 17, 40, 46, 63, 64, 105, 149, 154, 175, 176, 286, 291, 304, 306, 309, 403–405, 429
Alexithymia, 2, 44, 68, 107, 276, 291, 293, 294, 307, 384, 386, 387
Alternative DSM-5 Model
  antagonism, 20, 23
  detachment, 23, 26, 225–228, 233, 272, 352, 360
  disinhibition, 20, 23, 103, 149, 150, 177, 297, 304, 306, 422
  empathy, 19, 23, 208, 258, 259, 408
  intimacy, 23, 237
  negative affectivity, 1, 23, 64, 149, 289, 290, 292, 303–305
  psychoticism, 23, 290
Anger and aggression, 155, 310, 383, 405, 429
Anorexia nervosa (AN), 275, 377–384, 386–390
Anxiety disorders, 15, 37, 155, 186, 206, 248, 285, 286, 289, 302, 352, 359, 378, 379, 401, 421, 427, 433, 436
Attachment, 6, 16, 38, 39, 42, 44, 46–48, 75, 76, 106, 107, 147, 148, 228, 230, 232, 236, 237, 251, 256, 259, 275, 276, 287, 305, 307, 361, 362, 381
Attention, 4, 38, 62, 96, 125, 146, 166, 226, 251, 268, 351, 399, 430
Attention-deficit/hyperactivity disorder (ADHD), 15, 16, 40, 150, 151, 235, 236, 378, 399–411, 421
Autobiographical memory, 67, 68, 206, 207, 226
Avoidance, 2, 15, 66, 73, 103, 105, 106, 151, 158, 168, 173, 174, 177, 180, 181, 190, 210, 250, 252–254, 256, 258, 293, 294, 302, 314, 316–318, 352, 356, 359–362, 383, 384, 387, 390, 409

B

Behavioral dysregulation, 13, 22, 24, 46, 128, 151, 153, 165–167, 171, 175–177, 181, 182, 185–188, 191, 299, 305, 386
Binge-eating disorder (BED), 377, 378, 380, 381, 384, 386, 389
Binge-eating/purging type, 379
Biological vulnerability, 100, 108, 123, 124, 127–129, 147–149, 151, 155, 188, 314

M. Salavati, E. A. Selby, *Theories of Borderline Personality Disorder*, https://doi.org/10.1007/978-3-031-75503-3

Biosocial developmental model, 148, 157, 308, 310–313
Biosocial model, 102, 128, 145–147, 153, 165, 232, 283
Bipolar-borderline continuum, 424
Bipolar I and II disorders, 422–431
Borderline mothers, 38, 39
Borderline personality, 3
Borderline personality disorder (BPD), 1–7, 13–26, 37–48, 57–76, 95–109, 121–138, 145–158, 165–167, 171, 172, 175, 176, 178–191, 205–215, 225–237, 247–259, 268, 269, 271, 276, 277, 279, 286–289, 291, 292, 294–296, 298–318, 351–364, 377–390, 399–411, 421–436
BPD patients, 3
Bulimia nervosa (BN), 377–385, 387–390

C
Cascade of emotions, 185, 187
Child abuse, 58–61, 63, 64, 68, 72–74, 76, 135, 153, 154, 188, 317, 353, 357, 358, 423
Child emotional abuse, 74, 75
Childhood aversive experiences, 64, 236, 237
Childhood harmful experiences, 207
Childhood maltreatment, 48, 57–76, 206, 208, 215, 235, 236, 276, 279, 285, 286, 354, 357, 363, 431
Childhood trauma, 44, 47, 60, 71, 148, 234, 235, 352, 355, 357, 363, 410, 423, 424, 430, 431
Childhood traumatic experiences, 46, 76, 307, 431
Child neglect, 60, 62
Child physical abuse, 59
Child sexual abuse (CSA), 67, 70, 234, 357, 358, 410
Coercive/controlling behaviors, 40
Cognitive diffusion/fusion, 251, 253, 256, 259
Committed action, 251, 254, 255, 257, 259
Comorbidity, 3, 18, 25, 64, 69, 75, 165, 229, 230, 232, 234, 275, 278, 285, 300, 302, 303, 352–358, 362, 364, 377, 378, 381–383, 387, 390, 399, 402, 403, 411, 421–436
Complex post-traumatic stress disorder (c-PTSD), 235, 351–364
Constitutional vulnerability, 237
Contextual behavioral science (CBS), 248
Core emotional needs, 207, 208, 212

D
Deliberate self-harm (DSH), 14, 70, 269, 273, 278, 298, 314–316, 355, 356, 430
Depersonalization, 5, 67, 225–227, 229, 230, 232, 235, 301, 425
Derealization, 67, 225–227, 229, 230, 232, 235, 301
Developmental biosocial model, 102, 145, 311
Diagnostic and Statistical Manual of Mental Disorders (DSM), 4, 13–19, 25, 96, 121, 127–129, 152, 401, 402, 409
Dialectical behavior therapy (DBT), 99, 135–138, 146, 257, 390
Diathesis-stress model, 40, 123
Dimensional & categorical perspective, 18–22
Dimensional models, 19, 20, 25, 227, 361
Disinhibition, 20, 23, 103, 149, 150, 177, 297, 304, 306, 422
Dissociation, 15, 67, 213, 225, 301, 353, 382, 409, 426
Dissociative disorders (DDs), 225, 226, 229–231, 233–235
Dissociative experiences, 14, 63, 214, 227–230, 232, 233, 235, 300, 301
Dissociative identity disorder (DID), 206, 215, 225, 230, 233, 234
Distraction, 66, 103, 107, 170, 171, 181–186, 257, 259, 317, 429
Distress tolerance, 107, 134, 137, 153, 189, 258, 291–293, 316, 318
Disturbed control, 434
Disturbed interpersonal relationships, 1, 133, 156, 305, 351, 377, 426
Disturbed self-organization, 359, 361, 362
Domestic violence, 57–59, 76, 154, 358, 363
Dysregulated behaviors, 14, 152, 166, 167, 171–173, 175–189, 191, 303, 304, 317, 381, 384, 386, 390

E
Early maladaptive schemas (EMSs), 207–215
Eating disorders, 2, 107, 155, 187, 206, 236, 268, 377, 401, 421
Emotion, 1, 14, 38, 65, 95, 121, 146, 166, 206, 225, 248, 268, 355, 382, 400, 421
Emotional and interpersonal distress, 180
Emotional-based coping strategy, 277
Emotional cascade model (ECM), 105, 152, 165–191, 283, 308, 315, 317–318
Emotional cascades, 152, 166, 167, 171, 176, 178, 180–185, 187–191, 279, 317, 318

Emotional impulsivity, 400, 405
Emotional instability, 2, 14, 20, 24, 25, 37, 40, 62, 71, 75, 101, 105, 109, 121, 128, 133, 147–149, 152, 156, 165, 166, 184, 187, 212, 294, 295, 299, 303–306, 311, 351, 360, 361, 381–384, 386, 410, 425, 427
Emotional lability, 21, 23, 24, 26, 133, 148, 152, 377, 385, 400
Emotional vulnerability, 102, 106, 123, 129, 131, 134, 146, 147, 176, 180, 190
Emotional working memory (EWM), 66, 67
Emotion dysregulation, 39, 43, 62, 66, 68, 69, 73, 74, 76, 98, 121–124, 126, 127, 131, 133–135, 146–148, 150–156, 166, 174, 175, 178–182, 185, 232, 233, 258, 272, 276, 278–280, 291, 294–297, 300, 301, 304, 306, 308–311, 314, 315, 317, 318, 351, 355, 358–362, 364, 382–385, 387, 390, 400, 402, 403, 406–408, 410, 430, 436
Emotion regulation and dysregulation, 101
Emotion regulation models, 174, 309, 384, 386
Executive function, 97, 170, 175, 306, 351, 403
Experience sampling method (ESM), 407
Experiential avoidance, 106, 107, 180, 247, 251–253, 255–259, 293, 314–317
Experiential avoidance model (EAM), 180, 313–318

F

Five-Factor Model
  agreeableness, 2, 20–22, 232, 291, 293, 294, 296, 387, 409
  conscientiousness, 20–22, 149, 232, 293, 294, 387
  extraversion, 20–22, 232, 290, 294, 296, 387
  neuroticism, 2, 20–22, 146, 171, 176, 190, 232, 289–291, 293–296, 304, 305, 307, 318, 387, 436
  openness, 20–22, 232, 256, 291, 293, 294, 296
Fragile self-esteem, 38, 48
Functional contextualism, 247, 249, 259

G

GAD, 314, 352
Gene-environment interaction (G × E), 155

H

Harmful, 211
Hierarchical Taxonomy of Psychopathology (HiTOP) Primer, 25–26
Hostility, 7, 14, 23, 24, 26, 39, 40, 43–48, 423, 425
Hypervigilance, 38, 188, 352
Hypomanic, 422, 429–431

I

Identity issues, 14, 15, 24, 230, 363, 385
Impacts on themselves, 236
Impulsivity, 1, 13, 37, 63, 102, 121, 145, 165, 215, 235, 248, 272, 351, 381, 399, 424
Inattentiveness, 297, 402
Influences, 225
Insecure attachment, 39, 42, 44, 46, 67, 68, 75, 382, 385
Internalizing and externalizing behaviors, 24, 65, 206, 215, 404
Interpersonal difficulties, 37, 71, 102, 271, 305, 409
Interpersonal dysregulation, 45, 46, 128
Interpersonal effectiveness, 137, 430
Interpersonal instability, 13, 304
Interpersonal issues, 45, 68, 165, 176, 359, 360, 382, 409, 427
Intrinsic and extrinsic regulation, 98
Invalidated environment, 41, 123, 127
Invalidating environment, 63, 64, 75, 100, 102, 109, 124, 129–134, 146, 147, 152–154, 178, 180, 276
Invalidation, 41, 42, 48, 63, 127, 129–131, 136, 148, 152, 153, 167, 178, 305, 306, 314
Irritability, 14, 15, 23, 128, 138, 311, 361, 362, 400, 407, 408, 425, 428, 429

M

Major depressive disorder (MDD), 65, 71, 181, 225, 226, 229, 273, 303, 352, 425, 426, 431, 432, 436
Maladaptive coping modes, 211
Maladaptive coping strategies, 148, 149, 155–156, 311
Mania, 422, 425, 436
Maternal hostility, 45
Memory, 66, 126, 172, 173, 206, 207, 209, 210, 226–228, 252–257, 306, 314, 316, 351, 352, 355
Mentalization, 38, 236, 237
Mentalization-based treatment (MBT), 236, 237

Mentalizing issues, 74
Mindfulness, 103, 135, 137, 247, 254, 258, 259, 430
Mismatch model, 227
Modal model, 97, 127
Momentary events, 178
Mood, 2, 13, 71, 95, 125, 149, 165, 215, 231, 279, 352, 380, 400, 422
Mood fluctuations, 14, 109, 384, 425, 427

N
Negative affectivity, 154
Negative self-perception, 359
Neuroticism, 2, 20–22, 146, 171, 176, 190, 232, 289–291, 293–296, 304, 305, 307, 318, 387, 436
Non-suicidal self-harm (NSSH), 14, 65, 68, 69, 71–73, 76, 267–318, 361, 389
Non-suicidal self-injury (NSSI), 46, 63, 72, 73, 103, 109, 134, 152, 154, 157, 166, 171, 173, 175–178, 180–182, 184–186, 189–191, 206, 230, 232, 233, 235, 267–280, 285, 287–318, 355, 356, 358, 361, 378, 381, 388–390, 430, 432

O
Object relations, 5–7, 44, 205
Obsessive-compulsive disorder (OCD), 15, 171, 206, 226, 248, 285, 378, 379, 401, 433–434, 436

P
Parental emotional invalidation, 41
Parental separation, 46, 47, 57, 276, 307
Parent-child relationship, 39, 42, 44, 47, 72
Parenting styles, 1, 37–48, 133, 134, 207, 208
Perfectionism, 276, 289–291, 294, 387
Phobia, 15, 174, 288, 433
Post-traumatic stress disorder (PTSD), 65, 127, 156, 173, 225, 268, 352, 383, 421
Present moment awareness, 251, 254, 257–259
Problem solving, 15, 41, 48, 103, 105, 109, 128–131, 137, 153, 168, 169, 172–174, 176, 268, 286
Psychological flexibility, 247, 251–253, 258, 259
Psychotic symptoms, 15, 71, 134, 427, 430
Punishment, 39, 40, 42, 61, 63, 132, 147, 295

R
Reappraisal, 15, 103, 107, 108, 168, 170, 174, 184, 234, 287, 314, 386, 432
Re-experience, 360
Rejection, 15, 23, 38, 45, 48, 64, 106, 127, 208, 215, 234, 286, 291, 300, 382, 390, 428
Relational frame theory (RFT), 247, 249–251, 259
Risky use, 434
Rumination, 15, 103, 152, 166, 251, 268, 354, 384, 408, 428

S
Schema, 205–215, 275, 358, 423, 430
Schema mode, 209–215
Schema model, 205–215
Self-as-context, 251, 254, 258, 259
Self-control, 126, 135, 208, 212, 214, 430
Self-criticism, 23, 63, 68, 106, 171, 275, 276, 288, 428
Self-destructive behaviors, 1, 14, 15, 26, 62, 66, 76, 95, 100, 103, 105, 109, 126, 128, 129, 133–135, 145, 146, 154, 156, 165, 166, 168, 173, 189, 190, 210, 212, 215, 284, 297, 298, 300, 306, 355, 364, 404, 406, 407, 410
Self-destructive and self-harm behaviors, 14
Self-destructive patterns, 207, 215
Self-harm behaviors, 2, 15, 24, 68, 180, 278, 287–289, 295, 296, 298, 299, 301, 302, 304, 306, 307, 309, 317, 364, 383, 389
Self-inflicted behaviors, 24, 95, 100, 105, 134, 166, 175, 177, 289, 297
Self-inflicted injurious behaviors, 145, 148, 149, 156, 176, 297, 300, 307, 383, 425
Self-inflicted injury (SII), 68, 148, 149, 156, 157, 177, 269, 276, 287, 303, 304, 310–312, 318
Self-injurious behaviors, 14–17, 69, 107, 121, 137, 147–149, 153, 155–157, 190, 231, 233, 258, 259, 268, 272–279, 283, 288, 290–293, 295, 296, 298–300, 304, 306, 308–310, 315, 317, 355, 360, 362–364, 386, 401, 406, 426–428, 430, 435
Self-injurious thoughts and behaviors (SITBs), 269, 273, 277, 310
Self-punishment, 70, 180, 210, 275, 279, 287, 288, 294, 300, 307, 309, 310

Sensation-seeking, 177, 182, 290, 297, 307
Shame and guilt, 387
Social impairments, 165, 405, 434
Somatization, 71, 358
Stressful life events, 44, 65, 73, 107, 108, 168, 169
Stress-related dissociation, 229
Substance use and alcohol disorders, 421
Substance use disorders, 424, 434
Suicidal attempts, 76, 100, 146, 178, 179, 189, 233, 235, 278, 281, 283, 284, 301, 303, 308, 361, 364, 389, 428, 430, 431
Suicidality, 2, 15, 68, 73, 135, 137, 138, 281, 282, 285–287, 289, 296, 301, 303, 304, 361, 423–427, 430, 435
Suicidal thoughts/ideation, 15, 23, 39, 47, 65, 72, 109, 137, 138, 168, 171, 174, 233, 235, 268, 270–273, 275, 277, 281–286, 289, 290, 294, 298, 300, 304–306, 308–310, 313, 318, 351, 355, 356, 360, 378, 389, 404, 422, 424, 431, 432, 436
Suicide, 57, 105, 121, 149, 165, 231, 257, 267, 356, 378, 407, 423

T
Temperamental vulnerability, 64, 134
Thought suppression, 106, 166, 174, 182, 314
Trait-state model, 19
Trauma, 42, 61, 108, 124, 173, 207, 226, 277, 351, 404, 431
Trauma-related rumination, 173
Traumatic life events, 351, 353
Typological perspectives, 226, 227

U
Unwanted emotions, 63, 181, 185, 314, 316
Urgency, 175, 177, 182, 287, 293, 296, 297

V
Validation, 131, 136, 153, 189, 208
Values, 7, 20, 44, 57, 122, 247, 251, 253–255, 257–259, 359

W
Withdrawal, 3, 39, 41, 42, 155, 226, 276, 286, 434

www.ingramcontent.com/pod-product-compliance
Lightning Source LLC
Chambersburg PA
CBHW071720260826
50469CB00003B/51
9783031755026